ACCP Critical Care Medicine Board Review: 20th Edition

The American Board of Internal Medicine (ABIM) is not affiliated with, nor does it endorse, preparatory examination review programs or other continuing medical education. The content of the ACCP Critical Care Medicine Board Review: 20th Edition is developed independently by the American College of Chest Physicians (ACCP), which has no knowledge of or access to ABIM examination material.

The views expressed herein are those of the authors and do not necessarily reflect the views of the ACCP. Use of trade names or names of commercial sources is for information only and does not imply endorsement by the ACCP. The authors and the publisher have exercised great care to ensure that drug dosages, formulas, and other information presented in this book are accurate and in accord with the professional standards in effect at the time of publication. However, readers are advised to always check the manufacturer's product information sheet packaged with the respective products to be fully informed of changes in recommended dosages, contraindications, etc., before prescribing or administering any drug.

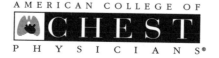

AMERICAN COLLEGE OF
CHEST
PHYSICIANS®

Published by the
American College of Chest Physicians
3300 Dundee Road
Northbrook, IL 60062-2348
Telephone: (847) 498-1400; Fax: (847) 498-5460
ACCP Web site: www.chestnet.org

Printed in the United States of America
First Printing
ISBN 978-0-916609-76-4

Contents

Authors

Joshua O. Benditt, MD, FCCP
Director of Respiratory Care Services
Division of Pulmonary and Critical Care
Medicine
University of Washington School of Medicine
Seattle, WA

Thomas P. Bleck, MD, FCCP
Chairman of Neurology, Evanston
Northwestern Healthcare and
Professor and Vice Chair for Academic
Programs
Department of Neurology
Northwestern University Feinberg School of
Medicine
Evanston, IL

R. Phillip Dellinger, MD, FCCP
Professor of Medicine
Robert Wood Johnson Medical School
Director, Division of Critical Care Medicine
Director, Medical/Surgical Intensive Care
Unit
Cooper University Hospital
Camden, NJ

David J. Dries, MD, MSE, FCCP
Assistant Medical Director for Surgical Care
HealthPartners Medical Group
John F. Perry, Jr., Professor of Surgery
University of Minnesota
Regions Hospital
St. Paul, MN

John W. Drover, MD
Associate Professor
Chair and Medical/Director
Critical Care Program
Queen's University
Kingston General Hospital
Kingston, ON Canada

Scott K. Epstein, MD, FCCP
Dean for Educational Affairs and Professor
of Medicine
Tufts University School of Medicine
Pulmonary, Critical Care and Sleep Medicine
Division
Tufts Medical Center
Boston, MA

Gregory T. Everson, MD
Professor of Medicine
Director of Hepatology
University of Colorado School of Medicine
Denver, CO

Brian K. Gehlbach, MD
Assistant Professor of Medicine
University of Chicago
Section of Pulmonary and Critical Care
Chicago, IL

Michael A. Gropper, MD, PhD, FCCP
Professor and Vice Chair
Department of Anesthesia and Perioperative
Care
Director, Critical Care Medicine
University of California, San Francisco
San Francisco, CA

Jesse B. Hall, MD, FCCP
Professor of Medicine
Anesthesia and Critical Care
The University of Chicago
The Pritzker School of Medicine
Chicago, IL

Steven M. Hollenberg, MD, FCCP
Professor of Medicine
Robert Wood Johnson Medical School
University of Medicine and Dentistry of New
Jersey
Director, Coronary Care Unit
Cooper University Hospital
Camden, NJ

George H. Karam, MD, FCCP
Paula Garvey Manship
Professor of Medicine
Louisiana State University
School of Medicine
New Orleans, LA
Head, Department of Internal Medicine
Earl Long Medical Center
Baton Rouge, LA

John P. Kress, MD, FCCP
Assistant Professor of Medicine
Section of Pulmonary and Critical Care
University of Chicago
Chicago, IL

James Kruse, MD
Chief, Critical Care Services
Bassett Healthcare
Cooperstown, NY

Richard S. Muther, MD
Medical Director
Division of Nephrology
Research Medical Center
Kidney Associates of Kansas City PC
Kansas City, MO

Michael S. Niederman, MD, FCCP
Chairman, Department of Medicine
Professor of Medicine
Winthrop University Hospital
Vice Chairman, Department of Medicine
SUNY at Stony Brook
Mineola, NY

James A. Roth, MD
Director of Electrophysiology
Associate Professor of Cardiovascular
Medicine
Medical College of Wisconsin
Milwaukee, WI

Gregory A. Schmidt, MD, FCCP
Professor, Division of Pulmonary,
Critical Care, and Occupational Medicine
Department of Internal Medicine
University of Iowa
Iowa City, IA

Jonathan S. Simmons, DO, MSc, FCCP
Clinical Assistant Professor
Co-Director, Critical Care Fellowship
Program
Chair, Disaster Preparedness and Emergency
Management
Departments of Anesthesia and Emergency
Medicine
Surgical Intensive Care Unit
University of Iowa Hospitals and Clinics
Iowa City, IA

Mary E. Strek, MD, FCCP
Associate Professor of Medicine
Section of Pulmonary and Critical Care
University of Chicago
Chicago, IL

Karl W. Thomas, MD, FCCP
Assistant Professor
Division of Pulmonary Diseases
Critical Care, and Occupational Medicine
University of Iowa
Iowa City, IA

Janice L. Zimmerman, MD, FCCP
Head, Division of Critical Care Medicine and
Director, Medical Intensive Care Unit
Department of Medicine
The Methodist Hospital
Houston, TX

DISCLOSURE OF AUTHORS' CONFLICTS OF INTEREST

The American College of Chest Physicians (ACCP) remains strongly committed to providing the best available evidence-based clinical information to participants of this educational activity and requires an open disclosure of any potential conflict of interest identified by our authors. It is not the intent of the ACCP to eliminate all situations of potential conflict of interest, but rather to enable those who are working with the ACCP to recognize situations that may be subject to question by others. All disclosed conflicts of interest are reviewed by the educational activity course director/chair, the Continuing Education Committee, or the Conflict of Interest Review Committee to ensure that such situations are properly evaluated and, if necessary, resolved. The ACCP educational standards pertaining to conflict of interest are intended to maintain the professional autonomy of the clinical experts inherent in promoting a balanced presentation of science. Through our review process, all ACCP CME activities are ensured of independent, objective, scientifically balanced presentations of information. Disclosure of any or no relationships will be made available on-site during all educational activities.

The following authors of the Critical Care Medicine Board Review: 20th Edition <u>have disclosed</u> to the ACCP that a relationship does exist with the respective company/organization as it relates to their presentation of material and should be communicated to the participants of this educational activity:

Authors	Relationship
Thomas P. Bleck, MD, FCCP	Grant monies (sources other than industry): NINDS, NIAD Grant monies (industry-related sources): ALSIUS, NovoNordisk, Actelion Consultant fee: USAMRICD Speakers bureau: PDL BioPharma
Steven M. Hollenberg, MD, FCCP	Speakers bureau: Novartis-Makers of Valsartan
Michael S. Niederman, MD, FCCP	Consultant fee, speaker bureau, advisory committee, etc: Pfizer, Inc., Merck & Co., Inc., Schering-Plough, Ortho-McNeil, Nektar, Cerexa Grant monies (from sources other than industry): Nektar to study aerosolized amikacin in VAP therapy. Brahms to study procalcitonin
James A. Roth, MD	Advisory committee: Medtronic Regional Advisory Board Member
Mary E. Strek, MD, FCCP	Grant monies (industry-related sources): AstraZeneca LP, GlaxoSmithKline

The following authors of the ACCP Critical Care Medicine Board Review: 20th Edition have disclosed to the ACCP that he or she may be discussing information about a product/procedure/technique that is considered research and is not yet approved for any purpose:

Thomas P. Bleck, MD, FCCP	Nicardipine for subarachnoid hemorrhage; several drugs for status epilepticus
John W. Drover, MD	Parenteral glutamine
Michael S. Niederman, MD, FCCP	Aerosolized amikacin

The following authors of the Critical Care Medicine Board Review: 20th Edition have indicated to the ACCP that <u>no potential conflict of interest</u> exists with any respective company/organization, and this should be communicated to the participants of this educational activity:

Joshua O. Benditt, MD, FCCP	Brian K. Gehlbach, MD	Richard S. Muther, MD
R. Phillip Dellinger, MD, FCCP	Michael A. Gropper, MD, PhD, FCCP	Gregory A. Schmidt, MD, FCCP
David J. Dries, MD, FCCP	Jesse B. Hall, MD, FCCP	Jonathan S. Simmons, DO, FCCP
John W. Drover, MD	George H. Karam, MD, FCCP	Karl W. Thomas, MD, FCCP
Scott K. Epstein, MD, FCCP	John P. Kress, MD, FCCP	Janice L. Zimmerman, MD, FCCP
Gregory T. Everson, MD	James A. Kruse, MD	

Needs Assessment

Rely on the ACCP Critical Care Medicine Board Review 2009 to review the type of information you should know for the Critical Care Subspecialty Board Examination of the American Board of Internal Medicine (ABIM). Designed as the best preparation for anyone taking the exam, this comprehensive, exam-focused review will cover current critical care literature and management strategies for critically ill patients.

The ABIM Critical Care Subspecialty Board Examination tests knowledge and clinical judgment in crucial areas of critical care medicine. This premier course will review the information you should know for the exam. Course content mirrors the content of the exam, as outlined by the ABIM, and includes the following topics:

Pulmonary disease	22.5%
Cardiovascular disorders	17.5%
Renal/Endocrine/Metabolism	15%
Infectious disease	12.5%
Neurologic disorders	7.5%
Surgical/Trauma/Transplantation	7.5%
Gastrointestinal disorders	5%
Hematologic/Oncologic disorders	5%
Pharmacology/Toxicology	5%
Research/Administration/Ethics	2.5%
Total	100%

Target Audience

Physicians in critical care and pulmonary medicine
Physicians in emergency departments
Physicians in anesthesiology
Physicians in surgery
Advanced critical care nurse practitioners
Advanced respiratory therapy practitioners
Physician assistants
Pharmacists

General Publications Disclaimer

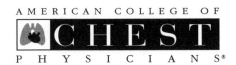

AMERICAN COLLEGE OF
CHEST
PHYSICIANS®

ACCP Member Benefits

So Many Reasons To Join. Find Yours Today.

Communications

- *CHEST*, for specialists in pulmonology, critical care, sleep medicine, thoracic surgery, cardiorespiratory interactions, and related disciplines

    Named one of the 100 most influential journals over the last 100 years in medicine and biology.

    Available at www.chestjournal.org

- *CHEST Physician,* the ACCP monthly news publication, featuring current chest medicine news from around the globe, plus updates on ACCP matters and events.

Health-care Advocacy

- A unified voice to policymakers on medical and payment issues

- Access to electronic tools for contacting Congress about issues affecting your patients, practice, and profession

- Timely alerts on legislation that impact the practice of medicine

Practice Resources

- Coding and reimbursement education

- Business of medicine resources

- Patient education tobacco cessation products

- ACCP Career Connection (online career service)

Educational Resources

- Discounted tuition for all CME courses and educational products

    Board review courses and preparation materials

    Hands-on clinical learning at the ACCP Simulation Center for Advanced Clinical Education

    Self-study tools, including ACCP-SEEK

- Discounted tuition for the annual CHEST meeting, offering essential updates in pulmonary, critical care, and sleep medicine

    CHEST benefits for ACCP members only:

    Free abstract submission

    Free topic proposal submission

- Interactive online resources, including free CME via Pulmonary and Critical Care Update (PCCU) articles

- Evidence-based practice guidelines and clinical resources, outlining new protocols in chest medicine

- Patient education tools and teaching materials

- Tools for making presentations to communities about lung health and smoking

Join the ACCP Today

Learn more about membership and apply online.

www.chestnet.org/membership/join

(800) 343-2227 or (847) 498-1400

Participation Opportunities

- ACCP NetWorks—special interest groups within the ACCP that focus on particular areas of chest medicine

- ACCP-Critical Care Institute, a center of excellence merging all programs and resources into a central organizational unit, providing the ACCP with a strong voice in the future of critical care medicine

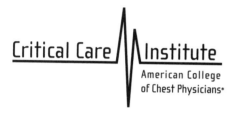

- Committee and leadership positions

- CHEST Foundation awards in clinical research, leadership in end-of-life care, and humanitarian service

- The CHEST Foundation's Ambassador's Group

Financial Benefits

- Discounts for ACCP courses and products

- Credit card programs

- Discounts for Apple and Dell computers and products

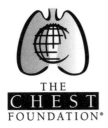

THE
CHEST
FOUNDATION®

Helping You Help Your Patients
Live and Breathe Easier

The CHEST Foundation is the philanthropic arm of the American College of Chest Physicians (ACCP), a 17,500-member international medical specialty society.

The CHEST Foundation mission is to provide resources to advance the prevention and treatment of diseases of the chest. In order to fulfill its mission to advance patient care in cardiopulmonary and critical care medicine, The CHEST Foundation has targeted the following four focus areas:

- Tobacco Prevention
- Humanitarian Service
- Clinical Research
- Critical Care/End-of-Life Care

Tobacco Prevention Education

- The 4th Edition CD-ROM: *Make the Choice: Tobacco or Health?* Speaker's Kit for presentations to health professionals and patients

- *Lung Lessons*^{SM} curriculum teaches elementary school children the negative health effects of smoking

- *Lung Lessons*^{SM}: *A Presenter's Guide* DVD demonstrates how to teach the *Lung Lessons*^{SM} curriculum to children

- *Evils of Tobacco* CD-ROM and video for children and women in India

Critical Care and End-of-Life Care

- The Critical Care Family Assistance Program and replication tool kit to improve coordination of care and communication with ICU staff, patients, and families

- *ICU – Frequently Asked Questions in the ICU* booklet, includes responses to questions that family members have when a family member is admitted to a hospital ICU

- *Stories at the End of Life* booklet series to comfort patients and their family members

Humanitarian Awards

Nearly $1.4 million awarded from 1998 to 2009 to recognize and support volunteer service in over 180 projects/services of ACCP members worldwide

Clinical Research Awards

- Over $5 million conferred from 1998 to 2009 to support promising clinical research

- Distinguished Scholar awards to foster innovation in clinical care to address public health related to chest and critical care medicine

    Eli Lilly and Company Distinguished Scholar in Critical Care Medicine

    GlaxoSmithKline Distinguished Scholar in Respiratory Health

    GlaxoSmithKline Distinguished Scholar in Thrombosis

- Clinical research awards in asthma, COPD, critical care, pulmonary fibrosis, thrombosis, and women's health

- Roger C. Bone Award for Advances in End-of-Life Care

- The CHEST Foundation and ACCP Grant in Venous Thromboembolism

- Alpha-1 Foundation and The CHEST Foundation Clinical Research Award in COPD and Alpha-1 Antitrypsin Deficiency

- The American Lung Association and CHEST Foundation Clinical Investigator Award

- The American Society of Transplantation and The CHEST Foundation Clinical Research Award in Lung Transplantation

- Association of Specialty Professors and The CHEST Foundation of the ACCP Geriatric Development Research Award

- The CHEST Foundation and the LUNGevity Foundation Clinical Research Award in Lung Cancer

- The CHEST Foundation California Chapter Clinical Research/Medical Education Award

- Scientific abstract-related awards

You can support these programs and projects through a tax-deductible donation to The CHEST Foundation. Your gift will help support these programs and resources that help you help your patients live and breathe easier.

Donate online at www.chestfoundation.org.

Solid Organ Transplantation

Joshua O. Benditt, MD, FCCP

Objectives:

- Review the main principals of solid organ transplantation, pertinent immunobiology and an approach to the major complications seen following the transplant procedure
- Identify the usual clinical course and major complications of liver transplantations
- Identify the usual clinical course and major complications of kidney and kidney-pancreas transplants
- Identify the usual clinical course and major complications of lung and heart transplantation

Key words: heart transplantation; kidney transplantation; kidney-pancreas transplantation; liver transplantation; lung transplantation

Overview of Solid Organ Transplantation

Solid organ transplantation has increased in frequency dramatically over the past 2 decades largely due to advances in the understanding and management of rejection immunobiology. Survival following solid organ transplantation has also increased with better antirejection medications, and an understanding that overimmunosuppression results in its own complications and is to be avoided. Currently, one of the major limitations to increasing the number of transplants performed is the imbalance between the limited supply of donor organs and the large and growing number of patients on organ-recipient waiting lists.

The major issues that are likely to be seen in the critical care setting regarding solid organ transplantation are complications in the postoperative period related to mechanical surgical procedure complications, infection, rejection, and complications related to the antirejection medicines themselves.

Rejection Immunobiology

A basic understanding of the immune system is important to understand the process of solid organ rejection as well as the antirejection medications that are used to try to prevent this problem. A brief review of the rejection immunobiology will be presented here. Reviews of this topic are referenced in the bibliography

The immune system is composed of the following two parts: natural immunity and adaptive immunity. Natural immunity refers to the nonspecific reaction whereby the recruitment of inflammatory cells such as macrophages, polymorphonuclear leukocytes, and lymphocytes are recruited to areas of infection or tissue injury is induced through nonspecific mechanisms of cellular response. Adaptive immunity involves the recognition of the presence of specific cell surface proteins on infectious agents or transplanted organs that results in the activation of T and B lymphocytes, which react to those foreign agents. This form of immunity is specific and results in the memory and specific recognition of foreign tissues and infectious agents. Although there is significant overlap and interaction between the innate and the adaptive systems, it is the latter that is more involved in solid organ transplant rejection.

The major response of the host to the transplanted organ is the activation of T-cell lymphocytes in the host that results in a cascade of reactions that are designed to destroy the transplanted foreign body. Key to this process is the recognition of the transplanted organ as "foreign." This occurs through cell surface recognition molecules known as the major histocompatibility complex (MHC) proteins on the cell surface of cells in the transplanted organ. These MHC proteins are recognized by antigen-presenting cells (APCs) that may be T cells or macrophages. A portion of the MHC molecule is usually then cleaved and processed by the APC, which then "presents" this foreign antigen fragment on its cell surface to T cells that are destined for activation. The APCs bind to the T cells through the foreign antigen fragment as well as a second costimulatory receptor on the T-cell surface. Once this binding of the two ligands occurs, activation of the T cell occurs. This T-cell activation leads to the rejection cascade that includes the following: (1) clonal expansion of B cells that produce antibodies to molecules on the transplanted organ cell surfaces; (2) induction of CD8-positive T cells that mediate cytotoxicity; and (3) help for macrophages to induce delayed type hypersensitivity responses. It is these processes that lead to the rejection and dysfunction of the transplanted solid organ. Modern immunosuppression regimens are designed to interfere with this process in a number of ways.

Several patterns of rejection have been described in solid organ transplantation. Hyperacute rejection is seen within minutes to hours of transplantation and is mediated by preformed antibodies that cause vascular injury. The kidney and heart are particularly susceptible. There is no specific treatment but this form of rejection usually can be avoided by pretransplant crossmatching. Accelerated rejection is an uncommon form of antibody-mediated rejection that is seen several days after transplantation and is characterized by vascular necrosis. Acute rejection is the most common cause of graft failure and is mediated by T-cell-mediated cytotoxicity. Acute rejection is defined as occurring between 1 week and 3 months following transplantation. Chronic rejection generally appears >3 months after the transplant procedure and is characterized by a slowly progressive course associated with the presence of fibrosis on histologic analysis of the transplanted organ.

Immunosuppression

Immunosuppression is required to prevent the rejection of the transplanted organ. The approaches to induction and maintenance immunosuppression, as well as the treatment of established rejection, vary significantly from one institution to another. Most centers use a combination of agents in low doses to minimize the toxicity of individual drugs. Cyclosporine is a fungal cyclic peptide that inhibits the transcription of interleukin (IL)-2 and the expression of IL-2 receptors, resulting in the blockade of T-cell activation. There are marked individual variations in the absorption and metabolism of cyclosporine; the precise timing of dosages

Table 1. *Drugs or Compounds That Affect Cyclosporine Levels*

Increase Levels	Decrease Levels
Diltiazem	Nafcillin
Nicardipine	Rifabutin
Verapamil	Rifampin
Fluconazole	Carbamazepine
Itraconazole	Phenobarbital
Ketoconazole	Phenytoin
Clarithromycin	Octreotide
Erythromycin	Ticlopidine
Lansoprazole	Oristat
Rabeprazole	St. John's wort
Cimetidine	
Methylprednisolone	
Allopurinol	
Bromocriptine	
Metoclopramide	
Colchicine	
Amiodarone	
Danazol	
Grapefruit juice	

and monitoring of drug levels are essential. Cyclosporine is metabolized by the hepatic cytochrome p450 system and is subject to many drug interactions (Table 1). Important side effects include nephrotoxicity, hypertension, neurotoxicity (*eg*, tremors, paresthesias, and seizures), gingival hyperplasia, hyperlipidemia, and hypertrichosis. Tacrolimus (FK506) is a macrolide that has essentially the same mechanism of action as cyclosporine. In liver, kidney, and lung transplant recipients, tacrolimus is more effective than cyclosporine in preventing acute and chronic rejection, and is effective in the treatment of acute rejection. In comparison with cyclosporine, tacrolimus is associated with more neurotoxicity, nephrotoxicity, and glucose intolerance, but less hypertension, dyslipidemia, gingival hyperplasia, or hirsutism. Sirolimus is a newer agent that has effects similar to those of cyclosporine and tacrolimus and is used more commonly in renal transplantation or in situations in which first-line immunosuppression protocols have not been entirely effective. Azathioprine is a purine analog that inhibits lymphocyte proliferation. Leukopenia, hepatitis, and cholestasis are important toxicities. Mycophenolate mofetil is a more selective inhibitor of purine synthesis that appears to be more effective than azathioprine at preventing acute rejection. Diarrhea, emesis, and leukopenia are the principal side effects of mycophenolate mofetil. Corticosteroids are nonspecific antiinflammatory agents that inhibit cytokine production, antigen recognition, and T-cell proliferation. The familiar side effects of corticosteroids include Cushing syndrome, hyperglycemia, hyperlipidemia, osteoporosis, myopathy, and cataracts. Polyclonal and monoclonal antibodies are used to deplete the T cells that mediate acute rejection. Antithymocyte and antilymphocyte globulin may cause serum sickness, thrombocytopenia, and leukopenia. Initial treatment with OKT3, a murine monoclonal antibody to the T-cell receptor, often elicits fever, chills, and a capillary leak syndrome resulting in hypotension and pulmonary edema. OKT3 also increases the risks of cytomegalovirus (CMV) infection and Epstein-Barr virus (EBV)-related posttransplant lymphoproliferative disorder (PTLD). Newer mouse/human chimeric monoclonal antibodies to IL-2 receptors (eg, basiliximab and daclizumab) are associated with less toxicity.

Complications of Solid Organ Transplantation

The complications of solid organ transplantation are most commonly divided into infectious and noninfectious complications. Each of these categories is then divided along temporal lines.

Infectious Complications: Infectious complications are most often divided into early and late infections. Nosocomial infections are prominent in the early posttransplant course, followed by the reactivation of latent infections in the graft or host, and new opportunistic infections related to the intensity and duration of immunosuppression. Staphylococci and Gram-negative bacilli are the most common early bacterial pathogens, followed later by infections caused by Legionella, Nocardia, Mycobacteria, and Listeria. Candidiasis and aspergillosis are the major fungal infections occurring in the first few months after transplantation, but the reactivation of endemic mycoses and cryptococcosis may present later. Herpes simplex virus (HSV) often reactivates in the initial weeks after transplantation, and herpesvirus-6 is increasingly recognized 2 to 4 weeks posttransplant. CMV and hepatitis C infections typically present after the first month. The peak incidence of EBV-related PTLD is 3 to 6 months after transplantation. Dermatomal reactivation of

varicella-zoster virus (VZV) also occurs in this time frame. Toxoplasmosis and *Pneumocystis carinii* pneumonia may develop after the first posttransplant month.

Pretransplant identification of latent infections in the donor and recipient is essential in defining risks. Routine testing includes serology testing for CMV; HSV; EBV; VZV; hepatitis A, B, and C; HIV, toxoplasmosis, and relevant endemic mycoses, such as histoplasmosis and coccidioidomycosis. A tuberculin test should be performed, and the chest radiograph evaluated for granulomatous disease. Indolent infection of the oral cavity and sinuses should be excluded, and immunizations should be brought up to date. Prophylaxis is effective against many latent and some acquired infections. Routine surveillance is helpful for the preemptive management of CMV infections, and possibly others. Suspected infection should be approached with an assessment of risks and an aggressive effort at specific diagnosis. CMV is the bane of transplantation. Primary infection occurs when a seronegative patient receives an organ from a seropositive donor; secondary or reactivation infection develops in seropositive recipients. Active infection (viral replication) will develop in most patients at risk, and is diagnosed by antigen detection, nucleic acid identification, or culture. Symptomatic disease develops in 40 to 60% of primary infections and approximately 20% of secondary infections. The manifestations of CMV disease vary with the organ transplanted. The risk of CMV disease is increased in patients who are treated with antithymocyte globulin or OKT3. CMV disease is treated with ganciclovir, with or without CMV Ig. CMV disease can be prevented by the use of screened blood products, oral valganciclovir prophylaxis, and by prophylactic or preemptive treatment (at the earliest sign of viral replication) with ganciclovir and hyper-Ig.

The PTLD is caused by EBV infection, and occurs in 6 to 9% of lung transplants, 3 to 5% of heart transplants, 2 to 4% of liver transplants, and <1% of kidney transplants. The risk of PTLD is increased by treatment with anti-T-cell antibodies. PTLD presents 6 to 24 weeks after transplantation with an infectious mononucleosis-like syndrome or diverse local manifestations that may involve any lymphatic tissue, the GI tract, lungs, kidneys, or brain. The diagnosis is made by demonstrating the EBV genome in association with benign or malignant lymphatic proliferation. Treatment strategies include reduced immunosuppression, interferon-α, and cytotoxic chemotherapy. Local resection may be helpful, and there is an uncertain role for acyclovir or ganciclovir.

Noninfectious Complications: Noninfectious complications consist of complications related to the surgical procedure itself, rejection, and those related to the toxicities of the immunosuppressant drugs. They also can be divided into early and late complications. Noninfectious problems in the first few weeks after solid organ transplantation include (1) surgical complications; (2) graft dysfunction related to ischemia, preservation, and reperfusion; and (3) rejection. After the first few months, chronic rejection is a significant problem as are the side effects of immunosuppressant medications, as noted above. These noninfectious complications will be discussed in more detail with each of the specific transplant types.

Liver Transplantation

Background

Liver transplantation is a treatment for both acute and chronic liver failure. In the acute setting, liver transplantation is used in cases of fulminant hepatic failure, which is defined as the onset of liver failure with encephalopathy within a short period of time (weeks). Cases of fulminant hepatic failure that may require transplant include acetaminophen toxicity, acute viral hepatitis, autoimmune hepatitis, and others. The criteria for transplantation have been difficult to evaluate as patients either survive to full recovery or die rapidly. The Kings College criteria (Table 2) are the most commonly used prognostic criteria to decide on the suitability of a patient for liver transplantation.

Chronic liver failure (cirrhosis) that is uncompensated is considered to be treatable by liver transplantation. The decision to consider liver transplantation will depend on the severity of the disease as well as the quality of life and the absence of contraindications. The system currently in place to characterize the severity of liver disease appropriate for transplantation is known as the Model for End-stage Liver Disease (or MELD) score. The score is calculated as 3.8 (Ln serum

Table 2. *King's College Hospital Criteria for Liver Transplantation in Patients With Fulminant Hepatic Failure*

Conditions	Criteria
Acetaminophen-induced disease	Arterial pH <7.3 (irrespective of the grade of encephalopathy) or grade III or IV encephalopathy, prothrombin time of >100 s, and serum creatinine level of >3.4 mg/dL (301 μmol/L)
All other causes of fulminant hepatic failure	Prothrombin time of >100 s (irrespective of the grade of encephalopathy) or any three of the following variables (irrespective of the grade of encephalopathy): (1) age <10 yr or >40 yr; (2) etiology of non-A, non-B hepatitis, halothane hepatitis, or idiosyncratic drug reactions; (3) duration of jaundice before onset of encephalopathy of <7 d; (4) prothrombin time of >50 s; and (5) serum bilirubin level of >18 mg/dL (308 μmol/L)

bilirubin [in milligrams per deciliter]) + 11.2 (Ln INR) + 9.6 (Ln serum creatinine [in milligrams per deciliter]) + 6.4. A score of ≥10 is the usual indication for referral to a liver transplant center. A listing for liver transplantation usually occurs at this point or with a higher score. The score is also used for prioritization on the waiting list.

Typical Postoperative ICU Course

Liver transplant recipients require ICU care for 1 to 4 days after surgery. The cardiac output is generally high, and the systemic vascular resistance is low; circulatory instability is common and usually volume-responsive. Myocardial depression is a poor prognostic sign. Calcium may be depleted by the citrate in blood products. Hyperglycemia is common, and potassium levels may be high or low. A mild metabolic acidosis may be present initially, but metabolic alkalosis develops as the liver metabolizes citrate. Deficient clotting factor levels and thrombocytopenia contribute to a significant bleeding diathesis. Blood products are usually replaced empirically (for evident bleeding and a fall in hematocrit), although many centers monitor coagulation with thromboelastography, which is a rapid measure of the time to the onset of clotting, the rate of clot formation, and maximum clot elasticity. Important signs of a functioning graft are the production of golden-brown bile, the restoration of clotting, the absence of metabolic acidosis, and the resolution of encephalopathy. Patients should be awake and alert within 12 h. The serum bilirubin level may rise initially because of hemolysis, but liver enzyme levels should fall each day. The prothrombin time and partial thromboplastin time should improve daily and should be normal within 72 h. Most patients can be extubated within 12 to 48 h.

Noninfectious Complications

Hemorrhage in the first 48 h usually is caused by diffuse oozing in the setting of a coagulopathy and is managed with blood products. Later, intraabdominal bleeding may be related to necrosis of a vascular anastamosis. GI hemorrhage may result from stress ulceration or the development of portal hypertension. Primary graft failure occurs in 1 to 5% of patients receiving liver transplants and usually is a consequence of ischemic injury. The signs of graft failure include poor bile formation, metabolic acidosis, and failure to resolve encephalopathy and coagulopathy. The treatment is retransplantation within 48 h, before brainstem herniation from cerebral edema occurs. Vascular complications include thromboses of the hepatic artery, hepatic vein, or portal vein. Hepatic artery thrombosis occurs in about 5% of patients and presents in one of the following four ways: massive liver necrosis (eg, fever, rising enzymes, deterioration in mental status, renal insufficiency, and shock); a bile leak with or without evidence of liver injury; recurrent bacteremia from hepatic abscesses; or as an asymptomatic finding on a routine ultrasound. The diagnosis is made by duplex ultrasonography, and the treatment is operative repair or retransplantation. Portal vein thrombosis is less common, and presents with ascites and variceal hemorrhage, with or without graft dysfunction. Hepatic vein thrombosis is rare, and presents with liver failure and massive ascites. Biliary complications occur in up to 28% of patients. Bile leaks are caused by traumatic or ischemic injury to the common bile duct. Biliary obstruction may be caused by the kinking of the bile duct or drainage tubes, dysfunction of the sphincter of Oddi,

or strictures. Biliary complications are diagnosed by cholangiography and are managed with surgical or endoscopic repair.

Acute rejection is the most common cause of liver dysfunction after transplantation. Most patients experience at least one episode, usually 4 to 14 days after transplantation. The clinical signs (eg, fever, tenderness, and enlargement of graft) and laboratory features (eg, elevated levels of hepatocellular enzymes and bilirubin) are nonspecific. The diagnosis is confirmed with a liver biopsy finding that demonstrates mononuclear cell portal infiltration, ductal injury, and venulitis. Most patients respond to therapy with pulse steroids or anti-T-cell antibodies. ICU readmission is rarely required. Common noninfectious pulmonary complications of liver transplantation include atelectasis, pleural effusions, and pulmonary edema. In most cases, preoperative shunting caused by the hepatopulmonary syndrome improves over days to months posttransplant. Respiratory muscle weakness, the abdominal wound, impaired mental status, and severe metabolic alkalosis may contribute to delayed weaning. ARDS occurs in <10% of liver graft recipients, usually as a consequence of sepsis. Neurologic dysfunction after liver transplantation may be caused by hepatic encephalopathy, hypoglycemia, intracranial hemorrhage, air embolism, drug toxicity, or infection.

Infection

Bacteria are the most important causes of infection after liver transplantation, particularly in the first 6 weeks after grafting. Gram-positive cocci and Gram-negative bacilli are the predominant pathogens, and the site of infection often involves the transplanted liver or the reconstructed biliary tree. Intraabdominal abscesses, peritonitis, cholangitis, and surgical wound infections are the most common foci of bacterial infection, followed by pneumonia, catheter sepsis, and urinary tract infections.

Prophylactic systemic and topical antibiotics are commonly used but are of unproven value. CMV infection will be evident in approximately 50% of liver transplant recipients, and half of these cases will be symptomatic. Seropositivity for CMV is the most important risk factor for CMV disease. The peak onset of CMV infection is

28 days after transplantation. The most common manifestation is a mononucleosis-like syndrome that is characterized by fever, malaise, myalgias, and neutropenia. Hepatitis is the most common involvement in the liver. Anecdotal reports have suggested that the treatment of CMV disease with ganciclovir is beneficial. CMV disease can be prevented in high-risk patients by long-term (100-day) ganciclovir prophylaxis or by preemptive treatment at the first sign of viral replication. HSV mucositis reactivates in 40 to 50% of seropositive patients and can be prevented or treated with acyclovir therapy. Fungal infections complicate 10 to 40% of liver transplants, usually in the first 2 months, and are more common in liver transplants than in the transplantation of other organs. Candidemia, from an abdominal or vascular source, is the leading mycosis, followed by pulmonary aspergillosis. Pneumocystis infections are rare in patients receiving prophylaxis.

Kidney Transplant

Background

Kidney transplantation is the treatment of choice for patients with end-stage renal disease. A successful kidney transplant improves the quality of life and reduces the mortality risk for most patients, when compared with maintenance dialysis. Unfortunately, the number of patients awaiting transplant far outstrips the supply of donor organs available and has resulted in many patients requiring ongoing dialysis with its associated morbidities. Sources for renal allografts include cadaveric donors, living related donors, and living unrelated donors. Human leukocyte antigen matching of the donor and the recipient is routinely performed, resulting in the high levels of graft survival that are seen. In the United States, diabetes or hypertension is the cause of chronic renal insufficiency in most recipients.

Typical Postoperative ICU Course

Patients who have undergone renal transplantation rarely, if ever, require ICU care in the immediate postoperative period. They are generally extubated in the recovery room and brought to a non-ICU hospital floor.

Noninfectious Complications

Serious noninfectious complications are uncommon after renal transplantation. Volume overload and graft dysfunction occasionally lead to pulmonary edema. Surgical complications such as renal artery thrombosis, renal vein thrombosis, urine leaks, and lymphoceles occur in <5% of patients. Hyperacute rejection from preformed antibodies causes immediate graft failure and is usually detected in the operating room. Acute rejection occurs in 50 to 60% of patients within the first 3 months and is suspected by a rise in creatinine level that is not attributable to cyclosporine toxicity. Acute rejection is empirically treated with corticosteroids; refractory cases are confirmed by renal biopsy. Chronic rejection develops in 8 to 10% of patients.

Infectious Complications

Urinary tract infections are common soon after renal transplantation and can be prevented with prophylaxis using antibiotics. Bacterial infections of the wound, IV catheter sites, and the respiratory tract also may complicate the early postoperative course. Opportunistic infections caused by Legionella, Nocardia, and Listeria usually occur 1 to 6 months after transplantation. Fungal infections are less common in renal graft recipients than in other organ transplant patients. Primary CMV infection develops in 70 to 90% of seronegative recipients of a kidney from a seropositive donor, and 50 to 60% of these patients will be symptomatic. CMV infection develops in 50 to 80% of seropositive recipients, and 20 to 40% of these patients will have clinical disease. The onset of infection is usually 1 to 6 months after transplant. The mononucleosis-like CMV syndrome is the most common manifestation of CMV disease in renal transplant recipients; CMV pneumonia will develop in about 25% of symptomatic patients. Ganciclovir appears to be effective in treating CMV disease in the setting of renal transplantation.

Kidney-Pancreas Transplant

Background

Kidney-pancreas transplant is considered for patients with renal failure and type I diabetes. The major reported benefit is an improved quality of life due to avoidance of the need for insulin and dialytic therapy. Most procedures are performed as simultaneous transplants, although sequential kidney then pancreas transplantation or pancreas transplantation alone is performed. For those patients with type I diabetes mellitus undergoing cadaveric transplantation (but not living donor transplantation), survival appears to be better with a simultaneous pancreas transplantation.

Typical Postoperative ICU Course

Patients require ICU monitoring of fluids and electrolytes, and tight glucose control with an insulin drip to keep the pancreas at rest. Glucose regulation may normalize within hours, but several days are often required for full graft function. Also, bicarbonate loss due to secretion by the pancreas into the bowel or bladder where the pancreas implant is placed can lead to metabolic acidosis.

Noninfectious Complications

Complications are more common after kidney-pancreas transplantation than after kidney transplantation alone. Surgical complications include vascular thrombosis, hematuria, perforation of the duodenal segment, and urethral stricture. Loss of sodium bicarbonate in the urine may cause significant dehydration and metabolic acidosis. Acute pancreatic rejection occurs in >85% of cases, more commonly than kidney rejection, and is more refractory to therapy with corticosteroids. Pancreatic rejection is diagnosed by an abrupt fall in urinary amylase levels; some centers confirm rejection histologically by cystoscopic biopsy. Most cases of pancreatic rejection fail to respond to corticosteroids and require repeated courses of OKT3.

Infectious Complications

Infections also are more common in patients who receive kidney-pancreas transplants than in recipients who receive kidney transplants alone because of the additional surgery and the need for more immunosuppression. Wound infections, urinary tract infections, and abdominal abscesses caused by bacteria or fungi are particularly

frequent in the first month after transplantation but may appear a year or more postoperatively. Active CMV infection will develop in most patients who are at risk, and the majority of these infections will be symptomatic with a viremic syndrome; the liver is the most common site of tissue infection in the form of hepatitis.

Heart Transplant

Background

Published recommendations for considering transplantation in patients with cardiac conditions are for those with advanced disease (generally, New York Heart Association class III or IV) that have not responded to maximal medical management. Underlying coronary artery disease and nonischemic cardiomyopathy each account for about 45% of cases, a distribution that has not changed appreciably in many years. Judging when in the course of chronic heart failure transplantation should be considered is difficult. In general, the peak oxygen uptake measured on cardiopulmonary exercise testing appears to provide the most objective assessment of functional capacity in patients with heart failure and may be the best predictor of when to list an individual patient for cardiac transplantation. The 2002 task force of the American College of Cardiology and the American Heart association recommended the use of exercise testing with ventilatory gas analysis for this purpose.

Usual Postoperative Course

Cardiac function is depressed for several days postoperatively, and the right ventricle recovers more slowly than the left. Cardiac output is initially rate-dependent in the denervated heart, and treatment with low-dose isoproterenol or pacing is often required for 2 to 4 days. Patients are routinely extubated within 24 h and discharged from the ICU within 48 h.

Noninfectious Complications

The early complications of heart transplantation include those of cardiac surgery in general. The development of left lower-lobe atelectasis and mediastinal fluid collection is common in most patients, but hemorrhage is unusual. Pulmonary edema is a frequent occurrence because of pretransplant congestion, postoperative left ventricular dysfunction, and volume overload; heparin-protamine reactions and reperfusion injury may alter lung permeability. Persistent pulmonary hypertension is an important early problem that may lead to right ventricular failure. Treatment with prostaglandin E1, nitric oxide, inotropes, and assist devices may be effective. Rejection may occur any time after heart transplantation and is diagnosed histologically from routine surveillance endomyocardial biopsies. Clinical signs of rejection such as fever, heart failure, arrhythmias, and pericardial friction rubs are unreliable. The severity of rejection is graded by the degree of lymphocytic infiltration and myocyte necrosis. Mild cases may resolve spontaneously; about one third of patients require treatment for rejection. Most episodes respond to treatment with pulse corticosteroids and/or increased doses of cyclosporine. Refractory patients usually respond to anti-T-cell treatment. Accelerated coronary atherosclerosis is the leading cause of death >1 year after heart transplantation. The cumulative incidence is approximately 10% per year. Calcium channel blockers and hydroxymethylglutaryl coenzyme A reductase inhibitors may slow the development of allograft vasculopathy.

Infectious Complications

Nosocomial bacterial pneumonia, mediastinitis, empyema, and catheter-related infections are common in the first month after transplantation. Gram-negative bacilli and *Staphylococcus aureus* are frequent pathogens. Legionella pneumonia and wound infections are important in the first 3 months after heart transplantation, particularly in hospitals with contaminated water supplies. Nocardia infection of the lung may present at any time after the first postoperative month and may disseminate to the brain or bone. Atypical mycobacterial infections have been reported in 3% of heart transplant recipients, usually involving the lung, mediastinum, or soft tissues. Aspergillosis is the most common fungal infection after heart transplantation, developing in 5 to 10% of recipients, usually in the first month. The lung is the primary site of infection, but dissemination is evident in half of the cases at diagnosis. Toxoplasmosis is an important consideration when a seronegative recipient receives a heart from a seropositive donor. Primary infection presents 4 to 6 weeks after transplantation with fever and nonspecific signs involving the heart, brain, eyes, lungs, and/or liver; myocardial infection may mimic rejection. The diagnosis is supported by seroconversion and confirmed by the demonstration of tachyzoites in tissue. Treatment with pyrimethamine and sulfadiazine is effective if instituted promptly. Pyrimethamine also may be effective in preventing primary infection. Reactivation of latent toxoplasmosis in seropositive recipients is not clinically significant. *P carinii* pneumonia develops in 3% of cardiac transplant patients without prophylaxis but is now rare. Active CMV infection will develop in most seropositive patients and seronegative recipients of hearts from seropositive donors. One third of these infections will be symptomatic, usually with a mononucleosis-like syndrome. CMV pneumonia develops in 10% of infected patients. Serious morbidity and mortality are largely limited to patients with primary infection. Ganciclovir appears to be effective in the treatment of CMV disease in heart transplant patients. The role of ganciclovir in prophylaxis is uncertain. The reactivation of oral and genital HSV infection is common in the first few months after heart transplantation. VZV typically reactivates in a dermatomal distribution 3 to 6 months after transplantation. HSV and VZV infections usually remain localized and respond to treatment with acyclovir. PTLD develops in 2 to 7% of heart transplant recipients, usually presenting 3 to 6 months after transplantation. PTLD is probably caused by EBV, and the risk is markedly increased by treatment with OKT3. Any lymphatic tissue may be involved, as well as the GI tract, lungs, kidneys, or brain. Most cases respond to a reduction in immunosuppressive therapy. The resection of localized tumors and treatment with acyclovir may be helpful.

Lung Transplant

Background

Lung transplantation is relatively infrequent compared to other transplants because of the pulmonary injury or infection that so often occurs in cadaveric donors. Because of this, lung transplantation after donation from a living related person, particularly for younger recipients, is currently being performed at a few centers. Lung transplantation is performed for a wide variety of diagnoses; however, the majority of individuals on the waiting list have COPD. Lung transplantation can be unilateral or bilateral. Currently, there is an increasing trend toward bilateral transplant for all diagnoses. Previously, time on the waiting list was used to order lung transplant recipient waiting lists; however, more recently a lung allocation score has been devised that includes the type and severity of disease, and other factors that predict mortality and prevent death while the patient is on the waiting list.

Usual Postoperative Clinical Course

Volume overload and pulmonary edema are common early problems. Cardiac function may be impaired if cardiopulmonary bypass was required (all heart-lung transplants and some lung transplants). Cardiac output is rate-dependent in denervated hearts, and responds to therapy with isoproterenol. Care must be taken to avoid airtrapping in an emphysematous native lung. Independent lung ventilation through a double-lumen endotracheal tube may be necessary in some single-lung transplant recipients to improve ventilation-perfusion matching or reduce airtrapping. Most patients can be extubated within 36 h. Patients receiving single-lung transplants for primary pulmonary hypertension often are heavily sedated for 48 to 72 h before extubation to reduce pulmonary arterial hypertensive crises. Reflexive coughing is lost in the denervated lung, and pulmonary toilet is critical for secretion management. The lymphatics are severed in the transplanted lung, impairing extravascular fluid clearance and rendering the graft particularly susceptible to edema.

Noninfectious Complications

Hemorrhage early after lung transplantation is usually from the mediastinum or pleura. Bleeding is particularly common in heart-lung transplants because of the extensive mediastinal dissection and the need for heparinization during bypass. Patients with cystic fibrosis also are at increased risk of hemorrhage because pleural adhesions often must be severed to remove the native lungs. Bilateral bronchial anastomoses require less mediastinal dissection and are associated with less bleeding than tracheal anastomoses. The pulmonary reimplantation response is evident in most patients. This is a form of reperfusion injury that results in noncardiogenic pulmonary edema. The clinical features include alveolar and interstitial infiltrates seen on a chest radiograph, a decline in lung compliance, and impaired gas exchange. The response peaks 2 to 4 days after transplantation and resolves gradually thereafter with careful fluid management and diuresis. The diagnosis is made by the clinical presentation and time course, and the exclusion of infection, rejection, and cardiogenic pulmonary edema.

Airway dehiscence, stenosis, and bronchomalacia were major causes of morbidity and mortality in the early years of lung transplantation. The use of telescoping bronchial anastomoses has markedly reduced the incidence of airway complications. Strictures now develop in about 10% of cases, and stents are occasionally required for the management of stenoses. Phrenic nerve paralysis resulting from thermal or mechanical injury occurs in <5% of patients. The injury is often temporary, with gradual recovery over several weeks. Acute rejection occurs as early as 3 days after lung transplantation, and most patients will experience at least one episode within the first postoperative month. Lung rejection is more common than heart rejection in heart-lung transplants. The clinical manifestations are nonspecific, and include low-grade fever, dyspnea, cough, fatigue, hypoxemia, a fall in FEV_1, and new or changing infiltrates seen on a chest radiograph (the chest radiograph is usually normal when rejection occurs >1 month after transplantation). Infection and edema are the major alternative considerations in the first few weeks after transplantation; later, CMV is the principal concern. Bronchoscopy is helpful in excluding infection and confirming rejection. Transbronchial biopsy specimens demonstrate the characteristic perivascular mononuclear infiltrates with a sensitivity of 70 to 90% and a specificity of >90%. There may be a role for identifying donor-sensitized lymphocytes by BAL. Most patients respond promptly to therapy with pulse corticosteroids; nonresponders are treated with anti-T-cell antibodies. Obliterative bronchiolitis is the major manifestation of chronic rejection in the transplanted lung and a leading cause of late mortality. The incidence of obliterative bronchiolitis increases over time and is found in 60 to 70% of patients who survive for 5 years after undergoing transplantation. Repeated episodes of acute rejection and CMV infection are possible risk factors. Obliterative bronchiolitis may present any time after the second postoperative month, with half of the cases presenting in the first year. Patients may complain of dyspnea or cough, and chest radiograph findings are usually normal. The clinical diagnosis hinges on a spirometric demonstration of significant declines in FEV_1 and the mid-expiratory phase of forced expiratory flow. Some centers have found transbronchial biopsies to be helpful. Treatment is administered with increased immunosuppression, but no strategy has been demonstrated to be effective. Pulmonary function may stabilize with treatment but rarely improves. The mortality rate of patients with obliterative bronchiolitis is 40% within 2 years of diagnosis.

Infectious Complications

Infection is the leading cause of death after lung transplantation, and most infections are located in the thorax. Most centers advocate an aggressive approach to etiologic diagnosis, relying heavily on bronchoscopy. In single-lung transplant recipients, infection in the native lung is a significant problem. Bacteria are the most common agents of infection after lung transplantation. Bacterial pneumonia is most frequent in the early postoperative period, but purulent bronchitis often presents weeks to months after transplantation; late bacterial infections are particularly common in patients with obliterative bronchiolitis. Typical nosocomial pathogens are the usual culprits, although native strains of *Pseudomonas cepacia* and *Pseudomonas aeruginosa* are problematic in patients with cystic fibrosis. Prophylactic broad-spectrum antibiotics are routinely administered for the first 48 to 72 h after transplantation, empirically or guided by cultures from the donor and recipient respiratory tracts; the validity of this practice has not been tested by controlled trial. Bacterial infections usually respond to treatment with antibiotics.

CMV disease is more common in lung allograft recipients than in other solid organ transplant patients. Positive blood and BAL cultures (active infection) will develop in most seropositive recipients a median of 40 days after transplantation in the absence of prophylaxis, but the risk and severity of symptomatic CMV disease are highest in seronegative patients who receive a lung from a seropositive donor (ie, those with a primary infection). Treatment with OKT3 is an additional risk for CMV, but CMV infection may increase the risk of acute and chronic rejection. Prophylaxis with ganciclovir may be effective in preventing or delaying CMV disease in at-risk patients, but the optimal regimen has not been defined. HSV mucositis develops in 30% of seropositive lung transplant recipients in the absence of acyclovir prophylaxis, and pneumonia develops in half of these patients.

Primary HSV infections are rare. Acyclovir appears to be effective in preventing the reactivation of HSV. EBV-related PTLD occurs in approximately 6% of lung allograft recipients. The typical case presents within the first 4 months after transplantation with nodular infiltrates in the lung allograft, although any lymphoid tissue may be involved. Most patients respond to a reduction in the immunosuppressive regimen. Fungal infections occur in 15 to 35% of lung transplant recipients. Candidiasis is the most common mycosis and may involve the mediastinum, the airway anastomosis, or dissemination from a cutaneous or vascular site. Invasive aspergillosis typically presents as a focal pneumonia or necrotizing airway infection. The reported mortality rate for patients with fungal infections after lung transplantation has ranged from 20 to 80%. The roles for antifungal prophylaxis and aggressive treatment of mucosal isolates are unclear. disease. CMV pneumonitis is the most common manifestation of CMV disease in lung allograft recipients. The chest radiograph is nonspecific, and a positive BAL culture finding is predictive of histologic evidence of infection only in the highest risk patients (ie, seronegative recipient/seropositive donor). Transbronchial biopsies are required to identify viral inclusions and to exclude rejection. The treatment of CMV pneumonitis in lung transplant recipients with ganciclovir is probably effective but has not been prospectively studied. The direct mortality rate from CMV disease in treated patients is about 1%,

Bibliography

Bakker NA, van Imhoff GW, Verschuuren EA, et al. Presentation and early detection of post-transplant lymphoproliferative disorder after solid organ transplantation. Transpl Int 2007; 20:207–218

Becker BN, Odorico JS, Becker YT, et al. Simultaneous pancreas-kidney and pancreas transplantation. J Am Soc Nephrol 2001; 12:2517–2527

Glanville AR, Estenne M. Indications, patient selection and timing of referral for lung transplantation. Eur Respir J 2003; 22:845–852

Knoop C, Estenne M. Acute and chronic rejection after lung transplantation. Semin Respir Crit Care Med 2006; 27:521–533

McGilvray ID, Greig PD. Critical care of the liver transplant patient: an update. Curr Opin Crit Care 2002; 8:178–182

Port FK, Dykstra DM, Merion RM, et al. Trends and results for organ donation and transplantation in the United States, 2004. Am J Transplant 2005; 5:843–849

Steinman TI, Becker BN, Frost AE, et al. Guidelines for the referral and management of patients eligible for solid organ transplantation. Transplantation 2001; 71:1189–1204

Notes

Infections in AIDS Patients and Other Immunocompromised Hosts

George H. Karam, MD, FCCP

Objectives:

- Propose an approach to the immunocompromised patient based on identification of defects in three major host defense systems
- Review the likely pathogens, their clinical presentations, and therapeutic options in patients with neutropenia
- Summarize the various limbs in humoral immunity, with particular attention to the clinical situations of asplenia and splenic dysfunction
- Outline the categories and clinical presentations of pathogens likely to be encountered with deficits of cell-mediated immunity
- Focus on the broadening number of clinical issues in patients whose cell-mediated immunity defect is on the basis of HIV infection

Key words: asplenia; cell-mediated immunity; HIV; humoral immunity; neutropenia

In the clinical approach to patients with fever presumed to be infectious in etiology, a basic consideration is whether the patient is a normal host or one who is immunocompromised. A traditional method has been to consider host defense in immunocompromised patients as being in one of two categories: (1) mechanical factors, including barrier systems such as skin and mucous membranes (which are protective against infection) or foreign bodies such as intravascular and urinary catheters (which predispose to infection); and (2) cellular host defense, which includes the three major categories of primary neutrophil defense, humoral immunity, and cell-mediated immunity. Use of an approach that identifies the defective limb of host defense allows for directed therapeutic decisions that are based on likely pathogens for the involved site.

Recent attention has been focused on the concept of type 1 and type 2 immunity as they interrelate with humoral and cell-mediated immunity.[1] Subpopulations of CD4+ lymphocytes are important in both humoral immunity and cell-mediated immunity, with T helper type 1 (Th1) and T helper type 2 (Th2) cells being the most relevant. All T helper lymphocytes start out as naive Th0 cells, which, after being activated, are capable of "polarizing" or differentiating into either Th1 or Th2 effector cells. Although multiple factors are involved, the key to polarization of Th0 cells into the Th1 phenotype is interleukin (IL)-12, whereas IL-4 is needed for Th2 polarization. These events may not occur until an activated T cell arrives at the site of danger and samples the local cytokine milieu to determine if an inflammatory or antibody response is appropriate. In questionable circumstances, the Th2 outcome is favored over the Th1 differentiation because IL-4 dominates IL-12. Th1 cells, which are involved with type 1 immunity, secrete interferon-gamma (IFN-γ), IL-2, and lymphotoxin-α as the cytokines chiefly responsible for their proinflammatory effect. The Th1 cell is associated with strong cell-mediated immunity and weak humoral immunity. Th2 cells are involved with type 2 immunity, are influenced by IL-4, IL-10, and IL-13, stimulate high titers of antibody production, and are associated with suppression of cell-mediated immunity and with strong humoral immunity. When integrated into the traditional approach of cell-mediated immunity and humoral immunity, type 1 and type 2 immunity have important therapeutic implications in the care provided for immunocompromised patients.

Primary Neutrophil Function

The polymorphonuclear leukocyte is the major phagocyte for both primary neutrophil defense and humoral immunity. Once a pathogen is ingested by these cells and is intracellular, killing is generally an easy process. Pathogens that classically infect patients with primary neutrophil problems are those that may be ingested without opsonization. The system of neutrophil defense has been described as being responsible for defending against organisms that are easy to eat and easy to kill.[2]

An important pathophysiologic consideration is that polymorphonuclear leukocytes may have either an extravascular or intravascular location. After leaving the bloodstream, these phagocytes go to two major sites: the subepithelial area of skin and the submucosal area of the GI tract. Recognition of this fact allows for an understanding of the organisms that classically infect neutropenic patients.

As represented in Table 1, neutrophil dysfunction may occur on either a qualitative or quantitative basis. Qualitative defects characteristically occur in children and are associated with polymorphonuclear leukocytes that are normal in number but abnormal in function. Classic qualitative defects of polymorphonuclear leukocytes are related to dysfunction in one of the following processes: (1) diapedesis (the ability to leave the intravascular space via endothelial channels); (2) chemotaxis (movement to the site of infection); (3) ingestion (the process of attaching to the pathogen and then getting that pathogen within the cell, where killing takes place); and (4) intracellular killing (which may occur via either oxygen-dependent or oxygen-independent mechanisms).

Quantitative defects, which are the more characteristic neutrophil problems in adults, clinically present as the entity interchangeably referred to as either granulocytopenia or neutropenia. Characteristic conditions that may lead to neutropenia are listed in Table 1. Although eosinophils are classified as granulocytes, for most clinical purposes the granulocyte count is calculated by adding the percentage of polymorphonuclear leukocytes and band forms, and then multiplying the total WBC count by that percentage. In the guidelines of the Infectious Diseases Society of America (IDSA) for management of febrile, neutropenic patients, a calculated granulocyte count of <500 cells/mm^3 indicates absolute neutropenia; a granulocyte count <1,000 cells/mm^3 with a predicted decline to <500 cells/mm^3 should be considered neutropenia.[3] In the setting of neutropenia and fever, the clinician must assume that the patient has impaired natural defense against the pathogens defended against by this limb of host defense.

The clinical course of patients with neutropenia is variable and may be explained in part by the integrity of the gut mucosa. In conditions such as aplastic anemia or HIV-associated neutropenia, the gut mucosa is usually intact, and those patients have a lower incidence of bacteremia. In contrast, patients who receive chemotherapeutic agents that cause mucositis have loss of both the mechanical barrier of gut mucosa and submucosal polymorphonuclear leukocytes. These patients are more likely to experience Gram-negative bacteremia and fungemia.

Infections due to bacteria are classically encountered when the neutropenia is either rapid in development or profound (especially with counts <100 cells/mm^3). The pathogens most likely to infect neutropenic patients are listed in Table 2. The bacteria characteristically involved are skin and gut flora, as might be predicted from the loss of subepithelial and submucosal polymorphonuclear leukocytes. Although any of the enterobacteriaceae (eg, Escherichia coli or Klebsiella) may cause infection in this setting, the most life-threatening

---

Table 1. *Conditions Causing Neutrophil Dysfunction*

Qualitative Defects
  Impaired diapedesis
  Impaired chemotaxis
  Impaired ingestion
  Impaired intracellular killing
Quantitative Defects (Neutropenia)
  Acute leukemia
  Invasion of bone marrow by neoplasms
  Treatment with agents toxic to marrow
  Drug idiosyncrasy
  Splenic sequestration syndromes
  HIV-associated neutropenia
  Idiopathic chronic neutropenia

Table 2. *Important Pathogens Causing Infection in Neutropenic Patients*

Gram-positive organisms
  Staphylococcus aureus
  Coagulase-negative staphylococci
  Viridans streptococci
  Enterococci
  Corynebacterium jeikeium
Enterobacteriaceae
Pseudomonas aeruginosa
Anaerobes, including *Bacteroides fragilis*
Fungi
  Yeasts, most notably Candida spp
  Filamentous fungi, most notably Aspergillus spp

Infections in AIDS Patients and Other Immunocompromised Hosts (Karam)

pathogen is *Pseudomonas aeruginosa*. Because of this (and despite the relative decline in the incidence of infection caused by this pathogen in neutropenic patients), a basic principle in empiric therapy of febrile neutropenic patients is coverage of *P aeruginosa*. The classic skin lesion that suggests such an infection is ecthyma gangrenosum. These lesions have a central area of hemorrhage surrounded by a halo of uninvolved skin with a narrow pink or purple rim. Histologically, the infection involves dermal veins, and clinically it may progress to bullae formation. Although other Gram-negative pathogens have been reported to cause such a process, the clinician should assume that ecthyma gangrenosum is caused by *P aeruginosa* until this pathogen has been excluded.

In recent years, infections caused by Gram-positive organisms have significantly increased in neutropenic patients. These pathogens, which are listed in Table 2, have increased in part because of the expanded use of invasive devices such as intravascular catheters, which breach the mechanical barrier of the skin. The important clinical finding of cavitary pulmonary infiltrates may be a clue to infection by either *Staphylococcus aureus* or *Corynebacterium jeikeium*. Notable among the Gram-positive pathogens is infection caused by viridans streptococci (eg, *Streptococcus mitis*), which may result in the viridans streptococcal shock syndrome. In a recent prospective study of 485 episodes of bacteremia in neutropenic patients with cancer,[4] viridans streptococci caused a total of 88 episodes (18%). Ten of these 88 cases (11%) were associated with serious complications, including ARDS plus septic shock (5 cases), ARDS (3 cases), and septic shock (2 cases). Of the patients with serious complications of their streptococcal bacteremia, 3 (30%) had a cutaneous rash, which in other reports has been associated on occasion with desquamation. Severe oral mucositis, high-dose chemotherapy with cyclophosphamide, and allogeneic bone marrow transplantation were the only variables found to be significantly associated with the development of complications. In patients with complications, 36% of these pathogens showed diminished susceptibility to penicillin, and approximately one half were resistant to ceftazidime. In a more recent review,[5] two additional risk factors for viridans streptococcal bacteremia in neutropenic patients were cytosine arabinoside and antimicrobial

prophylaxis with either trimethoprim/sulfamethoxazole or a fluoroquinolone.

The experience with antibiotic prophylaxis during the neutropenic period after autologous peripheral blood stem cell transplantation provides an important insight into a potential problem regarding viridans streptococci.[6] Despite the use of levofloxacin prophylaxis, viridans group streptococcal bacteremia developed in 6 of 37 patients (16.2%) who underwent transplantation over a 2-month period in 2001. All 6 patients presented with fever and mucositis after a mean of 4.5 days of neutropenia, and septic shock developed in 3 days. All six viridans group streptococcal isolates from these patients exhibited distinct patterns on pulsed-field gel electrophoresis. A conclusion of this paper was that the use of levofloxacin may select viridans group streptococci with diminished susceptibility to levofloxacin and other quinolones with enhanced activity against Gram-positive organisms and, therefore, may not be optimal for preventing viridans group streptococcal bacteremia in neutropenic patients.

A life-threatening complication that may occur in patients who have received chemotherapy is neutropenic enterocolitis. Previously referred to as typhlitis because of the cecum as the predominant site in many cases, neutropenic enterocolitis may involve the terminal ileum, the cecum, and the colon (with the ascending portion the most frequently involved). Pathogenetically, the process may occur on several bases including destruction of GI mucosa by chemotherapy, intramural hemorrhage due to severe thrombocytopenia, and alterations in GI tract flora. Patients characteristically present with the triad of fever, abdominal pain, and diarrhea, but these findings may be seen with other conditions including *Clostridium difficile* toxin–induced colitis and ischemic colitis. Ultrasound findings include echogenic thickening of the mucosa and bowel wall. Although isodense cecal wall thickening is the most notable CT finding, the distal ileum and remaining colon are also frequently involved. Although optimal therapy has not been definitively established, conservative medical management appears to be effective for most patients.[7]

Although the level of temperature elevation that mandates antimicrobial therapy in neutropenic patients may be influenced by the degree of neutropenia, fever in neutropenic patients has been defined as a single oral temperature of >38.5°C (101°F) or as a temperature of ≥38.0°C (100.4°F) over at least 1 h. In such patients, empiric antibiotics should be started after appropriate cultures are obtained. Because the patients do not have adequate neutrophils to provide natural host defense, all antimicrobial agents administered should be bactericidal. The classic regimen has been an antipseudomonal β-lactam antibiotic (*eg*, piperacillin or ceftazidime) in combination with an aminoglycoside. Although some centers acknowledge a decreasing prevalence of infection caused by *P aeruginosa*, the recommendation for coverage against this pathogen in febrile neutropenic patients is prompted by the higher rates of mortality that may occur when this pathogen infects neutropenic patients. According to a review of 410 episodes of Pseudomonas bacteremia in patients with cancer from 1972 to 1981, outcome was related to the interval between the onset of the bacteremia and the institution of appropriate therapy.[8] Of the neutropenic patients in this study who had *P aeruginosa* bacteremia and in whom therapy was delayed, 26% died within 24 h and 70% died within 48 h. In an update of these data from 1991 to 1995 in the same institution, the incidence of *P aeruginosa* bacteremia decreased between the two study periods from 4.7 to 2.8 cases per 1,000 admissions.[9] *P aeruginosa* bacteremia remained the most common in acute leukemia, where the frequency did not change. Overall cure rate was 80% in the latter study period vs 62% in the earlier study. The outcome among 230 patients who received appropriate therapy was related to the duration of bacteremia, with cure rates similar among patients who had bacteremia from 1 to 3 days (85%) but greater among patients with >3 days of bacteremia (for which the cure rate was only 50%.) A conclusion of the latter paper was that antibiotic regimens for empiric therapy in neutropenic patients and especially patients with acute leukemia should still provide coverage against *P aeruginosa*.[9]

Influenced by multiple factors, including the potential for acute mortality in neutropenic patients who are bacteremic with *P aeruginosa*, in its most recent recommendations for management of febrile neutropenic patients the IDSA has offered suggestions for empiric antimicrobial therapy.[3] In these recommendations, it was noted that the initial evaluation should determine (1) whether the patient is at low risk for complications (with the specifics defined in these guidelines), and (2) whether vancomycin therapy is needed. For low-risk adults only, an oral regimen using ciprofloxacin plus amoxicillin-clavulanate was suggested. Options in patients for monotherapy with vancomycin not being needed included one of the following agents: cefepime or ceftazidime; or imipenem or meropenem. Options for combination therapy were an aminoglycoside plus an antipseudomonal penicillin, cephalosporin (cefepime or ceftazidime), or carbapenem. In those patients in whom vancomycin is indicated (discussed in the following paragraph), three options were presented: cefepime or ceftazidime plus vancomycin, with or without an aminoglycoside; carbapenem plus vancomycin, with or without an aminoglycoside; or an antipseudomonal penicillin plus an aminoglycoside and vancomycin. Prior to the publication of the 2002 IDSA guidelines, a prospective, multicenter, double-blind, randomized clinical trial showed piperacillin-tazobactam given as monotherapy to be as effective as the combination of piperacillin-tazobactam plus amikacin for the treatment for adults who were febrile and neutropenic.[10] Even though an antipseudomonal penicillin was offered as an option in the 2002 IDSA guidelines for combination therapy without vancomycin and for therapy in which vancomycin was indicated, it was not presented as an option for monotherapy when vancomycin was not indicated.

An ongoing controversy remains regarding whether an agent like vancomycin, which would cover such pathogens as methicillin-resistant *S aureus*, penicillin- and cephalosporin-resistant *Streptococcus pneumoniae*, and *C jeikeium*, should be included in the initial regimen. Because of the risk of selecting vancomycin-resistant enterococci or vancomycin-resistant staphylococci with injudicious use of vancomycin, the IDSA guidelines for management of febrile neutropenic patients discouraged vancomycin use in routine empiric therapy for a febrile neutropenic patient and recommended that this agent be used in the following settings: (1) clinically suspected serious catheter-related infections (*eg*, bacteremia, cellulitis); (2) known colonization with methicillin-resistant *S aureus* or penicillin- and cephalosporin-resistant *S pneumoniae*; (3) positive results of blood cultures for Gram-positive bacteria before final identification and susceptibility testing; and (4) hypotension or other evidence of cardiovascular impairment.[3]

The guidelines of the American Society of Clinical Oncology (ASCO) for colony-stimulating factors were published in the *Journal of Clinical Oncology*.[11] Clinical situations for which recommendations were made in adults include the following: (1) when the expected incidence of neutropenia is ≥40% (although there are some special circumstances detailed in the ASCO guidelines that might be a valid exception); (2) as adjuncts to progenitor-cell transplantation; (3) after completion of induction chemotherapy in patients ≥55 years of age who have acute myeloid leukemia; and (4) after completion of the first few days of chemotherapy of the initial induction or first posttremission course in patients with acute lymphoblastic leukemia. In the 1996 ASCO guidelines, colony-stimulating factors were recommended after documented febrile neutropenia in a prior chemotherapy cycle to avoid infectious complications and maintain dose intensity in subsequent treatment cycles when chemotherapy dose reduction is not appropriate.[12] This was modified in the 2000 guidelines because there were no published regimens that have demonstrated disease-free or overall survival benefits when the dose of chemotherapy was maintained and secondary prophylaxis was instituted. Based on these data, it was recommended that, in the setting of many tumors but exclusive of curable tumors (*eg*, germ cell tumors), dose reduction after an episode of severe neutropenia should be considered as a primary therapeutic option. Colony-stimulating factors should be avoided in patients receiving concomitant chemotherapy and radiation therapy, particularly involving the mediastinum. Because no large-scale prospective, comparative trials evaluating the relative efficacy of granulocyte colony-stimulating factor vs granulocyte-macrophage colony-stimulating factor were available, guidelines about the equivalency of these preparations were not proposed. Certain patients with fever and neutropenia are at higher risk for infection-associated complications and have prognostic factors that are predictive of poor clinical outcome. The use of a colony-stimulating factor in such high-risk patients may be considered, but the benefits in

these circumstances have not been proven. Potential clinical factors mentioned in the 2000 guidelines include profound neutropenia (absolute neutrophil count <100/µL), uncontrolled primary disease, pneumonia, hypotension, multiorgan dysfunction (sepsis syndrome), and invasive fungal infection. Age > 65 years and posttreatment lymphopenia were mentioned as potentially being other high-risk factors, but it was acknowledged that these have not been consistently confirmed by multicenter trials.

Prolonged neutropenia is a major predisposition to fungal infection. Although the list of fungal organisms identified in neutropenic patients has increased significantly in recent years, the most important pathogens to consider are Candida spp and Aspergillus spp. On the basis of neutropenia, indwelling catheters, broad-spectrum antibiotics, and mucositis, neutropenic patients are at risk for candidemia. The clinical presentation may range from unexplained fever to a septic appearance. Autopsy series have suggested that as many as 50% of patients with evidence of metastatic candidal infections in visceral organs may have had negative antemortem blood cultures for Candida.[13] The characteristic clinical infection in this setting is chronic disseminated candidiasis, which has also been referred to as hepatosplenic candidiasis. This illness may present as unexplained fever, right upper quadrant tenderness, and elevated alkaline phosphatase. During the period of neutropenia, imaging studies may be negative, but as the granulocyte count improves, patients may demonstrate bull's-eye liver lesions on ultrasound and hypodense liver defects on abdominal CT scan.[14] In the 2004 guidelines of the IDSA for treatment of candidemia, the options for neutropenic patients included amphotericin B, liposomal amphotericin B, and caspofungin.[15] Noteworthy is that fluconazole, which was recommended in the treatment of candidemia in nonneutropenic patients, was not included as a treatment option in neutropenic patients. This recommendation is probably an acknowledgement of the evolving trend toward non-*albicans* species of Candida and of the potential role of azole therapy in selecting for such pathogens.

Aspergillus is a nosocomial pathogen that may be associated with vascular invasion and extensive tissue necrosis. The lungs are a prime site of infection, with a spectrum of disease that includes pulmonary infiltrates or cavitary lung lesions; infection of the paranasal sinuses and CNS may also occur.[16] Because of the nosocomial nature of this organism, it may be introduced into the skin with catheter insertion. With the lack of both intravascular and subepithelial polymorphonuclear leukocytes, and because of the vascular invasion, the skin lesions may be concentrically enlarging and necrotic. Blood cultures are not likely to reveal this pathogen. In a randomized trial comparing voriconazole with standard amphotericin B for primary treatment of invasive aspergillosis, voriconazole was demonstrated to be more effective than amphotericin B.[17] An evolving body of clinical data regarding this topic has led to the recent comment that voriconazole will likely become the drug of choice for treatment of invasive aspergillosis.[18]

There is not a consensus recommendation about when empiric antifungal therapy should be started for neutropenic patients who have persistent fever. The IDSA's clinical guidelines for treatment of infections caused by Candida suggest starting antifungal treatment when there is persistent unexplained fever despite 4 to 7 days of appropriate antibacterial therapy,[15] but the IDSA guidelines for therapy in febrile neutropenic patients suggest beginning empirical antifungal treatment when there is persistent fever for >3 days after antibacterial therapy is instituted in patients expected to have neutropenia for longer than 5 to 7 more days.[3] Because amphotericin B has activity against most Candida spp as well as Aspergillus, it has been the agent most often used. Liposomal amphotericin B has been shown to be as effective as conventional amphotericin B for empiric antifungal therapy in patients with fever and neutropenia, and it is associated with fewer breakthrough fungal infections, less infusion-related toxicity, and less nephrotoxicity.[19] More recently, a randomized, international, multicenter trial found that voriconazole (a new second-generation triazole with both Aspergillus and Candida activity) was comparable to liposomal amphotericin B for empiric antifungal therapy.[20] A statistically significant and noteworthy observation in this report was that patients receiving voriconazole had more episodes of transient visual changes (22%) than did those receiving liposomal amphotericin B (1%). In a blinded, randomized, international multicenter noninferiority study of caspofungin (50 mg daily; 70 mg on day 1) vs liposomal amphotericin B (3 mg/kg daily) for therapy of persistently febrile neutropenic patients, both agents were comparable in overall success; however, caspofungin was associated with more successful outcome in patients with baseline fungal infections (p = 0.043) and had fewer drug-related adverse events (p < 0.001).[21]

Humoral Immunity

To be ingested by polymorphonuclear leukocytes, there is a requirement that certain organisms undergo opsonization, a process in which those organisms are encased by a factor which then allows the phagocyte to attach. Once intracellular, these organisms are readily killed by the phagocyte. The humoral immune system provides for such opsonization through its major components of antibody and complement and may be summarized as providing protection against pathogens that are hard to eat but easy to kill.[2]

The antibody component of humoral immunity is dependent on the transformation of B lymphocytes into plasma cells, which produce as major opsonins IgG and IgM. A structural part of these antibodies is a component referred to as the Fc segment. Polymorphonuclear leukocytes have a receptor for this Fc segment. These Fc segments attach to the Fc receptor on the phagocyte, allowing the polymorphonuclear leukocyte to ingest the organism in a process that has been referred to as the "zipper" phenomenon of phagocytosis.

In addition to antibody, complement may serve as an opsonizer. Of the various complement components, the one most important for opsonization is C3b, which may be generated through two different pathways. In the classic complement pathway, the formation of antigen-antibody complexes turns on the complement cascade. Once C3 is activated, it is cleaved by C3 esterase to yield C3b. A limitation of the classic complement pathway is the requirement for antibody production, which may take hours to develop. In situations such as the acute development of pneumococcal infection, there is an immediate need for host defense that cannot wait for antibody production. It is in this setting that the alternative complement pathway (also known as the properdin system) becomes important. Instead of requiring an antigen-antibody complex to turn on the cascade, the alternative pathway is dependent on cell wall components such as teichoic acid and peptidoglycans found in Gram-positive organisms and lipopolysaccharides found in Gram-negative organisms. These lead to proteolytic cleavage of C3 to generate C3b, and this mechanism can lead to immediate opsonization. In addition to its opsonizing ability and its initiation of the membrane attack complex of complement, C3b can be joined by factors B and D to form a C3 convertase, which is highly labile. When bound by properdin, the C3 convertase is stabilized and can then cleave more C3 to generate more C3b, with a resultant amplification of the alternative complement pathway. Some clinical evidence exists that patients who have undergone splenectomy have a decrease in alternative pathway-mediated activation of C3.[22]

There are four clinically relevant situations within the category of defective humoral immunity: (1) disorders of immunoglobulin production; (2) asplenia or hyposplenic states; (3) hypocomplementemia; and (4) impaired neutralization of toxins.

The major clinical situations that result in disorders of immunoglobulin production are summarized in Table 3. Included in these processes is the lack of B-cell regulation, with its resultant production of abnormal immunoglobulins occurring on the basis of T-cell deficiency states in conditions such as HIV infection.

The characteristic pathogens infecting patients with impairment of immunoglobulin production are included in Table 4. Among the bacteria, the common feature is encapsulation, with the capsule essentially making them slippery and therefore dependent on opsonization for phagocyte attachment. Of the pathogens defended against by humoral immunity, the one that most frequently causes an acute life-threatening infection is *S pneumoniae*. In recent years, it has been noted that the severity of infection with *S pneumoniae* may be accentuated in patients with alcoholism or in those who are HIV-infected. In both patient groups, this pathogen may initially present as the etiologic agent of community-acquired pneumonia, which may be multilobar, with a high incidence of bacteremia and an increased risk of ARDS. An important consideration regarding infection with this pathogen is the increasing prevalence of penicillin resistance. Despite appropriate antibiotics and supportive care, the mortality in this setting remains high.

Also included among the pathogens that infect patients with defects in immunoglobulin production are certain viruses, including enteroviruses, influenza viruses, and arboviruses. Enteroviruses, particularly echovirus 24, have been associated with a clinical complex consisting of dermatomyositis-like skin lesions, edema, and neurologic problems. This has been referred to as chronic enteroviral meningoencephalitis.

Common variable immunodeficiency (CVI) is associated with functional abnormalities of both B and T cells but is usually classified as a primary antibody deficiency syndrome. Characterized by hypogammaglobulinemia and recurrent bacterial infections, CVI usually does not become clinically

Table 3. *Major Clinical Situations Resulting in Disorder of Immunoglobulin Production*

Congenital agammaglobulinemias
Common variable immunodeficiency (acquired hypogammaglobulinemia)
Heavy chain disease
Waldenström macroglobulinemia
Multiple myeloma
B-cell lymphomas
Chronic lymphocytic leukemia
T-cell deficiency states
Hyposplenic states

Table 4. *Pathogens in Patients With Defective Humoral Immunity*

Disorders of Immunoglobulin Production
  Streptococcus pneumoniae
  Haemophilus influenzae
  Encapsulated strains of Gram-negative bacilli
  Enteroviruses, particularly echovirus 24
  Influenza viruses
  Arboviruses
  Pneumocystis jiroveci (formerly *P carinii*)
  Giardia lamblia
Asplenic State or Splenic Dysfunction
  Streptococcus pneumoniae
  Capnocytophaga canimorsus
  Babesia microti
  Plasmodium spp
  Haemophilus influenzae
  Neisseria spp

---

apparent until the second or third decade of life. Affected patients have an increased risk of autoimmune, granulomatous, and lymphoproliferative diseases. Even though recurrent bacterial infections of the respiratory tract are the most common, diarrhea due to *Giardia lamblia* is frequently encountered. This reflects the importance of local immunoglobulin production in the GI tract as a component of defense against *G lamblia*. Because some of the common pathogens infecting the respiratory or GI tracts are dependent on antibody production for host defense, concomitant infection of these two body sites should raise the suspicion of immunoglobulin deficiency states such as CVI. IV immunoglobulin may be efficacious in patients with this clinical entity, but anaphylaxis with such therapy has been reported.

Anatomic asplenia, as well as the hyposplenic states that occur in persons with sickle cell disease (due to autoinfarction of the spleen) and in patients with Hodgkin disease (especially after therapy), are also important predispositions to infection. The propensity for infection in these patients occurs on the basis of impairment of several immunologic functions: (1) relative to other lymphoid organs, the spleen has a greater percentage of B lymphocytes and is therefore involved in the production of antibody to polysaccharide antigens; (2) the spleen participates as a phagocytic organ, removing opsonin-coated organisms or damaged cells from the circulation; and (3) alternative complement-mediated activation of C3 may be decreased in patients after splenectomy. An important clinical clue to heighten awareness of both functional and anatomic asplenia is the presence of Howell-Jolly bodies on the peripheral blood smear.

The important pathogens involved in infections in patients without a spleen or with splenic dysfunction are summarized in Table 4.[23] Responsible for about 80% of overwhelming infections in asplenic patients, *S pneumoniae* should be given a particularly high index of suspicion because the clinical entity of post-splenectomy pneumococcal sepsis may initially present as only a flu-like illness with fever and myalgias.[24] Within the course of a few hours, untreated patients may develop a fulminant course that includes disseminated intravascular coagulation, purpura fulminans, symmetrical peripheral gangrene, shock, and ultimately death. Although *S pneumoniae* and *Haemophilus influenzae* are pathogens encountered in patients with either disorders of immunoglobulin production or splenic dysfunction, the pathogens infecting the asplenic or hyposplenic patient are otherwise different. Also included are two pathogens, *Babesia microti* and Plasmodium spp, that infect erythrocytes to cause hemolytic states and that require removal of parasitized RBCs by the spleen as a protective defense. *Capnocytophaga canimorsus* produces an acute illness with eschar formation following dog bites to asplenic individuals.[25]

Patients with deficiencies in the late complement components (C5 through C8) may present with recurrent Neisseria spp infections. The total hemolytic complement (CH_{50}) is the best screening test for this population. If the assay is normal, one can essentially exclude complement deficiency. In addition, an X-linked properdin deficiency associated with absence of the alternative complement pathway may produce a similar picture of severe meningococcal disease.

Completing the spectrum of clinical problems that may occur on the basis of defective humoral immunity is less-than-optimal neutralization of toxins produced in diphtheria, tetanus, and botulism.

IV gammaglobulin is a polyvalent antibody product containing the IgG antibodies that regularly occur in the donor population as well as traces of IgA and IgM and immunoglobulin fragments. Its half-life of 3 weeks allows for once-monthly dosing for prophylaxis in patients with primary humoral immunodeficiency. For bone marrow transplant patients ≥20 years of age, it has been shown to decrease the risk of septicemia and certain other infections, interstitial pneumonia of infectious or idiopathic etiology, and acute graft-vs-host disease in the first 100 days posttransplant.[26] In this patient population, dosing is more frequent than in prophylaxis for primary humoral immunodeficiency. Contraindications to its use include selective IgA deficiency and severe systemic reactions to human immune globulin.

Prevention of disease with vaccine is important in patients with defects in humoral immunity, although responses to vaccine may be attenuated. The 23-valent pneumococcal vaccine is recommended for adults with functional or anatomic asplenia, chronic cardiovascular disease, chronic pulmonary disease, diabetes mellitus, alcoholism, chronic liver disease, cerebrospinal fluid (CSF) leaks, and immunocompromised states including malignancy and HIV infection. In the review by the Centers for Disease Control and Prevention (CDC),[27] revaccination once was recommended for two groups: (1) persons aged ≥2 years who are at highest risk for serious pneumococcal infection and those who are likely to have a rapid decline in pneumococcal antibody levels (*eg*, functional or anatomic asplenia, HIV infection, leukemia, lymphoma, Hodgkin disease, multiple myeloma, generalized malignancy, chronic renal failure, nephrotic syndrome, other conditions associated with immunosuppression [including transplantation], and those receiving immunosuppressive chemotherapy [including steroids]), provided that 5 years has elapsed since receipt of the first dose of pneumococcal vaccine; and (2) persons aged ≥65 years if they received the vaccine 5 years previously and were <65 years old at the time of the primary vaccination. In an overall analysis not limited to immunocompromised patients, the effectiveness of pneumococcal conjugate vaccine has been demonstrated to prevent disease in young children for whom the vaccine is indicated and may be reducing the rate of disease in adults.[28] This report noted that the vaccine provides an effective tool for reducing disease caused by drug-resistant strains. Routine vaccination with the quadrivalent *Neisseria meningitidis* vaccine is recommended for certain high-risk groups, including persons who have terminal complement component deficiencies and those who have anatomic or functional asplenia.[29] Although the need for revaccination of adults has not been determined, antibody levels to *N meningitidis* rapidly decline over 2 to 3 years, and revaccination may be considered 3 to 5 years after receipt of the initial dose. Prophylaxis options against meningococcal infection based on the patient population being treated include rifampin (600 mg orally q12h for 2 days), ciprofloxacin (500 mg orally as single dose in nonpregnant adults), or ceftriaxone (250 mg IM as a single dose). *H influenzae* B vaccines are immunogenic in splenectomized adults and may be considered for this group.[30] When elective splenectomy is planned, pneumococcal, meningococcal, and *H influenzae* B vaccination should precede surgery by at least 2 weeks, if possible.

Cell-Mediated Immunity

The cell-mediated immune system is dependent on the interrelationship of T lymphocytes with macrophages. In contrast to primary neutrophil defense and humoral immunity, in which the polymorphonuclear leukocyte is the major phagocyte, the predominant phagocytic cell in cell-mediated immunity is the macrophage. On initial exposure to an antigen, T lymphocytes become sensitized. When restimulated, these sensitized T lymphocytes produce a group of lymphokines, including macrophage activation factor. It is this substance that stimulates macrophages to better ingest and kill pathogens. In contrast to polymorphonuclear leukocytes, macrophages can readily ingest microorganisms but have a difficult time with intracellular killing. This system may be summarized as providing protection against pathogens that are easy to eat but hard to kill.[2]

Some of the disorders and clinical situations associated with defects in cell-mediated immunity are listed in Table 5. With aging alone, patients have a decrease in cell-mediated immunity. Pregnant women in their third trimester have a transient loss of cell-mediated immunity, which spontaneously reconstitutes itself within about 3 months of delivery.[31] Immunosuppressive drugs (including corticosteroids and cyclosporine) and HIV infection are associated with defects in this limb of host defense. Both steroids and HIV infection decrease total T lymphocyte numbers, resulting in production of abnormal amounts of lymphokines like macrophage activation factor. In contrast, cyclosporine does not decrease lymphocyte numbers but decreases the functional capacity of lymphocytes to produce lymphokines. Irrespective of the mechanism, a

Table 5. *Important Clinical Situations Associated With Defects in Cell-Mediated Immunity*

Aging
During and following certain viral illnesses
Thymic dysplasia
Congenital situations associated with defects in cell-mediated immunity
Third trimester of pregnancy
Lymphatic malignances of T-cell origin
Immunosuppressive therapy, especially corticosteroids and cyclosporine
AIDS and HIV-related disorders

Table 6. *Pathogens in Disorders of Cell-Mediated Immunity*

Bacteria	Fungi	Viruses	Parasites/Protozoa	Others
Mycobacteria	Cryptococcus	Herpes simplex	Pneumocystis	*Treponema pallidum*
Listeria	Histoplasma	Varicella-zoster	Toxoplasma	Chlamydiae
Nocardia	Coccidioides	Cytomegalovirus	Strongyloides	Rickettsiae
Rhodococcus	Blastomyces	Epstein-Barr virus	Giardia	
Salmonella	Candida	Polyoma viruses	Cryptosporidium	
Legionella	Aspergillus	Adenoviruses	Isospora	
Brucella		Measles virus	Trypanosoma	
Bartonella (formerly Rochalimaea)			Microsporidia	
			Leishmania	
			Amebae	

decrease in the production of macrophage activation factor decreases the stimulus for macrophages to optimally serve as the primary phagocytic cell in this host defense system.

The pathogens infecting patients with defects in cell-mediated immunity are summarized in Table 6 and can be divided into five categories: (1) bacteria (having as a common characteristic an intracellular location); (2) fungi (which often become clinically manifested in the setting of previous epidemiologic exposure); (3) viruses (most characteristically, DNA viruses); (4) parasites and protozoa; and (5) a miscellaneous group (some include spirochetes in this category).

Intracellular Bacteria

Mycobacterium tuberculosis

Although tuberculosis (TB) can be a problem in any patient with defective cell-mediated immunity, it has attracted recent attention because of the copathogenesis that may occur in individuals who are dually infected with the intracellular pathogens *M tuberculosis* and HIV-1. It has been suggested by some that mycobacteria and their products may enhance viral replication by inducing nuclear factor κ-B, the cellular factor that binds to promoter regions of HIV.[32] The presentation of TB in HIV-infected persons is variable and is influenced by the level of immunosuppression. With CD4$^+$ counts >300 cells/μL, the pattern of typical reactivation TB with cavitary disease or upper lobe infiltrates is more common. When CD4$^+$ cells fall to <200/μL, the pattern of disease is more

typically middle to lower lobe disease with or without intrathoracic lymphadenopathy.[33] In patients with CD4$^+$ counts at this level, extrapulmonary TB has been reported in at least 50%. Persons with serologic evidence of HIV infection and pulmonary TB fulfill the case definition for AIDS. These individuals with drug-susceptible strains tend to respond well to standard antituberculous therapy given as a short-course regimen for 6 months.[34] After initiation of antituberculosis therapy, some patients experience a paradoxical reaction, which is the temporary exacerbation of TB symptoms in the form of hectic fevers, lymphadenopathy, worsening of chest radiographic findings, and worsening of extrapulmonary lesions. These reactions are not associated with changes in *M tuberculosis* bacteriology, and patients generally feel well with no signs of toxicity. Such reactions have been attributed to recovery of delayed hypersensitivity response and an increase in exposure and reaction to mycobacterial antigens after bactericidal antituberculosis therapy is initiated. These reactions have been especially notable in individuals concurrently treated with antituberculosis and antiretroviral therapy. A noteworthy issue in HIV-infected patients is the interaction between antituberculosis drugs and antiretroviral therapy, including that with protease inhibitors. The rifamycins (*eg*, rifampin and rifabutin) accelerate the metabolism of protease inhibitors through induction of hepatic P$_{450}$ cytochrome oxidases. Rifabutin has comparable antituberculous activity but with less hepatic P$_{450}$ cytochrome enzyme-inducing effect than rifampin. The joint document of the American Thoracic Society, CDC, and IDSA on the treatment of tuberculosis includes recommendations for use of rifamycins in the treatment of TB.[34]

Two clinically relevant trends related to TB deserve comment. One is an apparent increase in TB reactivation associated with tumor necrosis factor-α inhibitors (eg, infliximab) used to treat rheumatoid arthritis and Crohn disease, with extrapulmonary TB being especially noted.[35] The other relates to the reports of liver failure and death after 2 months of therapy with rifampin and pyrazinamide.[36]

Some recent attention has focused on measures that foster type 1 immunity as a means of treating patients with TB, including those who may not have responded to initial therapy. Because IL-2 has a central role in regulating T-cell responses to M tuberculosis, a randomized, placebo-controlled, double-blinded trial in 110 HIV-negative, smear-positive, drug-susceptible pulmonary TB patients was conducted using adjunctive immunotherapy with recombinant IL-2.[37] In this trial, IL-2 did not enhance bacillary clearance or improvement in symptoms in HIV-seronegative adults with drug-susceptible TB.

A significant change has recently occurred regarding TB infection. For many decades, the terms "preventive therapy" and "chemoprophylaxis" were used to describe the status of persons with a positive tuberculin test but no symptoms or signs of active TB. The word *preventive* was inaccurate in that it referred to use of an agent such as isoniazid to prevent development of active TB in persons known or likely to be infected with M tuberculosis; it was not intended to imply prevention of true primary infection. To more accurately describe such therapy, in an official statement in 2000 the American Thoracic Society introduced the terminology "latent tuberculosis infection" (LTBI) as a substitute for "preventive therapy" and "chemoprophylaxis."[38] It acknowledged the role of LTBI as an important element in control of TB. It has been noted that HIV-infected persons with a positive tuberculin skin test have about a 7% chance per year of developing tuberculous disease, which exceeds the standard estimated lifetime risk of approximately 10% for the reactivation of LTBI in nonimmunocompromised persons with positive purified protein derivative tests.[39] In a prospective cohort study of persons with HIV infection in the United States, the annual risk of active TB among HIV-infected persons with a positive tuberculin test was 4.5 cases per 100 person-years of observation.[40] Based on such facts, it is recommended that HIV-infected persons with a tuberculin skin test with ≥5-mm induration be given treatment for latent tuberculosis. In the 2000 guidelines for treatment of LTBI, tuberculin positivity was also set at ≥5-mm induration for patients with organ transplants and other immunosuppressed patients receiving the equivalent of ≥15 mg/d of prednisone for 1 month or more. The risk of TB increases with a higher dose and longer duration of corticosteroids.

Mycobacterium avium *Complex*

Among individuals with defective cell-mediated immunity, *Mycobacterium avium* complex (MAC) classically infects HIV-infected persons when their CD4$^+$ cells are <50/μL. In patients with AIDS, there are several lines of evidence suggesting that most patients with disseminated MAC have recently acquired the organisms, in contrast to the reactivation that is common with TB.[41] Adherence of the organisms to the gut wall is the initial event in invasion, followed by entry into the lamina propria and then phagocytosis by macrophages. Local replication of organisms leads to the endoscopically visible 2- to 4-mm punctate lesions that are the hallmark of MAC disease in the gut. The clinical presentation is that of a wasting syndrome marked by fever, night sweats, weight loss, diarrhea, anorexia, and malaise. Despite positive sputum cultures, serious pulmonary infection is not common in HIV-infected patients. The organism is most characteristically isolated from blood, stool, respiratory secretions, bone marrow, GI tract mucosa, and lymph nodes (although granuloma formation is minimal or absent). A unique pathophysiologic abnormality seen in about 5% of AIDS patients with MAC disease is marked elevations (20 to 40 times normal) in serum alkaline phosphatase with little elevation of transaminases, bilirubin, or other parameters of hepatic function. This is believed to occur on the basis of interference with enzyme metabolism rather than because of hepatic tissue destruction.

In those patients with symptomatic disease, a multidrug regimen is recommended that should include either clarithromycin or azithromycin in combination with ethambutol.[42] With advanced immunosuppression (CD4$^+$ < 50/μL), with high mycobacterial loads, or in the absence of effective antiretroviral therapy, the treatment guidelines recommend that adding a third drug be considered. Additional drugs that may be added to this regimen include rifabutin (as an A-1 recommended agent) or ciprofloxacin, levofloxacin, or amikacin (as C-III recommendations). The response to therapy is variable among patients, and the acquisition of drug resistance is common, especially with monotherapy. Although rifabutin was the initial agent approved for prophylaxis against MAC infection, more recent recommendations for the prevention of opportunistic infections in HIV-infected persons have listed azithromycin or clarithromycin as the agent of choice when the CD4$^+$ count is <50/μL.[43]

Listeria monocytogenes

This intracellular Gram-positive rod characteristically infects persons with malignancy, diabetes mellitus, or renal transplantation followed by immunosuppressive therapy.[44] Neonates and pregnant women are also at risk, and the infection occurs with increased frequency with cirrhosis. About one third of patients in some series have no known risk factor, and Listeria has only recently been considered a cause of febrile GI illness in immunocompetent persons.[45] Listeria may be acquired via consumption of certain contaminated raw vegetables (with coleslaw as a source in some outbreaks), certain contaminated canned products (with sterile canned corn kernels as the source in one outbreak), raw food from animal sources (eg, beef, pork, or poultry), unpasteurized milk, or foods made from raw milk (notably, certain soft cheeses).

The most common clinical presentations are of CNS infection, sepsis, or a flu-like illness. When it causes acute meningitis, Listeria may be associated with a variable glucose level or with a CSF lymphocytosis or monocytosis. Gram stain of the CSF is positive in only about one fourth of patients. The infection has a predilection for the base of the brain with resultant focal neurologic signs, particularly cranial nerve involvement, in up to 40% of patients. Hydrocephalus may be a complication of this localization. Bacteremia is another common presentation, with cerebritis or brain abscess being less frequent.

Therapy is with high-dose IV ampicillin or penicillin.[46] Some favor the addition of a parenteral aminoglycoside with these agents even for treatment of meningitis, recognizing that the aminoglycosides administered parenterally in adults will not cross the blood-brain barrier but may help eradicate infectious sites outside the CNS.[47] For penicillin-allergic patients, trimethoprim-sulfamethoxazole is possibly effective. Extremely noteworthy is that cephalosporin therapy has no role in treating infection caused by Listeria. Because of the intracellular location of the organisms, 3 weeks of therapy is recommended for serious infections.

Nocardia asteroides

These filamentous aerobic Gram-positive rods are weakly acid-fast and characteristically produce disease in patients who have lymphoreticular neoplasms or have received long-term corticosteroid therapy. Because the organism most commonly infects humans through the respiratory tract, the classic pattern of infection is pulmonary disease, which may take the form of nodular infiltrates, cavitary lesions, or diffuse infiltrates with or without consolidation. Pustular skin lesions and neurologic disease in the form of encephalitis or brain abscess complete the triad of the most common presentations by this pathogen. The liver and kidneys are less likely to be involved. In the report from the Johns Hopkins Hospital of 59 patients diagnosed with nocardiosis over an 11-year time span, Nocardia was isolated most commonly from the respiratory tract (76%), followed by soft tissue (13%), blood (7%), and CNS (5%).[48] In this series, the infection was common in AIDS patients as well as in transplant recipients. In both groups of patients, disease developed in some despite prophylactic therapy against other pathogens with trimethoprim/sulfamethoxazole.

Standard therapy is with sulfonamides.[49] Trimethoprim-sulfamethoxazole is often used because of its convenient IV dosing; however, it has not been definitively proven that the combination is synergistic at the drug ratios that usually are achieved in serum or CSF.

Rhodococcus equi

Formerly called *Corynebacterium equi*, this partially acid-fast, aerobic, intracellular Gram-positive rod-coccus was first described in 1967 as the cause of disease in humans.[50] Even though the organism has been rarely reported to cause infection in immunocompetent patients, immunocompromised patients, especially those with HIV infection, are the ones most likely to develop clinical disease due to this pathogen. The most characteristic pattern of infection is described as a progressive pneumonia that may cavitate. Bacteremia is common in immunocompromised patients. Like Nocardia, it has also been associated with neurologic and skin lesions.

The intracellular location has made the organism difficult to treat, and principles of therapy include a prolonged duration of antibiotics, often in association with drainage. *In vitro*, *R equi* is usually susceptible to erythromycin, rifampin, fluoroquinolones, aminoglycosides, glycopeptides (*eg*, vancomycin), and imipenem; it has been suggested that immunocompromised patients and patients with serious infections receive IV therapy with two-drug or three-drug regimens that include vancomycin, imipenem, aminoglycosides, ciprofloxacin, rifampin, and/or erythromycin.[51] The choice of agents used and the duration of therapy are dependent on both the patient's host defense status and the site of infection. Oral antibiotics may be an option in certain immunocompetent patients with localized infection.

Salmonella spp

Patient populations with defective cell-mediated immunity that develop bacteremia with this intracellular Gram-negative rod include those with hematologic malignancies, systemic lupus erythematosus, and HIV infection. In those persons with HIV infection, a febrile typhoidal illness without diarrhea accounts for about 45% of the disease caused by this pathogen. More common is an illness associated with fever, severe diarrhea, and crampy abdominal pain. Compared with Shigella and Campylobacter, there is a lower incidence of bloody diarrhea and fecal leukocytes with Salmonella infection. Recurrent nontyphoidal bacteremia is considered an indication for secondary antibacterial prophylaxis in HIV-infected persons.[43]

Legionella spp

Legionella is a pathogen recognized to have the potential for causing acute mortality in patients with pulmonary infections, including even those who are not immunocompromised.[52] This pathogen causes more severe disease in transplant recipients, patients who receive corticosteroids, and HIV-infected persons. Immunocompromised patients with legionellosis may present with variable patterns of multisystem disease. Fever with a scanty productive cough is often described. In individuals receiving corticosteroids, cavitary lung lesions with abscess formation may occur. Dissemination seems to occur via bacteremic spread of the organism. In a review of Legionnaires disease, the most common extrapulmonary site was reported to be the heart (including myocarditis and pericarditis), and one would need to assume that such organ system involvement might be possible in immunocompromised patients.[53] Other patterns of extrapulmonary involvement by Legionella may take the form of sinusitis, cellulitis, pyelonephritis, and pancreatitis. Patients with hairy-cell leukemia, a disorder of monocyte deficiency and dysfunction, have an increased incidence of Legionella pneumonia. Legionella infection should be suspected in those individuals who do not respond to therapy with a β-lactam antibiotic. Useful in the acute diagnosis is the Legionella urinary antigen assay, which has been stated to be 70% sensitive and 100% specific in diagnosing infection caused by *Legionella pneumophila serogroup I*.

Erythromycin has traditionally been considered the agent of choice for treatment of this infection,[54] but recent reviews have suggested that the fluoroquinolones may be more efficacious.[53] Because of increased efficacy and the fact that macrolides such as erythromycin may have pharmacologic interactions with immunosuppressive agents used in transplant patients, some investigators feel that a fluoroquinolone should be added to the standard regimen for treating Legionnaires disease in transplant recipients with nosocomial pneumonia if the causative agent has not been identified. Some have suggested that rifampin be used as adjunctive therapy for severe Legionella infections, but this must be taken in context with the facts that (1) no prospective studies have evaluated such therapy, and (2) rifampin has the potential to induce the cytochrome P_{450} system and, therefore, cause a significant interaction with immunosuppressive therapy.

Brucella spp

Even though intracellular brucellae require cell-mediated immunity for eradication, the spectrum of brucellosis in immunocompromised hosts has not been frequently described. Because of the ability for splenic localization with the formation of suppurative lesions that might require splenectomy, this organism may cause further impairment of an otherwise compromised immune system.

Bartonella (Formerly Rochalimaea) spp

The small Gram-negative organisms in this genus may be demonstrated with Warthin-Starry staining or by electron microscopy. The patterns of infection in HIV-infected persons include the following: (1) bacteremia (in the absence of focal vascular proliferative response in tissue); (2) bacillary angiomatosis; and (3) peliosis hepatitis.[55] Bacillary angiomatosis presents in the later phases of HIV infection, usually with CD4+ counts <100 cells/μL. The condition is associated with a unique vascular lesion that may involve virtually every organ system, either alone or in association with other sites of involvement.[56] Of these, skin lesions are the most commonly recognized, with characteristic lesions being red and papular and therefore resembling Kaposi sarcoma. Lesions characteristically are associated with a long duration of symptoms or physical findings prior to diagnosis. Species causing such a process include Bartonella henselae and Bartonella quintana. Peliosis hepatitis refers to the blood-filled peliotic changes in the parenchyma of the liver or spleen that occur because of infection with these two species. Because these organisms are at present difficult to culture from blood or tissue, histopathology may be the study that directs further diagnostic evaluation. Erythromycin or doxycycline is considered the preferred agent.[42]

Fungi

Cryptococcus neoformans

Cryptococcal meningitis is an important infection in HIV-infected persons, particularly when CD4+ counts are <100 cells/μL, but may also occur in other populations, including elderly persons. The organism enters the body through the lungs, and the associated finding of pulmonary infiltrates in an HIV-infected person with meningitis should raise the suspicion of this diagnosis. The organism has a propensity to enter the bloodstream and may be detected in routine blood cultures. The resulting fungemia is often associated with multisegment pulmonary infiltrates and with skin lesions. Infection in the HIV population may present as a noninflammatory infection of the CNS, and the clinical features are therefore different from what one might expect in classic forms of meningitis caused by other pathogens. The history is frequently of a subacute or chronic illness associated mainly with headache. Physical examination may not reveal classic findings such as nuchal rigidity. Because of the lack of inflammation in the CNS, the CSF formula may include <20 WBC/mm³, normal glucose, and normal protein. These findings make CSF studies such as India ink stain, cryptococcal antigen, and fungal culture mainstays in the diagnosis.

The National Institute of Allergy and Infectious Diseases Mycoses Study Group and AIDS Clinical Trials Group reported their findings in 381 patients with cryptococcal meningitis treated in a double-blind multicenter trial.[57] Conclusions from this trial of AIDS-associated cryptococcal meningitis were that induction treatment for 2 weeks with the combination of amphotericin B (0.7 mg/kg/d) plus flucytosine (100 mg/kg/d in patients who were tolerant of this agent), followed by therapy with fluconazole (400 mg/d orally for 8 weeks) is safe and effective and should be considered the treatment of choice. The authors noted that high intracranial pressures have been associated with catastrophic neurologic deterioration and death in the absence of hydrocephalus. Of the patients in this study, 13 of 14 early deaths and 40% of deaths during weeks 3 through 10 were associated with elevated intracranial pressure. Based on the association between elevated intracranial pressure and mortality in patients with cryptococcal meningitis, it was suggested that measurement of intracranial pressure be included in the management of such patients. Included in the recommendations were daily lumbar punctures, use of acetazolamide, and ventriculoperitoneal shunts for asymptomatic patients with intracranial CSF pressure >320 mm H_2O and for symptomatic patients with pressures >180 mm H_2O. More recently, it was recommended that in the absence of focal lesions, opening pressures ≥250 mm H_2O should be treated with large-volume CSF drainage (defined in this report as allowing CSF to drain until a satisfactory closing pressure had been achieved, commonly <200 mm H_2O).[58] IDSA guidelines for the management of cryptococcal meningitis in HIV-infected persons with opening CSF pressure of >250 mm H_2O recommended lumbar drainage sufficient to achieve a closing pressure ≥200 mm H_2O or 50% of initial opening pressure.[59]

Maintenance therapy is required after completion of primary therapy, and studies have identified fluconazole as the agent of choice.[60,61] In an international observational study reported by the International Working Group on Cryptococcosis, discontinuation of maintenance therapy for cryptococcal meningitis was stated to be safe if the CD4+ cell count increases to >100 cells/μL while the patient is receiving highly active antiretroviral therapy (HAART).[62] These findings were consistent with previous recommendations by the US Public Health Service and the IDSA that discontinuation of secondary prophylaxis may be an option when CD4+ cells are >100 to 200 cells/μL for ≥6 months.[43] Recurrent cryptococcal infection should be suspected in patients whose serum cryptococcal antigen test results revert back to positive after discontinuation of maintenance therapy.[62]

Histoplasma capsulatum

The clinical entity of progressive disseminated histoplasmosis has become increasingly recognized because of HIV infection. The illness may occur on the basis of either reactivation or primary disease, making the epidemiologic history of travel to or residence in endemic areas crucial. Although patients may present with such nonspecific findings as fever, fatigue, weakness, and weight loss, a characteristic presentation in about half of patients is diffuse interstitial or miliary pulmonary infiltrates that are associated with hypoxemia and mimic *Pneumocystis jiroveci* (previously *Pneumocystis carinii*) pneumonia. These patients may concomitantly demonstrate reticuloendothelial involvement in the forms of hepatosplenomegaly, lymphadenopathy, and bone marrow involvement. A subgroup may present with a septic syndrome that can include disseminated intravascular coagulation. Small intracellular periodic acid-Schiff positive, yeast-like organisms are the characteristic morphologic form of the organism. Although the organism may be isolated from sputum, tissue, or blood, the *H capsulatum* polysaccharide antigen from blood, urine, or CSF may serve as a more rapid diagnostic study. In the IDSA guidelines for treating disseminated histoplasmosis, immunocompromised patients were divided into those with AIDS and those without AIDS.[63] In those without AIDS who were sufficiently ill to require hospitalization, amphotericin B (0.7 to 1.0 mg/kg/d) was recommended. It was noted that most patients respond quickly to amphotericin B and can then be treated with itraconazole (200 mg qd or bid) for 6 to 18 mo. For patients with AIDS, it was recommended that therapy be divided into an initial 12-week intensive phase to induce a remission in the clinical illness and then followed by a chronic maintenance phase to prevent relapse. Amphotericin B was recommended for patients sufficiently ill to require hospitalization, with replacement by itraconazole, 200 mg twice daily (when the patient no longer requires hospitalization for IV therapy), to complete a 12-week total course of induction therapy. Itraconazole (200 mg tid for 3 days and then bid for 12 weeks) was recommended for patients who have mild or moderately severe symptoms and do not require hospitalization. Maintenance therapy with itraconazole for life was included in the recommendations.

Coccidioides immitis

In HIV-infected persons as well as in transplant recipients, this fungal pathogen occurs most commonly in those individuals from endemic areas. The illness may resemble Pneumocystis pneumonia with diffuse reticulonodular infiltrates. The classic clinical pattern of disease, manifested as dissemination to sites such as meninges, skin, and joints, is not altered by HIV infection. In the IDSA guidelines for the treatment of coccidioidomycosis, it was noted that the presence of bilateral reticulonodular or miliary infiltrates produced by *C immitis* usually implies an underlying immunodeficiency state.[64] In such circumstances, therapy usually starts with amphotericin B. Several weeks of therapy is often required for improvement, at which point an oral azole may replace amphotericin. The IDSA guidelines for treatment of coccidioidomycosis offer recommendations for the management of meningitis, including a role for oral fluconazole in certain patients.

Candida spp

Host defense against Candida is provided by both neutrophils and cell-mediated immunity. In addition, the immunocompetent host may develop bloodborne infection with this pathogen, and notable risk factors for this include surgery (particularly of the GI tract), broad-spectrum antibiotics, hyperalimentation, and intravascular catheters.[15] With HIV infection, Candida may present in a hierarchical pattern. With $CD4^+$ counts in the 400 to 600 cells/μL range, women may develop recurrent vulvovaginal candidiasis. At $CD4^+$ levels of ~250 cells/μL, oral candidiasis is the expected clinical entity. The clinical presentation of odynophagia in a patient with oral candidiasis and a $CD4^+$ count of <100 cells/μL strongly raises the diagnosis of Candida esophagitis. These candidal infections generally respond well to therapy, and because of this, primary prophylaxis is not generally recommended. A recent trend has been toward non-*albicans* strains of Candida[65] and toward strains of *Candida albicans* that are fluconazole-resistant.[66] Patterns of azole use have probably contributed to such problems. Recurrent use of fluconazole in HIV-infected patients has been associated with an increasing number of reports of Candida spp resistant to this agent. In a bone marrow transplant unit in which patients were given fluconazole (400 mg/d, oral or IV) for the first 75 days after transplantation, 5% of patients became colonized with fluconazole-resistant strains of *C albicans*, and 53% of patients had at least one mouthwashing sample that yielded non-*albicans* species of Candida during the course of their bone marrow transplantation.[67]

Aspergillus spp

As is the case with Candida, Aspergillus may cause infection in patients with defects in either neutrophil function or cell-mediated immunity. In addition to being a nosocomial pathogen, infection with this agent may represent reactivation disease. This may be especially notable in patients who have received a bone marrow transplant or solid organ transplant. In AIDS patients with the concomitant problems of neutropenia, corticosteroid therapy, or ethanol use, invasive pulmonary or disseminated aspergillosis may occur. This tends to present in the later stages of HIV infection, especially when $CD4^+$ cells are <50/μL. Voriconazole is the preferred therapy for invasive aspergillosis in HIV-infected patients.[42]

Aspergillus infection and its treatment provide some important insights into the evolving clinical importance of type 1 immunity. Patients with chronic granulomatous disease have an increased incidence of infection with Aspergillus. Treatment of these patients with recombinant IFN-γ stimulates killing of this pathogen and reduces the frequency and severity of clinically apparent fungal infection.[1] This observation is important in that it conveys a treatment option for IFN-γ based on an understanding of the role of type 1 immunity in defending against certain fungal pathogens. The traditional treatment for Aspergillus has been amphotericin B given at maximum tolerated doses (*eg*, 1 to 1.5 mg/kg/d) and continued despite modest increases in serum creatinine.[68] Lipid formulations of amphotericin have noteworthy roles in two circumstances: (1) for the patient who has impaired renal function or develops nephrotoxicity while receiving amphotericin B deoxycholate[68] and (2) for patients who have undergone bone marrow transplantation.[69] The echinocandin caspofungin has been recently approved for patients in whom amphotericin fails. Itraconazole has been suggested as an alternative form of therapy in certain settings of Aspergillus infection. In a randomized trial comparing voriconazole with standard amphotericin B for primary treatment of invasive aspergillosis, voriconazole was demonstrated to be more effective than amphotericin B.[17] An evolving body of clinical data regarding this topic has led to the recent comment that voriconazole, which

Infections in AIDS Patients and Other Immunocompromised Hosts (Karam)

is available in both IV and oral formulations, will likely become the drug of choice for treatment of invasive aspergillosis.[18,42]

Viruses

Herpes Simplex Virus

The patterns of herpes simplex virus (HSV) infection vary according to the underlying immunosuppression status. Patients with hematologic or lymphoreticular neoplasms may develop disseminated mucocutaneous HSV lesions. In transplant patients, esophagitis, tracheobronchitis, pneumonitis, or hepatitis are characteristic presentations, with hepatitis caused by HSV presenting most classically as the triad of high fever, leukopenia, and markedly elevated aminotransferase levels.[70] HIV-infected persons can have a vast array of clinical conditions caused by HSV, including esophagitis, colitis, perianal ulcers (often associated with urinary retention), pneumonitis, and a spectrum of neurologic diseases. Acyclovir remains the drug of choice for these infections. However, acyclovir-resistant strains have emerged, for which foscarnet may be the alternative therapy.

Varicella-Zoster Virus

As is the case with HSV infection, varicella-zoster virus (VZV) may present differently according to the underlying type of immunosuppression. With both chickenpox and shingles in patients with solid and hematologic malignancies, cutaneous dissemination may occur and may be associated with such visceral involvement as pneumonitis, hepatitis, and meningoencephalitis. Herpes zoster may be multidermatomal in HIV-infected persons, and this may be the initial clue to the diagnosis of HIV infection. Treatment options for both varicella and zoster have been summarized.[71] Acyclovir, famciclovir, and valacyclovir are discussed according to the disease, the pattern of immunosuppression, and the requirement for IV vs oral therapy. With the depression of cell-mediated immunity that occurs during the third trimester of pregnancy,[31] there is increased risk of dissemination of VZV to the lungs during pregnancy. A recently published case-control analysis of 18 pregnant women with VZV pneumonia compared with 72 matched control subjects identified cigarette smoking and >100 skin lesions as markers for the development of varicella pneumonia in pregnancy.[72] In immunocompromised patients and pregnant women who are exposed to chickenpox and in whom there is no clinical or serologic evidence of immunity to VZV, administration of varicella-zoster immune globulin may prevent or significantly modify VZV infection.[71]

Cytomegalovirus

For perspective, it is important to recognize the three major consequences of cytomegalovirus (CMV) infection in solid organ transplantation recipients: (1) CMV disease, including a wide range of clinical illnesses; (2) superinfection with opportunistic pathogens; and (3) injury to the transplanted organ, possibly enhancing chronic rejection.[73] The virus may be present in the forms of latency (infection without signs of active viral replication), active infection (viral replication in blood or organs), and primary infection (active infection in a previously nonimmune seronegative person). A recent study addressed the impact of primary infection in bone marrow recipients who were CMV-seronegative and who received stem cells from CMV-seropositive recipients.[74] These patients died of invasive bacterial and fungal infections at a rate greater than that of patients who did not have primary infection, and it was hypothesized that primary CMV infection has immunomodulatory effects that predispose to such secondary infections.

The spectrum of clinically active CMV infection in immunocompromised patients is broad and may vary according to the immunosuppressive condition. In HIV-infected patients, the classic presentation has been chorioretinitis but may also include GI ulcerations, pneumonitis, hepatitis, encephalopathy, adrenalitis, and a painful myeloradiculopathy. Some immunosuppressed patients present with only a mononucleosis-like syndrome consisting of fever and lymphadenopathy.

New approaches in both hematopoietic stem cell or solid organ transplant recipients emphasize the use of prophylactic or preemptive therapy based on CMV monitoring.[75] Although serologic tests have previously been suggested to have a potential role in directing CMV therapy in bone marrow transplant patients and heart transplant patients, serologies are not the most reliable studies in predicting the presence of CMV infection or clinical disease. The appearance of CMV protein pp65 in peripheral blood leukocytes has proved to be superior to tests based on virus isolation[73] and has correlated with subsequent development of CMV disease. In addition to CMV antigenemia, DNA/RNAemia (especially quantitative polymerase chain reaction) is clinically useful, and detection tests for both are methods of choice for diagnosis and monitoring of active CMV infection after organ transplantation.

For the purpose of developing consistent reporting of CMV in clinical trials, definitions of CMV infection and disease were developed and published.[76] In addition, an approach to the management of CMV infection after solid organ transplantation has been recently published, and several clinically relevant messages provided it.[73] In managing CMV infection, the clinician needs to be aware of four types of treatment options: (1) therapeutic use (treatment based on the presence of established infection); (2) prophylactic use (use of antimicrobial therapy from the earliest possible moment); (3) preemptive use (antimicrobial therapy before clinical signs of infection); and (4) deferred therapy (initiation of therapy after onset of disease). In the therapeutic setting of CMV disease after solid organ transplantation, IV ganciclovir is the drug of choice, with anti-CMV hyperimmunoglobulin preparations being useful adjuncts in seronegative recipients of seropositive organs and with foscarnet (because of its inherent toxicity) being considered as rescue therapy. Although ganciclovir has for years been the mainstay of therapy for CMV retinitis in AIDS patients, valganciclovir (an oral prodrug of ganciclovir) has been approved as an effective treatment option. In addition, studies are ongoing using valganciclovir as both preemptive and definitive therapy of CMV infections in transplant patients. An immune reconstitution syndrome including visual blurring months after successful therapy of CMV retinitis has been described in AIDS patients who have started HAART.[77]

The role for prophylaxis against CMV was summarized based on the type of organ transplanted.[76] With detection of CMV antigenemia at a predefined level, IV ganciclovir may have a role in preventing CMV disease in certain patient populations. Secondary prophylaxis has been recommended but may be discontinued if the CD4+ cell count reaches >100 to 150 cells/µL and remains at this level for ≥6 months with no evidence of active CMV disease.[43]

Epstein-Barr Virus

The pathobiology of Epstein-Barr virus (EBV) is important in understanding the evolution of EBV-associated disease in immunocompromised patients. Although early studies indicated that EBV replicated in epithelial cells in the oropharynx, more recent studies suggest that B cells in the oropharynx may be the primary site of infection.[78] This has led to the thought that resting memory B cells are the site of persistence of EBV within the body, with the number of latently infected cells remaining stable for years.[79] What has not been definitively elucidated at the present time is the role of oral epithelial cells in the transmission and latency of EBV. Even though the finding of antibodies against EBV viral proteins and antigens is consistent with the fact that there is some degree of humoral immunity to the virus, it is the cellular immune response that is the more important for controlling EBV infection. Important among the proteins produced by EBV is latent membrane protein 1, which acts as an oncogene and whose expression in an animal model has resulted in B-cell lymphomas. In patients who have AIDS or have received organ or bone marrow transplants, an inability to control proliferation of latently EBV-infected cells may lead to EBV lymphoproliferative disease, which in tissue may take the form of plasmacytic hyperplasia, B-cell hyperplasia, B-cell lymphoma, or immunoblastic lymphoma.[78] It has been suggested that therapy for EBV lymphoproliferative disease should include reduction in the dose of immunosuppressive medication when possible. More specific, definitive recommendations for therapy are not available, but potential options have been reviewed.[78]

Completing the spectrum of EBV disease in immunocompromised patients is oral hairy leukoplakia, a common, nonmalignant hyperplastic lesion of epithelial cells seen most characteristically in HIV-infected patients. In its classic presentation, hairy leukoplakia presents as raised white lesions of the oral mucosa, especially on the lateral aspect of the tongue. Contributing to the ongoing attempts to elucidate the pathobiology of EBV, a study of serial tongue biopsy specimens from HIV-infected patients demonstrated EBV replication in normal tongue epithelial cells (in contrast to the lack of active viral replication in certain EBV-associated malignancies) and suggested that the tongue may be a source of EBV secretion into saliva.[80] In this clinical trial, valacyclovir treatment completely abrogated EBV replication, resulting in resolution of hairy leukoplakia when it was present, but EBV replication returned in normal tongue epithelial cells after valacyclovir treatment. These findings are consistent with clinical experience that the lesions of hairy leukoplakia respond to antiviral therapy but recur once therapy is stopped. Topics not evaluated in this study, but important in the understanding of EBV, are whether other oral epithelial cells support viral replication and whether oral epithelial cells participate with B cells in viral latency.

Polyoma Viruses (Including JC Virus and BK Virus)

Clinically important members of this class of double-stranded DNA viruses include BK virus and JC virus. Primary infection with BK virus is generally asymptomatic and occurs in childhood. Following primary infection, the virus can remain latent in many sites, with the most notable being the kidney. With cellular immunodeficiency, the virus can reactivate and cause clinical disease. Although the kidney, lung, eye, liver, and brain are sites of both primary and reactivated BK virus-associated disease, the most characteristic disease entities are hemorrhagic and nonhemorrhagic cystitis, ureteric stenosis, and nephritis, and these occur most often in recipients of solid organ or bone marrow transplants.[81]

JC virus is the etiologic agent in progressive multifocal leukoencephalopathy (PML). In this primary demyelinating process involving the white matter of the cerebral hemispheres, patients present subacutely with confusion, disorientation, and visual disturbances, which may progress to cortical blindness or ataxia. CSF is characteristically acellular. A feature on neuroradiology imaging studies is lack of mass effect. No definitive therapy

is presently available for this infection, and clinical efforts have recently focused on the role of immune reconstitution in modifying the clinical course of the illness. In a multicenter analysis of 57 consecutive HIV-positive patients with PML, neurologic improvement or stability at 2 months after therapy was demonstrated in 26% of patients who received HAART in contrast to improvement in only 4% of patients who did not receive HAART (p = 0.03).[82] In this study, decreases in JC virus DNA to undetectable levels predicted a longer survival. In the context that untreated PML may be fatal within 3 to 6 months, such potential for preventing neurologic progression and improving survival by controlling JC virus replication becomes clinically relevant.

Adenoviruses

In immunocompromised patients, these DNA viruses may produce generalized illness that classically involves the nervous system, respiratory system, GI tract, and liver. This class of viruses has recently emerged as a major problem in some bone marrow transplant units. The infections may have a fulminant course, which may result in death. No drug has been shown to be definitively beneficial in these patients, although IV ribavirin may be effective in some.

Measles Virus

Because individuals are protected against measles by cell-mediated immunity and since measles may cause severe illness in HIV-infected persons, protection via vaccine is an important consideration. A basic tenet in infectious diseases has been that live-virus vaccines should not be administered to immunocompromised patients. An exception has been use of measles vaccine, a live-virus vaccine, in asymptomatic HIV-infected individuals and potentially in those with symptomatic HIV infection. Fatal giant-cell pneumonitis has been described in a young male measles vaccine recipient with AIDS.[83] Even with the overwhelming success of measles immunization programs, this case has prompted reappraisal of recommendations and some have suggested that it may be prudent to withhold measles-containing vaccines from HIV-infected persons with evidence of severe immunosuppression.

Emerging Viral Pathogens in Persons With Defects in Cell-Mediated Immunity

There have been increasing reports of infections caused by respiratory syncytial virus or parainfluenza virus, particularly in persons who have received bone marrow or solid organ transplantation. The spectrum of disease caused by these pathogens is evolving, with the lung being an important target organ. These viruses should be considered to be among the pathogens that may cause pneumonia in patients with defects in cell-mediated immunity.

Parasites and Protozoa

P jiroveci (*Previously* P carinii)

In recognition of its genetic and functional distinctness, the organism that causes human Pneumocystis pneumonia has been recently renamed *P jiroveci*, but despite this change, the use of the acronym *PCP* is not precluded because it can be read Pneumocystis pneumonia.[84] The clinical setting in which *P jiroveci* pneumonia (PCP) develops continues to evolve. In the pre-AIDS era, this pathogen was described as a cause of rapidly progressive infection in patients with malignant diseases, especially during the time of steroid withdrawal. Following the onset of the AIDS epidemic in the early 1980s, PCP was most often diagnosed in HIV-infected persons. Following the widespread use of HAART in the mid-1990s, HIV-associated PCP has decreased, and it has been recently reported that PCP may in certain settings be diagnosed more often in non-HIV immunocompromised patients than in those with HIV infection.[85] Host defense against Pneumocystis includes humoral immunity; however, because of the overwhelming predominance of infection by this pathogen in HIV-infected persons, it has been included in this section of pathogens that infect patients with defective cell-mediated immunity.

Although diffuse interstitial infiltrates are the most characteristic pulmonary finding with PCP, patients may present with focal infiltrates, cavitary lesions, or nodular lung lesions. Findings that support, but do not prove, the diagnosis of PCP in an HIV-infected patient with pulmonary infiltrates include a CD4+ cell count <250 cells/μL, a WBC count <8,000 cells/mm^3, and an elevated serum lactate dehydrogenase. PCP may occur as part of the presentation of the acute retroviral syndrome. In the review of PCP from the Clinical Center at the National Institutes of Health,[85] diagnostic studies for PCP were reviewed. It was noted that traditional stains on sputum or from BAL specimens for the cyst form of *P jiroveci* have been the mainstay of diagnosis in most settings. Direct immunofluorescent staining using monoclonal antibody 2G2 (which detects both cysts and trophozoites) has been used for many years in the algorithm of the National Institutes of Health Clinical Center for diagnosing PCP. This stain is performed first on induced sputum, and if that smear is negative, then a BAL specimen is obtained for the same study. Ongoing investigation has been focused on the development of a quantitative polymerase chain reaction assay that can be performed on oral washes or gargles and that might allow a clinician not only to diagnose PCP at an earlier stage than has traditionally been possible, but also to distinguish between colonization and disease with *P jiroveci*.

Trimethoprim-sulfamethoxazole is the current first-line therapeutic agent. As alternative therapy, pentamidine has been recommended for severe PCP.[42] Clindamycin/primaquine has been compared with trimethoprim-sulfamethoxazole in a clinical trial and found to be a reasonable alternative therapy for mild to moderate PCP.[42] Also listed as alternative therapy for mild to moderate disease are dapsone plus trimethoprim, atovaquone, or trimetrexate with leucovorin. Adjunctive corticosteroid therapy is recommended for patients with PCP whose room air Pao$_2$ is <70 mm Hg or whose arterial-alveolar oxygen gradient is >35 mm Hg.[86] It is important that steroids are started at the time antipneumocystis therapy is initiated in an attempt to prevent the lung injury that may occur when this pathogen is killed. The dramatic decrease in the number of cases of PCP relative to the number of patients with HIV infection has been attributable to prophylaxis, which is recommended for those patients with a CD4+ cell count <200 cells/μL,

CD4[+] cells <14% of total lymphocyte count, constitutional symptoms such as thrush or unexplained fever >100°F for ≥2 weeks (regardless of the CD4[+] count), or a previous history of PCP. Based on several clinical investigations, it seems that discontinuing prophylaxis in patients with adequate immune recovery is a useful strategy that should be widely considered.[43,87–89]

Toxoplasma gondii

Patient populations at higher risk for toxoplasmosis include those with hematologic malignancies (particularly patients with lymphoma), bone marrow transplant, solid organ transplant (including heart, lung, liver, or kidney), or AIDS.[90] In the vast majority of immunocompromised patients, toxoplasmosis results from reactivation of latent infection, but in heart transplant patients and in a small number of other immunocompromised patients, the highest risk of developing disease is in the setting of primary infection (ie, a seronegative recipient who acquires the parasite from a seropositive donor via a graft).[91]

Although pulmonary disease due to this pathogen is associated with nonspecific radiographic findings of which bilateral pulmonary interstitial infiltrates are most common, neurologic disease is the classic pattern. In HIV-infected persons, it classically presents as fever, headache, altered mental status, and focal neurologic deficits, especially in individuals whose CD4[+] count falls below 100 cells/μL. Because the disease is due to reactivation of latent infection in about 95% of cases, IgG antibody to Toxoplasma is generally present. Imaging studies of the brain show multiple (usually ≥3) nodular contrast-enhancing lesions, found most commonly in the basal ganglia and at the gray-white matter junction. Mass effect is characteristic with these lesions.[92]

In the classic setting, empiric therapy with sulfadiazine and pyrimethamine is recommended; the total duration of acute therapy should be at least 6 weeks.[42] Clindamycin-containing regimens may have a role in sulfa-allergic patients. Brain biopsy should be considered in immunocompromised patients with presumed CNS toxoplasmosis if there is a single lesion on MRI, a negative IgG antibody test result, or inadequate clinical response to an optimal treatment regimen or to what the physician considers to be an effective prophylactic regimen against T gondii.[90] Trimethoprim-sulfamethoxazole given for PCP prophylaxis serves as primary prophylaxis for toxoplasmosis, but should not be used for therapy. After acute therapy for toxoplasmic encephalitis, maintenance therapy is recommended but may be discontinued when the CD4[+] cell count is >200/μL for ≥6 months.[43]

Strongyloides stercoralis

Infection with this parasite has often been described in patients with COPD who have been receiving chronic steroid therapy and who present with Gram-negative bacteremia. Among patients with defects in cell-mediated immunity, bacteremia secondary to the hyperinfection is uncommon in two groups: (1) transplant recipients who receive cyclosporine (because of the anthelminthic properties of this rejection agent); and (2) HIV-infected patients, unless the CD4[+] cell count is ≤200 cells/mm[3] and the patient is concomitantly receiving corticosteroids.[91] The bacteremia occurs because of this organism's hyperinfection cycle, during which filariform larvae penetrate the intestinal mucosa, pass to the lungs by way of the bloodstream, break into alveolar spaces, and ascend to the glottis where they are swallowed into the intestinal tract to continue their process of autoinfection. Infection with this pathogen should be suspected in a patient with a defect in cell-mediated immunity who presents with clinical features that include generalized abdominal pain, diffuse pulmonary infiltrates, ileus, shock, and meningitis. Eosinophilia is often absent in steroid-treated patients.

In recent years, recommendations for therapy have changed based on the recognition that thiabendazole may not be consistently efficacious and that albendazole may be superior. Ivermectin may also be more effective than thiabendazole.

Cryptosporidium parvum

Although self-limited diarrhea associated with waterborne outbreaks has been noted in normal hosts, the clinical presentation of watery diarrhea, cramping, epigastric pain, anorexia, flatulence, and malaise in an HIV-infected patient suggests the diagnosis of cryptosporidiosis. Four clinical syndromes have been identified[93]: chronic diarrhea (in 36% of patients); cholera-like disease (33%); transient diarrhea (15%); and relapsing illness (15%). Biliary tract symptoms similar to cholecystitis have been noted in 10% of cases. Diagnosis is confirmed by finding characteristic acid-fast oocysts on examination of feces.

No predictably effective antimicrobial therapy is available, and management consists largely of symptomatic treatment of diarrhea. Effective antiretroviral therapy (to increase CD4$^+$ count to >100 cells/μL) has been noted to result in complete, sustained clinical, microbiologic, and histologic resolution of HIV-associated cryptosporidiosis.[42]

Isospora belli

Like cryptosporidiosis, this pathogen is acid-fast and can cause a very similar diarrheal illness. In contrast to cryptosporidiosis, the pathogen is larger, oval, and cystic, and very importantly, responds to therapy with trimethoprim-sulfamethoxazole.[42]

Microsporidia

These obligate intracellular protozoa are probably transmitted to humans through the ingestion of food contaminated with its spores, which are resistant to environmental extremes. *Enterocytozoon bienuesi* produces a protracted diarrheal illness accompanied by fever and weight loss similar to that caused by Cryptosporidium; it is reported to occur in 20 to 30% of patients with chronic diarrhea not attributable to other causes. *Enterocytozoon cuniculi* has been described as an etiologic agent for hepatitis, peritonitis, and keratoconjunctivitis.

Transmission electron microscopy with observation of the polar filament is considered the gold standard for diagnosis, but the Brown-Brenn stain and the Warthin-Starry silver stain are commonly used for detecting microsporidia in tissue culture. The modified trichrome stain has been used in clinical diagnostic laboratories to detect microsporidia in fluids.[94]

Treatment guidelines have recommended the initiation and optimization of antiretroviral therapy with immune reconstitution to a CD4$^+$ count >100 cells/μL.[42] Albendazole may be the most effective drug to treat disseminated (not ocular) and intestinal infection attributed to microsporidia other than *E bienuesi*.[42] For GI infections caused by *E bienuesi*, fumagillin has been suggested as being effective. For ocular infection, fumidil in saline eye drops and albendazole for management of systemic infection have been recommended.

Amoebae

Naegleria and Acanthamoeba are free-living amoebae that have the potential to infect humans. Of these, Acanthamoeba spp may infect individuals with defects in cell-mediated immunity (including patients who have AIDS or have undergone organ transplantation) and result in granulomatous amebic encephalitis. Clinical manifestations include mental status abnormalities, seizures, fever, headache, focal neurologic deficits, meningismus, visual disturbances, and ataxia. An important clinical clue may be preexisting skin lesions that have been present for months before CNS disease is clinically manifested, lesions may take the form of ulcerative, nodular, or subcutaneous abscesses. Pneumonitis may also be a part of the clinical presentation.

There are few data regarding therapy for granulomatous amebic encephalitis, but it appears that the diamidine derivatives pentamidine, propamidine, and dibromopropamidine have the greatest activity against Acanthamoeba.

Leishmania spp

In endemic areas of the world, these pathogens infect patients with defective cell-mediated immunity and cause a febrile illness with visceral involvement, most notably hepatomegaly and splenomegaly. Recently, leishmaniasis has been increasingly described in HIV-infected persons from endemic regions and may take a chronic relapsing course. Pentavalent antimonials (with sodium stibogluconate as the representative agent) may be useful for this infection. Notable is that the drug may cause dose-related QT prolongation on ECG, with arrhythmias (atrial and ventricular) and sudden death occasionally. It is contraindicated in patients with myocarditis, hepatitis, or nephritis.

Antimony resistance has been noted in some HIV-infected patients; in such situations, liposomal amphotericin B has been shown to be potentially effective because it targets infected macrophages and reaches high levels in plasma and tissues.

Of the relevant disease models influencing the understanding of the clinical significance of type 1 and type 2 immunity, leishmaniasis is important. Biopsy specimens from patients with localized infection with *Leishmania braziliensis* were consistent with a protective type 1 immune response that included prominent messenger RNA coding for IL-2 and IFN-γ.[95] As the lesions in patients became more destructive, there was a switch to a marked increase in the level of IL-4 messenger RNA, which is consistent with a failed type 2 immune response. Such data have been interpreted as an eloquent demonstration of the facts that type 1 immunity is the key to protection against Leishmania infections in humans and that a high infectious burden suppresses the human immune system from mounting type 1 responses. This has implications for therapy, which has included the use of IFN-γ as an adjunctive agent for visceral leishmaniasis.

Trypanosoma cruzi

With immunosuppression including HIV infection, reactivation of this pathogen can occur. In both posttransplantation infection and HIV-associated infection, patients may present with headache, cognitive changes, seizures, and hemiparesis.[42] In addition to the characteristic lesions seen with Chagas disease, immunosuppressed patients have an increased incidence of neurologic disease, with neuroimaging studies showing large solitary or multiple ring-enhancing lesions with surrounding edema.[42]

Miscellaneous Pathogens

Chlamydiae

This group of intracellular pathogens has been listed in some recent reviews of pathogens defended against by cell-mediated immunity. Although patients with a defect in this host defense system may be at increased risk for chlamydial infections, such problems have not been classically described.

Rickettsiae

As with chlamydiae, rickettsiae are intracellular pathogens defended against by cell-mediated immunity. Recent reviews have not described immunocompromised patients as being at increased risk for infection by pathogens in this group.

Treponema pallidum

Defense against this pathogen may include a role for macrophages and other antigen-presenting cells, such as dendritic cells, that process and present treponemal antigens to helper T cells. HIV-infected patients can have abnormal serologic test results, including unusually high, unusually low, or fluctuating titers. However, aberrant serologic responses are uncommon, and most specialists believe that both treponemal and nontreponemal serologic tests for syphilis can be interpreted in the usual manner for patients who are infected with both HIV and *T pallidum*.[95] With HIV infection, treponemal infection is more likely to have an atypical clinical presentation, be aggressive, or invade sites, such as the CNS. A reactive CSF-VDRL and a CSF WBC count $\geq$10 cells/mm^3 support the diagnosis of neurosyphilis.[42] Although the VDRL test on CSF is the standard serologic test for neurosyphilis, it may be nonreactive when neurosyphilis is present. The CSF fluorescent treponemal antibody absorption test is less specific for neurosyphilis than the VDRL-CSF, but the high sensitivity of the study has led some experts to believe that a negative CSF fluorescent treponemal antibody absorption test excludes neurosyphilis.[96] Such considerations are important, since HIV-1 infection might be associated with mild mononuclear CSF pleocytosis (5–15 cells/mm^3), particularly among persons with peripheral blood CD4$^+$ counts >500 cells/mm^3.[42] In addition to meningitis, a characteristic clinical presentation of syphilis in the CNS is stroke in a young person.

The recommended regimen for the treatment of patients with neurosyphilis is aqueous penicillin G (18 to 24 million U/d, administered as 3 to 4 million U IV q4h or as continuous infusion) for

10 to 14 days.[42,95] If compliance with therapy can be insured, an alternative regimen is procaine penicillin (2.4 million U IM once daily) plus probenecid (500 mg orally 4 times a day), both for 10 to 14 days. Because the duration of treatment recommended for neurosyphilis is shorter than for latent syphilis, some experts recommend administering benzathine penicillin (2.4 million IM once weekly) for up to 3 weeks on completion of the neurosyphilis regimen to provide a comparable total duration of therapy. It is recommended that all HIV-infected persons be tested for syphilis and that all persons with syphilis be tested for HIV. Spinal fluid examination has been recommended for all HIV-infected persons with latent syphilis or with neurologic abnormalities. Some experts have recommended spinal fluid examination for any HIV-1-infected person with syphilis, regardless of stage.[42]

Summary

The identification of a defect in neutrophil function, humoral immunity, or cell-mediated immunity allows the clinician to better focus on the most likely pathogens involved in an infectious process. An approach to the immunocompromised patient based on pathogenesis of disease should result in more directed, cost-effective therapy and in improved patient outcome.

References

1. Spellberg B, Edwards JE Jr. Type 1/type 2 immunity in infectious diseases. Clin Infect Dis 2001; 32:76–102

2. Karam GH, Griffin FM. An approach to diagnosing and treating infections in immunocompromised patients. In: Parrillo JE, ed. Current therapy in critical care medicine. St Louis, MO: Mosby–Year Book, 1997; 281–288

3. Hughes WT, Armstrong D, Bodey GP, et al. 2002 guidelines for the use of antimicrobial agents in neutropenic patients with cancer. Clin Infect Dis 2002; 34:730–751

4. Marron A, Carratalà J, González-Barca E, et al. Serious complications of bacteremia caused by viridans streptococci in neutropenic patients with cancer. Clin Infect Dis 2000; 31:1126–1130

5. Tunkel AR, Sepkowitz KA. Infections caused by viridans streptococci in patients with neutropenia. Clin Infect Dis 2002; 34:1524–1529

6. Razonable RR, Litzow MR, Khaliq Y, et al. Bacteremia due to viridans group streptococci with diminished susceptibility to levofloxacin among neutropenic patients receiving levofloxacin prophylaxis. Clin Infect Dis 2002; 34:1469–1474

7. Gomez L, Martino R, Rolston KV. Neutropenic enterocolitis: spectrum of the disease and comparison of definite and possible cases. Clin Infect Dis 1998; 27:695–699

8. Bodey GP, Jadeja L, Elting L. Pseudomonas bacteremia. Arch Intern Med 1985; 145:1621–1629

9. Chatzinikolaou I, Abi-Said D, Bodey GP, et al. Recent experience with *Pseudomonas aeruginosa* bacteremia in patients with cancer: retrospective analysis of 245 episodes. Arch Intern Med 2000; 160:501–509

10. Del Favero A, Menichetti F, Martino P, et al. A multicenter, double-blind, placebo-controlled trial comparing piperacillin-tazobactam with and without amikacin as empiric therapy for febrile neutropenia. Clin Infect Dis 2001; 33:1295–1301

11. Ozer H, Armitage JO, Bennett CL, et al. 2000 update of recommendations for the use of hematopoietic colony-stimulating factors: evidence-based, clinical practice guidelines. J Clin Oncol 2000; 18: 3558–3585

12. American Society of Clinical Oncology. Update of recommendations for the use of hematopoietic colony-stimulating factors: evidence-based clinical practice guidelines. J Clin Oncol 1996; 14: 1957–1960

13. Armstrong D. Treatment of opportunistic fungal infections. Clin Infect Dis 1993; 16:1–9

14. Thaler M, Pastakia B, Shawker TH, et al. Hepatic candidiasis in cancer patients: the evolving picture of the syndrome. Ann Intern Med 1988; 108:88–100

15. Pappas PG, Rex JH, Sobel JD, et al. Guidelines for treatment of candidiasis. Clin Infect Dis 2004; 38:161–189

16. Patterson TF, Kirkpatrick WR, White M, et al. Invasive aspergillosis: disease spectrum, treatment practices, and outcomes. Medicine (Baltimore) 2000; 79:250–260

17. Herbrecht R, Denning DW, Patterson TF, et al. Voriconazole versus amphotericin B for primary therapy of invasive aspergillosis. N Engl J Med 2002; 347:408–415

18. Johnson LB, Kauffman CA. Voriconazole: a new triazole antifungal agent. Clin Infect Dis 2003; 36:630–637

19. Walsh TJ, Finberg RW, Arndt C, et al. Liposomal amphotericin B for empirical therapy in patient with persistent fever and neutropenia. N Engl J Med 1999; 340:764–771

20. Walsh RJ, Pappas P, Winston DJ, et al. Voriconazole compared with liposomal amphotericin B for empirical antifungal therapy in patients with neutropenia and persistent fever. N Engl J Med 2002; 346:225–234

21. Walsh T, Teppler H, Donowitz G, et al. Caspofungin versus liposomal amphotericin B for empirical antifungal therapy in patients with persistent fever and neutropenia. N Engl J Med 2004; 351: 1391–1402

22. de Ciutiis A, Polley MJ, Metakis LJ, et al. Immunologic defect of the alternate pathway-of-complement activation postsplenectomy: a possible relation between splenectomy and infection. J Natl Med Assoc 1978; 70:667–670

23. Barza MJ, Schooley RT. Case records of the Massachusetts General Hospital (Case 29-1986). N Engl J Med 1986; 315:241–249

24. Norris RP, Vergis EN, Yu VL. Overwhelming postsplenectomy infection: a critical review of etiologic pathogens and management. Infect Med 1996; 13:779–783

25. Parsonnet J, Baluta A, Versalovic J. Case records of the Massachusetts General Hospital (Case 17-1999). N Engl J Med 1999; 340:1819–1826

26. Sullivan KM, Kopecky KJ, Jocom J, et al. Immunomodulatory and antimicrobial efficacy of intravenous immunoglobulin in bone marrow transplantation. N Engl J Med 1990; 323:705–712

27. Centers for Disease Control and Prevention. Prevention of pneumococcal disease: recommendations of the Advisory Committee on Immunization Practices (ACIP). MMWR Recomm Rep 1997; 46(RR-8):1–24

28. Whitney CG, Farley MM, Hadler J, et al. Decline in invasive pneumococcal disease after the introduction of protein-polysaccharide conjugate vaccine. N Engl J Med 2003; 348:1737–1746

29. Centers for Disease Control and Prevention. Prevention and control of meningococcal disease: recommendations of the Advisory Committee on Immunization Practices (ACIP). MMWR Recomm Rep 2000; 49(RR-7):1–20

30. Centers for Disease Control and Prevention. Recommendations of the Advisory Committee on Immunization Practices (ACIP): use of vaccines and immune globulins for persons with altered immunocompetence. MMWR Recomm Rep 1993; 42(RR-4):1–12

31. Weinberg ED. Pregnancy-associated depression of cell-mediated immunity. Rev Infect Dis 1984; 6:814–831

32. Havlir DV, Barnes PF. Tuberculosis in patients with human immunodeficiency virus infection. N Engl J Med 1999; 340:367–373

33. Haas DW, Des Prez RM. Tuberculosis and acquired immunodeficiency syndrome: a historical perspective on recent developments. Am J Med 1994; 96:439–450

34. American Thoracic Society/Centers for Disease Control and Prevention/Infectious Diseases Society of America. Treatment of tuberculosis. Am J Respir Crit Care Med 2003; 167:603–662

35. Keane J, Gershon S, Wise RP, et al. Tuberculosis associated with infliximab, a tumor necrosis factor α-neutralizing agent. N Engl J Med 2001; 345: 1098–1104

36. Update: fatal and severe liver injuries associated with rifampin and pyrazinamide for latent tuberculosis infection, and revisions in American Thoracic Society/CDC recommendations—United States, 2001. MMWR Morb Mortal Wkly Rep 2001; 50:733–735

37. Johnson JL, Ssekasanvu E, Okwera A, et al. Randomized trial of adjunctive interleukin-2 in adults with pulmonary tuberculosis. Am J Respir Crit Care Med 2003; 168:185–191

38. American Thoracic Society. Targeted tuberculin testing and treatment of latent tuberculosis infection. Am J Respir Crit Care Med 2000; 161:S221–S247

39. Selwyn PA, Hartel D, Lewis VA, et al. A prospective study of the risk of tuberculosis among intravenous drug users with human immunodeficiency virus infection. N Engl J Med 1989; 320: 545–550

40. Markowitz N, Hansen NI, Hopewell PC, et al. Incidence of tuberculosis in the United States among HIV-infected persons. Ann Intern Med 1997; 126:123–132

41. Horsburgh CR. The pathophysiology of disseminated *Mycobacterium avium* complex disease in AIDS. J Infect Dis 1999; 179(suppl 3):S461–S465

42. Centers for Disease Control and Prevention, National Institutes of Health, HIV Medicine

Association/Infectious Diseases Society of America. Treating opportunistic infections among HIV-infected adults and adolescents. MMWR Recomm Rep 2004;53(RR-15):1–112

43. Guidelines for preventing opportunistic infections among HIV-infected persons—2002: recommendations of the U.S. Public Health Service and the Infectious Diseases Society of America. MMWR Recomm Rep 2002; 52(RR-8):1–52

44. Wing EJ, Gregory SH. *Listeria monocytogenes*: clinical and experimental update. J Infect Dis 2002; 185(suppl 1):S18–S24

45. Aureli P, Fiorucci GC, Caroli D, et al. An outbreak of febrile gastroenteritis associated with corn contaminated by *Listeria monocytogenes*. N Engl J Med 2000; 342:1236–1241

46. Lorber B. Listeriosis. Clin Infect Dis 1997; 24:1–11

47. Tunkel AR, Hartman BJ, Kaplan SL, et al. Practice guidelines for the management of bacterial meningitis. Clin Infect Dis 2004; 39:1267–1284

48. Walensky RP, Moore RD. A case series of 59 patients with nocardiosis. Infect Dis Clin Pract 2001; 10:249–254

49. Lerner PI. Nocardiosis. Clin Infect Dis 1996; 22:891–905

50. Verville TD, Huycke MM, Greenfield RA, et al. *Rhodococcus equi* infections of humans: 12 cases and a review of the literature. Medicine 1994; 73:119–132

51. Weinstock DM, Brown AE. *Rhodococcus equi*: an emerging pathogen. Clin Infect Dis 2002; 34:1379–1385

52. Torres A, Serra-Batlles J, Ferrer A, et al. Severe community-acquired pneumonia: epidemiology and prognostic factors. Am Rev Respir Dis 1991; 144:312–318

53. Stout JE, Yu VL. Legionellosis. N Engl J Med 1997; 337:682–687

54. Edelstein PH. Antimicrobial chemotherapy for Legionnaires' disease: a review. Clin Infect Dis 1995; 21(suppl 3):S265–S276

55. Koehler JE, Sanchez MA, Garrido CS, et al. Molecular epidemiology of bartonella infections in patients with bacillary angiomatosis-peliosis. N Engl J Med 1997; 337:1876–1883

56. Koehler JE, Sanchez MA, Tye S, et al. Prevalence of *Bartonella* infection among human immunodeficiency virus-infected patients with fever. Clin Infect Dis 2003; 37:559–566

57. van der Horst CM, Saag MS, Cloud CA, et al. Treatment of cryptococcal meningitis associated with the acquired immunodeficiency syndrome. N Engl J Med 1997; 337:15–21

58. Graybill JR, Sobel J, Saag M, et al. Diagnosis and management of increased intracranial pressure in patients with AIDS and cryptococcal meningitis. Clin Infect Dis 2000; 30:47–54

59. Saag MS, Graybill RJ, Larsen RA, et al. Practice guidelines for the management of cryptococcal disease. Clin Infect Dis 2000; 30:710–718

60. Powderly WG, Saag MS, Cloud GA, et al. A controlled trial of fluconazole or amphotericin B to prevent relapse of cryptococcal meningitis in patients with acquired immunodeficiency syndrome. N Engl J Med 1992; 326:793–798

61. Saag MS, Cloud GA, Graybill JR, et al. A comparison of itraconazole versus fluconazole as maintenance therapy for AIDS-associated cryptococcal meningitis. Clin Infect Dis 1999; 28:291–296

62. Mussini C, Pezzotti P, Miro JM, et al. Discontinuation of maintenance therapy for cryptococcal meningitis in patients with AIDS treated with highly active antiretroviral therapy: an international observational study. Clin Infect Dis 2004; 38:565–571

63. Wheat J, Sarosi G, McKinsey D, et al. Practice guidelines for the management of patients with histoplasmosis. Clin Infect Dis 2000; 30:688–695

64. Galgiani JN, Ampel NM, Catanzaro A, et al. Practice guidelines for the treatment of coccidioidomycosis. Clin Infect Dis 2000; 30:658–661

65. Pfaller MA, Diekema DJ, Jones RN, et al. International surveillance of bloodstream infections due to Candida species: frequency of occurrence and in vitro susceptibilities to fluconazole, ravuconazole, and voriconazole of isolates collected from 1997 through 1999 in the SENTRY antimicrobial surveillance program. J Clin Microbiol 2001; 39: 3254–3259

66. Rex JH, Rinaldi MG, Pfaller MA. Resistance of Candida species to fluconazole. Antimicrob Agents Chemother 1995; 39:1–8

67. Marr KA, Seidel K, White TC, et al. Candidemia in allogeneic blood and marrow transplant recipients: evolution of risk factors after adoption of prophylactic fluconazole. J Infect Dis 2000; 181:309–316

68. Stevens DA, Kan VL, Judson MA, et al. Practice guidelines for diseases caused by Aspergillus. Clin Infect Dis 2000; 30:696–709

69. Wingard JR, Kubilis P, Lee L, et al. Clinical significance of nephrotoxicity in patients treated with amphotericin B for suspected or proven aspergillosis. Clin Infect Dis 1999; 29:1402–1407

70. Farr RW, Short S, Weissman D. Fulminant hepatitis during herpes simplex virus infection in apparently immunocompetent adults: report of two cases and review of the literature. Clin Infect Dis 1997;24:1191–1194

71. Cohen JI, Brunell PA, Staus SE, et al. Recent advances in varicella-zoster virus infection. Ann Intern Med 1999; 130:922–932

72. Harger JH, Ernest JM, Thurnau GR, et al. Risk factors and outcome of varicella-zoster virus pneumonia in pregnant women. J Infect Dis 2002; 185:422–427

73. van der Bij, Speich R. Management of cytomegalovirus infection and disease after solid-organ transplantation. Clin Infect Dis 2001; 33(suppl 1): S33–S37

74. Nichols WG, Corey L, Gooley T, et al. High risk of death due to bacterial and fungal infection among cytomegalovirus (CMV)-seronegative recipients of stem cell transplants from seropositive donors: evidence for indirect effects of primary CMV infection. J Infect Dis 2002; 185:273–282

75. Dykewicz CA. Summary of the guidelines for preventing opportunistic infections among hematopoietic stem cell transplant recipients. Clin Infect Dis 2001; 33:139–144

76. Ljungman P, Griffiths P, Paya C. Definitions of cytomegalovirus infection and disease in transplant recipients. Clin Infect Dis 2002; 34:1094–1097

77. Karavellas MP, Azen SP, MacDonald JC, et al. Immune recovery vitritis and uveitis in AIDS: clinical predictors, sequelae, and treatment outcomes. Retina 2001; 21:1–9

78. Cohen JI. Epstein-Barr virus infection. N Engl J Med 2000; 343:481–492

79. Babcock GJ, Decker LL, Volk M, et al. EBV persistence in memory B cells in vivo. Immunity 1998; 9: 395–404

80. Walling DM, Flaitz CM, Nichols CM, et al. Persistent productive Epstein-Barr virus replication in normal epithelial cells *in vivo*. J Infect Dis 2001; 184:1499–1507

81. Reploeg MD, Storch GA, Clifford DB. BK virus: a clinical review. Clin Infect Dis 2001; 33:191–202

82. De Luca A, Giancola ML, Ammassari A, et al. The effect of potent antiretroviral therapy and JC virus load in cerebrospinal fluid on clinical outcome of patients with AIDS-associated progressive multifocal leukoencephalopathy. J Infect Dis 2000; 182:1077–1083

83. Angel JB, Walpita P, Lerch RA, et al. Vaccine-associated measles pneumonitis in an adult with AIDS. Ann Intern Med 1998; 129:104–106

84. Stringer JR, Beard CB, Miller RF, et al. A new name (*Pneumocystis jiroveci*) for Pneumocystis from humans. Emerg Infect Dis 2002; 8:891–896

85. Kovacs JA, Gill VJ, Meshnick S, et al. New insights into transmission, diagnosis, and drug treatment of *Pneumocystis carinii* pneumonia. JAMA 2001; 286:2450–2460

86. Bozzette SA. The use of corticosteroids in *Pneumocystis carinii* pneumonia. J Infect Dis 1990; 162:1365–1369

87. de Quiros JCLB, Miro JM, Peña JM, et al. A randomized trial of the discontinuation of primary and secondary prophylaxis against *Pneumocystis carinii* pneumonia after highly active antiretroviral therapy in patients with HIV infection. N Engl J Med 2001; 344:159–167

88. Ledergerber B, Mocroft A, Reiss R, et al. Discontinuation of secondary prophylaxis against *Pneumocystis carinii* pneumonia in patients with HIV infection who have a response to antiretroviral therapy. N Engl J Med 2001; 344:168–174

89. Trikalinos TA, Ioannidis JPA. Discontinuation of *Pneumocystis carinii* prophylaxis in patients infected with human immunodeficiency virus: a meta-analysis and decision analysis. Clin Infect Dis 2001; 33:1901–1909

90. Montoya JG. Laboratory diagnosis of *Toxoplasma gondii* infection and toxoplasmosis. J Infect Dis 2002; 185(suppl 1):S73–S82

91. Walker M, Zunt JR. Parasitic central nervous system infections in immunocompromised hosts. Clin Infect Dis 2005; 40:1005–1015

92. Walot I, Miller BL, Chang L, et al. Neuroimaging findings in patients with AIDS. Clin Infect Dis 1996; 22:906–919

93. Manabe YC, Clark DP, Moore RD, et al. Cryptosporidiosis in patients with AIDS: correlates of disease and survival. Clin Infect Dis 1998; 27:536–542

94. Didier ES. Microsporidiosis. Clin Infect Dis 1998; 27:1–8

95. Pirmez C, Yamamura M, Uyemura K, et al. Cytokine patterns in the pathogenesis of human leishmaniasis. J Clin Invest 1993; 91:1390–1395

96. Centers for Disease Control and Prevention. Sexually transmitted diseases treatment guidelines 2002. MMWR Recomm Rep 2002; 51(RR-6): 1–8

Notes

Nervous System Infections and Catheter Infections

George H. Karam, MD, FCCP

Objectives:

- Review clinical presentations of nervous system infections that may present as serious or life-threatening processes
- Outline principles influencing diagnosis and management of nervous system infections
- Present an approach to infections related to catheters placed in the vasculature, urinary bladder, or peritoneum
- Summarize existing opinions and data about management of catheter-related infections

Key words: botulism; brain abscess; catheter-related infections; cavernous sinus thrombosis; encephalitis; meningitis; rabies; spinal epidural abscess

Introduction

Infection affecting various parts of the nervous system has the potential to be life-threatening or to result in severe sequelae if the infection is not appropriately diagnosed and treated. Although infections such as meningitis, encephalitis, and brain abscess are the most frequently encountered, processes such as spinal epidural abscess, septic intracranial thrombophlebitis, rabies, and botulism may present as emergent problems that require a high level of clinical suspicion for prompt diagnoses to be made. Infections associated with catheters placed in the vasculature, urinary bladder, or peritoneum can also result in morbidity and create diagnostic or therapeutic dilemmas for the clinician. This review will attempt to summarize these infections as they relate to the critical care setting.

Nervous System Infections

Meningitis

From 1986 to 1995, the median age of persons with bacterial meningitis increased from 15 months to 25 years, making meningitis in the United States predominantly a disease of adults rather than of infants and young children.[1]

The basic diagnostic tool in the diagnosis of meningitis is examination of cerebrospinal fluid (CSF). When such fluid is obtained, important clinical studies include (1) stains and cultures, (2) glucose, (3) protein, and (4) cell count with differential. Gram stain and culture of CSF are highly specific but may have a median sensitivity of about 75%. Helpful in understanding the pathogenesis of meningitis due to varied processes is the CSF glucose level. Glucose enters the CSF by facilitated transport across choroid plexuses and capillaries lining the CSF space.[2] Normally, the CSF-to-blood glucose ratio is 0.6. Although consumption of glucose by white blood cells and organisms may contribute to low CSF glucose levels (which is referred to as *hypoglycorrhachia*), the major mechanism for low glucose is impaired transport into the CSF; this classically occurs because of acute inflammation or with infiltration of the meninges by granulomas or malignant cells. Protein is usually excluded from the CSF but levels rise after disruption of the blood-brain barrier. Levels are lower in cisternal and ventricular CSF than in lumbar CSF. Usual elevations in patients with meningitis are in the 100 to 500 mg/dL range. Extreme elevations (*ie*, >1,000 mg/dL) are often indicative of subarachnoid block. When protein levels exceed 150 mg/dL, the fluid may appear xanthochromic.

The diagnosis of meningitis is made by the finding of a CSF pleocytosis and may occur on the basis of both infectious and noninfectious processes. In the absence of a positive stain on the CSF, the most helpful study in the initial approach to the patient with meningitis is a cell count with differential on the CSF. As summarized in Table 1, an approach for diagnosing the etiology of meningitis based on the CSF analysis would include three common categories: (1) polymorphonuclear meningitis, (2) lymphocytic meningitis with a normal glucose, and (3) lymphocytic meningitis with a low glucose. In addition, on rare occasions patients may have a predominance of eosinophils in the CSF, but eosinophilic meningitis is uncommon.

Table 1. *An Approach to CSF Pleocytosis**

Polymorphonuclear	Lymphocytic With Normal Glucose	Lymphocytic With Low Glucose
Bacterial (see Table 2)	Viral meningitis	Fungal
Early meningitis	Enteroviruses, including poliovirus	Tuberculous
Tuberculosis	Herpes simplex virus (usually type 2)	Certain forms of meningoencephalitis (*eg*, herpes
		simplex) or viral meningitis
Fungal	HIV	Partially treated bacterial meningitis
Viral	Adenovirus	Carcinomatous meningitis
Drug-induced	Tick-borne viruses	Subarachnoid hemorrhage
Parameningeal foci	Meningoencephalitis, including viral causes	Chemical meningitis
Brain abscess	Parameningeal foci	
Subdural empyema	Partially treated bacterial meningitis	
Epidural abscess	Listeria meningitis	
Sinusitis	Spirochetal infections	
Mastoiditis	Syphilis	
Osteomyelitis	Leptospirosis	
Persistent neutrophilic meningitis	Lyme disease	
	Rickettsial infections	
	Rocky Mountain spotted fever	
	Ehrlichiosis	
	Infective endocarditis	
	Immune-mediated diseases	
	Sarcoidosis	
	Drug-induced	

*Although not clinically common in the United States, eosinophilic meningitis can occur, and the characteristic pathogens causing such a process are *Angiostrongylus cantonesis, Trichinella spiralis, Taenia solium, Toxocara canis, Gnathostoma spinigerum, Paragonimus westwermani*, and *Baylisascaris procyonis*.

Polymorphonuclear Meningitis: Because of the acute inflammation, this process is usually associated with a low CSF glucose owing to impaired transport across the meninges. This is most notable with bacterial meningitis. In the differential diagnosis of polymorphonuclear meningitis, there are four major groups of disease: (1) bacterial infection, (2) the early meningeal response to any type of infection or inflammation, (3) parameningeal foci, and (4) persistent neutrophilic meningitis. Because of the sequelae that may be associated with a delay in therapy, the single most important cause of a polymorphonuclear meningitis is bacterial infection. Discussion in this syllabus will be limited to this topic.

Likely etiologic agents for bacterial meningitis are summarized in Table 2 from the perspectives of (1) the age of the patient and (2) underlying predispositions to meningitis. Presented in a different manner, rates of meningitis per 100,000 population in 22 counties in four states revealed the following: *Streptococcus pneumoniae*, 1.1; *Neisseria meningitidis*, 0.6; group B streptococci, 0.3; *Listeria monocytogenes*, 0.2; and *Haemophilus*

influenzae, 0.2.[1] The most notable change in etiologic agents over the past decade has been the dramatic decrease in the incidence of *H influenzae* meningitis, which has occurred as a result of vaccination against this pathogen.

Although pneumococci are the most common pathogens in bacterial meningitis, the problematic strains of *S pneumoniae* are those that are penicillin-resistant. Strains with relative, or intermediate, resistance will have a penicillin minimal inhibitory concentration (MIC) of 0.12 to 1.0 µg/mL. High-level resistance to penicillin is defined as an MIC ≥2 µg/mL.[3] Compounding this problem is the inability of certain antibiotics to cross the blood-brain barrier effectively enough to yield CSF levels significantly above the MIC for the infecting organism. For pneumococcal meningitis caused by penicillin-susceptible strains, penicillin G and ampicillin are equally effective. Although high-dose penicillin (150,000 to 250,000 U/kg/d) has been useful in patients with pneumonia caused by strains of pneumococci with intermediate resistance, such high doses do not predictably lead to CSF levels of

Table 2. *Likely Pathogens in Bacterial Meningitis Based on Patient's Age or Underlying Conditions*

Neonates	Enterobacteriaceae Group B streptococci *Listeria monocytogenes*
<6 yr	*Neisseria meningitidis, Streptococcus pneumoniae Haemophilus influenzae*
6 yr to young adult	*N meningitidis, S pneumoniae*
Adults <50 yr	*S pneumoniae, N meningitidis*
Alcoholic and elderly	*S pneumoniae, N meningitidis* Enterobacteriaceae *L monocytogenes*
Closed skull fracture	*S pneumoniae, H influenzae* *Staphylococcus aureus* Coagulase-negative staphylococci Gram-negative bacilli
Open skull fracture	Gram-negative bacilli, including *Klebsiella pneumoniae* and *Acinetobacter calcoaceticus* (when meningitis develops from a contiguous postoperative traumatic wound infection) *S aureus*
Penetrating trauma; Postneurosurgery	*S aureus* Coagulase-negative staphylococci Aerobic Gram-negative bacilli (*including Pseudomonas* *aeruginosa*)
CSF leak	*S pneumoniae, H influenzae* Gram-negative bacilli Staphylococci
CSF shunt–associated	Coagulase-negative staphylococci *S aureus* Aerobic Gram-negative bacilli (including *P aeruginosa*) *Propionibacterium acnes*
Diabetes	*S pneumoniae* Gram-negative bacilli *S aureus*
Defects in cell-mediated immunity	*L monocytogenes*
Concern of bioterrorism	*Bacillus anthracis*

penicillin that exceed the MIC of intermediately resistant strains.[4]

In 2002, the National Committee for Clinical Laboratory Standards began offering differing cephalosporin breakpoints for pneumococcal susceptibility based on the site of infections.[5] For *S pneumoniae* from a meningeal source, the ceftriaxone and cefotaxime breakpoints were listed as follows: susceptible, 0.5 μg/mL; intermediate susceptibility, 1 μg/mL; and resistant, 2 μg/mL. This was in contrast to nonmeningeal breakpoints, which were stated as follows: susceptible, 1 μg/mL; intermediate susceptibility, 2 μg/mL; and resistant, 4 μg/mL.[5] These recommendations have been repeated in subsequent National Committee for Clinical Laboratory Standards reports.[3] To assess the effect of these new criteria on reporting of nonsusceptible *S pneumoniae* isolates, the Centers for Disease Control and Prevention (CDC) analyzed cefotaxime MIC data from the Active Bacterial Core Surveillance of the Emerging Infections Program Network from 1998 to 2001.[6] This analysis indicated that after the new criteria were applied, the number of isolates defined as nonsusceptible to cefotaxime decreased 52.1 to 61.2% each year. Even though cefotaxime or ceftriaxone has been recommended for pneumococci with intermediate susceptibility to penicillin, clinical failures have been reported when these agents have been used for such strains. For isolates with high-level resistance, vancomycin is the drug of choice. The less-than-optimal penetration of vancomycin into CSF has an impact on this therapeutic option. Steroids given concomitantly for meningitis may further decrease vancomycin's penetration.

In December 2004, the Infectious Diseases Society of America (IDSA) published recommendations for the management of bacterial meningitis[7] to update recommendations that have been available since 1997.[8] A summary of the empiric therapy recommendations from those guidelines is included in Table 3. Because of the importance of *S pneumoniae*, including those strains demonstrating antibiotic resistance, the guidelines provided an approach to therapy of proven pneumococcal meningitis based on *in vitro* susceptibility. For penicillin-susceptible isolates, penicillin or ampicillin was suggested. With intermediate susceptibility to penicillin (MIC, 0.1 to 1.0 μg/mL), a third-generation cephalosporin was recommended. It was suggested that the regimen of a broad-spectrum cephalosporin plus vancomycin be used if the *S pneumoniae* isolate is resistant to penicillin (MIC ≥2 μg/mL) and to ceftriaxone and cefotaxime (MIC ≥1 μg/mL). Clinical data on the efficacy of rifampin in patients with bacterial

Table 3. *CSF Recommendations for Empiric Therapy of Meningitis When Lumbar Puncture Is Delayed or in Patients With a Nondiagnostic CSF Gram Stain***

Patient Group	Recommended Drugs
Age 2 to 50 yr	Vancomycin plus a third-generation cephalosporin
Age >50 yr	Vancomycin plus ampicillin plus a third-generation cephalosporin
Penetrating head trauma, or postneurosurgery, or CSF shunt	Vancomycin plus ceftazidime or vancomycin plus cefepime[†], or vancomycin plus meropenem[‡]

*Adapted from Tunkel and colleagues.[7]
[†]Not approved by the Food and Drug Administration (FDA) for meningitis.
[‡]FDA-approved for bacterial meningitis in pediatric patients ≥3 mo old.

meningitis are lacking, but some authorities would use this agent in combination with a third-generation cephalosporin, with or without vancomycin, in patients with pneumococcal meningitis caused by highly penicillin- or cephalosporin-resistant strains.[7] This statement was qualified in the IDSA guidelines for treatment of bacterial meningitis with the comment that rifampin should be added only if the organism is shown to be susceptible and there is a delay in the expected clinical or bacteriologic response. The usual duration of therapy for pneumococcal meningitis is generally stated to be 10 to 14 days.[7]

The role of steroids in adults with meningitis has not been definitively established. An early opinion by experts in the field suggested that adult patients who might be candidates for steroid therapy in meningitis are those with a high CSF concentration of bacteria (*ie*, demonstrable bacteria on Gram stain of CSF), especially if there is increased intracranial pressure.[9] A prospective, randomized, double-blind, multicenter trial assessed the value of adjuvant treatment with dexamethasone compared with placebo in adults 17 years of age or older with suspected meningitis who had cloudy CSF, bacteria in CSF on Gram staining, or a CSF leukocyte count of $>1,000/mm^3$.[10] Early treatment with dexamethasone was shown to improve the outcome and did not increase the risk of GI bleed. The dose of dexamethasone used in this study was 10 mg IV q6h for 4 days. In the 2004 IDSA guidelines for the treatment of bacterial meningitis in adults, it was recommended that dexamethasone (0.15 mg/kg q6h for 2 to 4 days, with the first dose administered 10 to 20 min before, or at least

concomitant with, the first dose of antimicrobial therapy) be given in adults with suspected or proven pneumococcal meningitis.[7] It was stated that adjunctive dexamethasone should not be given to adult patients who have already received antimicrobial therapy, because administration of dexamethasone in this circumstance is unlikely to improve patient outcome. Even though the data are inadequate to recommend adjunctive dexamethasone in adults with meningitis caused by bacterial pathogens other than *S pneumoniae*, it was acknowledged that some authorities would initiate dexamethasone in all adults because the etiology of meningitis is not always ascertained at initial evaluation.[7]

The infectious syndromes caused by *N meningitidis* are somewhat broad and include meningococcal meningitis, meningococcal bacteremia, meningococcemia (purpura fulminans and the Waterhouse-Friderichsen syndrome), respiratory tract infections (pneumonia, epiglottitis, otitis media), focal infection (conjunctivitis, septic arthritis, urethritis, purulent pericarditis), and chronic meningococcemia.[11] Important in the pathogenesis of the clinical illnesses caused by the meningococcus is the organism's natural reservoir in the nasopharynx. It is this site from which disease may develop. The epidemiology of meningococcal meningitis is evolving. The traditional groups of patients at risk have included children and young adults, especially college students or military recruits who live in relatively confined quarters. A report from Argentina described epidemic meningococcal disease in the northeastern part of that country associated with disco patronage, supporting the pathogenetic point that close confinement allows aerosolization and spread of the organism from the nasopharynx.[12] An additional observation from this study, which has been raised in previous studies, is the association with passive or active cigarette smoking. This report, which was titled "Disco Fever," expanded the closed settings in which meningococcal meningitis originates to include dance clubs and discos. Air travel–associated meningococcal disease has also been described and is defined as a patient who meets the case definition of meningococcal disease within 14 days of travel on a flight of at least 8-h duration.[13] Pneumonia, sinusitis, and tracheobronchitis are important sources of bacteremic meningococcal disease. Although meningitis is the characteristic infection caused by N meningitidis, a report from Atlanta noted that only 14 (32%) of the 44 adult patients with meningococcal infection had meningitis.[14] When it occurs, meningococcal meningitis is usually acute and often associated with purpuric skin lesions (although the Atlanta report noted that only 10 of the 14 adults with meningitis [71%] had a generalized rash). During the very early stages of infection, the CSF analysis may be relatively normal even though the clinical course is hyperacute with fever, nuchal rigidity, and coma. Although variably reported through the years, the potential for N meningitidis to cause purulent pericarditis should be noted. The illness may progress to acidosis, tissue hypoxia, shock, disseminated intravascular coagulopathy, and hemorrhagic adrenal infarction. The potential for β-lactamase-producing strains remains a concern, as does the existence of relatively resistant strains, presumably caused by alterations in the penicillin-binding proteins; however, active surveillance among a large, diverse population in the United States has failed to identify any such strains.[15] Penicillin or ampicillin, therefore, remains a drug of choice for treating meningitis caused by this pathogen. The usual duration of therapy is generally 7 days.[7]

With meningococcemia, a fulminant complication is acute, massive adrenal hemorrhage with the resultant clinical entity of the Waterhouse-Friderichsen syndrome. However, not all patients who die of meningococcemia have evidence of adrenal hemorrhage at autopsy, and many steroid-treated patients succumb despite therapy, implying that adrenal insufficiency may not be the primary cause of circulatory collapse. Because of the implications of such a complication, it would be helpful to have definitive recommendations about the role, if any, of steroids in management of patients with meningococcal meningitis. There are anecdotal reports in the literature of improved outcome in such patients treated with corticosteroids. In some patients with meningococcal infection, cortisol levels may be elevated. In contrast, other reports have noted that not all patients with severe meningococcal infection who have been given adrenocorticotropic hormone have responded to adrenocorticotropic hormone stimulation of cortisol production, and this raises the issues of whether adrenal reserves may be decreased in certain patients and whether steroids may have a role. In 1992, IDSA published a review of the role of steroids in patients with infectious diseases.[16] There were 10 infections for which steroids were strongly supported or suggested as having a role, and meningococcemia was not one of those listed. At the present time, the role of steroids in meningococcemia is unresolved. Because fulminant meningococcal septicemia represents an extreme form of endotoxin-induced sepsis and coagulopathy, with clinical consequences that include amputations and organ failure, investigators have addressed other potential therapeutic modalities that may be beneficial in patients with overwhelming meningococcal infection. The dual function of protein C as an anticoagulant and as a modulator of the inflammatory response was recently reviewed in the context of experimental data showing that activated protein C replacement therapy reduces the mortality rate for fulminant meningococcemia.[17] Such data become especially noteworthy given the efficacy and safety data about recombinant human activated protein C in patients with severe sepsis.[18]

In patients treated with penicillin for meningococcal meningitis, posttreatment with rifampin, ciprofloxacin, or ceftriaxone has been recommended to eradicate the nasal carrier state, as penicillin will not eliminate organisms at this site.[19] These recommendations are similar to those for chemoprophylaxis for individuals exposed to a

Table 4. *Schedule for Administering Chemoprophylaxis Against Meningococcal Disease**

Drug	Age Group	Dosage	Duration/Route of Administration[†]
Rifampin[‡]	Children <1 mo	5 mg/kg q12h	2 d
	Children ≥1 mo	10 mg/kg q12h	2 d
	Adults	600 mg q12h	2 d
Ciprofloxacin[§]	Adults	500 mg	Single dose
Ceftriaxone	Children <15 yr	125 mg	Single IM dose
	Adults	250 mg	Single IM dose

* Reprinted from the Centers for Disease Control and Prevention. MMWR Recomm Rep 2000; 49(RR-7):1–10.
† Oral administration unless indicated otherwise.
‡ Rifampin is not recommended for pregnant women because the drug is teratogenic in laboratory animals. Because the reliability of oral contraceptives may be affected by rifampin therapy, consideration should be given to using alternative contraceptive measures while rifampin is being administered.
§ Ciprofloxacin generally is not recommended for persons aged <18 yr or for pregnant and lactating women, because the drug causes cartilage damage in immature laboratory animals. However, ciprofloxacin can be used for chemoprophylaxis in children when no acceptable alternative is available.

person with known meningococcal disease. Those recommendations are summarized in Table 4. Prophylaxis is recommended for close contacts, which include household members, day-care center contacts, and anyone directly exposed to the patient's oral secretions (*eg*, kissing, mouth-to-mouth resuscitation, endotracheal intubation, endotracheal tube management). Because the rate of secondary disease for close contacts is highest during the first few days after the onset of disease in the primary patient, antimicrobial chemoprophylaxis should be administered as soon as possible (ideally within 24 h after the case is identified). Chemoprophylaxis administered >14 days has been stated to be of limited or no value.[13]

Since 1991, there have been increased numbers of outbreaks of serogroup C meningococcal disease in the United States. Meningococcal polysaccharide vaccine has been shown to be effective against serogroup C meningococcal disease in a community outbreak, with a vaccine efficacy among 2- to 29-year-olds of 85%.[20] Based on this observation, it has been recommended that emphasis be placed on achieving high vaccination coverage in future outbreaks, with special efforts to vaccinate young adults. The Advisory Committee on Immunization Practices and the American Academy of Pediatrics have recommended that health-care providers and colleges educate freshmen college students—especially those who live in dormitories—and their parents about the increased risk of

meningococcal diseases and the potential benefits of immunization so that informed decisions about vaccination can be made.[21] A predisposing factor for neisserial infections is deficiency in the late complement components (*ie*, C5 to C8). Because previous studies have demonstrated an incidence as high as 39% in populations of patients with meningococcal infections, at a minimum, a screening test for complement function (CH_{50}) has been suggested for all patients who have invasive meningococcal infections[22]; it was also noted that direct assessment of complement (C5, C6, C7, C8, and C9) and properdin proteins should be considered.

Like the meningococcus, *H influenzae* may be isolated from the nasopharynx, and this may be the immediate source of invading pathogens. Rates of infection caused by this pathogen have decreased because of vaccination against *H influenzae*. In patients with meningitis due to this organism, a contiguous focus of infection such as sinusitis or otitis media should be investigated. In adults without these underlying processes, a search for a CSF leak, which may be the basis for the meningitis, is necessary. Because about one third of *H influenzae* isolates are β-lactamase producers, agents that are stable in the presence of these enzymes and that cross the blood-brain barrier should be used. The third-generation cephalosporins cefotaxime and ceftriaxone have had the most successful record of use in this regard. Even though the second-generation cephalosporin cefuroxime is active against *H influenzae*, it has been shown to result in delayed sterilization of the CSF when compared with ceftriaxone.[23] A lower incidence of sensorineural hearing loss was demonstrated in children who adjunctively received dexamethasone (3.3%) vs those who did not receive steroids (15.5%). Similar findings have not been corroborated in adults. The usual duration of therapy for *H influenzae* meningitis is generally 7 days.[7]

Meningitis due to Gram-negative bacilli occurs most characteristically after neurosurgical procedures, with head trauma being a less likely predisposition. Medical conditions, including urosepsis, account for about 20% of episodes of this infection. In certain patient populations in which Gram-negative meningitis develops in the setting of impaired cell-mediated immunity, one should exclude *Strongyloides stercoralis* infection as the underlying predisposing cause. Of note, hyperinfection with the resultant predisposition to Gram-negative meningitis is uncommon in two groups of patients with defects in cell-mediated immunity: (1) transplant recipients who receive cyclosporine, because of the anthelminthic properties of this rejection agent; and (2) HIV-infected patients, unless the CD4+ cell count is ≤200 cells/mm^3 and the patient is concomitantly receiving corticosteroids.[24] Parenterally administered aminoglycosides do not cross the blood-brain barrier after the 28th day of life. For these antibiotics to be useful beyond the neonatal period, they need to be administered intrathecally or intraventricularly. Chloramphenicol has activity against some Gram-negative bacilli, and it crosses the blood-brain barrier. Concern about toxicity issues such as aplastic anemia has decreased the use of this agent over the years, although it still plays an important role in persons with meningitis and type I (IgE-mediated) hypersensitivity to penicillins. Third-generation cephalosporins have become the mainstay of therapy for Gram-negative meningitis because of their spectrum and their penetration into the CSF. All of the presently available third-generation agents except for cefoperazone have an indication for meningitis due to susceptible pathogens. For meningitis due to *Pseudomonas aeruginosa*, ceftazidime is an efficacious agent. It is usually administered with a parenteral aminoglycoside, recognizing that this latter agent will not cross the blood-brain barrier in adults but that it might help to eradicate the site of infection outside the CNS that served as the focus for the meningitis. According to the recent IDSA guidelines for the management of bacterial meningitis, cefepime has greater *in vitro* activity than the third-generation cephalosporins against *Enterobacter* spp and *P aeruginosa*, and it has been used successfully in some patients with meningitis caused by these bacteria.[7] The guidelines summarized these observations by stating that they support cefepime as a useful agent in the treatment of patients with bacterial meningitis. This should be taken within the context that as of 2005, cefepime does not have an FDA-approved indication for the treatment of bacterial meningitis.[25] For meningitis due to Gram-negative pathogens, the IDSA guidelines list 21 days as the duration of therapy.[7]

Pharmacologic and microbiologic issues are important for two important pathogens that cause meningitis. *L monocytogenes* is an intracellular Gram-positive rod that characteristically infects persons with defects in cell-mediated immunity. It may also cause disease in diabetics and elderly persons, and about 30% of infected adults have no apparent risk. Acquisition has been associated with consumption of contaminated coleslaw, milk, and cheese. Although the CSF cellular response is usually polymorphonuclear, some patients present either with lymphocytes or with a normal glucose. Like fungal and tuberculous meningitis, Listeria meningitis has a predilection for involving the meninges at the base of the brain. This may lead to hydrocephalus. Ampicillin or penicillin is the drug of choice, and there is no significant activity by third-generation cephalosporins against this pathogen.[26] Some experts suggest the addition of an aminoglycoside given parenterally because of *in vitro* synergy. For those patients who are allergic to penicillin, trimethoprim-sulfamethoxazole is the agent of choice. Because of the intracellular location of this pathogen, 21 days of therapy has been recommended.[7] A review of *Staphylococcus aureus* meningitis divided this disease entity into two categories: (1) hospital-acquired and (2) community-acquired.[27] It was noted that hospital-acquired infection occurred as an occasional complication of neurosurgical procedures, with the presence of medical devices, or with certain skin infections; it generally had a favorable prognosis and a relatively low mortality rate. In contrast, community-acquired *S aureus* meningitis was associated with valvular heart disease, diabetes mellitus, or drug or alcohol abuse, and the mortality rate was significantly higher than for nosocomial infection. In this review of 28 patients with community-acquired *S aureus* meningitis, 8 had negative or no CSF culture. Of these 8 patients, 4 had received antibiotics prior to lumbar puncture. This finding is consistent with the observation that an important presentation of *S aureus* is in patients with addict-associated infective endocarditis. For *S aureus*, nafcillin or oxacillin has better activity against methicillin-sensitive strains than does vancomycin. In addition, the penetration of vancomycin into CSF may be variable, even in the setting of meningeal inflammation.

Beginning with the September 11, 2001, episode of terrorism in the United States, anthrax is an important consideration in the differential diagnosis of patients with a life-threatening illness that includes a meningeal component. Inhalational anthrax is a biphasic clinical syndrome with initial nonspecific flu-like symptoms (fatigue, malaise, myalgia, headache, nonproductive cough, and nausea/vomiting) followed by a second phase with hemodynamic collapse, septic shock/multiorgan dysfunction syndrome, and rapid death with overwhelming bacterial spread. It is during the stage of bacteremia that there is a strong likelihood of meningitis, which some sources cite as occurring in 50% of cases. The index case of bioterrorism anthrax in Florida presented with hemorrhagic meningitis,[28] which is characteristic of disseminated anthrax; however, meningitis without hemorrhage can occur with anthrax. In patients in whom infection with *Bacillus anthracis* is suspected to be the cause of meningitis, some have suggested adding either penicillin or chloramphenicol to the multidrug regimen that would be given for inhalational anthrax.[29]

Empiric therapy for meningitis has changed in recent years. In previously healthy, nonallergic individuals with acute pyogenic community-acquired meningitis in whom little information is available, ampicillin was suggested in a 1993 review as a reasonable empiric agent.[30] For patients with a type I (IgE-mediated) penicillin allergy, chloramphenicol was offered in that review as appropriate therapy. In 1997, recommendations suggested a broad-spectrum cephalosporin (*eg,* cefotaxime or ceftriaxone) as empiric therapy for individuals aged 18 to 50 years who have a nondiagnostic Gram stain.[8] As summarized in Table 3, the 2004 IDSA guidelines suggested vancomycin plus a third-generation cephalosporin as empiric therapy of meningitis when lumbar puncture is delayed or in patients with a nondiagnostic CSF Gram stain.[7] This evolution from 1993 to 2004 in the recommendations for empiric therapy of meningitis is influenced by penicillin resistance in pneumococci. The addition of ampicillin to a broad-spectrum cephalosporin plus vancomycin is reasonable empiric therapy for polymorphonuclear meningitis undiagnosed by Gram stain in patient populations with the following underlying conditions: (1) advanced age; (2) alcoholism; and (3) immunocompromised states. The activity by ampicillin against Listeria is an important component of the coverage in this regimen.

Certain epidemiologic situations may exist that influence the acquisition of specific pathogens, which may then cause meningitis. Those conditions (including skull fractures and shunt-associated infections), and the pathogens likely to occur in their setting, are summarized in Table 2.

Lymphocytic Meningitis With Normal Glucose: The meningeal response to infection or inflammation may be less marked in certain conditions, and the response may therefore be less associated with the inability to transport glucose across the meninges. Those conditions associated with the findings of lymphocytes and normal glucose in the CSF are listed in Table 1. The classic consideration in this differential has been viral meningitis. Enteroviruses, which are recognized causes of pleurodynia and pericarditis, are the most common cause of aseptic meningitis and characteristically cause a self-limited form of meningitis that presents with fever, headache, and lymphocytic pleocytosis, most often in the late summer or early fall. Recently, however, two other viruses have gained importance in the differential diagnosis of viral meningitis. With initial episodes or flares of genital herpes simplex virus infection, patients may develop meningitis as a systemic manifestation of their herpes infection. This process is distinctly different from the life-threatening entity of herpes encephalitis in that it is self-limited and does not require therapy. Because of the propensity for herpes genitalis to recur, this form of meningitis may similarly present as a recurrent form of lymphocytic meningitis. HIV has a predilection for neural tissue, and patients, including those with the acute retroviral syndrome, may present with viral meningitis that may resolve spontaneously. In those individuals who have risk factors for HIV and present with an illness consistent with viral meningitis, HIV infection is an important consideration.

Encephalitis may occur on the basis of both infectious and noninfectious causes. When these conditions are associated with WBCs in the CSF, the diagnosis of meningoencephalitis may be made. The traditional teaching has been that meningoencephalitis, like viral encephalitis, will give a normal glucose level in association with lymphocytes. As outlined in Table 1, herpes encephalitis may result in a low glucose level.

Spirochetal infections are an important cause of lymphocytic meningitis with normal glucose level. *Treponema pallidum*, the etiologic agent of syphilis, is a recognized cause of asymptomatic infection of the CNS in nonimmunocompromised hosts. Meningovascular syphilis has been increasingly diagnosed in the era of HIV infection; it may take the form of syphilitic meningitis or a stroke syndrome. In December 2004, new guidelines were published for the management of infections in HIV-infected persons.[31] Several important points were made regarding neurosyphilis. Because CNS disease can occur during any stage of syphilis, a patient who has clinical evidence of neurologic involvement with syphilis (*eg*, cognitive dysfunction, motor or sensory deficits, ophthalmic or auditory symptoms, cranial nerve palsies, and symptoms or signs of meningitis) should undergo a CSF examination. Because it is highly specific (although insensitive), the VDRL test in CSF (VDRL-CSF) is the standard serologic test for CSF. When reactive in the absence of substantial contamination of CSF with blood, it is considered diagnostic of neurosyphilis. However, with syphilitic meningitis, patients may present without symptoms of nervous system disease and analysis of their CSF may reveal only a few lymphocytes and a negative VDRL-CSF. The fluorescent treponemal antibody absorption test on CSF is less specific for neurosyphilis than the VDRL-CSF, but the high sensitivity of the study has led some experts to believe that a negative CSF fluorescent treponemal antibody absorption test excludes neurosyphilis.[31] The guidelines now state that a reactive CSF-VDRL and a CSF WBC count ≥ 10 cells/mm³ support the diagnosis of neurosyphilis. An analysis of laboratory measures after treatment for neurosyphilis revealed that HIV-infected patients were less likely than non-HIV-infected patients to normalize their CSF-VDRL reactivity with higher baseline titers, even though the CSF WBC count and serum rapid plasma reagin reactivity in both populations were likely to normalize.[32] Neurosyphilis can present as cerebrovascular insufficiency, often in young patients with a stroke syndrome caused by an endarteritis, which most characteristically involves the middle cerebral artery.

According to guidelines,[31] the recommended regimen for patients with neurosyphilis is 18 to 24 million U/d of aqueous crystalline penicillin G, administered as 3 to 4 million U IV q4h or continuous infusion, for 10 to 14 days. If compliance with therapy can be ensured, patients may be treated with procaine penicillin (2.4 million U IM once daily) plus probenecid (500 mg orally 4 times a day), both for 10 to 14 days. Because these durations are shorter than the regimen used for late syphilis in the absence of neurosyphilis, some specialists administer benzathine penicillin (2.4 million U IM once per week for up to 3 weeks after completion of these neurosyphilis treatment regimens) to provide a comparable total duration of therapy. The CSF leukocyte count has been stated to be a sensitive measure of the effectiveness of therapy.

The classic presentation of neurologic Lyme disease, which is caused by *Borrelia burgdorferi*, is seventh nerve palsy (which may be bilateral) in association with a lymphocytic meningitis.

Leptospirosis, caused by *Leptospira interrogans*, is epidemiologically linked to such factors as infected rat urine or exposure to infected dogs. It presents as two distinct clinical syndromes.[33] Anicteric leptospirosis is a self-limiting illness, which progresses through two well-defined stages: a septicemic stage and an immune stage. The septicemic stage occurs after a 7- to 12-day incubation period and is primarily manifested as fever, chills, nausea, vomiting, and headache. The most characteristic physical finding during this stage is conjunctival suffusion. The causative organism can be isolated from blood or CSF at this point. Following a 1- to 3-day asymptomatic period, the immune stage develops; it is characterized by aseptic meningitis. Leptospira are present in the urine during this stage and may persist for up to 3 weeks. Icteric leptospirosis, or Weil syndrome, is a less common but potentially fatal syndrome that occurs in 5 to 10% of cases. Jaundice, renal involvement, hypotension, and hemorrhage are the hallmarks of this form of leptospirosis; however, the severity of these manifestations can vary greatly, and renal involvement is not universal. In icteric leptospirosis, the biphasic nature of the disease is somewhat obscured by the persistence of jaundice and azotemia throughout the illness, but septicemic and immune stages do occur. Leptospires can be isolated from blood or CSF during the first week and from the urine during the second week of illness. Additionally, the diagnosis can be made by demonstrating rising antibody titers. Treatment of leptospirosis involves intense supportive care as well as antibiotic coverage. The use of IV penicillin (1.5 million U every 6 h) has been shown to shorten the duration of fever, renal dysfunction, and hospital stay. In a prospective, open-label, randomized trial, ceftriaxone and penicillin G were shown to be equally effective for the treatment of severe leptospirosis.[34]

Over the years, Rocky Mountain spotted fever, which is caused by *Rickettsia rickettsii*, has been considered the classic rickettsial infection in the United States. Results of CSF analysis are usually normal unless patients have stupor or coma, in which case there may be a lymphocytic pleocytosis with normal glucose and elevated protein levels. An important emerging infection in the United States is ehrlichiosis. The clinical illness attributable to this infection is discussed in this syllabus in the section on encephalitis. The characteristic CSF abnormalities in patients with ehrlichiosis have been a lymphocytic pleocytosis with elevated protein. In a recent review of the subject, the CSF glucose level was normal in the majority of patients, with 24% of the patients having borderline low CSF glucose concentrations.[35] In this review, morulae were seen in CSF white cells in only a small minority of the patients. Clinical features supporting the diagnosis of ehrlichiosis are leukopenia (because of the intracellular location of the organism), thrombocytopenia, and elevated liver enzymes. From the limited clinical data available, it appears that chloramphenicol or tetracycline is the agent most frequently used for this infection.

Certain infectious diseases, such as infective endocarditis, may cause a lymphocytic pleocytosis with normal glucose that is the result of a vasculitis, which the infectious process causes in the CNS. A review of a 12-year experience at the Cleveland Clinic included the results of lumbar punctures done on 23 of 175 patients with endocarditis.[36] There was a CSF pleocytosis in 14 and no CSF WBCs in 9. Of the 14 patients who had a pleocytosis, the etiology was attributed to a stroke in 8 and to encephalopathy in 5; the remaining patient only had isolated headaches. No positive CSF cultures were reported in any of these 14 patients. Such information underscores a dilemma for the clinician managing a patient with endocarditis who has a CSF pleocytosis: Is the pleocytosis due to secondary bacterial seeding of the meninges, or is it due to other events associated with endocarditis that lead to a CNS response that is associated with a secondary cellular response?

A group of noninfectious causes of lymphocytic meningitis with a normal glucose level are described in Table 1.

Lymphocytic Meningitis With Low Glucose: With chronic processes, it is not surprising that the cellular CSF response would be lymphocytes. Low CSF glucose has been described in this syllabus as occurring due to impaired transport based on acute inflammation of the meninges. In certain conditions, glucose transport may be associated with infiltration of the meninges by either granulomatous processes or malignant cells. Such is the situation for several of the conditions summarized in Table 1 that cause lymphocytic meningitis with a low glucose level.

Viral meningitis due to mumps and lymphocytic choriomeningitis has characteristically been associated with a low CSF glucose. As previously discussed, certain forms of meningoencephalitis, including that due to herpes simplex virus, may present in this manner. Partially treated bacterial meningitis and certain chemical-induced meningitides may have similar findings. Four other groups of conditions are important in this setting are tuberculous meningitis, fungal meningitis, carcinomatous meningitis, and subarachnoid hemorrhage.

A review of 48 adult patients with tuberculous meningitis who were admitted to an ICU demonstrates the potential for this infectious process to cause serious disease.[37] It also emphasizes the difficulty often encountered in establishing the diagnosis. Repeated large volumes (10 to 20 mL) of CSF have a higher yield for acid-fast bacilli.[38] When four CSF smears for acid-fast bacilli are obtained, positive findings may occur in up to 90% of patients with tuberculous meningitis. Some studies have shown that elevated CSF titers of adenosine deaminase[39] or CSF chloride levels <110 mEq/L in the absence of bacterial infection support the diagnosis of tuberculous meningitis. Enzyme-linked immunosorbent assays (ELISAs) are felt by some to be helpful with this diagnosis. Polymerase chain reaction (PCR) for *Mycobacterium tuberculosis* may be helpful when performed on CSF, but false-negative results have been reported. Because of a predilection for tuberculous meningitis to involve the base of the brain, imaging studies of the CNS may reveal an obstructing hydrocephalus. In addition to antituberculous therapy with agents such as isoniazid, rifampin, pyrazinamide, and ethambutol, corticosteroids may play a role, especially in situations of increased intracranial pressure or obstruction resulting from the infection. The most recent guidelines of the American Thoracic Society give steroids in the treatment of tuberculous meningitis an A-1 recommendation.[40] A randomized, double-blind, placebo-controlled trial in Vietnam in patients >14 years of age with tuberculous meningitis showed that adjunctive treatment with dexamethasone improved survival but probably did not prevent severe disability.[41] From the series of patients with tuberculous meningitis admitted to an ICU, several important clinical points can be extracted[37]: (1) Ischemic lesions with signs of localization may be present. (2) Extrameningeal tuberculous infection may support the diagnosis. (Overall, the rate has been stated to be 40 to 45%, but in this review it was 66%.) (3) Clinical features and CSF profiles did not appear to be modified in the HIV-infected patients. (4) Delay to onset of treatment and the neurologic status at admission were identified as the main clinical prognostic factors. In low-incidence geographic areas, clinicians should suspect tuberculous meningitis in members of immigrant groups from high-incidence areas, as well as in patients who abuse alcohol or drugs and those with immunosuppression from any cause.[42]

Although fungal meningitis may be due to several etiologic agents, the two most common ones are *Cryptococcus neoformans* and *Coccidioides immitis*. Although both of these pathogens have been increasingly diagnosed as a cause of meningitis because of HIV infection, both caused meningitis in normal hosts prior to the AIDS era. Both organisms gain access to the body via the lungs. In HIV-infected persons with cryptococcal meningitis, there may be a lack of inflammation in the CSF, and therefore findings may include <20 CSF WBCs/mm^3 and a normal glucose level. The India ink stain, latex agglutination test, and fungal culture of the CSF are, therefore, important in the diagnosis. Potentially helpful in establishing the diagnosis are other sites of involvement, including lung, skin, and blood. Based on data from the Mycoses Study Group of the National Institutes of Health (NIH), it appears that therapy for cryptococcal meningitis in HIV-infected patients should begin with amphotericin B (0.7 mg/kg/d) in combination with flucytosine (100 mg/kg/d in persons with normal renal function) for the initial 2 weeks of therapy followed by fluconazole (400 mg/d orally) for an additional 8 to 10 weeks.[43] In the 381 patients with cryptococcal meningitis treated in this double-blind, multicenter trial, 13 of 14 early deaths and 40% of deaths during weeks 3 through 10 were associated with elevated intracranial pressure. Based on the association of elevated intracranial pressure and mortality in patients with cryptococcal meningitis, it was suggested that measurement of intracranial pressure be included in the management of such patients. Included in the recommendations were daily lumbar punctures, use of acetazolamide, and ventriculoperitoneal shunts for asymptomatic patients with intracranial CSF pressure >320 mm H$_2$O and for symptomatic patients with pressure >180 mm H$_2$O. More recently, it was recommended that in the absence of focal lesions, opening pressures ≥250 mm H$_2$O should be treated with large-volume CSF drainage (defined in this report as allowing CSF to drain until a satisfactory closing pressure had been achieved, commonly <200 mm H$_2$O).[44] The IDSA guidelines for the management of cryptococcal meningitis in

HIV-infected persons with opening CSF pressure of >250 mm H_2O recommended lumbar drainage sufficient to achieve a closing pressure ≤200 mm H_2O or 50% of initial opening pressure.[45] Maintenance therapy is required after completion of primary therapy, and studies have defined fluconazole (200 mg/d orally) as the agent of choice.

Meningitis due to *C immitis* commonly presents with headache, vomiting, and altered mental status. Although the CSF formula is usually one of lymphocytes with a low glucose level, eosinophils are occasionally present. In addition to direct examination and culture of CSF, complement-fixing antibodies in the CSF may be an especially important aid to the diagnosis of coccidioidal meningitis. As with cryptococcal meningitis, the epidemiologic history and the other body sites of involvement (including lung, skin, joints, and bone) are important in making the diagnosis. In contrast to cryptococcal meningitis, management strategies for coccidioidal meningitis may vary from patient to patient. Recent IDSA guidelines noted that oral fluconazole is currently the preferred therapy, with itraconazole being listed as having comparable efficacy.[46] It was acknowledged that some physicians initiate therapy with intrathecal amphotericin B in addition to an azole on the basis of their belief that responses may be more prompt with this approach. Because Coccidioides has a predilection for the basilar meninges, hydrocephalus may occur. Regardless of the regimen being used, this potential complication nearly always requires a shunt for decompression.

Other fungi have the capability of causing meningitis, but they are less likely to do so. Because CNS involvement may be clinically recognized in 5 to 10% of cases of progressive disseminated histoplasmosis, the diagnosis and management of CNS histoplasmosis has been recently reviewed.[47] As a general rule, fungal meningitis, like tuberculous meningitis, may involve the base of the brain and cause obstruction of CSF flow with resulting hydrocephalus.

Eosinophilic Meningitis: The subject of eosinophilic meningitis has been recently reviewed.[48]

Angiostrongylus cantonensis is a nematode that can infect humans who ingest poorly cooked or raw intermediate mollusk hosts, such as snails, slugs, and prawns. Infection can also occur when fresh vegetables contaminated with infective larvae are eaten. Once ingested, the infective larvae penetrate the gut wall and migrate to the small vessels of the meninges to cause a clinical picture of fever, meningismus, and headache. CSF analysis reveals an eosinophilic pleocytosis; larvae are usually not found. Such a process has been most characteristically described in Asia and the South Pacific. A recent report described an outbreak of meningitis due to *A cantonensis* that developed in 12 travelers who traveled to the Caribbean and whose clinical illness was strongly associated with the consumption of a Caesar salad at a meal.[49] From this outbreak, it was suggested that *A cantonensis* infection should be suspected among travelers at risk who present with headache, elevated intracranial pressure, and pleocytosis, with or without eosinophilia, particularly in association with paresthesias or hyperesthesias.

Less classic infectious causes of eosinophilic meningitis include *Trichinella spiralis*, *Taenia solium*, *Toxocara canis*, *Gnathostoma spinigerum*, *Paragonimus westermani*, and *Baylisascaris procyonis*. Important noninfectious causes include malignancy (*eg*, Hodgkin disease, non-Hodgkin lymphoma, and eosinophilic leukemia), medications (*eg*, ciprofloxacin, ibuprofen), and intraventricular medications or shunts.

Meningitis Caused by Protozoa or Helminth: Of the causes, five deserve special comment. The most common is due to *Toxoplasma gondii* and presents most often as multiple ring-enhancing lesions in HIV-infected patients. These lesions may be associated with a CSF pleocytosis, but meningitis is not the most likely presentation of CNS toxoplasmosis. Because this infection usually represents reactivation disease, the IgG antibody to Toxoplasma is positive in about 95% of these individuals. Therapy is with sulfadiazine and pyrimethamine.

Naegleria fowleri is a free-living amoeba that enters the CNS by invading the nasal mucosa at the level of the cribriform plate. The classic presentation is of an acute pyogenic meningitis in a person who recently swam in fresh water.[50] The CSF analysis shows a polymorphonuclear pleocytosis, many RBCs, and hypoglycorrhachia. The diagnosis is confirmed by identifying the organism on CSF wet mount as motile amoeba, or it can be made by biopsy of brain tissue. Amphotericin B administered systemically and intraventricularly is the drug of choice. Another amoebic pathogen infecting the nervous system is Acanthamoeba, which may infect individuals with defects in cell-mediated immunity (including patients with AIDS or after organ transplantation) and result in a granulomatous amoebic encephalitis. Clinical manifestations include mental status abnormalities, seizures, fever, headache, focal neurologic deficits, meningismus, visual disturbances, and ataxia. An important clinical clue may be preexisting skin lesions that have been present for months before CNS disease and may take the form of ulcerative, nodular, or subcutaneous abscesses. Pneumonitis may also be a part of the clinical presentation.

Neurocysticercosis, which is caused by the pork tapeworm *T solium*, is the most common cause of acquired epilepsy in the world and is highly endemic in all parts of the developing world where pigs are raised, especially Latin America, most of Asia, sub-Saharan Africa, and parts of Oceania.[24] Even though seizures are the most common manifestation of neurocysticercosis, other symptoms include headache, hemiparesis, and ataxia. Symptoms typically begin years after the initial infection, when a host inflammatory response develops against *T solium* antigens released after the death of the parasite. Although not the most classic presentation of neurocysticercosis, eosinophilic meningitis may be part of the clinical presentation. Brain imaging studies may reveal intracranial lesions, which may be cystic or calcified; because of chronic inflammation at the base of the brain, hydrocephalus may be present. The epidemiologic history, combined with brain imaging studies and serologies (serum enzyme-linked immunoelectrotransfer blot or CSF ELISA), helps make the diagnosis. The drug treatment of choice for neurocysticercosis includes albendazole or praziquantel; steroids should be given concomitantly to reduce edema produced by medical treatment, especially for meningeal infection.[24] Most experts agree that the inflammatory response produced by the death of the cyst produces symptomatic neurocysticercosis and that inactive infection (ie, presence of calcified or ring-enhancing lesions) does not require anthelminthics.[24]

As previously noted, *A cantonensis* may be a cause of eosinophilic meningitis.

Miscellaneous Issues in the Diagnosis and Management of Meningitis: The timing of diagnostic studies in patients with meningitis is of critical importance. An important issue is focality. Over the last several decades, many have limited the designation of focality to such processes as hemiparesis, isolated abnormalities on an imaging study of the brain, or an abnormal focus on an EEG. More recently, it has been stated that altered mental status indicates bilateral hemispheric or brainstem dysfunction and severely compromises the ability to determine whether the patient's neurologic assessment is nonfocal.

Because of the potential for severe neurologic sequelae in individuals with bacterial meningitis who are treated in a suboptimal manner, attention has been focused in recent years on the appropriate sequencing of diagnostic studies. A prospective study of 301 adults with suspected meningitis was conducted to determine whether clinical characteristics present before CT of the head was performed could be used to identify patients who were unlikely to have abnormalities on CT.[51] Thirteen baseline clinical characteristics were used to predict abnormal findings on head CT: age ≥60 years; immunocompromised state; history of CNS disease; seizure within 1 week before presentation; abnormal level of consciousness; inability to answer two questions correctly; inability to follow two commands correctly; gaze palsy; abnormal visual fields; facial palsy; arm drift; leg drift; and abnormal language (ie, aphasia, dysarthria, and extinction). From the results of the study, the authors concluded that adults with suspected meningitis who have none of the noted baseline features are good candidates for immediate lumbar puncture since they have a low risk of brain herniation as a result of lumbar puncture. It was acknowledged that such an approach would have resulted in a 41% decrease in the frequency of CT scans performed in the study cohort. When imaging is indicated, the following sequence of evaluation and management has been suggested: (1) obtain blood cultures; (2) institute empiric antibiotic therapy; and (3) perform lumbar puncture immediately after the imaging study if no intracranial mass lesion is present.[8]

Supporting the importance of the timing of antibiotics in patients with meningitis are the findings of a retrospective, observational cohort study of patients with community-acquired bacterial meningitis.[52] In this study, patients with microbiologically proven, community-acquired bacterial meningitis were stratified into three groups based on the clinical findings of hypotension, altered mental status, and seizures. Patients with none of these three predictor variables were in stage I; those with one predictor variable, stage II; and those with two or more predictor variables, stage III. Delay in therapy after arrival in the emergency department was associated with adverse clinical outcome when the patient's condition advanced from stage I or II to stage III before the initial antibiotic dose was given, a finding that underscores the need for prompt administration of antibiotics in patients with bacterial meningitis. This study was further interpreted as suggesting that the risk for adverse outcome is influenced more by the severity of illness than the timing of initial antibiotic therapy for patients who arrive in the emergency department at stage III.

A recent analysis of the causes of death in adults hospitalized with community-acquired bacterial meningitis provides some important insights.[53] Although 50% of the 74 patients had meningitis as the underlying and immediate cause of death, 18% of patients had meningitis as the underlying but not immediate cause of death, and 23% had meningitis as neither the underlying nor immediate cause of death. A 14-day survival end point discriminated between deaths attributable to meningitis and those with another cause. It was concluded that such an end point will facilitate greater accuracy of epidemiologic statistics and will assist investigations of the impact of new therapeutic interventions.

For many years, clinicians have relied on a CSF pleocytosis for diagnosing meningitis. Because of implications in both therapy and prophylaxis of meningitis, rapid and accurate diagnostic tests for bacterial meningitis are important. A recent report describes the potential role for broad-range bacterial PCR in excluding the diagnosis of meningitis and in influencing the decision to initiate or discontinue antimicrobial therapy.[54]

In the *Medical Knowledge Self-Assessment Program IX* of the American College of Physicians, it was acknowledged that there are at least four clinical entities in which patients may have fever, coma, and nuchal ridigity but a normal CSF analysis: (1) early bacterial meningitis; (2) cryptococcal meningitis with concomitant HIV infection; (3) parameningeal foci; and (4) herpes simplex encephalitis.[55]

Encephalitis

Characteristic of processes involving cortical brain matter are alterations of consciousness and/or cognitive dysfunction. A representative clinical entity with such findings is acute viral encephalitis, which occurs on the basis of direct infection of neural cells with associated perivascular inflammation, neuronal destruction, and tissue necrosis.[56] Pathologically, the involvement in acute viral encephalitis is in the gray matter. This may be associated with evidence of meningeal irritation and CSF mononuclear pleocytosis, in which the process is referred to as meningoencephalitis. In addition to infectious agents, which may cause direct brain injury, there are indirect mechanisms including induction of autoimmune diseases. This process is referred to as postinfectious encephalomyelitis and is characterized by widespread perivenular inflammation with demyelination localized to the white matter of the brain. The list of infectious and noninfectious processes causing encephalitis is lengthy and is partially summarized in Table 5. An additional process, which represents the sequelae of an infection, is production of neurotoxins as occurs with shigellosis, melioidosis, and cat-scratch disease.

Of all the mechanisms by which an infectious process leads to involvement of the brain, direct viral invasion of neural cells is the most classic. Although the most common cause of acute viral meningitis is enteroviral infection (notably coxsackie A and B viruses and echoviruses), it has been stated that <3% of the CNS complications from such infections would be classified as encephalitis. Diagnostic studies should include viral pharyngeal, rectal, and urine cultures, but confirmation using acute- and convalescent-phase serology is important because viral shedding from the sites of culture may occur without clinical disease. No specific therapy is available for enteroviral encephalitis.

Table 5. *Encephalitis**

Infectious	Postinfectious Encephalomyelitis	Noninfectious Diseases Simulating Viral Encephalitis
Viral		
Rabies	Vaccinia virus	Systemic lupus erythematosus
Herpes viruses: HSV 1 and 2, varicella-zoster, herpes B	Measles virus	Granulomatous angiitis
(simian herpes), Epstein-Barr, CMV, human herpes 6	Varicella-zoster virus	Behçet disease
Arthropod-borne (Table 6)	Rubella virus	Neoplastic diseases, including carcinomatous meningitis
Mumps	Epstein-Barr virus	Sarcoid
Lymphocytic choriomeningitis	Mumps virus	Reye syndrome
Enteroviruses: coxsackievirus, echovirus, hepatitis A	Influenza virus	Adrenal leukodystrophy
HIV	Nonspecific respiratory disease	Metabolic encephalopathies
Bacterial (including Brucella, Listeria, Nocardia,	...	Cerebrovascular disease
Actinomyces, relapsing fever, cat scratch disease,		
Whipple disease, infective endocarditis, parameningeal foci)		
M tuberculosis	...	Subdural hematoma
Mycoplasma pneumoniae	...	Subarachnoid hemorrhage
Spirochetes: syphilis, Lyme disease, leptospirosis		Acute multiple sclerosis
Fungal: including Cryptococcus, Coccidioides,	...	Toxic encephalopathy, including cocaine-induced
Histoplasma, Blastomyces, Candida		
Rickettsial: RMSF, typhus, Ehrlichia, Q fever	...	Drug reactions
Parasites: Toxoplasma, Naegleria, Acanthamoeba,	...	
Plasmodium falciparum, Trichinella, Echinococcus,		
Cysticercus, *Trypanosoma cruzii*		

*CMV = cytomegalovirus; RMSF = Rocky Mountain spotted fever.

From the clinical perspective, the most emergent encephalitis to diagnose is that due to herpes simplex virus (HSV).[57] This infection is characteristically caused by HSV type 1 and results in inflammation or necrosis localized to the medial-temporal and orbital-frontal lobes. Although it may have an insidious onset, in its most classic form HSV encephalitis presents as an acute, febrile, focal illness. Because of the temporal lobe localization, personality change may be prominent for a few days to as long as a week before other manifestations. Headache is also a prominent early symptom. Patients may progress rapidly from a nonspecific prodrome of fever and malaise, to findings such as behavioral abnormalities and seizures, to coma. A hallmark of the diagnosis is focality, which may be demonstrated with history (*eg*, changes in personality or in olfaction), physical examination, imaging studies of the brain, or EEG. These findings most characteristically involve the temporal lobes. Subtle clues to focality may include abnormalities such as changes in olfaction, which may be influenced by the fact that HSV might access the brain via the olfactory tract. CSF analysis may initially be unrevealing even in some acutely ill patients who have fever, nuchal rigidity, and coma. Characteristic features with lumbar puncture include increased intracranial pressure, CSF lymphocytosis, and the presence of RBCs in the CSF. Although CSF glucose is characteristically normal, patients may have hypoglycorrhachia. For many years, brain biopsy with viral culture was considered the gold-standard diagnostic study. In suspected cases, such pathologic examination of brain tissue often yielded another treatable diagnosis. Because of the invasiveness of the procedure and because neurosurgical services are not available at all hospitals, there has been attention to noninvasive diagnostic procedures. PCR analysis of CSF (when performed with optimal techniques in an experienced laboratory) has been reported to be 100%

specific and 75 to 98% sensitive. In a decision model comparing a PCR-based approach with empiric therapy, the PCR-based approach yielded better outcomes with reduced acyclovir use.[58] Prompt initiation of IV therapy with acyclovir is critical in management of patients in whom this infection is suspected because prognosis is influenced by the level of consciousness at the time therapy is begun. It has been stated that one cannot anticipate an accuracy of >50% in the diagnosis of HSV encephalitis in the early course of the infection, even when one uses physical examination, spinal fluid analysis without PCR, and neuroimaging studies. Relapse of HSV encephalitis has been stated to occur in some patients 1 week to 3 months after initial improvement and completion of a full course of acyclovir therapy. Retreatment may be indicated in these patients.

The arthropod-borne encephalitides are a group of CNS infections in which the viral pathogen is transmitted to humans via a mosquito or tick vector. Of those described in Table 6, all are mosquito-borne except for Powassan encephalitis, which is transmitted by the tick *Ixodes cookei*. The distinguishing features of these illnesses are summarized in this table. Of these, Eastern equine encephalitis is associated with the highest mortality rate (30 to 70%), and this fulminant process results in neurologic sequelae in >80% of survivors. St. Louis encephalitis (SLE) is caused by a flavivirus, which induces clinical disease in about 1% of those infected. Following a nonspecific pro-

drome, patients may experience the abrupt onset of headache, nausea, vomiting, disorientation, and stupor. Common laboratory findings include inappropriate secretion of antidiuretic hormone and pyuria. In contrast to Eastern equine encephalitis, the overall mortality related to SLE is about 2%, with the highest mortality rate occurring in elderly persons. Emotional disturbances are the most common sequelae.

The outbreak of arboviral encephalitis described in metropolitan New York City in the late summer and fall of 1999 was caused by West Nile virus (WNV), a flavivirus that is serologically closely related to SLE virus and that was responsible for 61 human cases, including 7 deaths.[59] In 2002, the virus became much more widespread in its prevalence across the United States, making WNV an important diagnostic consideration in patients with an acute viral illness. In the summary of pertinent information on this virus,[60] several important points were made. It was noted that 1 in 5 infected persons had developed a mild febrile illness, with 1 in 150 developing meningitis, encephalitis, or both. Advanced age was the greatest risk factor for severe neurologic disease, long-term morbidity, and death. The most efficient diagnostic method noted in that review was IgM antibody-capture ELISA for IgM antibody to WNV in serum or CSF. Important bases for using this diagnostic study are that IgM antibody does not cross the blood-brain barrier and that 90% of serum samples obtained within 8 days of symptom onset had been positive for IgM antibody. A feature clinicians need to be familiar with is that related flaviviruses—such as those causing SLE or dengue—may produce a false-positive assay for WNV. The cited review presents a concise summary of the criteria for making possible, probable, and confirmed diagnoses of WNV based on the US national case definitions for WNV encephalitis. Recently reported is the experience with WNV infection in 28 patients, 54% of whom had a focal neurologic deficit at presentation.[61] In 47% of these patients with focal deficits, a meningitis or encephalitis syndrome was absent. During the outbreak of WNV in the summer of 2002, several patients were described who presented with acute flaccid paralysis syndrome.[62] Noteworthy features in these patients included an asymmetrical weakness without pain or sensory loss in association with

Table 6. *Arthropod-Borne Encephalitis*

Encephalitis	Mortality	Neurologic Sequelae
Eastern equine encephalitis	30–70%	80%
St. Louis encephalitis	2–20%	20%
California encephalitis	*	*
West Nile encephalitis	11%[†]	[‡]
Western equine encephalitis	5–15%	30%
Venezuelan equine encephalitis	1%	Rare
Powassan encephalitis	15%	…

*Uneventful recovery in most patients; abnormal EEGs in 75%, with seizures in 6 to 10%.

[†]Based on the 1999 outbreak in metropolitan New York, NY (MMWR Morb Mortal Wkly Rep 2000; 49:25–28).[59]

[‡]The limited data available suggest that many patients have substantial morbidity (Ann Intern Med 2002; 137:173–179).[60]

a CSF pleocytosis. Although some of these patients were initially thought to have Guillain-Barré syndrome, they did not have the symmetric pattern with sensory changes, paresthesias, and CSF protein elevation in the absence of CSF pleocytosis that are typical of Guillain-Barré syndrome. Preliminary interpretation of the findings of acute flaccid paralysis in WNV-infected patients is that the pattern is a polio-like syndrome with involvement of the anterior horn cells of the spinal cord and motor axons. Treatment for WNV encephalitis is supportive. Several approaches, including interferon-α2b and immunoglobulin with high titer against WNV, offer promise based on animal models and limited clinical experience.[63] Like SLE virus, WNV is transmitted principally by Culex mosquitoes.

Health-care providers should consider arboviruses in the differential diagnosis of aseptic meningitis and encephalitis cases during the summer months. According to recommendations by the CDC, serum (acute and convalescent) and CSF samples should be obtained for serologic testing, and cases should be reported promptly to state health departments.[64] Diagnosis of arbovirus encephalitis may be rapidly facilitated by testing acute serum or spinal fluid for virus-specific IgM antibody. Unfortunately, no effective specific therapy is available for any of these infections. Supportive measures should focus on cerebral edema, seizures, or ventilation if problems related to any of these occur.

HIV has tropism for neural tissue, and a significant number of patients will develop involvement of the CNS. As a part of the acute retroviral syndrome that follows initial infection with HIV, patients may develop an acute encephalitis that can include seizures and delirium and from which patients may spontaneously recover with few, if any, neurologic sequelae. On a chronic basis and occurring later in the course of HIV infection, patients may develop an encephalopathy associated with cerebral atrophy and widened sulci on CT studies of the brain. Clinical features may initially include forgetfulness and impaired cognitive function; these may progress to include weakness, ataxia, spasticity, and myoclonus.

The DNA polyoma virus JC is the etiologic agent in progressive multifocal leukoencephalopathy (PML). In this primary demyelinating process involving white matter of the cerebral hemispheres, patients present subacutely with confusion, disorientation, and visual disturbances, which may progress to cortical blindness or ataxia. CSF is characteristically acellular. A feature on neuroradiology imaging studies is lack of mass effect. No definitive therapy is presently available for this infection, and clinical efforts have recently focused on the role of immune reconstitution in modifying the clinical course of the illness. In a multicenter analysis of 57 consecutive HIV-positive patients with PML, neurologic improvement or stability at 2 months after therapy was demonstrated in 26% of patients who received highly active antiretroviral therapy, in contrast to improvement in only 4% of patients who did not receive this therapy (p = 0.03).[65] In this study, decreases in JC virus DNA to undetectable levels predicted a longer survival. In the context that untreated PML may be fatal within 3 to 6 months, the potential for preventing neurologic progression and improving survival by controlling JC virus replication becomes clinically relevant.

In recent months, there have been increasing reports of human rabies in the United States. Although this infection does not occur very often, it raises some important points about epidemiology, transmission, clinical presentation, and prevention. Rabies is probably best considered to be an encephalomyelopathy. After inoculation, the virus replicates in myocytes and then enters the nervous system via unmyelinated sensory and motor nerves. It spreads until the spinal cord is reached, and it is at this point in the clinical course that paresthesias may begin at the wound site. The virus then moves from the CNS along peripheral nerves to skin and intestine as well as into salivary glands, where it is released into saliva.[66] Knowledge of these factors allows an understanding of both clinical presentation and prevention. A review of the topic by the CDC stated that "… this infection should be considered in the differential diagnosis of persons presenting with unexplained rapidly progressive encephalitis."[67] A recent report acknowledges the potential for rabies to be spread through organ transplantation[68] and provides further support for the contention that rabies should be considered in any patient with unexplained encephalitis. It is the CNS involvement that leads to the cognitive dysfunction characteristic in encephalitis. Because the rabies virus may in the early stages localize to limbic structures, changes in behavior may result. Although an ascending paralysis simulating the Guillain-Barré syndrome has been described, the most classic presentation is of encephalitis associated with hypertonicity and hypersalivation. Noteworthy in Table 7 is that 13 of the 15 patients had pain and/or weakness, explainable since rabies is a myelopathic infection.[67-77]

Of the cases of bat-related rabies reported in the United States since 1980, the minority is definitively related to an animal bite. Only 3 of the 15 cases reported in the recent *Morbidity and Mortality Weekly Reports* cited in Table 7 were bite-related.

When the management of rabies in humans was reviewed in 2003,[78] it was acknowledged that the only survivors of the disease had received rabies vaccine before the onset of illness. In 2004, a previously healthy 15-year-old girl developed rabies after being bitten by a bat approximately 1 month before symptom onset. Her case represented the sixth known occurrence of human recovery after rabies infection; however, the case was unique because the patient received no rabies prophylaxis either before or after illness onset.[77] Despite this very rare occurrence, there is still a strong impetus for postexposure prophylaxis, which is discussed in the following paragraph. The cited review notes that the normal management of patients with rabies should be palliative. In those individuals who might be candidates for aggressive management, a combination of specific therapies was listed for consideration, including rabies vaccine, rabies immunoglobulin, monoclonal antibodies, ribavirin, interferon-α, and ketamine. A summary of the potential role of each of these agents was included. Because severe brain edema with herniation has been rare in patients with rabies and because corticosteroids have been associated with increased mortality and shortened incubation period in mouse models of rabies, the review stated that corticosteroids should not be used.

Rabies prophylaxis has been recently reviewed.[79] In individuals who were not previously vaccinated against rabies but have an indication for rabies postexposure prophylaxis, the treatment regimen includes local wound cleansing, human rabies immune globulin, and vaccine.

Table 7. *Clinical Presentation of Rabies**

Clinical Feature	Encephalitis Symptoms	Pain and Weakness	Findings of CI	Myoclonus	Paralysis	Autonomic Instability
Case 1[67]	Hallucinations	Left arm	Yes	Yes	Total body	No
Case 2[67]	Hypersalivation	Left arm	Yes	Yes	No	Yes
Case 3[69]	Confusion	Left face, ear	Yes	Yes	Vocal cord, ocular	No
Case 4[70]	Hallucinations	Right shoulder	Yes	No	No	Yes
Case 5[71]	Confusion	Right wrist	No	Yes	No	Yes
Case 6[71]	Confusion; hypersalivation	Right arm	No	Yes	Dysphagia	Yes
Case 7[71]	Disorientation; hypersalivation	No	No	No	No	Yes
Case 8[71]	No	Right arm	Yes	No	Flaccid paralysis	No
Case 9[71]	Delirium	Left arm	Yes	Yes	Dysphagia	Yes
Case 10[72]	Agitation	Both legs	Yes	No	No	Yes
Case 11[73]	Agitation; hypersalivation	Right arm	Yes	No	Dysphagia	Yes
Case 12[74]	Hallucinations; intractable seizures	Abdominal	No	No	Respiratory dysfunction	No
Case 13[75]	Ataxia; confusion	No	Yes	Yes	No	No
Case 14[76]	Confusion	Right arm	Yes	No	No	No
Case 15[77]	Hypersalivation	Left arm	Yes	Yes	Sixth nerve palsy	Yes

*CI = cerebrovascular insufficiency.

Nervous System Infections and Catheter Infections (Karam)

The doses of human rabies immune globulin and vaccine have been summarized.[79] The administration of rabies immune globulin has been modified, and recommendations now are that as much as anatomically feasible of the 20 IU/kg body weight dose should be infiltrated into and around the wound(s), with the remainder administered IM in the deltoid or quadriceps at a location other than that used for vaccine inoculation, to minimize potential interference. An important consideration is the prevention of rabies infection after exposure of family members or health-care providers to an index case. Possible percutaneous or mucous membrane exposure to a patient's saliva or CSF is an indication for postexposure prophylaxis. In the reports of the 15 patients summarized in Table 7, the following numbers of persons received postexposure prophylaxis: case 1, 46; case 2, 50; case 3, 60; case 4, 53; case 5, 48; case 6, 37; case 7, 71; case 8, 20; case 9, 27; case 10, 23; case 11, 46; case 12, 53; case 13, 8; case 14, 6; and case 15, 5. For persons in whom preexposure prophylaxis is indicated, only vaccine is recommended.[79]

A group of viruses, including dengue virus, enteroviruses, adenoviruses, and cytomegalovirus, may cause direct infection that results in encephalitis. In addition to viruses producing direct infection of the brain, certain viruses may cause a postinfectious encephalomyelitis. At one time, this form of CNS pathology accounted for about one third of fatal cases of encephalitis (with acute viral encephalitis being the major cause of infectious mortality in this category). With the elimination of vaccinia virus by vaccination for smallpox, the mortality attributable to postinfectious encephalomyelitis is now estimated to be 10 to 15% of cases of acute encephalitis in the United States. The pathogenesis of this process has not been definitively elucidated. The pathologic changes have been compared with those occurring in persons in whom acute encephalomyelitis developed following rabies immunization using vaccine prepared in CNS tissue. It has been suggested that certain viral infections may cause a disruption of normal immune regulation, with resultant release of autoimmune responses. The viruses that have been associated with postinfectious encephalomyelitis are summarized in Table 4. Treatment of patients with such problems is limited to supportive care.

Two common infections that usually have benign courses in adolescents and young adults may progress to serious disease, which may include involvement of the CNS. Mononucleosis due to Epstein-Barr virus may, on rare occasions, cause direct infection of the brain and an encephalitic process, which is the most common cause of death resulting from this infection. CNS infection is the most significant extrarespiratory manifestation of infection caused by *Mycoplasma pneumoniae*. Even though this organism has been isolated from the CSF, the mechanism by which it causes encephalitis is thought to be an autoimmune one.

Rickettsiae have the ability to produce infection of the CNS. Of these, the most characteristic is Rocky Mountain spotted fever (RMSF), caused by *R rickettsii*. After being transmitted to humans via a tick bite, this intracellular pathogen can produce a constellation of symptoms and signs that includes fever, petechial skin lesions (involving the palms, soles, wrists, and ankles), and a meningoencephalitis. Because of the skin lesions and neurologic involvement, acute forms of this infection may mimic disease caused by *N meningitidis*. Chloramphenicol is effective against both of these pathogens, but tetracycline is considered the usual first-line drug when only RMSF is suspected. In contrast to the distal skin lesions that progress centrally in RMSF, epidemic typhus caused by *Rickettsia prowazekii* is characterized by central lesions that move distally. This infection is more likely to occur during the winter months than is RMSF, which usually occurs during the late summer and early fall. The emerging rickettsial pathogen identified as a cause of nervous system involvement is Ehrlichia. Pathogens within the genus Ehrlichia have the propensity to parasitize either mononuclear or granulocytic leukocytes, with the resultant infections referred to as human monocytic ehrlichiosis or human granulocytic ehrlichiosis, respectively. The epidemiology of ehrlichiosis, including outdoor activity and exposure to ticks, is similar to that of RMSF, but in contrast to RMSF, ehrlichiosis is associated with rash in only about 20% of cases. In addition to causing the characteristic findings of fever, leukopenia, thrombocytopenia, and abnormal liver enzymes, nervous system involvement in ehrlichiosis may include severe headache, confusion, lethargy, broad-based gait, hyperreflexia, clonus, photophobia, cranial nerve palsy, seizures, blurred vision, nuchal rigidity, and ataxia. The characteristic CSF abnormalities have been a lymphocytic pleocytosis with an elevated protein level. In a recent review of the subject, the CSF glucose level was normal in the majority of patients, with 24% of the patients having borderline low CSF glucose concentrations. In this review, morulae were seen in CSF white cells in only a small minority of the patients. Radiographic and encephalographic studies did not reveal any lesions that supported a specific diagnosis. Although the definitive agent for treating this infection has not been established by clinical trials, it appears that chloramphenicol or tetracycline is the agent most frequently used. The clinical experience with this process has been limited, and the outcome in patients with nervous system involvement is not well established.

As summarized in Table 5, certain noninfectious diseases may mimic viral encephalitis.

Brain Abscess

Among bacterial infections of the CNS, brain abscess is the second most common. On a pathogenetic basis, this infection may develop after hematogenous dissemination of organisms during systemic infection (which often occurs in the context of such conditions as infective endocarditis, cyanotic congenital heart disease, and lung abscess), with extension from infected cranial structures (eg, sinuses or middle ear) along emissary veins, or as a consequence of trauma or neurosurgery. The classic presentation may include recent onset of severe headache, new focal or generalized seizures, and clinical evidence of an intracranial mass. In the nonimmunocompromised host, brain abscess represents a deviation from the classic tenet that Bacteroides fragilis is not a significant pathogen above the diaphragm. In the patient without predisposing factors, streptococci (including the Streptococcus intermedius [milleri] group) along with anaerobes (including B fragilis) are the predominant pathogens.[80] Excision or stereotactic aspiration of the abscess is used to identify the etiologic agents and has been recommended for lesions >2.5 cm.[81] Some experts have advocated using empiric antimicrobial therapy without aspiration of the abscess in patients who are

neurologically stable and have an abscess <3 cm in diameter that is not encroaching on the ventricular system; however, if such a decision is made, they have advised that the patient must be followed meticulously with a brain imaging study such as CT or MRI, and enlargement of the abscess during therapy mandates surgery. Because of the lack of consistent efficacy of metronidazole against streptococci and upper airway anaerobic cocci, penicillin or a third-generation cephalosporin (eg, cefotaxime or ceftriaxone) is usually combined with this agent. An alternative to metronidazole in this regimen would be chloramphenicol. In the settings of penetrating head trauma, following neurosurgical procedures, or with acute bacterial endocarditis, therapy for S aureus should be included. Those patients with a presumed otic or sinus origin for their abscess should have coverage against enterobacteriaceae and H influenzae using a third-generation cephalosporin.

In HIV-infected persons, T gondii classically presents as fever, headache, altered mental status, and focal neurologic deficits, especially in individuals whose CD4+ count falls below 100 cells/mm³. Because the disease is due to reactivation of latent infection in about 95% of cases, IgG antibody to Toxoplasma is generally present. A review of neuroimaging studies in patients with AIDS is summarized in Table 8, with a key point being whether or not mass effect is present.[82] Imaging studies of the brain in AIDS patients with Toxoplasma brain abscess show multiple (usually ≥3) nodular contrast-enhancing lesions with mass effect found most commonly in the basal ganglia and at the gray-white matter junction. In the clas-

Table 8. *Approach to Mass Lesions In HIV-Infected Persons**

Focal Lesions With Mass Effect in HIV-Infected Persons	Focal Lesion Without Mass Effect in HIV-Infected Persons
Toxoplasmosis	Progressive multifocal leukoencephalopathy
Primary lymphoma of the CNS	
Cerebral cryptococcosis†	
Neurotuberculosis†	
Syphilitic gumma‡	

*CNS=central nervous system. Adapted from Clin Infect Dis 1996; 22:906–919.[82]
† Rarely present as abscesses.
‡ Rare presentation of neurosyphilis.

Nervous System Infections and Catheter Infections (Karam)

sic setting described above, empiric therapy with sulfadiazine and pyrimethamine is recommended. Clindamycin-containing regimens may be considered in sulfa-allergic patients. Brain biopsy is reserved for atypical presentations and for patients who do not respond to initial therapy. After acute therapy for toxoplasmic encephalitis, prophylaxis to prevent recurrence has been recommended with a regimen like sulfadiazine plus pyrimethamine plus leucovorin, but may be discontinued once CD4+ cells are >200/μL for ≥6 months.[83] The lesions of toxoplasmosis may be confused with primary CNS lymphoma, which also causes a mass effect due to surrounding edema and which may undergo central necrosis and present as ring-enhancing masses.

Spinal Epidural Abscess and Subdural Empyema

A review of spinal epidural abscess provides the basis for understanding two common threads included in literature published about this infection: reports of poor prognosis and appeals for rapid treatment.[84] Spinal epidural abscess represents a neurosurgical emergency because neurologic deficits may become irreversible when there is a delay in evacuating the purulent material. Although the basis for this irreversibility has not been definitively established, mechanisms for the associated spinal cord necrosis include a decrease in arterial blood flow, venous thrombosis, or direct compression of the spinal cord. The triad of findings that supports the diagnosis is fever, point tenderness over the spine, and focal neurologic deficits. The predisposing factors to this infection shed light on the likely pathogens. Skin and soft tissue are the most probable source of infection and provide an understanding of why S aureus is the most common pathogen in this infection. Spinal epidural abscess has been reported to follow surgery, trauma, urinary tract infections, and respiratory diseases. Of increasing importance are the reports of this infection occurring as a complication of lumbar puncture and epidural anesthesia. In 16% of cases, the source of infection may be unknown. Usual pathogens include S aureus, streptococci (both aerobic and anaerobic), and Gram-negative bacilli.

Gadolinium-enhanced MRI has replaced myelography as the diagnostic study of choice because it identifies not only mass lesions, but also signal abnormalities that are consistent with acute transverse myelopathy and spinal cord ischemia.[85]

Subdural empyema is an infection that occurs between the dura and arachnoid and that results as organisms are spread via emissary veins or by extension of osteomyelitis of the skull. The paranasal sinuses are the source in over half the cases, with otitis another likely predisposing condition. In young children, it is usually a complication of meningitis. The clinical features include fever, headache, vomiting, signs of meningeal irritation, alteration in mental status, and focal neurologic deficits that progress to focal seizures. The usual pathogens are aerobic streptococci (including S pneumoniae), staphylococci, H influenzae, Gram-negative bacilli, and anaerobes (including B fragilis). The diagnosis is often made using MRI, but CT scan with contrast enhancement may offer the advantage of imaging bone. Antibiotics directed against the likely pathogens and surgical interventions are mainstays of therapy.

Septic Intracranial Thrombophlebitis

Thrombosis of the cortical vein may occur as a complication of meningitis and is associated with progressive neurologic deficits, including hemiparesis, bilateral weakness, or aphasia. Thrombosis of the intracranial venous sinuses classically follows infections of the paranasal sinuses, middle ear, mastoid, face, or oropharynx, although the process may be metastatic from lungs or other sites. The most frequent pathogens are S aureus, coagulase-negative staphylococci, streptococci, Gram-negative bacilli, and anaerobes. Five anatomic sites may be involved with varying clinical presentations.[86] Superior sagittal sinus thrombosis results in bilateral leg weakness or in communicating hydrocephalus. Lateral sinus thrombosis produces pain over the ear and mastoid, with possible edema over the mastoid. Superior petrosal sinus thrombosis causes ipsilateral pain, sensory deficit, or temporal lobe seizures. Inferior petrosal sinus thrombosis may produce the syndrome of ipsilateral facial pain and lateral rectus weakness that is referred to as Gradenigo's syndrome.

Of the forms of venous sinus thrombosis, cavernous sinus thrombosis is the most frequently discussed. Within this sinus lie the internal carotid artery with its sympathetic plexus and the sixth cranial nerve. In the lateral wall of the sinus are the third and fourth cranial nerves, along with the ophthalmic and sometimes maxillary divisions of the trigeminal nerve. The clinical presentation is influenced by these anatomic considerations. The process, which is considered life-threatening, begins unilaterally but usually becomes bilateral within hours. High fever, headaches, malaise, nausea, and vomiting are the predominant findings. Patients progress to develop proptosis, chemosis, periorbital edema, and cyanosis of the ipsilateral forehead, eyelids, and root of the nose. Ophthalmoplegia may develop, with the sixth cranial nerve usually involved first. Trigeminal nerve involvement may manifest itself as decreased sensation about the eye. Ophthalmic nerve involvement may present as photophobia and persistent eye pain. Papilledema, diminished pupillary reactivity, and diminished corneal reflexes may also develop. The disease may be relentless in its progression to alteration in level of consciousness, meningitis, and seizures. The mainstays of therapy include broad-spectrum antibiotics and surgical drainage with removal of infected bone or abscess. The issue of anticoagulation in patients with suppurative intracranial thrombophlebitis is controversial. It is the opinion of some experts in the field that heparin followed by warfarin may be beneficial,[87] but heparin-induced thrombocytopenia has been noted as a potential complication. Steroids may be necessary if involvement of the pituitary gland leads to adrenal insufficiency and circulatory collapse.

Neuritis

Infection of nervous tissue outside of the CNS can take place on the basis of several pathogenetic mechanisms. Certain pathogens, such as *Borrelia burgdorferi* (the etiologic agent of Lyme disease), HIV, cytomegalovirus, HSV type 2, and varicella-zoster virus, can produce peripheral neuropathy. Direct infection of nerves may occur with *Mycobacterium leprae* and Trypanosoma spp. *Corynebacterium diphtheriae*, *Clostridium tetani*, and *Clostridium botulinum* can produce toxins that can injure peripheral nerves.

C diphtheriae produces a toxin that directly involves nerves to cause a noninflammatory demyelination. Clinical sequelae of such a process initially include local paralysis of the soft palate and posterior pharyngeal wall, followed by cranial nerve involvement, and culminating in involvement of peripheral nerves. Myocarditis occurs in as many as two thirds of patients, but <25% develop clinical evidence of cardiac dysfunction. Antitoxin is indicated in infected patients, along with antibacterial therapy. Both penicillin and erythromycin have been recommended as treatment of diphtheria by the World Health Organization. In a study in Vietnamese children with diphtheria that compared IM benzylpenicillin with erythromycin, both antibiotics were efficacious, but slower fever clearance and a higher incidence of GI side effects were associated with erythromycin.[88] Erythromycin resistance was noted in some of the isolates tested, but all were susceptible to penicillin. Both *C tetani* and *C botulinum* cause indirect nerve involvement on the basis of toxin production. The epidemiology of tetanus has changed somewhat in recent years. Joining elderly patients as a patient population at risk for tetanus are injection drug users who inject drugs subcutaneously (ie, "skin pop"). The toxin of *C tetani* is transported up axons and binds to presynaptic endings on motor neurons in anterior horn cells of the spinal cord. This blocks inhibitory input and results in uncontrolled motor input to skeletal muscle and tetanic spasm. Antitoxin is not available for this disorder, but tetanus immune globulin and tetanus toxoid are given for clinical disease. Prevention plays a pivotal role in controlling the number of cases of tetanus. A population-based serologic survey of immunity to tetanus in the United States revealed protective levels of tetanus antibodies ranging from 87.7% among those 6 to 11 years of age to 27.8% among those 70 years of age or older.[89] Although there is an excellent correlation between vaccination rates (96%) and immunity (96%) among 6-year-olds, antibody levels decline over time such that one fifth of older children (10 to 16 years of age) do not have protective antibody levels. Such data argue strongly for ongoing tetanus immunization throughout a person's life in an attempt to prevent this potentially fatal disease.

The toxin of *C botulinum* binds to the presynaptic axon terminal of the neuromuscular junction with inhibition of acetylcholine release. This results in a symmetric, descending, flaccid paralysis of motor and autonomic nerves, usually beginning with the cranial nerves. Recent reports of botulism

Nervous System Infections and Catheter Infections (Karam)

have noted not only foodborne outbreaks associated with consumption of contaminated fish, commercial cheese sauce, and baked potatoes held in aluminum foil for several days at room temperature, but also wound botulism in injection drug users who injected Mexican black tar heroin subcutaneously. The classic presentation includes neurologic and GI findings. Nausea and vomiting may be followed by diminished salivation and extreme dryness of the mouth, and by difficulty in focusing the eyes that occurs due to interruption of cholinergic autonomic transmission. Patients progress to cranial nerve palsies (with common presentations being diplopia, dysarthria, or dysphagia) and then to a symmetrical descending flaccid voluntary muscle weakness that may progress to respiratory compromise. Normal body temperature and normal sensory nerve examination findings are typical, as is an intact mental status despite a groggy appearance. A large outbreak occurred in 1994 in El Paso, TX, and was traced to a dip prepared in a restaurant from potatoes that had been baked in aluminum foil and then left at room temperature for several days.[90] In that report, the following criteria were used for making the diagnosis of botulism: (1) an electromyographic (EMG) study showing an increase of ≥50% in the evoked train of compound muscle action potentials with rapid repetitive stimulation (20 to 50 Hz); (2) stool culture positive for C botulinum; and (3) blurred vision, dysphagia, or dysarthria in a person who did not have EMG findings indicating botulism and who did not have C botulinum detected in stool (findings consistent with the diagnosis of "suspected case"). In addition, the mouse inoculation test for toxin using serum, stool, or food may be positive. In a recent review of laboratory findings in foodborne botulism, the following were listed: normal CSF values; specific EMG findings (normal motor conduction velocities; normal sensory nerve amplitudes and latencies; decreased evoked muscle action potential; facilitation following rapid repetitive nerve stimulation); and standard mouse bioassay positive for toxin from clinical specimens and/or suspect food.[91] Researchers from the CDC and the Republic of Georgia's National Center for Disease Control studied 706 cases of botulism in Georgia, which has the highest reported rate of foodborne botulism of any country.[92] They discovered that the patients at highest risk of dying were

those who reported to the hospital with shortness of breath and impaired gag reflex but no diarrhea. This constellation of symptoms, if validated in the United States and other countries as predictors of death, would allow doctors to give first consideration to patients who are at highest risk of dying in a botulism outbreak.[92]

Intestinal botulism, which occurs most commonly in infants and is rare in children and adults, is the most common form of human botulism in the United States.[93] Along with the traditional forms of botulism, there are two additional forms of importance. Since 1978, the CDC has recorded cases of botulism in which extensive investigation failed to implicate a specific food as the cause. These have been referred to as cases of "undetermined origin." Investigation has shown that some of these cases were caused by colonization of the GI tract by C botulinum or Clostridium baratii with in vivo production of toxin, analogous to the pathogenesis of infant botulism. In some cases of botulism strongly suspected to represent intestinal colonization, the patients had a history of GI surgery or illnesses such as inflammatory bowel disease, which might have predisposed them to enteric colonization. This form of botulism has been referred to as intestinal colonization botulism (also termed by some as adult-type infant botulism). Of more recent interest is inhalational botulism, which could occur as a component of bioterrorism with intentional release of aerosolized botulinum toxin.

As summarized in Table 9, antitoxin is indicated for adult botulism, which occurs on the

Table 9. *Toxin-Mediated Peripheral Neuritis*

Direct toxin injury
  *Corynebacterium diphtheriae**
Indirect toxin injury
  Clostridium tetani
  Clostridium botulinum
    Traditional categories
      Adult botulism*
      Infant (intestinal) botulism†
      Wound botulism*
      Intestinal colonization botulism‡
    New category
      Inhalational botulism‡

*Antitoxin indicated.
†Role for botulism immune globulin IV (human) [BIG-IV].
‡See text.

basis of ingestion of preformed toxin, and for wound botulism, in which toxin is produced locally at the infected wound. A review of botulism has noted that antitoxin is released from the CDC for cases of intestinal colonization botulism.[94] With inhalational botulism, it has been suggested that antitoxin be given as early as possible based on clinical suspicion and should not be delayed while awaiting microbiologic testing.[95] It has been noted with this form of botulism that antitoxin might only prevent progression of disease but not reverse paralysis once it has occurred. It is important to be aware that skin testing should be performed to assess for sensitivity to serum or antitoxin prior to administration of antitoxin. In contrast, infant botulism, which occurs when the ingested organism produces toxin within the GI tract, does not respond to antitoxin. A human-derived human botulism immune globulin has been administered to infants with botulism and has been shown to reduce length of stay with this pattern of disease. Although this product is not yet commercially available, it may be obtained for the treatment of infant botulism under a Treatment Investigational New Drug protocol by contacting the California Department of Health Services (telephone (510) 540-2646). The acute, simultaneous onset of neurologic symptoms in multiple individuals should suggest a common source for the problem and increase the suspicion of botulism.

Certain toxins produced by fish and shellfish have been associated with neurologic involvement. Ciguatera fish poisoning follows consumption of marine fish (most characteristically grouper, red snapper, and barracuda) that have been contaminated with toxins produced by microalgae known as dinoflagellates. The classic constellation of findings involves GI, cardiovascular, and neurologic systems. The characteristic neurologic findings include paresthesias (which may be chronic) periorally and in distal extremities, often associated with a debilitating hot-to-cold reversal dysesthesia. Taste sensation is often altered. Implicated toxins include ciguatoxin (which induces membrane depolarization by opening voltage-dependent sodium channels), maitotoxin (which opens calcium channels), and palytoxin (which causes muscle injury). Therapy is primarily symptomatic and supportive. Paralytic shellfish poisoning is caused by consumption of shellfish (most characteristically butter clams, mussels, cockles, steamer clams, sea snails, or razor clams) or broth from cooked shellfish that contain either concentrated saxitoxin (a heat-stable alkaloid neurotoxin) or related compounds, with resultant sensory, cerebellar, and motor dysfunction. Characteristic neurologic findings include paresthesias of the mouth and extremities, ataxia, dysphagia, muscle paralysis, coma, and total muscular paralysis. Treatment is supportive.

The ascending paralysis that comprises the Guillain-Barré syndrome characteristically follows respiratory infection, GI infection (notably, Campylobacter infection), or immunization. The pathology is segmental inflammation with perivascular mononuclear cells and demyelination. An exact etiology for this process has not been elucidated.

Catheter-Related Infections

Urinary Bladder Catheters

A clinical situation frequently associated with injudicious use of antibiotics in the critical care setting is asymptomatic bacteriuria. In March 2005, the IDSA published guidelines for the diagnosis and treatment of asymptomatic bacteriuria in adults.[96] In that document, the diagnosis of asymptomatic bacteruria was based on results of a culture of a urine specimen collected in a manner that minimizes contamination. For asymptomatic women, *bacteriuria* was defined as two consecutive voided urine specimens with isolation of the same bacterial strain in quantitative counts $\geq 10^5$ cfu/mL. *Asymptomatic bacteriuria* was defined as (1) a single, clean-catch voided urine specimen with one bacterial species isolated in a quantitative count $\geq 10^5$ cfu/mL in men, or (2) a single catheterized urine specimen with one bacterial species isolated in a quantitative count $\geq 10^2$ cfu/mL in women or men. Of note is that pyuria accompanying asymptomatic bacteriuria was not considered to be an indication for antimicrobial therapy. In adults, two A-1 recommendations were made regarding treatment of asymptomatic bacteriuria in adults: (1) pregnant women, and (2) men scheduled to undergo transurethral resection of the

Table 10. *Treatment of Asymptomatic Bacteriuria in Adults*

Adults in Whom Therapy Is Recommended

Pregnant women[97-99]

Men about to undergo transurethral resection of the prostate or other urologic procedures for which mucosal bleeding is anticipated[96,100]

Adults in Whom Therapy May Be Considered

Women with catheter-acquired bacteriuria that persists 48 h after indwelling catheter removal

Persons in Whom Definitive Recommendations Are Not Available but for Whom Some Provide Therapy

Certain immunocompromised patients, especially those who are neutropenic or who have undergone renal transplantation (see comments in text about renal transplant patients[101])

Elderly persons with obstructive uropathy[102-105]

Patients with diabetes mellitus[106]

Persons with positive urine cultures both at the time of catheter removal and then again 1–2 wk after catheter removal[107]

Those undergoing certain types of surgery, particularly when prostheses or foreign bodies (notably vascular grafts) may be left in place

Some patients with struvite stones

Persons with spinal cord injury[96]

Catheterized patients while the catheter remains *in situ*[96]

---

prostate. An A-III recommendation was given for treatment of asymptomatic bacteriuria before urologic procedures (other than transurethral resection of the prostate) for which mucosal bleeding is anticipated. The guidelines stated that antimicrobial treatment of asymptomatic women with catheter-acquired bacteriuria that persists 48 h after indwelling catheter removal may be considered for treatment. Table 10 summarizes those situations where therapy for asymptomatic bacteriuria was not recommended and reviews situations where the data are evolving but not conclusive.[96-107]

A clinically important area, but one in which there are no definitive data, relates to renal transplant recipients. It has been acknowledged that urine culture surveillance and periodic renal scan or ultrasound examinations are recommended by some authors, at least during the first months after transplantation. Based on cited references that treatment of asymptomatic urinary tract infections in renal transplant recipients are largely unsuccessful and that such therapy may not have an observable effect on graft function, it was noted that asymptomatic urinary tract infections in this immunocompromised patient population may be left untreated.[101] Frequent or inappropriate use of antibiotics exerts selective pressures that are responsible for the increasing prevalence of bacterial resistance. Because of this, it is important to use antibiotics in situations where the clinical

benefits exceed risks such as adverse effects and the selection of resistant organisms. A recent report of the NIH-sponsored Mycoses Study Group evaluated the issue of treatment for candiduria that was asymptomatic or minimally symptomatic.[108] Patients were randomly assigned to receive fluconazole (200 mg/d) or placebo for 14 days. In 50% of cases, the isolate was *Candida albicans*. At the end of treatment, urine was cleared in 50% of patients given fluconazole vs 29% of those given placebo. However, cure rate was about 70% in both groups at 2 weeks posttreatment. Although these data represented short-term eradication of candiduria (especially following catheter removal), the long-term eradication rates were not associated with clinical benefit. Notable in this study were the observations in the placebo group that candiduria resolved in about 20% of chronically catheterized patients when their catheter was only changed and in 41% of untreated patients when the catheter was removed.

Peritoneal Dialysis Catheters

Abdominal pain and/or fever and/or cloudy peritoneal fluid are the clinical features usually found in patients who are undergoing either continuous ambulatory peritoneal dialysis or automated peritoneal dialysis and who develop peritonitis. The organisms most frequently isolated in such processes have been coagulase-negative staphylococci (eg, *Staphylococcus epidermidis*) or *S aureus*, but the incidence of Gram-negative pathogens has increased in patients utilizing disconnect systems. When caused by *S aureus*, a toxic shock–like syndrome has been occasionally noted. The finding of >100 WBCs/mm^3, of which at least 50% are polymorphonuclear neutrophils, is supportive of the diagnosis of peritonitis. Recent trends in the management of this infection have been affected by the emergence of vancomycin resistance, both in enterococci as well as in *S aureus*. Vancomycin use has influenced this resistance. In a review of vancomycin-intermediate *S aureus*, it was noted that of the first 6 patients reported in the United States with this pathogen, all but 1 had had exposure to dialysis for renal insufficiency, with the resultant potential for recurrent vancomycin use.[109] In recognition of the contribution of injudicious use of vancomycin to the development of vancomycin resistance in Gram-positive organisms, the Advisory Committee on Peritonitis Management of the International Society for Peritoneal Dialysis recommended that traditional empiric therapy of catheter-associated peritonitis be changed from the regimen of vancomycin and gentamicin to a first-generation cephalosporin (eg, cefazolin or cephalothin in a loading dose of 500 mg/L and a maintenance dose of 125 mg/L) in combination with an aminoglycoside.[110] The committee stated further that modifications to this regimen could be made based on the organism isolated or on sensitivity patterns. In its more recent iteration of recommendations for treatment of adult peritoneal dialysis-related peritonitis,[111] the International Society for Peritoneal Dialysis suggested the substitution of ceftazidime for the aminoglycoside. Residual renal function is an independent predictor of patient survival. It is especially noteworthy that use of any aminoglycoside,[112] even when given for short periods, and the rate of peritonitis[113] are independent risk factors for the decline of residual renal function in patients using continuous ambulatory peritoneal dialysis. A concern about ceftazidime is its risk of selecting resistant Gram-negative organisms, including those that produce type I β-lactamases or extended-spectrum β-lactamases.[114] The role of empiric therapy with cefazolin has also been reported in potentially infected hemodialysis patients,[115] with vancomycin

being reserved for confirmed resistant organisms.[116] Many episodes of catheter-associated peritonitis may be managed without removal of the catheter, but peritonitis that does not respond to antibiotic therapy and peritonitis associated with tunnel infections may be indications for catheter removal. Infection with Pseudomonas, a fungal pathogen, or mycobacteria often requires catheter removal for cure.[117] Another entity that influences the decision for catheter removal is relapsing peritonitis, defined as an episode of peritonitis caused by the same genus/species that caused the immediately preceding episode, occurring within 4 weeks of completion of the antibiotic course. If no clinical response is noted after 96 h of therapy for relapsing peritonitis, catheter removal is indicated; if the patient responds clinically, but subsequently relapses an additional time, catheter removal and replacement are recommended.[111]

Vascular Catheters

Of the 200,000 nosocomial bloodstream infections that occur each year in the United States, most are related to different types of intravascular devices. The IDSA, the Society of Critical Care Medicine, and the Society for Healthcare Epidemiology of America have recently published guidelines for management of intravascular catheter–related infections.[118] In their review, the following recommendations were made regarding blood cultures in cases of suspected catheter-associated bacteremia: (1) two sets of blood samples for culture, with a least one drawn percutaneously, should be obtained with a new episode of suspected central venous catheter–related bloodstream infection; and (2) paired quantitative blood cultures or paired qualitative blood cultures with a continuously monitored differential time to positivity should be collected for the diagnosis of catheter-related infection, especially when the long-term catheter cannot be removed. The recommendation regarding blood cultures noted in the preceding statement is different from those recommended in a recent *New England Journal of Medicine* review,[119] in which it was stated that "Two cultures of blood from peripheral sites should be evaluated because it is difficult to determine whether a positive culture of blood from a central venous catheter indicates contamination of the hub, catheter colonization, or a catheter-related bloodstream infection." Quantitative blood cultures simultaneously obtained through a central venous catheter and a peripheral vein and demonstrating a five- to 10-fold increase in concentration of an organism in catheter blood compared with peripheral blood have been reported to correlate well with catheter-related infections; however, some studies have not supported such a correlation. For tunneled catheters, a quantitative culture of blood from the central venous catheter that yields at least 100 cfu/mL may be diagnostic without a companion culture of a peripheral blood sample.[120] A new diagnostic method has been made possible by continuous blood culture monitoring systems and compares the time to positive cultures of blood drawn from the catheter and from a peripheral vein. One study has shown a sensitivity of 91% and a specificity of 94% in determining catheter-related infection when a blood culture drawn from a central venous catheter became positive at least 2 h earlier than the culture drawn from a peripheral vein.[121] These data have most applicability to tunneled catheters.

Over the past two decades, the medical literature has proposed several predictors of sepsis from a catheter. Although Gram stain of material from the tip of a catheter may be helpful with diagnosis of local infection, it is significantly less sensitive than quantitative methods. The most traditionally quoted study regarding predictors of catheter-related infection suggests that the presence of ≥15 colonies on a semiquantitative roll culture of the tip of a catheter or needle is most useful.[122] Although such techniques are relied on at present to assist in the determination of an infected catheter, some data have suggested that the semiquantitative culture may not be predictive of clinical outcome. When compared with qualitative cultures, quantitative methods—which include either (1) flushing the segment with broth or (2) vortexing or sonicating the segment in broth, followed by serial dilutions and surface plating on blood agar—have greater specificity in the identification of catheter-related infections. In the recently published guidelines for management of intravascular catheter-related infections,[104] the sensitivities of these three methods were listed as

follows: sonication, 80%; roll plate method, 60%; and flush culture, 40 to 50%.

A review of 51 English-language studies published from 1966 to July 2004 studied the eight diagnostic methods that are most frequently used in clinical practice and for which performance data have been published: qualitative catheter segment culture, semiquantitative catheter segment culture (roll-plate method), or quantitative catheter segment culture, each combined with demonstrated concordance with results of concomitant blood cultures; qualitative blood culture drawn through an intravascular device (IVD); paired quantitative peripheral and IVD-drawn blood cultures; acridine orange leukocyte cytospin testing of IVD-drawn blood; and differential time to positivity of concomitant qualitative IVD-drawn and peripheral blood cultures (>2 h).[123] In this analysis, paired quantitative blood culture was the most accurate test for diagnosis of IVD-related bloodstream infection. However, most other methods studied showed acceptable sensitivity and specificity (both >0.75) and negative predictive value.

In the IDSA guidelines for the management of catheter-related infections, alternative routes of antibiotic administration were also discussed.[118] An important consideration is whether the infection is intraluminal or extraluminal. Catheters that have been in place for <2 weeks are most often infected extraluminally, whereas catheters in place for a longer duration were more likely to have intraluminal infection. Antibiotic solutions that contain the desired antimicrobial agent in a concentration of 1 to 5 mg/mL are usually mixed with 50 to 100 U of heparin (or normal saline) and are installed or "locked" into the catheter lumen during periods when the catheter is not used (eg, for a 12-h period each night). The volume of installed antibiotic is removed before infusion of the next dose of an antibiotic or IV medication or solution, and the most often used duration of such therapy is 2 weeks. Summarized in this review are some reports of cure of patients with infected tunneled catheters who were treated with both parenteral and lock therapy.

Of the pathogens most characteristically isolated as a complication of indwelling vascular catheters, coagulase-negative staphylococci, *S aureus*, and Candida spp have been most frequently reported. In immunocompromised patients with long-term indwelling catheters, *Corynebacterium jeikeium* and Bacillus spp are important, and notably both have vancomycin as the drug of choice for therapy. Gram-negative bacilli and atypical mycobacteria are also included as possible pathogens in this setting.

An important and common clinical question is whether a catheter-related intravascular infection can be cured with a long-term indwelling catheter left in place. The medical literature suggests that catheter-related coagulase-negative staphylococcal bacteremia may be successfully treated without recurrence in up to 80% of patients whose catheters remained in place and who received antibiotics.[124] In the 20% of patients who remained bacteremic while taking antibiotics with their catheters in place, metastatic infection was not a significant problem. For patients with vascular catheter-associated coagulase-negative staphylococcal bacteremia, the following recommendations have been made:[118] (1) if a central venous catheter is removed, appropriate systemic antibiotic therapy is recommended for 5 to 7 days; (2) if a nontunneled central venous catheter is retained and intraluminal infection is suspected, systemic antibiotic therapy for 10 to 14 days and antibiotic lock therapy are recommended; and (3) if a tunneled central venous catheter or an IVD is retained in patients with uncomplicated, catheter-related, bloodstream infection, patients should be treated with systemic antibiotic therapy for 7 days and with antibiotic lock therapy for 14 days.

Although some authors have suggested that infections caused by *S aureus* in the setting of a vascular catheter may respond to treatment with the catheter left in place, there are increasing reports of metastatic sites of infection by this organism when the catheter is not removed. As a result, it seems most prudent to remove the catheter when *S aureus* is isolated from the bloodstream.[125] A scoring system based on the presence or absence of four risk factors (community acquisition, skin examination findings suggesting acute systemic infection, persistent fever at 72 h, and positive follow-up blood culture results at 48 to 96 h) has been suggested as a means of clinically identifying complicated *S aureus* bacteremia.[126] With this system, the strongest predictor was a positive follow-up blood culture at 48 to 96 h. Because of the potentially devastating complications that may occur when

S aureus seeds heart valves or bone, the issue of duration of therapy for bacteremia due to this pathogen in catheter-associated bacteremia is exceedingly important. It is well accepted that individuals with endocarditis or osteomyelitis occurring as complications of metastatic *S aureus* infection should receive a prolonged course of parenteral antimicrobial therapy, with 6 weeks as the frequently stated duration in these settings. The duration of therapy for patients with *S aureus* bacteremia that is catheter-related may be similar to that for *S aureus* bacteremia due to a drainable focus. Discussed frequently in the medical literature, therapy for this clinical problem has not been definitively established by clinical trials.

Based on the available data, the most frequently noted minimum duration of parenteral therapy in such settings is 2 weeks. However, before one makes the decision to limit parenteral therapy to this short course, all four of the following criteria should probably be met: (1) there is removal of the intravascular catheter or drainage of the abscess that was presumed to be the source of the bacteremia; (2) the bacteremia is demonstrated to promptly resolve with the removal or drainage; (3) there is prompt clinical response, including resolution of fever; and (4) heart valves are demonstrated to be normal. Some have suggested that transesophageal echocardiography (TEE) may be a cost-effective means of stratifying patients with catheter-associated *S aureus* bacteremia to a specific duration of therapy.[127] With infectious disease consultation as one of the six components of the evaluation, it was suggested that a 7-day course of antibiotics may be appropriate for patients with what has been termed "simple bacteremia" with *S aureus* if all of the other criteria are met: (1) TEE on day 5 to 7 of therapy was negative for both vegetations and predisposing valvular abnormalities; (2) negative surveillance culture of blood obtained 2 to 4 days after beginning appropriate antibiotic therapy and removal of focus; (3) removable focus of infection; (4) clinical resolution (afebrile and no localizing complaints attributable to metastatic staphylococcal infections within 72 h of initiating therapy and removal of focus); and (5) no indwelling prosthetic devices.[128] Even in such settings, patients with diabetes mellitus may still be at an increased risk for developing *S aureus* endocarditis, and some experts have suggested 4 weeks of therapy in this patient population even if heart valves are normal. Removal is suggested in the following settings of *S aureus* bacteremia: (1) nontunneled central vascular catheters; and (2) tunneled central vascular catheters or IVDs when there is evidence of tunnel, pocket, or exit-site infection.[118] In the recommendations just cited, it was noted that tunneled central vascular catheters or IVDs with uncomplicated intraluminal infection and *S aureus* bacteremia should be removed or, in selected cases, retained and treated with appropriate systemic and antibiotic lock therapy for 14 days. For patients who remain febrile and/or have bacteremia for >3 days after catheter removal and/or initiation of antibiotic therapy, a longer course of therapy and an aggressive workup for septic thrombosis and infective endocarditis should be instituted. Because the sensitivity of transthoracic echocardiography is low, it is not recommended for excluding a diagnosis of catheter-related endocarditis if TEE can be done.[118] It is important to reiterate that not all of the recommendations listed in this discussion of *S aureus* bacteremia have been definitively validated by clinical trials.

In a retrospective review of 51 patients with prosthetic heart valves in whom *S aureus* bacteremia developed, 26 (51%) had definite endocarditis using the modified Duke criteria for the diagnosis of endocarditis.[129] The risk of endocarditis was independent of the type, location, or age of the prosthetic valve. Because of the high mortality of prosthetic valve endocarditis, it has been recommended that all patients with a prosthetic valve in whom *S aureus* bacteremia develops should be aggressively screened and followed for endocarditis.[129]

Like *S aureus* and enterococci, Candida spp have a predilection to cause metastatic infection on heart valves and in bone when these organisms are bloodborne. In addition to the complications of endocarditis and osteomyelitis, Candida may seed the retina of the eye to cause retinal abscesses that proliferate into the vitreous and result in the clinical entity of Candida endophthalmitis. Because of the significant complications associated with candidemia, there are now two basic recommendations for patients with a positive blood culture for Candida: (1) the patient should receive a course of antifungal therapy[130]; and (2) intravascular lines should be removed.[131]

Risk factors cited for candidemia vary by reports, but the following is a representative list from international experts in the field: antibiotics; indwelling catheters; hyperalimentation; cancer therapy; immunosuppressive therapy after organ transplantation; hospitalization in ICUs; candiduria; and colonization with Candida spp.[132]

A clinical trial conducted by the Mycoses Study Group of the NIH compared amphotericin B with fluconazole in the treatment of candidemia in nonneutropenic and nonimmunocompromised patients.[133] In the 194 patients who had a single species of Candida isolated, 69% of the organisms were *C albicans*. The study concluded that fluconazole and amphotericin B were not significantly different in their effectiveness in treating candidemia. Since that study was performed, there has been an increasing prevalence of non-*albicans* strains of Candida in the bloodborne isolates from certain hospitals, and some of these strains may not respond to traditional doses of fluconazole. In their guidelines for the treatment of candidemia, the IDSA presented options for the treatment of candidemia based on the presence or absence of neutropenia.[134] In nonneutropenic patients, fluconazole, amphotericin B, and caspofungin were offered as options for therapy. In neutropenic patients, amphotericin B, a lipid preparation of amphotericin B, or caspofungin were recommended, with the absence of fluconazole in this patient population acknowledging the role of azole exposure as a risk factor for non-*albicans* strains of Candida. In a trial comparing the echinocandin caspofungin to amphotericin B in patients with Candida infection involving blood or another sterile body site, caspofungin was shown to be superior with significantly fewer drug-related adverse events than in the amphotericin B group.[135] Because echinocandins are more likely to have activity against non-*albicans* strains of Candida, they are potentially useful in patients who have previously been exposed to azole therapy or in whom empiric therapy is needed for presumed life-threatening fungal infection.

Other clinical situations for which catheter removal is necessary for cure of a catheter-related infection include the following: (1) bacteremia due to *C jeikeium* and Bacillus spp; (2) bacteremia with Gram-negative bacilli; (3) fungemia; (4) persistence of fever or bacteremia during therapy; (5) evidence of tunnel infection; and (6) rapid relapse after treatment. Currently available data do not support the need for scheduled replacement of short-term central venous catheters, either by guidewire exchange or through insertion at a new site.[136]

References

1. Schuchat A, Robinson K, Wenger JD, et al. Bacterial meningitis in the United States in 1995. N Engl J Med 1997; 337:970–976

2. Greenlee JE. Approach to diagnosis of meningitis: cerebrospinal fluid evaluation. Infect Dis Clin North Am 1990; 4:583–598

3. National Committee for Clinical Laboratory Standards. Performance standards for antimicrobial susceptibility testing: 14th informational supplement (vol 24). Wayne, PA: National Committee for Clinical Laboratory Standards, January 2004; M100S14

4. Friedland IR, McCracken GH Jr. Management of infections caused by antibiotic-resistant Streptococcus pneumoniae. N Engl J Med 1994; 331:377–382

5. National Committee for Clinical Laboratory Standards. Performance standards for antimicrobial susceptibility testing: 12th informational supplement (vol 22, no 1). Wayne, PA: National Committee for Clinical Laboratory Standards, January 2002; M100-S12

6. Centers for Disease Control and Prevention (CDC). Effect of new susceptibility breakpoints on reporting of resistance in Streptococcus pneumoniae—United States, 2003. MMWR Morb Mortal Wkly Rep 2004; 53:152–154

7. Tunkel AR, Hartman BJ, Kaplan SL, et al. Practice guidelines for the management of bacterial meningitis. Clin Infect Dis 2004; 39:1267–1284

8. Quagliarello V, Scheld WM. Treatment of bacterial meningitis. N Engl J Med 1997; 336:708–716

9. Quagliarello VJ, Scheld WM. New perspectives on bacterial meningitis. Clin Infect Dis 1993; 17:603–610

10. de Gans J, van de Beek D; European Dexamethasone in Adulthood Bacterial Meningitis Study Investigators. Dexamethasone in adults with bacterial meningitis. N Engl J Med 2002; 347:1549–1556

11. Rosenstein NE, Perkins BA, Stephens DS, et al. Meningococcal disease. N Engl J Med 2001; 344: 1378–1388

12. Cookson ST, Corrales JL, Lotero JO, et al. Disco fever: epidemic meningococcal disease in northeastern Argentina associated with disco patronage. J Infect Dis 1998; 178:266–269

13. Centers for Disease Control and Prevention. Exposure to patients with meningococcal disease on aircrafts—United States, 1999–2001. MMWR Morb Mortal Wkly Rep 2001; 50:485–489

14. Stephens DS, Hajjeh RA, Baughman WS, et al. Sporadic meningococcal disease in adults: results of a 5-year population-based study. Ann Intern Med 1995; 123:937–940

15. Rosenstein NE, Stocker SA, Popovic T, et al. Antimicrobial resistance of Neisseria meningitidis in the United States, 1997. Clin Infect Dis 2000; 30:212–213

16. McGowan JE, Chesney PJ, Crossley KB, et al. Guidelines for the use of systemic glucocorticosteroids in the management of selected infections. J Infect Dis 1992; 165:1–13

17. Alberio L, Lämmle B, Esmon CT. Protein C replacement in severe meningococcemia: rationale and clinical experience. Clin Infect Dis 2001; 32:1338–1346

18. Bernard GR, Vincent JL, Laterre PF, et al. Efficacy and safety of recombinant human activated protein C for severe sepsis. N Engl J Med 2001; 344: 699–709

19. Centers for Disease Control and Prevention. Prevention and control of meningococcal disease: recommendations of the Advisory Committee on Immunization Practices (ACIP). MMWR Recomm Rep 2000; 49[RR-7]:1–10

20. Rosenstein N, Levine O, Taylor JP, et al. Efficacy of meningococcal vaccine and barriers to vaccination. JAMA 1998; 279:435–439

21. Centers for Disease Control and Prevention. Meningococcal disease and college students: recommendations of the advisory committee on immunization practices (ACIP). MMWR Recomm Rep 2000; 49[RR-7]:13–20

22. Overturf GD. Indications for the immunological evaluation of patients with meningitis. Clin Infect Dis 2003; 36:189–194

23. Schaad UB, Suter S, Gianella-Borradori, et al. A comparison of ceftriaxone and cefuroxime for the treatment of bacterial meningitis in children. N Engl J Med 1990; 322:141–147

24. Walker M, Zunt JR. Parasitic central nervous system infections in immunocompromised hosts. Clin Infect Dis 2005; 40:1005–1015

25. Maxipime (cefepime hydrocholoride), product labeling. In: Physicians' desk reference. 59th ed. Montvale, NJ: Thomson PDR, 2005; 1207–1212

26. Lorber B. Listeriosis. Clin Infect Dis 1997; 24:1–11

27. Lerche A, Rasmussen N, Wandall JH, et al. *Staphylococcus aureus* meningitis: a review of 28 consecutive community-acquired cases. Scand J Infect Dis 1995; 27:569–573

28. Bush LM, Abrams BH, Beall A, et al. Index case of fatal inhalational anthrax due to bioterrorism in the United States. N Engl J Med 2001; 345:1607–1610

29. Mayer TA, Bersoff-Matcha S, Murphy C, et al. Clinical presentation of inhalational anthrax following bioterrorism exposure: report of 2 surviving patients. JAMA 2001; 286:2549–2553

30. Durand ML, Calderwood SB, Weber DJ, et al. Acute bacterial meningitis in adults: a review of 493 episodes. N Engl J Med 1993; 328:21–28

31. Centers for Disease Control and Prevention, National Institutes of Health, HIV Medicine Association/Infections Diseases Society of America. Treating opportunistic infections among HIV-infected adults and adolescents. MMWR 2004; 53[RR-15]: 1–112

32. Marra CM, Maxwell CL, Tantalo L, et al. Normalization of cerebrospinal fluid abnormalities after neurosyphilis therapy: does HIV status matter? Clin Infect Dis 2004; 38:1001–1006

33. Farr RW. Leptospirosis. Clin Infect Dis 1995; 21:1–6

34. Panaphut T, Domrongkitchaiporn S, Vibhagool A, et al. Ceftriaxone compared with sodium penicillin G for treatment of severe leptospirosis. Clin Infect Dis 2003; 36:1507–1513

35. Ratnasamy N, Everett ED, Roland WE, et al. Central nervous system manifestations of human ehrlichiosis. Clin Infect Dis 1996; 23:314–319

36. Salgado AV, Furlan AJ, Keys TF, et al. Neurologic complications of endocarditis: a 12-year experience. Neurology 1989; 39:173–178

37. Verdon R, Chevret S, Laissy J-P, et al. Tuberculous meningitis in adults: review of 48 cases. Clin Infect Dis 1996; 22:982–988

38. Kent SJ, Crowe SM, Yung A, et al. Tuberculous meningitis: a 30-year review. Clin Infect Dis 1993; 17:987–994

39. Lopez-Cortes LF, Cruz-Ruiz M, Gomez-Mateos J, et al. Adenosine deaminase activity in the CSF of patients with aseptic meningitis: utility in the diagnosis of tuberculous meningitis or neurobrucellosis. Clin Infect Dis 1995; 20:525–530

40. American Thoracic Society/Centers for Disease Control and Prevention/Infectious Diseases Society of America. Treatment of tuberculosis. Am J Respir Crit Care Med 2003; 167:603–662

41. Thwaites GE, Bang ND, Dung NH, et al. Dexamethasone for the treatment of tuberculous meningitis in adolescents and adults. N Engl J Med 2004; 351:1741–1751

42. Donald PR, Schoeman JF. Tuberculous meningitis. N Engl J Med 2004; 351:1719–1720

43. van der Horst CM, Saag MS, Cloud CA, et al. Treatment of cryptococcal meningitis associated with the acquired immunodeficiency syndrome. N Engl J Med 1997; 337:15–21

44. Graybill JR, Sobel J, Saag M, et al. Diagnosis and management of increased intracranial pressure in patients with AIDS and cryptococcal meningitis. Clin Infect Dis 2000; 30:47–54

45. Saag MS, Graybill RJ, Larsen RA, et al. Practice guidelines for the management of cryptococcal disease. Clin Infect Dis 2000; 30:710–718

46. Galgiani JN, Ampel NM, Catanzaro A, et al. Practice guidelines for the treatment of coccidioidomycosis. Clin Infect Dis 2000; 30:658–661

47. Wheat LJ, Musial CE, Jenny-Avital EJ. Diagnosis and management of central nervous system histoplasmosis. Clin Infect Dis 2005; 40:844–852

48. Lo Re V 3rd, Gluckman SJ. Eosinophilic meningitis. Am J Med 2003; 114:217–223

49. Slom TJ, Cortese MM, Gerber SI, et al. An outbreak of eosinophilic meningitis caused by *Angiostrongylus cantonensis* in travelers returning from the Caribbean. N Engl J Med 2002; 346:668–675

50. Centers for Disease Control and Prevention. Primary amebic meningoencephalitis—Georgia, 2002. MMWR Morb Mortal Wkly Rep 2003; 52:962–964

51. Hasbun R, Abrahams J, Jekel J, et al. Computed tomography of the head before lumbar puncture in adults with suspected meningitis. N Engl J Med 2001; 345:1727–1733

52. Aronin SI, Peduzzi P, Quagliarello VJ. Community-acquired bacterial meningitis: risk stratification for adverse clinical outcome and effect of antibiotic timing. Ann Intern Med 1998; 129:862–869

53. McMillan DA, Lin CY, Aronin SI, et al. Community-acquired bacterial meningitis in adults: categorization of causes and timing of death. Clin Infect Dis 2001; 33:969–975

54. Saravolatz LD, Manzor O, VanderVelde N, et al. Broad-range bacterial polymerase chain reaction

for early detection of bacterial meningitis. Clin Infect Dis 2003; 36:40–45

55. Karchmer AW, Barza M, Drew WL, et al. Infectious disease medicine. In: American College of Physicians' Medical Knowledge Self-Assessment Program IX (MKSAP IX). 1991; 307–353

56. Johnson RT. Acute encephalitis. Clin Infect Dis 1996; 23:219–226

57. Whitley RJ, Lakeman F. Herpes simplex virus infections of the central nervous system: therapeutic and diagnostic considerations. Clin Infect Dis 1995; 20:414–420

58. Tebas P, Nease RF, Storch GA. Use of the polymerase chain reaction in the diagnosis of herpes simplex encephalitis: a decision analysis model. Am J Med 1998; 105:287–295

59. Centers for Disease Control and Prevention. Guidelines for surveillance, prevention, and control of West Nile virus infection—United States. MMWR Morb Mortal Wkly Rep 2000; 49:25–28

60. Petersen LR, Marfin AA. West nile virus: a primer for the clinician. Ann Intern Med 2002; 137:173–179

61. Watson NK, Bartt RE, Houff SA, et al. Focal neurological deficits and West Nile virus infection. Clin Infect Dis 2005; e59–e62

62. Centers for Disease Control and Prevention. Acute flaccid paralysis syndrome associated with West Nile virus infection—Mississippi and Louisiana. MMWR Morb Mortal Wkly Rep 2002; 51:825–828

63. Gea-Banacloche J, Johnson RT, Bagic A, et al. West nile virus: pathogenesis and therapeutic options. Ann Intern Med 2004; 140:545–553

64. Centers for Disease Control and Prevention. Arboviral disease—United States, 1994. MMWR Morb Mortal Wkly Rep 1995; 44:641–644

65. De Luca A, Giancola ML, Ammassari A, et al. The effect of potent antiretroviral therapy and JC virus load in cerebrospinal fluid on clinical outcome of patients with AIDS-associated progressive multifocal leukoencephalopathy. J Infect Dis 2000; 182:1077–1083

66. Plotkin SA. Rabies. Clin Infect Dis 2000; 30:4–12

67. Centers for Disease Control and Prevention. Human rabies—Montana and Washington, 1997. MMWR Morb Mortal Wkly Rep 1997; 46:770–774

68. Srinivasin A, Burton EC, Kuehnert MJ, et al. Transmission of rabies virus from an organ donor to four transplant recipients. N Engl J Med 2005; 352:1103–1111

69. Centers for Disease Control and Prevention. Human rabies—Texas and New Jersey, 1997. MMWR Morb Mortal Wkly Rep 1998; 47:1–5

70. Centers for Disease Control and Prevention. Human rabies—Virginia, 1998. MMWR Morb Mortal Wkly Rep 1999; 48:95–97

71. Centers for Disease Control and Prevention. Human rabies—California, Georgia, Minnesota, New York, and Wisconsin, 2000. MMWR Morb Mortal Wkly Rep 2000; 49:1111–1115

72. Centers for Disease Control and Prevention. Human rabies—California, 2002. MMWR Morb Mortal Wkly Rep 2002; 51:686–688

73. Centers for Disease Control and Prevention. Human rabies—Tennessee, 2002. MMWR Morb Mortal Wkly Rep 2002; 51:828–829

74. Centers for Disease Control and Prevention. Human rabies—Iowa, 2002. MMWR Morb Mortal Wkly Rep 2003; 51:47–48

75. Centers for Disease Control and Prevention. First human death associated with raccoon rabies—Virginia, 2003. MMWR Morb Mortal Wkly Rep 2003; 52:1102–1103

76. Centers for Disease Control and Prevention. Human death associated with bat rabies—California, 2003. MMWR Morb Mortal Wkly Rep 2004; 53:33–35

77. Centers for Disease Control and Prevention. Recovery of a patient from clinical rabies—Wisconsin, 2004. MMWR Morb Mortal Wkly Rep 2004; 53:1171–1173

78. Jackson AC, Warrell MJ, Rupprecht CE, et al. Management of rabies in humans. Clin Infect Dis 2003; 36:60–63

79. Rupprecht CE, Gibbons RV. Prophylaxis against rabies. N Engl J Med 2004; 351:2626–2635

80. Tattevin P, Bruneel F, Clair B, et al. Bacterial brain abscesses: a retrospective study of 94 patients admitted to an intensive care unit (1980 to 1999). Am J Med 2003; 115:143–146

81. Tunkel AR, Wispelwey B, Scheld WM. Brain abscess. In: Mandell GL, Bennett JE, Dolin R, eds. Mandell, Douglas, Bennett's principles and practice of infectious diseases. 5th ed. Philadelphia, PA: Churchill Livingstone, 2000; 1016–1028

82. Walot I, Miller BL, Chang L, Mehringer CM. Neuroimaging findings in patients with AIDS. Clin Infect Dis 1996; 22:906–919

83. Centers for Disease Control and Prevention. Guidelines for preventing opportunistic infections among HIV-infected persons—2002: recommendations of

the U.S. Public Health Service and Infectious Diseases Society of America. MMWR Recomm Rep 2002; 51[RR-8]:1–52

84. Darouiche RO, Hamill RJ, Greenberg SB, et al. Bacterial spinal epidural abscess: review of 43 cases and literature survey. Medicine 1992; 71:369–385

85. Stabler A, Reiser MF. Imaging of spinal infection. Radiol Clin North Am 2001; 39:115–135

86. Southwick FS, Richardson EP, Swartz MN. Septic thrombosis of the dural venous sinuses. Medicine 1986; 65:82–106

87. Bleck TP, Greenlee JE. Suppurative intracranial phlebitis. In: Mandell GL, Bennett JE, Dolin R, eds. Mandell, Douglas, Bennett's principles and practice of infectious diseases. 5th ed. Philadelphia, PA: Churchill Livingstone, 2000; 1034–1036

88. Kneen R, Pham NG, Solomon T, et al. Penicillin vs erythromycin in the treatment of diphtheria. Clin Infect Dis 1998; 27:845–850

89. Gergen PJ, McQuillan GM, Kiely M, et al. A population-based serologic survey of immunity to tetanus in the United States. N Engl J Med 1995; 332:761–766

90. Angulo FJ, Getz J, Taylor JP, et al. A large outbreak of botulism: the hazardous baked potato. J Infect Dis 1998; 178:172–177

91. Centers for Disease Control and Prevention. Outbreak of botulism type E associated with eating a beached whale—Western Alaska, July 2002. MMWR Morb Mortal Wkly Rep 2003; 52:24–26

92. Varma JK, Katsitadze G, Moiscrafishvili M, et al. Signs and symptoms predictive of death in patients with foodborne botulism—Republic of Georgia, 1980–2002. Clin Infect Dis 2004; 39:357–362

93. Centers for Disease Control and Prevention. Infant botulism—New York City, 2001–2002. MMWR Morb Mortal Wkly Rep 2003; 52:21–24

94. Shapiro RL, Hatheway C, Swerdlow DL. Botulism in the United States: a clinical and epidemiologic review. Ann Intern Med 1998; 129:221–228

95. Arnon SS, Schechter R, Inglesby TV, et al. Botulism toxin as a biological weapon: medical and public health management. JAMA 2001; 285:1059–1070

96. Nicolle LE, Bradley S, Colgan R, et al. Infectious Diseases Society of America guidelines for the diagnosis and treatment of asymptomatic bacteriuria in adults. Clin Infect Dis 2005; 40:643–654

97. Kaitz AL, Hodder EW. Bacteriuria and pyelonephritis of pregnancy: a prospective study of 616 pregnant women. N Engl J Med 1961; 265:667–672

98. Mittendork R, Williams MA, Kas EH. Prevention of preterm delivery and low birth weight associated with asymptomatic bacteriuria. Clin Infect Dis 1992; 14:927–932

99. Gratacos E, Torres PJ, Vila J, et al. Screening and treatment of asymptomatic bacteriuria in pregnancy prevents pyelonephritis. J Infect Dis 1994; 169:1390–1392

100. Stamm WE, Stapleton AE. Approach to the patient with urinary tract infection: asymptomatic bacteriuria. In: Gorbach SL, Bartlett JG, Blacklow NR, eds. Infectious diseases. 3rd ed. Philadelphia, PA: Lippincott Williams & Wilkins, 2004; 868–869

101. Munoz P. Management of urinary tract infections and lymphocele in renal transplant recipients. Clin Infect Dis 2001; 33[suppl 1]:S53–S57

102. Nordenstam GR, Brandberg CA, Oden AS, et al. Bacteriuria and mortality in an elderly population. N Engl J Med 1986; 314:1152–1156

103. Nicolle LE, Bjornson J, Harding GK, et al. Bacteriuria in elderly institutionalized men. N Engl J Med 1983; 309:1420–1425

104. Abrutyn E, Mossey J, Berlin JA, et al. Does asymptomatic bacteriuria predict mortality and does antimicrobial treatment reduce mortality in elderly ambulatory women? Ann Intern Med 1984; 120:827–833

105. Boscia JA, Abrutyn E, Kaye D. Asymptomatic bacteriuria in elderly persons: treat or do not treat? Ann Intern Med 1987; 106:764–766

106. Zhanel GG, Harding GK, Nicolle LE. Asymptomatic bacteriuria in patients with diabetes mellitus. Rev Infect Dis 1991; 13:150–154

107. Warren JW. Catheter-associated urinary tract infections. Infect Dis Clin North Am 1987; 1:823–824

108. Sobel JD, Kauffman CA, McKinsey D, et al. Candiduria: a randomized, double-blind study of treatment with fluconazole and placebo. Clin Infect Dis 2000; 30:19–24

109. Fridkin SK. Vancomycin-intermediate and -resistant *Staphylococcus aureus*: what the infectious disease specialist needs to know. Clin Infect Dis 2001; 32:108–115

110. Keane WF, Alexander SR, Bailie GR, et al. Peritoneal dialysis-related peritonitis treatment recommendations. Perit Dial Int 1996; 16:557–573

111. Keane WF, Bailie GR, Boeschoten E, et al. Adult peritoneal dialysis-related peritonitis treatment recommendations: 2000 update. Perit Dial Int 2000; 20:396–411

112. Shemin D, Maaz D, St Pierre D, et al. Effect of aminoglycoside use on residual renal function in peritoneal dialysis patients. Am J Kidney Dis 1999; 34:14–20

113. Shin SK, Noh H, Kang SW, et al. Risk factors influencing the decline of residual renal function in continuous ambulatory peritoneal dialysis patients. Perit Dial Int 1999; 19:138–142

114. Paterson DL, Ko WC, Von Gottberg A, et al. International prospective study of *Klebsiella pneumoniae* bacteremia: implications of extended-spectrum β-lactamase production in nosocomial infections. Ann Intern Med 2004; 140:26–32

115. Marx MA, Frye RF, Matzke GR, et al. Cefazolin as empiric therapy in hemodialysis-related infections: efficacy and blood concentrations. Am J Kidney Dis 1998; 32:410–414

116. Tokars JI. Vancomycin use and antimicrobial resistance in hemodialysis centers. Am J Kidney Dis 1998; 32:521–523

117. Johnson CC, Baldessarre J, Levison ME. Peritonitis: update on pathophysiology, clinical manifestations, and management. Clin Infect Dis 1997; 24:1035–1047

118. Mermel LA, Farr BM, Sherertz RJ, et al. Guidelines for the management of intravascular catheter-related infections. Clin Infect Dis 2001; 32:1249–1272

119. McGee DC, Gould MK. Preventing complications of central venous catheterization. N Engl J Med 2003; 348:1123–1133

120. Capdevila JA, Planes AM, Palomar M, et al. Value of differential quantitative blood cultures in the diagnosis of catheter-related sepsis. Eur J Microbiol Infect Dis 1992; 11:403–407

121. Blot F, Schmidt E, Nitenberg G, et al. Earlier positivity of central-venous- versus peripheral-blood cultures is highly predictive of catheter-related sepsis. J Clin Microbiol 1998; 36:105–109

122. Maki DG, Weise CE, Sarafin HW. A semiquantitative culture method for identifying intravenous-catheter-related infection. N Engl J Med 1977; 296:1305–1309

123. Safdar N, Fine JP, Maki DG. Meta-analysis: methods for diagnosing intravascular device-related bloodstream infection. Ann Intern Med 2005; 142:451–466

124. Raad I, Davis S, Khan A, et al. Impact of central venous catheter removal on the recurrence of catheter-related coagulase-negative staphylococcal bacteremia. Infect Control Hosp Epidemiol 1992; 13:215–221

125. Raad I. Intravascular-catheter-related infections. Lancet 1998; 351:893–898

126. Fowler VG, Olsen MK, Corey R, et al. Clinical identifiers of complicated *Staphylcoccus aureus* bacteremia. Arch Intern Med 2003; 163:2066–2072

127. Rosen AB, Fowler VG, Corey R, et al. Cost-effectiveness of transesophageal echocardiography to determine the duration of therapy for intravascular catheter-associated *Staphylococcus aureus* bacteremia. Ann Intern Med 1999; 130:810–820

128. Fowler VG Jr, Sanders LL, Sexton DJ, et al. Outcome of *Staphylococcus aureus* bacteremia according to compliance with recommendations of infectious diseases specialists: experience with 244 patients. Clin Infect Dis 1998; 27:478–486

129. El-Ahdab F, Benjamin DK, Wang A, et al. Risk of endocarditis among patients with prosthetic valves and *Staphylococcus aureus* bacteremia. Am J Med 2005; 118:225–229

130. Edwards JE Jr, Filler SG. Current strategies for treating invasive candidiasis: emphasis on infections in nonneutropenic patients. Clin Infect Dis 1992; 14(suppl 1):S106–S113

131. Rex JH. Editorial response: catheters and candidemia. Clin Infect Dis 1996; 22:467–470

132. Edwards JE Jr, Bodey GP, Bowden RA, et al. International conference for the development of a consensus on the management and prevention of severe candidal infections. Clin Infect Dis 1997; 25:43–59

133. Rex JH, Bennett JE, Sugar AM, et al. A randomized trial comparing fluconazole with amphotericin B for the treatment of candidemia in patients without neutropenia. N Engl J Med 1994; 331:1325–1330

134. Pappas PG, Rex JH, Sobel JD, et al. Guidelines for treatment of candidiasis. Clin Infect Dis 2004; 38:161–189

135. Mora-Duarte J, Betts R, Rotstein C, et al. Comparison of caspofungin and amphotericin B for invasive candidiasis. N Engl J Med 2002; 347:2020–2029

136. O'Grady NP, Alexander M, Dellinger EP, et al. Guidelines for the prevention of intravascular catheter-related infections. Clin Infect Dis 2002; 35:1281–1307

Bradycardias: Diagnosis and Management

James A. Roth, MD

Objectives:

- Understand the mechanisms that govern the normal regulation of heart rate
- Understand the forms of sinus node dysfunction and indications for pacemaker implantation
- Understand the forms of atrioventricular block and the indications for pacemaker implantation
- Understand the significance of atrioventricular conduction disturbances complicating acute myocardial infarction

Key words: atrioventricular block; bradycardia; chronotropic incompetence; myocardial infarction; pacemaker; sinus node dysfunction

Bradycardia Overview

All bradycardia is a consequence of the impairment of sinus node function, atrioventricular (AV) block, or, occasionally, the combination of both processes. It is important to recognize that isolated sinus node dysfunction generally results only in severe symptomatic bradycardia in the setting of concomitant failure of normal subsidiary escape mechanisms usually at the level of the AV junction. Therefore, symptomatic sinus node dysfunction is usually a sign of an extensive process affecting not only the sinus node but subsidiary escape mechanisms as well. Clinically significant bradycardia or pauses may occur as a consequence of autonomic disturbances, the use of drugs, chronic intrinsic conduction system disease, or acute cardiac damage as might occur with endocarditis or infarction.

Normal Conduction System: Anatomy and Physiology

Heart rate is normally determined by the intrinsic automaticity of the sinus node. Although it is common to refer to the sinus node as a discrete structure, it is in fact a large complex of pacemaker cells extending for several centimeters along the superior lateral right atrium extending downward from the superior vena cava atrial junction within the sulcus terminalis. Blood supply is derived from the sinus node artery, which arises from the proximal right coronary artery in 65% of cases, from the distal circumflex artery in 25% of cases, and both in the remainder of cases. Within this complex, the dominant pacemaker activity migrates depending on autonomic tone, with faster rates originating in the more superior portions of the complex and slower rates in more inferior portions.

Activation then proceeds through the right atrium to the AV node located in the low interatrial septum adjacent to the tricuspid annulus. The AV node is also a complex structure with at least three preferential atrial insertions. The anterior atrial insertion has a short conduction time and generally determines the normal AV conduction time in sinus rhythm. There are also posterior right and left atrial insertions that have long conduction times and are important in mediating paroxysmal supraventricular tachycardia. The AV node derives its blood supply from the AV nodal artery, which is a branch of the proximal posterior descending artery that is supplied by the right coronary artery in the majority of patients.

Following entry into the AV node, conduction becomes electrocardiographically silent and proceeds to the His bundle through the fibrous annulus and along the membranous septum before splitting into a leftward Purkinje branch, which ramifies over the LV endocardium and rightward branch, which similarly ramifies over the right ventricular endocardium. The leftward branch may be damaged proximally, resulting in full left bundle branch block or more distally in its anterior or posterior divisions, resulting in fascicular hemiblock patterns. Only following the completion of AV node, His bundle, and Purkinje system activation does activity emerge from the conduction system and become electrocardiographically apparent with the onset of ventricular muscle activation and the QRS complex.

Normal Autonomic Regulation of Heart Rate

Normal heart rate is a consequence of tonic and phasic autonomic modulation of intrinsic sinus node automaticity. The intrinsic heart rate in the absence of autonomic modulation ranges between 85 and 105 beats/min and is somewhat faster than normal resting heart rates. That the normal heart rate is slower than the intrinsic rate is a consequence of the dominance of parasympathetic tone over adrenergic tone in the resting state. Based on a review of Holter recordings in a healthy population, normal resting heart rate ranges between 46 and 93 beats/min in men and 51 to 95 beats/min in women.[1] Based on this, it has been proposed that 50 to 90 beats/min is a clinically more accurate working definition of normal heart rate in adults than the traditional 60 to 100 beats/min commonly used by consensus. However, heart rates well below these estimates may be seen in healthy subjects, especially during the hours of sleep. In athletes, a resting heart rate below 40 beats/min may be seen; nocturnal second-degree AV block and sinus pauses are common and are related to autonomic adaptations. For these reasons, defining a cutoff value for pathologic bradycardia in the absence of symptoms is problematic in an otherwise healthy patient.

The maximum stress-induced heart rate is related to maximal sympathetic stimulation accompanied by the withdrawal of parasympathetic tone. This is commonly estimated as HRMax = (220 − age), where HRMax is maximum heart rate. Because exercise entails both sympathetic stimulation and simultaneous parasympathetic withdrawal, age-predicted maximal heart rates are only observed when both arms of the autonomic nervous system are affected. As a consequence, the use of pharmacologic catecholamine stimulation will result in modest tachycardia with the patient at rest. However, if parasympathetic tone is also reduced by autonomic dysfunction, physiologic stress, or drug effects, the resultant tachycardia from modest sympathetic stimulation can be more labile and dramatic.

Sinus Node Dysfunction

Sick sinus syndrome or, equivalently, sinus node dysfunction is a common clinical syndrome that increases in prevalence with age. Its prevalence is estimated at 1 in 600 patients over the age of 65 years, and it accounts for about half of all pacemaker implantations. Sinus node dysfunction is a consequence of the following two distinct processes: the failure of intrinsic automaticity; or the failure of the propagation of sinus node impulses to the surrounding atrial tissue, which is also referred to a *sinus exit block*.

Sinus node dysfunction presents clinically as one of the following several patterns: persistent or episodic sinus bradycardia; the inability to appropriately augment heart rate with exercise, usually referred to as *chronotropic incompetence*, and sinus pauses; or, commonly, a combination of these patterns. It is important to recognize that the sinus node is at the top of a cascade of automaticity and is normally backed up by a competent AV junctional escape mechanism. Therefore, severe symptoms due to sinus node dysfunction always imply both sinus node dysfunction and accompanying simultaneous failure of normal subsidiary escape mechanisms. In the presence of a competent escape, even severe sinus node dysfunction may be completely asymptomatic and clinically well tolerated, and may require no specific therapy.

Resting Sinus Bradycardia

As noted above, there is no set rate at which sinus bradycardia can be labeled as pathologic, but it is best defined as significant bradycardia associated with symptoms that are plausibly attributable to bradycardia. Modest persistent bradycardia is often asymptomatic. When symptoms are present, they are commonly nonspecific ones, such as fatigue, listlessness, or dyspnea, making the attribution of symptoms to resting bradycardia difficult. Sinus bradycardia may also exacerbate congestive heart failure as well as limit the effective use of β-blocker therapy, which is one of the modern cornerstones of therapy. When inappropriate sinus bradycardia is persistent, especially when severe, plausible symptoms are present, and alternate causes of symptoms have been excluded, pacemaker implantation is reasonable. Asymptomatic sinus bradycardia should rarely be treated with pacing unless the need for medical therapy expected to further exacerbate bradycardia is expected.

Chronotropic Incompetence

Cardiac output during exercise is increased by both an augmentation in stroke volume and an increase in heart rate. If the rise in heart rate with exercise is inadequate, then exertional symptoms such as fatigue or dyspnea may ensue. As in the case of resting sinus bradycardia, unless severe, the attribution of symptoms to chronotropic incompetence is difficult. Various criteria for this condition have been proposed, ranging from the inability to reach 85% of the age-predicted maximum heart rate (likely an excessively inclusive definition) to the inability to achieve a heart rate of >100 beats/min with exercise, which is a much more conservative definition. As is the case for resting sinus bradycardia, the decision to implant a pacemaker for chronotropic incompetence is a matter of judgement more than criteria.

Sinus Pauses or Arrest: An abrupt failure of sinus node automaticity will result in a pause in atrial activity; P-waves will be absent; and, if of adequate duration and not accompanied by a competent escape mechanism, will result in abrupt symptoms. Pauses of <3 s are commonly seen in healthy subjects and are rarely symptomatic. Pauses exceeding 3 s and not occurring during sleep are often pathologic and may result in symptoms. Pauses associated with simultaneous symptoms, or the documentation of pauses of ≥3 s in the presence of a history of symptoms plausibly related to bradycardia are indications for pacemaker therapy.

Sinoatrial Exit Block

Bradycardia due to sinus node dysfunction may also result, not from the failure of automaticity, but from the failure of propagation from the sinus node complex to the atrium. As sinus node activity is not apparent from a surface ECG, the diagnosis is made indirectly by the observation of an abrupt halving in sinus P-wave rate followed by an abrupt return of the baseline sinus rate. Although other patterns may be observed as well, a 2:1 exit block is the most common. Except for its intriguing physiology, the symptoms of and therapy for sinoatrial exit block are identical to that of intermittent sinus bradycardia discussed in a previous section.

Bradycardia: Tachycardia Syndrome as a Consequence of Sinus Node Dysfunction

An additional common syndrome is the *bradycardia-tachycardia syndrome*, constituting the presence of intermittent pathologic atrial arrhythmias, most commonly intermittent atrial fibrillation, with concomitant sinus node dysfunction resulting in long pauses or symptomatic sinus bradycardia when the patient's heart is in sinus rhythm. A common manifestation of this syndrome is a prolonged period of asystole following the termination of atrial fibrillation due to the slow recovery of sinus node automaticity with resultant presyncope or syncope. The common combination of these two seemingly independent processes is in part a consequence of the high prevalence of both atrial fibrillation and sinus node dysfunction in the elderly, as well as the need to use potent drugs to decrease ventricular response during atrial fibrillation, which may result in unintended iatrogenic secondary sinus node dysfunction between periods of atrial arrhythmias. It has also been proposed, although it is unproven, that sinus bradycardia itself may promote atrial fibrillation. This form of bradycardia-tachycardia syndrome represents an important form of clinical sinus node dysfunction and is a common indication for pacemaker implantation. This form of sinus node dysfunction should be distinguished from a common unrelated form of bradycardia-tachycardia syndrome. This is the presence of chronic atrial fibrillation, as opposed to intermittent atrial fibrillation, with periods of both rapid and slow ventricular response. This condition is often incorrectly referred to as *sick sinus syndrome* as well. However, in this syndrome, the atrium chronically fibrillates, and hence the sinus node has no influence on heart rate. Bradycardia in the presence of chronic atrial fibrillation is a consequence of impaired AV conduction and is unrelated to sinus node dysfunction.

Primary and Secondary Causes of Sinus Node Dysfunction

Sinus node dysfunction may be primarily related to intrinsic dysfunction of the sinus node complex, or secondarily related to extrinsic and transient causes of sinus node dysfunction.

Intrinsic chronic dysfunction of the sinus node is rarely difficult to suspect and diagnose as sinus bradycardia; pauses are usually frequent, if not continuous, and are readily documented by monitoring or ambulatory recording even when the patient is asymptomatic. However, transient sinus pauses and bradycardia are frequently seen in the hospital setting as well as in patients with intermittent symptoms such as syncope. Between such episodes, sinus node function behaves normally with normal resting heart rates and no apparent pauses. The most common factor causing such intermittent sinus node dysfunction is an autonomic disturbance. In the ambulatory patient, the observation of intermittent pauses, severe bradycardia, or transient asystole associated with syncope or presyncope with otherwise normal sinus node function between episodes is usually related to the syndrome of neurocardiogenic or vasovagal syncope. As this syndrome is common in otherwise healthy patients and has a favorable prognosis in the absence of pacing, it is important to recognize this syndrome. Often, the diagnosis is suggested by the relatively young age of the patient, recognizing that intrinsic sinus node dysfunction is mostly a disorder of the elderly. In addition, symptoms in this syndrome are due to a combination of vasodilation and subsequent bradycardia, and often precede the development of bradycardia, excluding the bradycardia as a primary cause of symptoms. At other times, symptoms may occur in the absence of or be out of proportion to the degree of bradycardia observed. Finally, profound noncardiac autonomic symptoms including dysphoria, nausea, and diaphoresis may accompany these episodes, suggesting an autonomic process and not primarily an arrhythmic process. The following are ACC/AHA/NASPE guidelines for pacemaker implantation in sinus node dysfunction.[2]

Guidelines for Pacemaker Implantation in Sinus Node Dysfunction

Class I: conditions for which there is evidence and/or general agreement that a given procedure or treatment is beneficial, useful, and effective;

Class II: conditions for which there is conflicting evidence and/or a divergence of opinion about the usefulness/efficacy of a procedure or treatment;

Class IIA: the weight of evidence/opinion is in favor of usefulness/efficacy;

Class IIB: usefulness/efficacy is less well established by evidence/opinion; and

Class III: conditions for which there is evidence and/or general agreement that a procedure/treatment is not useful/effective and in some cases may be harmful.

Recommendations for Permanent Pacing in Sinus Node Dysfunction

Class I

1. Sinus node dysfunction with documented symptomatic bradycardia; and
2. Symptomatic chronotropic incompetence.

Class IIA

1. Sinus node dysfunction occurring spontaneously or as a result of necessary drug therapy, with a heart rate of < 40 beats/min without association of symptoms with bradycardia; and
2. Syncope of unexplained origin when major abnormalities of sinus node function are discovered or provoked in electrophysiologic studies.

Class IIB

In minimally symptomatic patients, the long-term heart rate is <40 beats/min while awake.

Class III

1. Sinus node dysfunction in asymptomatic patients;
2. Sinus node dysfunction in patients with symptoms suggestive of bradycardia that are clearly documented as not associated with a slow heart rate; and
3. Sinus node dysfunction with symptomatic bradycardia due to nonessential drug therapy.

AV Conduction Disturbances

Disturbances of AV conduction result in delay, or intermittent or persistent failure of AV conduction. The PR interval encapsulates three distinct phases of AV conduction. Although the individual components of AV conduction can be readily recorded by a His bundle catheter in an electrophysiology laboratory, the salient features of AV conduction disturbances can usually be elucidated by the careful interpretation of the surface ECG without the need to resort to invasive recording techniques. The right atrial conduction time from the area of the sinus node where the P-wave begins to the region of the AV node occupies a short first portion of the PR interval, usually no >30 ms. As the atrial conduction time is short and does not change much over time in a given patient, it can conveniently be ignored when assessing AV conduction. The second portion of the PR interval is the propagation time through the AV node itself, which is normally 50 to 120 ms. The last component of the PR interval is the time for propagation through the His bundle and bundle branches, which is typically 30 to 55 ms. Although this last portion, constituting His-Purkinje conduction is short, it is the major prognostic component of AV conduction and hence is very important clinically. This last interval, as it is the time from the onset of His bundle to the time of ventricular activation is commonly referred to as the *HV interval*.

First-Degree AV Block

First-degree AV block is defined as a PR interval exceeding 0.2 s (or 200 ms) in the presence of otherwise preserved AV conduction. The presence of first-degree AV block implies the presence of conduction delay in one of the components of AV conduction, usually at the level of the AV node or His-Purkinje System (ie, the infranodal conduction system). First-degree AV block is usually asymptomatic but is a sign of the presence of AV conduction system disease and as such may be a diagnostic clue to the mechanism of intermittent symptoms undocumented by ECG in a patient with unexplained syncope. Rarely, first-degree AV block alone may exacerbate heart failure due to the maladaptive timing of atrial contraction relative to the onset of ventricular systole. The use of conventional AV pacing to rectify this problem has been attempted but has generally been unrewarding. This is likely due to the adverse hemodynamic consequences of pacing the right ventricle in a patient with preexisting congestive heart failure. The development of biventricular pacing has addressed this potential issue and may be appropriate when dual-chamber

pacing is undertaken for the purpose of first-degree AV block in the setting of congestive heart failure.

Second-Degree AV Block

Second-degree AV block is defined as the intermittent failure of AV conduction with interspersed periods of intact AV conduction. Second-degree AV block may be seen commonly in athletes with high parasympathetic tone and resting sinus bradycardia as well as during hours of sleep, and is hence not, in and of itself, an indication of the presence of AV conduction system disease. Second-degree AV block may be asymptomatic or associated with mild symptoms such as palpitations, or, if resulting in protracted pauses or persistent bradycardia, may result in hemodynamic symptoms including lightheadedness, syncope, and fatigue. AV block at the level of the AV node is usually indolent and gradually progressive. Because of stable junctional escape mechanisms that are associated with progression to complete heart block at the level of the AV node, second-degree AV block at the level of the AV node tends to have a benign prognosis and in the absence of symptoms can be followed up safely without intervention. By contrast, a block in the infranodal conduction system composed of the His bundle and bundle branches can be malignant with a tendency to progress abruptly and unpredictably to higher degrees of AV block accompanied by unstable or absent subsidiary escape mechanisms. Once symptomatic, infranodal block may progress to complete heart block and in some cases sudden death. Despite its malignant nature, sudden cardiac death is rarely attributable to complete heart block, suggesting that most patients will present with symptoms permitting intervention before progression to sudden death. Because of the profound difference in the natural history of second-degree AV block at the AV nodal vs infranodal levels, the major clinical task in evaluating patients with second-degree AV block is to establish the probable level of block. In this regard, the surface ECG and pattern of the block are useful in establishing the probable level of block.

Mobitz I AV Block

Also referred to as *Wenkebach block*, Mobitz I AV block is defined as a progressive prolongation in

PR interval prior to the development of AV block, usually for one cycle, followed by the recovery of conduction with a return to baseline PR interval. As the degree of prolongation of the PR interval is less with each successive beat before block, the RR intervals actually tend to paradoxically shorten in the final beats before block. Mobitz I AV block is almost always associated with block at the level of the AV node. But very rarely this pattern can be seen with advanced infranodal disease in the His and bundle branches. As the block is at the level of the AV node, infranodal conduction is commonly normal and is associated with a narrow conducted QRS complex. In ambiguous cases, other clues may be helpful. As AV node function is improved with exercise, Mobitz I block tends to normalizes with activity and return at rest. Second-degree block at the level of the AV node is improved with the use of atropine and is exacerbated by carotid sinus massage. If associated with periods of complete heart block, block at the level of the AV node is associated with a junctional escape with a QRS morphology similar to that in conducted sinus rhythm.

Mobitz II AV Block

Mobitz II AV block is defined as the intermittent failure of AV conduction during stable atrial rates without antecedent PR prolongation followed by the recovery of AV conduction. Mobitz II AV block is always a sign of block in the infranodal tissues including the His bundle and bundle branches. Whereas infranodal block may rarely display Mobitz I/Wenkebach periodicity, it is generally held that AV block at the level of the AV node never results in true Mobitz II AV block. Therefore, the finding of Mobitz II AV block is always reason for concern. Although Mobitz II AV block may result from block in either the His bundle or subsidiary bundle branches, block at the level of the His bundle is rare, and, in practice, the vast preponderance of cases of Mobitz II AV block is due to intermittent conduction failure within the main bundle branches or the hemifascicles of the left bundle. In order for intermittent failure of conduction in a bundle branch or hemifascicle to result in AV block, it is also necessary to have fixed block in all the remaining branches antecedent to the intermittent failure resulting in

block. For example, for intermittent failure in the right bundle to result in second-degree AV block, the patient must already have a full left bundle branch block present between episodes of block. As a consequence, patients with Mobitz II AV block will generally display a wide conducted QRS complex between episodes of second-degree AV block. In ambiguous cases, other clues may be helpful. As infranodal function improves relatively little with exercise, infranodal block tends to worsen with increasing heart rates associated with exercise or stress. Atropine therapy is not helpful for the treatment of infranodal block, and because it may accelerate sinus rates, it may cause a patient to progress to higher degrees of AV block with a consequent decrease in conducted ventricular rate. Therapy with catecholamines may be helpful but should not be relied on. Because of its malignant potential, hemodynamically significant Mobitz II AV block should be addressed with early temporary or permanent pacing.

2:1 and High-Degree AV Block

2:1 AV block is defined as conduction of every other P wave. This pattern is most commonly seen with infranodal block in the His bundle or bundle branches. However, as two consecutive conducted P-waves are not available to assess Mobitz pattern, 2:1 AV block is neither Mobitz I nor Mobitz II. High-degree AV block is defined as second-degree AV block with conduction failure of two or more consecutive P-waves. Again, high-degree AV block is neither Mobitz I nor Mobitz II. Although Mobitz periodicity cannot be assigned, like other forms of second-degree AV block, the level of block may still be established to assess prognosis and guide therapy. In this case, the ancillary clues described above under Mobitz block remain useful.

Third-Degree AV Block

Third-degree AV block, or, equivalently, complete heart block, is defined as the complete failure of AV conduction. In the presence of underlying sinus rhythm, this is defined as an atrial rate that is faster than the ventricular rate associated with AV dissociation. However, when the underlying rhythm is atrial fibrillation, the definition of complete heart block cannot rely on the demonstration of AV dissociation. As conducted atrial fibrillation always results in an irregular ventricular response, the finding of a regular and a slow ventricular response during atrial fibrillation implies the presence of associated complete heart block. As is the case for second-degree AV block, the level of block determines the clinical behavior and prognosis of complete heart block. Complete heart block at the level of the AV node is associated with a generally stable junctional escape with heart rates between 40 and 50 beats/min and usually a narrow QRS complex. If the patient had an antecedent bundle branch block prior to the development of complete heart block, block at the level of the AV node would be associated with a wide QRS escape identical to the conducted QRS complex prior to the development of the block. By contrast, complete heart block at an infranodal level is associated with a wide and slow ventricular escape, often slower than 40 beats/min with a QRS complex that is different from the antecedent conducted morphology. Unfortunately, infranodal escape rhythms may be absent entirely, leading to the troubling observation of consecutive P-waves alone with accompanying asystole and loss of consciousness. When infranodal complete heart block is suspected, regardless of the toleration of the ventricular escape rhythm, the prompt institution of either temporary or permanent ventricular pacing is mandatory. Whereas a junctional escape may be quite reliable and trustworthy, a ventricular escape rhythm, no matter how seemingly benign and well tolerated, should not be relied on. The following are ACC/AHA/NASPE guidelines for pacemaker implantation in acquired AV block.

Recommendations for Permanent Pacing in Acquired AV Block in Adults

Class I

1. Third-degree and advanced second-degree AV block at any anatomic level, associated with any one of the following conditions;
2. Bradycardia with symptoms presumed to be due to AV block;
3. Arrhythmias and other medical conditions that require drugs that result in symptomatic bradycardia;

4. Documented periods of asystole of ≥3.0 s or any escape rate of <40 beats/min in awake, symptom-free patients;
5. After catheter ablation of the AV junction;
6. Postoperative AV block that is not expected to resolve after cardiac surgery;
7. Neuromuscular diseases with AV block; and
8. Second-degree AV block regardless of the type or site of the block, with associated symptomatic bradycardia.

Class IIA

1. Asymptomatic third-degree AV block at any anatomic site with average awake ventricular rates of ≥40 beats/min, especially if cardiomegaly or LV dysfunction is present;
2. Asymptomatic type II second-degree AV block with a narrow QRS complex. When type II second-degree AV block occurs with a wide QRS complex, pacing becomes a class I recommendation;
3. Asymptomatic type I second-degree AV block at intra-His or infra-His levels found on electrophysiologic study performed for other indications; and
4. First-degree or second-degree AV block with symptoms similar to those of pacemaker syndrome.

Class IIB

1. Marked first-degree AV block (>0.30 s) in patients with LV dysfunction and symptoms of congestive heart failure in whom a shorter AV interval results in hemodynamic improvement, presumably by decreasing left atrial filling pressure; and
2. Neuromuscular diseases with any degree of AV block (including first-degree AV block), with or without symptoms, because there may be an unpredictable progression of AV conduction disease.

Class III

1. Asymptomatic first-degree AV block;
2. Asymptomatic type I second-degree AV block at the supra-His level (AV node) or not known to be at intra-His or infra-His level; and
3. AV block expected to resolve and/or unlikely to recur (eg, drug toxicity, Lyme disease, or

Sinus Bradycardia and AV Block Complicating Acute Myocardial Infarction

Sinus bradycardia occurs frequently, constituting 30% to 40% of acute myocardial infarction (AMI)-associated cardiac arrhythmias. Heart block may develop in approximately 6 to 14% of patients with ST-segment elevation myocardial infarction (STEMI). Intraventricular conduction delay has been reported in about 10 to 20% of patients with STEMI in past reviews. The development of AV and intraventricular blocks during STEMI is generally related to the extent of the ischemic/infarcted segment. As such, AV block predicts an increased risk of in-hospital mortality but is less predictive of long-term mortality in those who survive to hospital discharge. In the acute reperfusion era, the risk of developing heart block has decreased.[3]

AMI may result in transient dysfunction as well as persistent dysfunction of the AV conduction system. Block may occur due to infarction or ischemia of the AV node and the infranodal conduction system including the bundle branches. Transient bradycardia may also occur due to hypervagotonia, especially during infarction involving the inferior and posterior walls of the LV. As myocardial infarction is an acute event where transient changes may occur, the decision regarding the institution of long-term pacing vs simple monitoring with our without short-term temporary pacing arises. As is the case with other causes of AV block, prognosis and management are related to the presence of symptoms and the level of the block.

Acute inferior wall infarction may spare the AV node entirely if due to occlusion within the posterior descending artery. However, more proximal occlusion of the right coronary artery (or circumflex artery in the minority of patients with a left-dominant circulation) will involve the AV nodal artery and may result in complete heart block at the level of the AV node. Such block is often well tolerated, may be responsive to atropine therapy, and my be associated with a stable escape rhythm;

in the vast majority of patients, it will resolve over time following infarction and not require permanent pacing. Temporary pacing is only required in the presence of hemodynamic compromise related to bradycardia. With the recovery of AV conduction after the acute phase of infarction, the long-term prognosis is excellent, and recurrent AV block does not tend to occur.

Acute anterior wall infarction due to occlusion within the left anterior descending coronary artery may result in septal infarction and associated damage to the branches of the infranodal conduction system. The risk of developing AV block is highest when there is new bilateral bundle branch involvement such as right bundle branch block with an associated left hemiblock. New bundle branch block presents a higher risk than the presence of old preexisting bundle branch block. Before the era of readily available transcutaneous pacing, these findings in the setting of acute anterior wall infarction were indications for prophylactic temporary pacing. In the current era, the ready availability of transcutaneous pacing has made the need for prophylactic pacing in the absence of second-degree or third-degree AV block during the acute phase of infarction less of an issue in such patients. However, even transient second-degree or third-degree infranodal AV block with an associated bundle branch block presents both a short-term risk as well as a long-term risk of progression to complete heart block. Therefore, unlike the case with block at the level of the AV node complicating inferior wall infarction, even transient infranodal block complicating anterior infarction is an indication for long-term permanent pacing, which should be instituted before hospital discharge. The following are ACC/AHA guidelines for pacemaker implantation following the acute phase of myocardial infarction.[3]

Recommendations for Permanent Pacing After the Acute Phase of Myocardial Infarction

Class I

1. Persistent second-degree AV block in the His-Purkinje system with bilateral bundle branch block or third-degree AV block within or below the His-Purkinje system after AMI;

2. Transient advanced (second-degree or third-degree) infranodal AV block and associated bundle branch block; and
3. Persistent and symptomatic second-degree or third-degree AV block.

Class IIB

Persistent second-degree or third-degree AV block at the AV node level.

Class III

1. Transient AV block in the absence of intraventricular conduction defects;
2. Transient AV block in the presence of isolated left anterior fascicular block;
3. Acquired left anterior fascicular block in the absence of AV block; and
4. Persistent first-degree AV block in the presence of bundle branch block that is old or age indeterminate.

Summary and Conclusions

All instances of bradycardia are a consequence of the impairment of sinus node function, of AV conduction, or both. Sinus and AV nodal function are strongly influenced by autonomic tone. Parasympathetic tone dominates at rest, and significant bradycardia as well as second-degree AV block may be observed in healthy subjects due to increased parasympathetic tone, especially during sleep or in the setting of athletic training. Clinical sinus node dysfunction presents as one of several syndromes, including sinus bradycardia, chronotropic incompetence, exit block, and bradycardia-tachycardia syndrome due to sinus pauses and bradycardia when concomitant atrial arrhythmias terminate to sinus rhythm.

AV conduction disturbances may occur at the AV nodal level or infranodal level. Block at the level of the AV node tends to be indolent and characterized by gradual progression, and competent subsidiary escapes usually protect the patient from catastrophic bradycardia. This permits asymptomatic patients to be followed up clinically for the development of symptoms before intervention. By contrast, second-degree or third-degree infranodal block at the level of the bundle branches is potentially malignant, is often not accompanied by stable escape mechanisms,

and, if not managed aggressively, can eventuate in sudden death. Clues to an infranodal level of block are Mobitz II periodicity, associated bundle branch block, worsening heart block with tachycardia or exercise, and a wide QRS escape rhythm that is different from the conducted QRS in the presence of high-degree or third-degree AV block.

Sinus bradycardia and heart block occurring in the setting of AMI have a natural history related to the location of the infarction and the natural evolution of acute infarction. Inferior infarction commonly results in sinus bradycardia and impairment of AV conduction at the level of the AV node. These processes tend to be well tolerated and usually resolve following infarction. By contrast, anterior infarction may affect the infranodal conduction system at the level of the bundle branches. Even transient second-degree or third-degree block associated with anterior infarction and bundle branch block is associated with a high risk of future progression as well as death, and pacemaker implantation is indicated even if the block appears to have resolved before hospital discharge.

References

1. Spodick DH. Normal sinus heart rate: appropriate rate thresholds for sinus tachycardia and bradycardia. South Med J 1996; 89:666–667
2. Gregoratos G, Abrams J, Epstein AE, et al. ACC/AHA/NASPE 2002 guideline update for implantation of cardiac pacemakers and antiarrhythmia devices: a report of the American College of Cardiology/American Heart Association Task Force on Practice Guidelines (ACC/AHA/NASPE Committee on Pacemaker Implantation); 2002. Available at: http://www.acc.org/qualityandscience/clinical/guidelines/pacemaker/incorporated/index.htm. Accessed March 10, 2007
3. Antman EM, Anbe DT, Armstrong PW, et al. ACC/AHA guidelines for the management of patients with ST-elevation myocardial infarction: executive summary: a report of the ACC/AHA Task Force on Practice Guidelines (Committee to Revise the 1999 Guidelines on the Management of Patients With Acute Myocardial Infarction). J Am Coll Cardiol 2004; 44:671–719

Notes

Upper and Lower GI Bleeding in the ICU

Gregory T. Everson, MD

Objectives:

- Clinically distinguish upper from lower GI hemorrhage
- Define the common etiologies of GI hemorrhage occurring in the ICU
- Develop strategies for rapid diagnosis and management for both upper and lower GI hemorrhage
- Discuss prophylactic regimens for prevention of GI hemorrhage
- Compare therapeutic options for treatment of GI hemorrhage

Key words: angiography; diverticulosis coli; endoscopy; GI hemorrhage; hematemesis; hematochezia; melena; nonsteroidal antiinflammatory drugs; peptic ulcer disease; resuscitation; varices

Upper GI Hemorrhage

Upper GI (UGI) hemorrhage accounts for 0.1 to 1% of all admissions to the hospital, occurs twice as frequently in men, is more common in the elderly, and remains a significant cause of ICU morbidity and mortality. For unknown reasons, UGI bleeding from peptic ulcer disease is more common during the winter months. The current mortality rate from transfusion-requiring hemorrhage ranges from 5 to 15%. The mortality rate increases with age; hemodynamic instability; volume of transfusion requirement (≥ 6 U packed RBCs [pRBCs]); evidence of organ dysfunction, particularly renal failure; underlying cardiopulmonary disease; and underlying liver disease. The risk of death increases threefold if the patient is already hospitalized at the time of the initial bleed. The following three principles underline management: volume and blood product resuscitation; emergent endoscopy for diagnosis; and prompt definition and institution of therapy targeted to the underlying etiology. Surgical consultation should be obtained in the early stages of resuscitation and evaluation.

Case Presentation 1

A 48-year-old woman experienced sudden hematemesis at work while performing her usual secretarial duties. She was noted by coworkers to be pale, diaphoretic, and faint. Emergency medical technicians started peripheral IV lines and administered saline solution. On arrival at the emergency department, she was alert and oriented, pale, with a BP of 95/55, a pulse of 120 beats/min, a respiratory rate of 22 breaths/min, and a temperature of 37°C. She passed a melenic stool, and examination revealed only a few scattered spider telangiectasias with mild hepatosplenomegaly. Two units of pRBCs were infused and a nasogastric (NG) tube was placed revealing dark blood with clots in the stomach; the patient was admitted to the medical ICU. She described the recent use of ibuprofen for headaches but denied alcohol use or any knowledge of underlying liver disease. Her medical history was unremarkable except for the receipt of a blood transfusion at age 23 years for postpartum hemorrhage.

Resuscitation

The initial assessment of severity of bleeding requires a critical evaluation of vital signs. Hematocrit is not a reliable indicator of the degree of hemorrhage because it does not decrease immediately with acute bleeding. The decrease in hematocrit that occurs with bleeding is due to the reequilibration of body fluid and may take 24 to 72 h to manifest. The patient who has sustained a UGI hemorrhage typically exhibits features of hypovolemia or hypovolemic shock.

Immediate measures are focused at restoring intravascular volume and maintaining tissue oxygenation. Two large-bore indwelling IV catheters should be placed early in the resuscitation effort, and BP should be immediately corrected with a bolus infusion of normal saline solution. The ideal hematocrit guiding the transfusion of blood or pRBCs is somewhat controversial, although most investigators have recommended a target hematocrit of 25 to 30%. Because elderly patients (*ie*, age >60 years) and those patients with underlying cardiovascular disease are prone to myocardial infarction during significant GI hemorrhage, a higher target hematocrit may be recommended for these populations. The determination of hematocrit/hemoglobin from the sampling if peripheral venous blood is preferable to use of portable bedside hemoglobin monitoring using capillary blood.

Oxygen delivery to tissues is ensured by volume replacement to restore BP, the maintenance of RBC volume to restore oxygen-carrying capacity, and the administration of nasal oxygen to saturate the carrying capacity of the blood. Coagulopathic patients may require platelets, fresh-frozen plasma, or cryoprecipitate (to replace fibrinogen). Calcium infusion may be required in those patients receiving massive units of citrate-treated stored blood since citrate may chelate calcium and lower its plasma concentration.

During resuscitative efforts, the patient should be evaluated for underlying organ dysfunction due to the hemorrhage and examined for the presence of chronic liver disease. Lactic acidosis, renal failure, myocardial ischemia and infarction, bowel ischemia, cerebral ischemia, and limb ischemia may all complicate hemorrhagic shock. UGI hemorrhage in the setting of chronic liver disease is related to portal hypertension in approximately 50% of cases (varices or portal hypertensive gastropathy). Management is influenced significantly by the presence of underlying chronic liver disease and its etiology.

Etiology

The causes of UGI bleeding are given in Table 1. Endoscopy or radiologic imaging is required to establish the cause of bleeding. The most common etiology is duodenal ulcer disease, representing 30 to 35% of all cases of UGI bleeding. Bleeding from gastric ulcers is the next most common diagnosis, followed by Mallory-Weiss lesions, portal hypertensive gastropathy, and varices. However, a wide array of conditions may present with UGI hemorrhage.

Table 1. *Causes of UGI Hemorrhage*

Site	% of All UGI Bleeds
Esophageal	
Varices	10
Erosive esophagitis	2
Mallory-Weiss lesion	5–15
Medication-induced ulceration	≤1
Caustic ingestion	≤1
Infectious esophagitis	≤1
Herpes	
CMV	
HIV	
Candida infection	
Carcinoma	≤1
Gastric	
Peptic lesions	15–20
Gastric ulcer	
Gastritis	
NSAID ulcers	
Dieulafoy lesion	≤1
Varices	1–3
Portal hypertensive gastropathy	10–15
Vascular malformations	≤1
Neoplastic lesions	≤1
Carcinoma	
Lymphoma	
Leiomyoma	
Duodenal	
Peptic ulcer	30–35
Vascular malformation	≤1
Aortoenteric fistula	≤1
Hemobilia	≤1
Hemosuccus pancreatitis	≤1

Nonsteroidal Antiinflammatory Drugs and Risk of Bleeding

The risk of bleeding with use of nonselective nonsteroidal antiinflammatory drugs (NSAIDs) is approximately 0.5% after 6 months of ongoing treatment. Risk increases with age, history of ulcer disease, and history of cardiovascular disease, and is related to the dose of NSAID. Risk is reduced, but not eliminated, by the use of the more selective cyclooxygense-2 inhibitors (*eg*, celecoxib and rofecoxib). The coadministration of nonselective NSAIDs to patients receiving steroids or anticoagulation therapy (*eg*, heparin or warfarin) increases the relative risk of bleeding up to 12-fold. *Helicobacter pylori*, although proven to increase the risk for ulcer disease, is not an independent risk factor for UGI bleeding. ICU patients who have experienced UGI hemorrhage may have a higher

Upper and Lower GI Bleeding in the ICU (Everson)

prevalence of *H pylori*. A number of studies have demonstrated the effectiveness of proton pump inhibitors (PPIs) for preventing gastroduodenal ulcers in patients receiving NSAIDs.

Diagnosis

The initial findings of a physical examination may be useful in providing clues to the location of the bleeding lesion in the GI tract. The evaluation of vital signs, an abdominal examination, and the appearance of the bowel movement may localize the bleeding site. A patient passing bright red blood via the rectum with stable vital signs and a benign abdomen is most likely bleeding from a lower, left-sided colonic lesion. A hemodynamically stable patient passing purplish clots and darker blood may be bleeding from the right colon or small bowel. Mild-to-moderate UGI bleeding is characterized by loose, black bowel movements (melena). The development of melena requires a minimum bleed of ≥100 mL and prolonged residence in the gut (≥12 h). Massive bleeding from varices or an artery in an ulcer base, is often characterized by hemodynamic instability or shock, and hematemesis. With brisk bleeding from a UGI source (≥1,000 mL), one may observe the passage of red blood via the rectum; almost always mixed with darker blood or clots and characterized by hypotension. Approximately 5 to 15% of cases, initially thought to be bleeding from a lower GI (LGI) source, are actually bleeding from a UGI source.

NG tubes can be helpful diagnostically in some cases, but hemoccult testing of aspirates is not useful and not recommended. If the aspirate lacks blood and contains bile, a UGI source for ongoing active bleeding is less likely. However, 16% of UGI bleeds from duodenal ulcer disease are associated with a clear NG aspirate. The major role for NG tubes is to allow lavage and the clearance of blood from the stomach for the purpose of performing endoscopy or other diagnostic studies. Other clues to a UGI source are the elevation of BUN levels, hyperactive bowel sounds, and physical findings (*eg*, spider telangiectasias, jaundice, hepatosplenomegaly, acanthosis nigricans, pigmented lip lesions, and palpable purpura). Some gastroenterologists also use the NG tube to assess the patient for activity of ongoing bleeding and to determine prognosis. A patient admitted

Table 2. *Prediction of Outcome After Upper Gastrointestinal Bleed From Peptic Lesions*

Increased risk of mortality is associated with
  Age >60 yr
  Hemodynamic instability with initial bleed
  Onset of bleeding during hospitalization for unrelated co-
    morbid condition
  History of cancer
  Underlying comorbid conditions
  Endoscopic finding of giant ulcer
  Endoscopic finding of visible vessel in base of ulcer
Endoscopic features predictive of rebleeding
  Spurting artery (actively bleeding)
  Nonbleeding but elevated visible vessel
  Adherent clot
  Flat cherry red or black spot with oozing

to the hospital for melena, who has a clear NG aspirate, has a predicted mortality rate of ≤5%. In contrast, a patient admitted to the hospital with hematochezia, who has a red NG aspirate, has a predicted mortality rate of approximately 30%. A recent analysis of ICU mortality (Mortality Probability Model, MPM0-III) indicated that ICU mortality related to GI hemorrhage has diminished in recent years.

Emergent endoscopy, after resuscitation of the patient and the clearance of blood and clots from the stomach, is indicated for nearly all acute UGI bleeders. Not only is endoscopy diagnostic in >90% of cases, it can also be used to provide definitive therapy (*eg*, variceal ligation or sclerotherapy, electrocautery, alcohol or sclerosant injection, and biopsy for *H pylori*, which in some cases may lead to antibiotic treatment). In addition, endoscopy is useful in identifying patients who are at high risk of rebleeding and may benefit from early surgical intervention (*eg*, a visible vessel not responding to endoscopic management, giant ulcer, diffuse hemorrhagic gastritis, or miscellaneous lesions) (Table 2).

Case 1 (Continued)

Our patient underwent endoscopy, which revealed esophageal varices with stigmata of a recent hemorrhage (*ie*, cherry red spot over a varix) and minimal erosive gastritis. She was treated with endoscopic ligation of the varices, had no further bleeding, and was discharged from the hospital 72 h after admission. Subsequent evaluation revealed cirrhosis due to chronic hepatitis C. Varices were eradicated by repeated ligation treatments, and she underwent evaluation for liver transplantation.

Imaging studies may also be useful in localizing a bleeding source. If endoscopic studies are nondiagnostic and bleeding persists, a nuclear medicine ^{99m}Tc-RBC scan may indicate the site of bleeding. This scan is more sensitive than angiography, and when sequential scans are performed the bleeding site may be localized in 60 to 80% of cases. Although the scan can localize bleeding to a site in the bowel, etiology is rarely, if ever, defined from this study. Angiography is used in patients with higher bleeding rates and may be therapeutic if embolization of the bleeding site is performed. Angiography can be diagnostic for vascular lesions of the bowel. A Meckel scan (with technetium pertechnetate) is usually performed only after all other studies have failed to provide a diagnosis. Barium studies are not recommended in the initial evaluation of UGI bleeding.

Specific Therapeutic Approaches

Peptic Lesions

Bleeding from peptic lesions of the UGI tract is treated as follows:

1. Gastric acid suppression (PPIs are favored over H2-blockers but are not effective in the setting of active bleeding). High-dose antisecretory therapy (IV PPIs) significantly decrease the risk of rebleeding in patients with bleeding ulcers. Both H2-blockers and PPIs are preferable to sucralfate.

2. Octreotide, a 50-μg bolus followed by 50 μg/h infusion. The use of octreotide for this indication is controversial, but some studies have suggested that the rebleeding rate is reduced by 30 to 50%.

3. Correction of coagulopathy.

4. Therapeutic endoscopy (ie, electrocautery and injection of sclerosant). The effectiveness of endoscopic therapy is limited by arterial size. Arterial bleeders with a diameter of ≥2 mm usually do not respond to therapy and require surgery. Rebleeding after initial control with endoscopic treatment is best managed by repeat endoscopic therapy or radiologic intervention. Surgery is only necessary in approximately 10% of rebleeds.

5. Surgery for those patients who do not respond to endoscopic management.

6. After resolution of the acute bleed, all patients with duodenal ulcers should be considered for triple therapy against *H pylori*. After an acute bleed, *H pylori* status should be determined before initiating triple therapy. The incidence of non-*H pylori*-related duodenal ulcer is increasing, and these patients have significantly worse outcomes if treated empirically for *H pylori*. Other peptic lesions may also require this therapy if the patient is *H pylori*-positive.

Varices

The risk of bleeding from esophageal varices is directly related to portal pressure (≥12 mm Hg), variceal size and appearance on endoscopy, advanced Child-Pugh score (Table 3), and coincident gastric varices. The mortality rate from UGI hemorrhage from varices ranges from 30 to 50%.

Table 3. *Prognostic Models for Patients With Cirrhosis**

Child-Pugh Criteria	1 Point	2 Points	3 Points
Bilirubin, mg/dL	<2	2–3	>3
Albumin, g/dL	>3.5	2.8–3.5	<2.8
Prothrombin time, s prolonged	1–3	4–6	>6
Ascites	None	Slight	Moderate
Encephalopathy	None	1–2	3–4

*Grades: A = 4–6 points; B = 7–9 points; C = 10–15 points. See Pugh's modification of the Child-Turcotte prognostic classification (Pugh RN, Murray-Lyon IM, Dawson JL, et al. Transection of the esophagus for bleeding of esophageal varices. Br J Surg 1973; 60:646–649).

Upper and Lower GI Bleeding in the ICU (Everson)

Cirrhotic patients with three or more failing organ systems have a 90% mortality rate. The most common failing organ systems were hepatic, renal, and cardiovascular. The model end-stage liver disease (or MELD) score (calculated as 0.957[Ln creatinine] + 0.378[Ln bilirubin] + 1.120[Ln international normalized ratio] + 0.643) [Table 3] is a better predictor of survival than either acute physiology and chronic health evaluation (APACHE) II score or Child-Turcotte-Pugh score, although APACHE II and III scores have been more predictive than the Child-Turcotte-Pugh score.

The treatment of bleeding from esophageal varices is aimed at the control of portal hypertension using pharmacologic agents and the direct application of endoscopic treatment to the bleeding variceal channels. A number of pharmacologic agents can lower portal hypertension (eg, β-blockers, nitroglycerin, vasopressin, and somatostatin). We currently favor the use of octreotide or vapreotide since they are effective, well-tolerated, and have few side effects. A loading dose of octreotide of 50 µg is administered initially and is followed by continuous infusion at 50 µg/h. As noted above, patients with variceal hemorrhage typically have portal pressures of >12 mm Hg. Studies using transjugular hepatic vein pressure measurements indicate that a reduction of portal pressure to <12 mm Hg or a ≥20% reduction in portal pressure controls bleeding and reduces the risk of rebleeding.

The conditions of the majority of patients bleeding from esophageal varices can be controlled by endoscopic ligation, especially if it is performed with the coadministration of a long-acting somatostatin analog. Endoscopic ligation treatment (banding) is associated with fewer complications than endoscopic sclerotherapy and is currently the preferred modality of treatment.

Bleeding gastric varices are more difficult to manage endoscopically; ligation/banding is associated with a very high risk for rebleeding, and sclerotherapy, although preferred over banding as a single modality, obtains suboptimal control. Many experienced endoscopists have used combined modalities, such as combination ligation/banding with sclerotherapy or a high-volume injection of cyanoacrylate. Still, management is compromised by relatively high rates of rebleeding and significant morbidity and mortality.

Patients bleeding from gastric varices or those who rebleed from esophageal varices despite endoscopic treatment may require the placement of a Sengstaken-Blakemore tube and the performance of either transjugular intrahepatic portal-systemic shunt (TIPS) or surgical shunt (Table 4). TIPS placement is successful in 90 to 95% of cases, but TIPS may thrombose or stenose and require repeated radiologic interventions. In addition, TIPS is costly, and 15 to 30% of patients undergoing TIPS experience post-TIPS encephalopathy. Other interventional procedures include balloon-occluded retrograde transvenous obliteration and partial splenic embolization; these procedures are reserved for patients with thrombosis of the main portal vein or for those patients who are not candidates for TIPS. Interestingly, in one series of 32 patients, fundic varices were eradicated in 97% of patients by balloon-occluded retrograde transvenous obliteration without the recurrence of either varices or bleeding. Mortality rates from bleeding varices are directly related to Childs-Pugh score, ongoing alcohol use, and comorbid illness. The mortality rate is >50% in Childs class C cirrhotic patients (Table 5).

Lower GI Hemorrhage

The principles of management for LGI bleeding are similar to those mentioned for UGI bleeding, as

Table 4. *Indications for and Contraindications to TIPS**

Indications	Contraindications
Accepted	Absolute
Gastroesophageal variceal hemorrhage	Heart failure with elevated CVP
Refractory acute variceal bleeding	Polycystic liver disease
Refractory recurrent variceal bleeding	Severe hepatic failure
Bleeding from intestinal varices	Relative
Cirrhotic hydrothorax	Active intrahepatic or systemic infection
Promising	Portal vein occlusion
Refractory ascites	Hypervascular hepatic neoplasms
Hepatorenal syndrome	Poorly controlled hepatic encephalopathy
Budd-Chiari syndrome	Stenosis of celiac trunk

*CVP = central venous pressure.

Table 5. *Risk of Death From Variceal Hemorrhage According to Severity of Liver Disease*

Child-Pugh Class	%
A	≤5
B	≤25
C	>50

Table 6. *Causes of Significant Acute LGI Bleeding*

Causes	%
Diverticulosis	30
Postpolypectomy	7
Ischemic colitis	6
Colonic ulcerations	6
Neoplasm (cancer and polyps)	5
Angiodysplasia	4
Radiation proctitis	2
Inflammatory bowel disease	2
Miscellaneous lesions	12
Undiagnosed LGI bleeding	26

follows: resuscitation; diagnosis; and planning for specific therapy. One initial consideration in evaluating the LGI bleeder is to exclude a UGI source. A negative result for NG lavage may obviate the need for upper endoscopy, but nearly 5 to 15% of patients who were thought to have LGI bleeding actually receive a diagnosis of an UGI source, and about 5% are from the small bowel. The average age of LGI bleeders is 65 years. The causes of LGI bleeding include the following: hemorrhoids; angiodysplasia; diverticular disease; neoplastic lesions; inflammatory bowel disease; and other vascular lesions or tumors of the LGI tract (Table 6).

Diagnosis

Colonoscopy

The primary diagnostic test in LGI bleeding is colonoscopy after purgation of the bowel by use of a bowel evacuant (Colyte; Schwarz Pharma; Milwaukee, WI). Studies comparing colonoscopy to air-contrast barium enema indicate that colonoscopy is far superior, identifying the source in approximately 70% of cases compared to only approximately 30% for air-contrast barium enema. One series of ICU patients indicated that bedside

colonoscopy after purgation was diagnostic in two thirds of cases. Another advantage of colonoscopy is the ability to provide treatment (*eg*, cautery, polypectomy, or sclerotherapy), although endoscopic treatment is required in less than one third of cases. However, there is a 2% risk of perforation with endoscopic treatments when administered in the setting of acute bleeding. Sigmoidoscopy should be reserved for the evaluation of minor LGI bleeding in relatively young patients (≤40 years).

Angiography

Angiography can be diagnostic in up to 75% of cases if the rate of bleeding is ≥0.5 mL/min. This diagnostic and therapeutic modality is usually restricted to cases in which endoscopy is not possible due to large amounts of blood in the gut lumen or when certain treatments are planned (*eg*, vasopressin infusion or embolization). Angiography is particularly useful in the diagnosis and management of isolated vascular malformation. A study compared angiography to urgent colonoscopy and found that colonoscopy had a higher diagnostic yield, but that both were comparable in terms of the control of bleeding, transfusion requirement, rebleeding, need for surgery, length of ICU stay, and patient survival.

Other Techniques

Technetium-labeled RBC scans are often ordered because of the ease of performance of the test and the perception that valuable information is gained. However, these scans rarely provide definitive information regarding the cause or localization of bleeding and cannot provide therapy. The usefulness of RBC scans is quite limited.

Etiology

Diverticular Disease

Diverticuli are the cause of LGI bleeding in 30% of all cases and in 50% of those patients with active hemorrhage who are undergoing angiography. However, diverticuli are very common, and prevalence increases with advancing age.

Upper and Lower GI Bleeding in the ICU (Everson)

Overall, only 3% of patients with diverticulosis coli ever experience LGI bleeding. When bleeding occurs, it is usually sudden, painless, and often from the right colon (in up to 70% of cases). Acute bleeding stops spontaneously in 80% of cases, but 20 to 25% of patients rebleed. The localization of the site of bleeding is essential to plan appropriately for treatment, which may include segmental colonic resection or even subtotal colectomy.

A list of other relatively common causes of LGI bleeding is given in Table 6. Additional rare causes of LGI bleeding include infectious colitis, NSAID ulcers, rectal varices, vasculitis, and juvenile polyps. As with other causes of GI bleeding, treatment is directed at the underlying etiology.

Bibliography

Portal Hypertension

Cales P, Masliah C, Bernard B, et al. Early administration of vapreotide for variceal bleeding in patients with cirrhosis. N Engl J Med 2001; 344:23–28

Cholongitas E, Senzolo M, Patch D, et al. Risk factors, sequential organ failure assessment and model for end-stage liver disease scores for predicting short term mortality in cirrhotic patients admitted to intensive care unit. Aliment Pharmacol Ther 2006; 23:883–893

Cholongitas E, Senzolo M, Patch D, et al. Review article: scoring systems for assessing prognosis in critically ill adult cirrhotics. Aliment Pharmacol Ther 2006; 24:453–464

Corley DA, Cello JP, Adkisson W, et al. Octeotide for acute esophageal variceal bleeding: a meta-analysis. Gastroenterology 2001; 120:946–954

D'Amico G, Garcia-Pagan JC, Luca A, et al. Hepatic vein pressure gradient reduction and prevention of variceal bleeding in cirrhosis: a systemic review. Gastroenterology 2006; 131:1611–1624

Grace ND. Diagnosis and treatment of gastrointestinal bleeding secondary to portal hypertension. Am J Gastroenterol 1997; 92:1081–1091

Grace ND, Bhattacharya K. Pharmacologic therapy of portal hypertension and variceal hemorrhage. Clin Liver Dis 1997; 1:59–75

Pagliaro L, D'Amico G, Sorrenson TA, et al. Prevention of first bleeding in cirrhosis: a meta-analysis of randomized trials of non-surgical treatment. Ann Intern Med 1992; 117:59–70

Yoshida H, Mamada Y, Taniai N, et al. New methods for the management of gastric varices. World J Gastroenterol 2006; 12:5926–5931

UGI Bleeding

Bytzer P, Teglbjaerg PS. *Helicobacter pylori*-negative duodenal ulcers: prevalence, clinical characteristics, and prognosis–results from a randomized trial with 2-year follow-up. Am J Gastroenterol 2001; 96:1409–1416

Ciociola AA, McSorley DJ, Turner K, et al. *Helicobacter pylori* infection rates in duodenal ulcer patients in the United States may be lower than previously estimated. Am J Gastroenterol 1999; 94:1834–1840

Cook D, Heyland D, Griffith L, et al. Risk factors for clinically important upper gastrointestinal bleeding in patients requiring mechanical ventilation. Crit Care Med 1999; 27:2812–2817

Dara SI, Afessa B, Bajwa AA, et al. Outcome of patients with end-stage renal disease admitted to the intensive care unit. Mayo Clin Proc 2004; 79:1385–1390

Ekstrom P, Carling L, Wetterhus S, et al. Prevention of peptic ulcer and dyspeptic symptoms with omeprazole in patients receiving continuous non-steroidal anti-inflammatory drug therapy: a Nordic multicentre study. Scand J Gastroenterol 1996; 31:753–758

Garnett WR. History of acid suppression: focus on the hospital setting. Pharmacotherapy 2003; 23:56S–60S

Gostout CJ, Wang KK, Ahlquist DA. Acute gastrointestinal bleeding: experience of a specialized management team. J Clin Gastroenterol 1992; 14:260–267

Graham DY, Agrawal NM, Campbell DR, et al. Ulcer prevention in long-term users of nonsteroidal anti-inflammatory drugs: results of a double-blind, randomized, multicenter, active- and placebo-controlled study of misoprostol vs lansoprazole. Arch Intern Med 2002; 162:169–175

Higgins TL, Teres D, Copes WS, et al. Assessing contemporary intensive care unit outcome: an updated Mortality Probability Admission Model (MPM0-III). Crit Care Med 2007; 35:827–835

Kaviani MJ, Hashemi MR, Kazemifar AR, et al. Effect of oral omeprazole in reducing re-bleeding in bleeding peptic ulcers: a prospective, double-blind, randomized, clinical trial. Aliment Pharmacol Ther 2003; 17:211–216

Lai KC, Lam SK, Chu KM, et al. Lansoprazole for the prevention of recurrences of ulcer complications from long-term low-dose aspirin use. N Engl J Med 2002; 346:2033–2038

Lau JYW, Sung JJY, Lam YH, et al. Endoscopic retreatment compared with surgery in patients with recurrent bleeding after initial endoscopic control of bleeding ulcers. N Engl J Med 1999; 340:751–756

Lau JY, Sung JJ, Lee KK, et al. Effect of intravenous omeprazole on recurrent bleeding after endoscopic treatment of bleeding peptic ulcers. N Engl J Med 2000; 343:310–336

Maury E, Tankovic J, Ebel A, et al. An observational study of upper gastrointestinal bleeding in intensive care units: is *Helicobacter pylori* the culprit? Crit Care Med 2005; 33:1513–1518

Prendergast HM, Sloan EP, Cumpston K, et al. Myocardial infarction and cardiac complications in emergency department patients admitted to the intensive care unit with gastrointestinal hemorrhage. J Emerg Med 2005; 28:19–25

Rockall TA, Logan RF, Devlin HB, et al. Selection of patients for early discharge or outpatient care after acute upper gastrointestinal haemorrhage: national audit of acute upper gastrointestinal haemorrhage. Lancet 1996; 347:1138–1140

Rockall TA, Logan RFA, Devlin HB, et al. Incidence and mortality from acute gastrointestinal hemorrhage in the United Kingdom. BMJ 1995; 311:222–226

Rockey DC, Koch J, Cello JP, et al. Relative frequency of upper gastrointestinal and colonic lesions in patients with positive fecal occult-blood tests. N Engl J Med 1998; 339:153–159

Van de Louw A, Lasserre N, Drouhin F, et al. Reliability of HemoCue in patients with gastrointestinal bleeding. Intensive Care Med 2007; 33:355–358

Zimmerman J, Siguencia J, Tsvang E. Predictors of mortality in patients admitted to hospital for acute gastrointestinal hemorrhage. Scand J Gastroenterol 1995; 30:327–331

LGI Bleed

Bokhari M, Vernava AM, Ure T, et al. Diverticular hemorrhage in the elderly: is it well-tolerated? Dis Colon Rectum 1996; 39:191–195

Green BT, Rockey DC, Portwood G, et al. Urgent colonoscopy for evaluation and management of acute lower gastrointestinal hemorrhage: a randomized controlled trial. Am J Gastroenterol 2005; 100: 2395–2402

Lin C-C, Lee Y-C, Lee H, et al. Bedside colonoscopy for critically ill patients with acute lower gastrointestinal bleeding. Intensive Care Med 2005; 31:743–746

Richter JM, Christensen MR, Kaplan LM, et al. Effectiveness of current technology in the diagnosis and management of lower gastrointestinal hemorrhage. Gastrointest Endosc 1994; 41:93–98

Tachycardias: Diagnosis and Management

James A. Roth, MD

Objectives:

- Understand the basic mechanisms underlying arrhythmogenesis
- Recognize and understand the mechanism of the common paroxysmal supraventricular tachycardia syndromes
- Understand the mechanisms and management of atrial arrhythmias, including focal atrial tachycardia, atrial flutter, and atrial fibrillation
- Understand the management of ventricular tachycardia and ventricular fibrillation in the setting of structural heart disease
- Understand and recognize the various ventricular tachycardia syndromes that occur in the absence of evident structural heart disease, including idiopathic ventricular tachycardia, occult arrhythmogenic right ventricular cardiomyopathy/dysplasia, and the cardiac ion channel diseases including long QT syndrome

Key words: atrial fibrillation; atrial flutter; idiopathic ventricular tachycardia; long QT syndrome; sudden cardiac death; supraventricular tachycardia; ventricular fibrillation; ventricular tachycardia

Tachyarrhythmias

Tachycardia presents a different range of clinical problems than bradycardia. Whereas bradycardias may be amenable to pharmacologic palliation, clinically significant bradycardia can always be addressed definitively by electrical pacing. As a consequence, bradycardia rarely presents an ongoing management conundrum. By contrast, the management of pathologic tachycardia requires an assessment of mechanism and selection of appropriate management based on this assessment. In the case of tachyarrhythmias, identifying the underlying tachycardia mechanism, its associated pathophysiology, and exploitation of the likely vulnerabilities of the tachycardia is the key to successful management. Consequently, tachycardia management is more complex and challenging than the management of bradycardia. Although the mechanisms of tachyarrhythmias encountered in critically ill patients are the same as those encountered in other settings, acute arrhythmias in the ICU often can be traced to a proximate cause related to the acute illness requiring intensive care. New arrhythmias presenting in the ICU setting are always secondary to either some aspect of the patient's critical illness itself, or alternatively the therapy being used, with good intention, to manage that acute illness. As such, the intensivist is at a potential advantage, being in a position to potentially identify the proximate cause of the arrhythmia and, if possible, remove that cause.

The range of tachyarrhythmias is wide and classified broadly into supraventricular arrhythmias and ventricular arrhythmias. Supraventricular arrhythmias are defined as those in which the mechanism depends on the atrium, the atrioventricular (AV) node, or both. By contrast, ventricular arrhythmias are defined as those in which the mechanism is not dependent on either the atrium or AV node. Although it is commonly believed that ventricular arrhythmias are more dangerous than atrial arrhythmias, this is not necessarily true.

Pathologic tachycardias are attributable to three mechanisms: abnormal automaticity, triggered automaticity, and reentry. Although cells in the specialized conduction system are normally capable of intrinsic automaticity, the working myocardium does not normally exhibit automaticity. However under some conditions, cells may exhibit abnormal automaticity, which may result in either salvos or continuous rapid activity. A related phenomenon is triggered automaticity. Triggered arrhythmias are initiated by afterdepolarizations. Afterdepolarizations that reach threshold will result in a propagated beat. Afterdepolarizations occurring before complete repolarization are referred to as *early afterdepolarizations*. Early afterdepolarizations are promoted by long-action potential durations, hypokalemia, and hypomagnesemia. They can be triggered by pauses that further prolong repolarization and are, therefore, bradycardia-dependent. They are believed to be causal in the premature beats, which initiate torsades de pointes in long QT syndrome. Afterdepolarizations occurring after full repolarization are referred to as *delayed afterdepolarizations* (DADs). DADs are promoted by intracellular calcium overload and are triggered by tachycardia or rapid pacing. DADs are the cause of ventricular arrhythmias in digitalis toxicity and are likely causal in various calcium-channel blocker-responsive arrhythmias including focal atrial tachycardia (AT) and some forms of idiopathic ventricular tachycardia (VT). Automatic mechanisms are generally self-reinitiating and hence not responsive to electrical cardioversion.

Reentry is a distinct arrhythmia mechanism that because of its propensity to cause sustained rapid arrhythmias is the major mechanism of clinically significant tachyarrhythmias. Whereas abnormal automaticity and triggered automaticity are cellular phenomena, reentry is a macroscopic tissue phenomenon requiring large populations of cells. The normal heart is designed to prevent reentry by maintaining adequate propagation velocities, long-enough refractory periods, and small-enough chamber sizes to discourage reentry from occurring. However under appropriate conditions, reentry can promote continuous and often sustained tachycardia. The requirements for reentry are unidirectional block, a region of slowed conduction, and either an anatomic or functional obstacle that forms an anchor point for the reentrant wave front to circulate around or through. Reentry is initiated by a premature beat that finds one path refractory or blocked, and finds a second functioning alternate pathway available. The functioning pathway must conduct with adequate delay to permit the previously refractory muscle to recover and be reactivated later in the cardiac cycle. Reentrant arrhythmias are inducible by rapid stimulation or ectopic beats, and may also be terminated by the same methods. They are amenable to electrical cardioversion or defibrillation.

Supraventricular Tachycardias

Supraventricular arrhythmias may be broadly classified as the syndrome of paroxysmal supraventricular tachycardia (SVT), and a distinct group of atrial arrhythmias including atrial fibrillation (AF), atrial flutter (AFL), and AT. The term *SVT* is usually reserved for the common paroxysmal SVT syndrome and atrial arrhythmias are considered separately. The syndromes are distinguished both by mechanism and by clinical presentation. Paroxysmal SVT is commonly seen in otherwise normal patients with recurrent, abrupt, and often sustained palpitations due to stable SVT. Atrial arrhythmias may be paroxysmal or persistent and are often associated with underlying structural heart disease or atrial enlargement. As their mechanism and clinical implications are distinct, atrial arrhythmias will be addressed separately.

Paroxysmal SVT

The incidence of SVT is 35 cases per 100,000 persons per year, and prevalence is approximately 2.5/1,000.[1] The syndrome is characterized by recurrent bouts of rapid palpitations often leading to emergency department or physician visits. Symptoms related to unremitting tachycardia, in addition to palpitations, may include dyspnea, diaphoresis, lightheadedness and, occasionally, especially at tachycardia onset before vascular adaptations to tachycardia, syncope, or presyncope. It is important to emphasize that anginal chest pain is frequent, especially during persistent and rapid tachycardia. Ischemic ST-segment depression is commonly observed on initial ECG and is related to markedly augmented myocardial oxygen demand combined with loss of normal diastolic coronary perfusion time. Such changes are common in patients with SVT, are not a sign of underlying coronary artery disease, and resolve quickly with termination of the tachycardia.

Diagnosis

SVT may present in childhood, commonly in adolescence when the heart achieves adult size, as well as later in life. Although commonly associated with an otherwise normal heart, certain forms of congenital malformations may predispose to SVT. Most types of tachycardia have a reentrant mechanism, with a few well-understood

Tachycardias: Diagnosis and Management (Roth)

conditions accounting for the vast preponderance of episodes. In patients with normal ECG findings in sinus rhythm (ie, with no evidence of a delta wave), the most common cause of paroxysmal SVT is AV nodal reentry, accounting for at least 60% of all patients with SVT. Approximately 30% of cases of paroxysmal SVT are related to an accessory AV pathway that, due to poor antegrade conduction, is not evident on ECG. This condition is usually referred to as *concealed Wolff Parkinson White* (WPW) syndrome. The remaining 10% are related to an assortment of mechanisms, including focal AT and physiologically inappropriate sinus tachycardia. The other important group of patients are those with the ECG pattern of WPW, which is related to an accessory AV connection with visible antegrade conduction in sinus rhythm. Although the most common arrhythmia seen in WPW is clinically very similar to other forms of paroxysmal SVT, WPW allows for several other more complex arrhythmias and additionally carries a small but real risk of sudden death.

As the underlying mechanism of SVT is rarely known at the time of clinical presentation, it is helpful to develop an approach to such arrhythmias to guide management. The most convenient strategy is to assess the AV relationship during tachycardia. If the P-wave is embedded (and hence difficult or impossible to perceive during tachycardia) or follows close on the heels of the preceding QRS complex, the arrhythmia is classified as a *short RP tachycardia*. By contrast, if the P-wave follows long after the preceding QRS, in particular when the RP is comparable to or longer than the next PR interval during tachycardia, the arrhythmia is classified as a *long RP tachycardia*.

Short RP Tachycardias: Tachycardias exhibit a short RP pattern when retrograde VA conduction time is short relative to antegrade AV conduction time. This is the case in the two most common paroxysmal forms of SVT: typical AV nodal reentry tachycardia, and reciprocating AV tachycardia related to WPW.

Long RP Tachycardias: Tachycardias exhibit a long RP pattern on ECG if retrograde conduction time back to the atrium is long due to a slowly conducting retrograde pathway during tachycardia. The most common cause of this is atypical

AV node reentry, in which retrograde conduction is via the slow AV nodal pathway, resulting in a long RP interval. Slower ATs may also give a long RP interval appearance on ECG, due to a normal short PR during tachycardia.

AV Nodal Reentry Tachycardia

Far and away the most common form of paroxysmal SVT, atrioventricular nodal reentry tachycardia (AVNRT), is seen frequently in young healthy patients but also commonly presents later in life. Long before the advent of curative ablation or identification of the anatomic substrate of this arrhythmia, the mechanism was recognized to be related to two distinct pathways at the level of the AV node: one with a long conduction time but short refractory period (the "slow pathway"), and the other with a short conduction time but longer refractory period (the "fast pathway"). With the insights gained with catheter ablation, it has become apparent that these pathways actually correspond to the posterior and anterior atrial insertions into the AV node. The posterior insertions needing to traverse the entire compact AV node to activate the His bundle account for the long conduction time, and the anterior insertion bypassing much of the compact AV node account for a shorter conduction time to the His bundle. The existence of these dual pathways is believed to be a normal feature of the AV node. Patients with tachycardia appear to differ from normal subjects by the presence of more robust conduction down the slow pathway than the fast. Under these conditions, a spontaneous and unrelated premature atrial contraction may block in the fast pathway and conduct exclusively down the slow pathway, generating a long PR interval and, if delay is adequate, permitting recovery of fast pathway conduction in time to permit retrograde conduction back to the atrium and initiating reentry down the slow pathway and up the fast pathway. As retrograde conduction time up the fast pathway is short, and antegrade conduction time down the slow pathway is long, this tachycardia is characterized by a very short RP interval. In fact RP is so short during typical slow-fast AVNRT that the P-wave is entirely

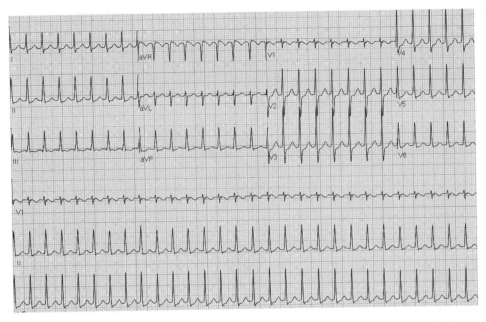

Figure 1. Typical AVNRT. This is a "short-RP" tachycardia mediated by conduction down the AV node slow pathway and retrograde up the AV node fast pathway. As is common for this arrhythmia, the P-wave during tachycardia is not apparent because it begins within and is mostly, if not completely, obscured by the QRS complex. Sometimes a careful comparison with a sinus rhythm ECG on the same patient will reveal subtle changes in the QRS morphology such as a small "pseudo" R or S wave, which is the only reflection of the P-wave in the QRS during tachycardia. EP testing confirmed the mechanism of this tachycardia, which was cured by slow pathway ablation.

obscured by the QRS in the majority of patients, making it entirely unapparent by ECG (Fig 1). As ongoing tachycardia is dependent on AV nodal conduction, either spontaneous or drug-induced failure of AV nodal conduction, for even a single beat generally results in immediate termination of tachycardia. Drug therapy of this tachycardia is directed at the AV node. When symptoms are problematic or drug therapy not tolerated or desired, catheter ablation of the slow pathway at the posterior AV node is highly successful in elimination of the arrhythmia with a >90% success rate and a low risk of complications. Typical AVNRT is due to conduction down the slow pathway and up the fast. As might be suspected, it is also possible for patients to have tachycardia mediated by conduction down the fast pathway and up the slow, and this is referred to as *atypical AVNRT*. Atypical is considerably less common than typical AVNRT and leads to a long RP pattern on ECG with very obvious deeply inverted retrograde P-waves in leads 2, 3, and aVF. A sample of this tachycardia is shown in Figure 2. It is responsive to similar drugs and interventions as the much more common typical slow-fast AVNRT.

Reciprocating AV Tachycardia

The second most common cause of paroxysmal SVT is reciprocating AV tachycardia. Reciprocating tachycardia is an AV arrhythmia requiring participation of both the atrium and ventricle in the tachycardia. It is dependent on the presence of an extranodal AV connection, referred to as an *accessory pathway* or equivalently a *Kent bundle*. Accessory pathways are AV muscle fibers with behavior similar to working myocardium. They are a consequence of incomplete development of the AV annulus, which normally results in a complete fibrous annulus throughout the AV groove with the exception of the penetrating His bundle. If capable of antegrade conduction, the presence of early activation of the ventricle in sinus rhythm, prior to conduction through the normal AV conduction system, results in shortening of the PR interval and slurring of the QRS onset referred to as a *delta wave* (Fig 3). By contrast, if the pathway is not capable of antegrade conduction, the ECG in sinus rhythm will lack a delta wave and appear totally normal; however, the patient may still be susceptible to AV tachycardia due to the presence

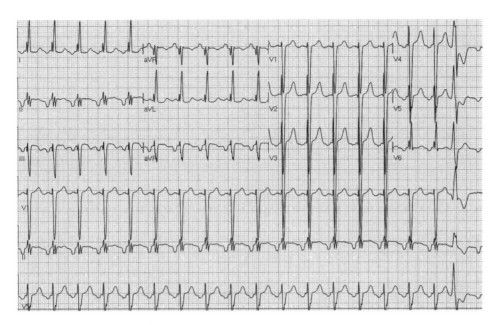

Figure 2. Atypical AVNRT. This is a "long-RP" tachycardia. This example is relatively slow, at approximately 115/min. It is mediated by antegrade conduction down the fast pathway, resulting in a normal PR interval during tachycardia, followed by retrograde conduction back up the slow AV nodal pathway, resulting in a very long RP interval in this patient. The P-wave during this tachycardia is characteristically deeply inverted in the inferior leads. This ECG could also be compatible with a focal AT but, in this patient's case, the arrhythmia was readily initiated by PVCs and terminated abruptly with AV block, both features which are unexpected with AT. EP testing confirmed the mechanism of this tachycardia, which was cured by ablation of the slow pathway.

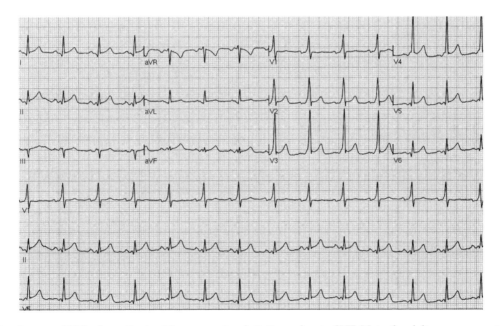

Figure 3. WPW pattern on ECG of a patient with recurrent palpitations due to SVT. Note the delta waves most obvious as a positive going slur of the QRS onset in V_1 to V_4. A positive delta wave in V_1 indicated a left-sided pathway, a strongly negative delta wave in V_1 indicates a right-sided pathway, and an indeterminate/isoelectric delta wave indicates a paraseptal or septal location. The ECG showing SVT in Figure 4 is the same patient in ORT. Note the absence of delta waves when in tachycardia. At EP testing, this pathway was confirmed to be left sided and treated by catheter ablation.

of retrograde conduction up the pathway. The presence of a functioning pathway capable of good retrograde conduction and hence able to support tachycardia but unapparent on ECG as it lacks antegrade conduction is referred to as *concealed* WPW.

Whether manifest or concealed WPW, the most common tachycardia associated with an accessory pathway is mediated by conduction down the AV node to the ventricle followed by retrograde conduction up the accessory pathway to the atrium and back down the AV node.

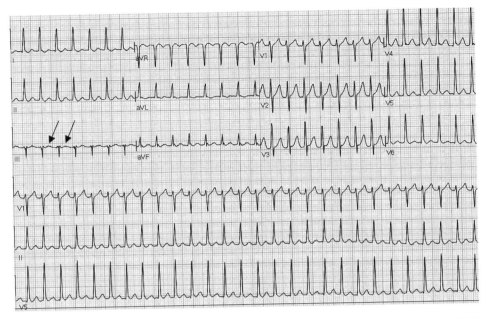

Figure 4. ORT related to underlying WPW. This tachycardia occurred in the patient whose sinus rhythm ECG is shown in Figure 3. This is also a "short-RP" tachycardia like AV nodal reentry. However in WPW, activation must traverse the His-Purkinje system, then the ventricular myocardium before arriving at the accessory pathway and propagating back to the atrium. This results in a retrograde P-wave that is usually easily visible in the ST segment following the QRS (arrows) and not buried within it as is the case in typical AV node reentry. Also note that the delta waves are absent during the most common form of tachycardia in WPW. As the patient was symptomatic and had manifest WPW on ECG, he was subjected to EP testing and underwent ablation that eliminates the clinical tachycardia as well as any risk of sudden death from future rapidly conducted AF.

This tachycardia is referred to as *orthodromic reciprocating AV tachycardia* (ORT) because it conducts in the normal antegrade or "orthodromic" direction down the normal conduction system. Like AV nodal reentry, this tachycardia results in a "short RP" pattern on ECG and is absolutely dependent on 1:1 AV conduction. A single failure to conduct either antegrade via the AV node or retrograde up the accessory pathway will result in immediate termination of the tachycardia. It is very important to emphasize that this tachycardia is almost identical in appearance and clinical behavior to typical AVNRT. Both are "short-RP" tachycardias, and because the accessory pathway is monopolized serving retrograde conduction during tachycardia, the QRS complex in ORT is usually narrow and the delta wave absent during tachycardia regardless of its presence or absence in sinus rhythm (Fig 4). However, whereas the most common tachycardia in WPW is clinically similar to typical AVNRT, if the accessory pathway is also capable of antegrade conduction as evidenced by a delta wave on ECG in sinus rhythm, special considerations apply.

Special Considerations in Patients With SVT and Delta Waves on Sinus Rhythm ECG

Patients with delta waves on ECG without symptoms are said to have *WPW pattern* and generally have an excellent prognosis. Further evaluation and therapy are not generally indicated. Rarely, such patients may be subjected to electrophysiologic testing and ablation if they participate in activities in which a poorly tolerated arrhythmia would entail undo risk. Patients with delta waves on ECG and associated SVT or symptoms compatible with tachycardia such as palpitations or syncope are said to have *WPW syndrome*. All patients with WPW and associated symptoms are at potential risk for sudden death and require additional evaluation, commonly electrophysiology (EP) testing and, if a competent accessory pathway is identified, catheter ablation. Because of the common need to perform EP testing to stratify risk in WPW syndrome and the high efficacy of ablation, it has become very rare to carry adults with symptomatic WPW on medical therapy and not proceed with ablation.

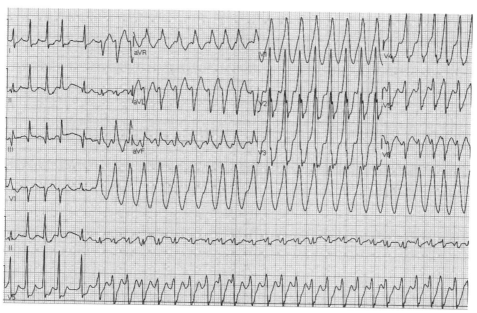

Figure 5. Preexcited AF with underlying WPW. The term *preexcited* means that the ventricle is activated before activation via the normal conduction system. This is the arrhythmia that one worries about in any patient with manifest WPW on ECG and symptoms. The salient features are the presence of a very wide QRS combined with rapid conduction. In this patient, because of relatively good AV node conduction, there are periods of narrow QRS conduction as well, when conduction was predominantly down the AV node instead of the accessory pathway. Also note how wide the QRS is during preexcited AF. This is because conduction is directly into the ventricular myocardium bypassing the conduction system entirely (like a PVC or VT would activate the ventricle). Because the QRS is often so wide with preexcited AF, it is common for this to be misdiagnosed as VT in the emergency setting. Note also that the shortest preexcited (*eg,* down the Kent bundle) RR interval is quite short, at approximately 240 ms (see the third to last cycle on the ECG), indicating that the pathway is capable of very rapid conduction. Conduction >250 ms predicts a risk for sudden death if the pathway is not ablated. This patient underwent ablation and was found to have a left free wall accessory pathway with rapid conduction. Ablation of the pathway in WPW not only eliminates the risk of sudden death but also usually eliminates the AF as well.

WPW Syndrome and AF

The mechanism of sudden death in WPW syndrome has been associated with the degeneration of reciprocating tachycardia into AF, followed by rapid antegrade conduction down the accessory pathway and resultant ventricular fibrillation (VF). The risk of sudden death is eliminated by successful catheter ablation of the accessory pathway, as is the risk of AF in most patients. Because of the malignant potential of AF in the setting of WPW, special considerations apply to its therapy. As WPW syndrome, once symptomatic, is commonly subjected to curative ablation, it is uncommon in this era for a patient with known WPW to present with rapidly conducted AF. In most cases, the presence of underlying WPW will not be known at the time of presentation. The clinician will usually be confronted with an unknown rapid and worrisome ECG and need to suspect WPW in the absence of a sinus rhythm ECG showing delta waves. Therapy for AF in the setting of WPW is quite different from ordinary AF. Therefore, it is important to recognize the ECG signature of AF in the presence of underlying WPW solely from the presenting ECG.

The key feature of rapidly conducted AF due to underlying WPW is the presence of a wide QRS complex during AF (Fig 5). AV conduction via an accessory pathway results in ventricular activation outside of the normal AV conduction system and results in a wide QRS similar to a ventricular focus. No matter how fast AF may conduct, if the QRS complex is narrow, conduction is unrelated to rapid conduction down an accessory pathway, and conventional therapy directed at AV node conduction is safe as in any other patient with AF. However, when conduction is rapid and the QRS is either intermittently or continuously wide, then the possibility of AF with rapid conduction down an accessory pathway must be considered. During AF with underlying WPW, the presence of competing conduction down the AV node paradoxically moderates conduction down the accessory pathway by concealed retrograde activation of the accessory pathway. If AV nodal conduction is impaired by the use of drugs with selective effects on the AV node, antegrade conduction down the accessory pathway may be facilitated leading to hemodynamic collapse or VF. Therefore, when rapidly conducted AF presents with wide QRS conduction, digoxin and calcium-channel blockers should be avoided. As β-blockers have favorable effects on both AV node and accessory pathway conduction, β-blockers may be used with caution in this setting but are commonly avoided as well. The recommended medical therapy is the use of drugs that prolong the refractory period of working myocardium, including IV ibutilide, procainamide or, occasionally, in the setting of left ventricular dysfunction, IV amiodarone.

Atrial Arrhythmias

Atrial arrhythmias are defined as arrhythmias that are entirely dependent on the atria and mechanistically independent of AV conduction. As a consequence, intraatrial arrhythmias will persist despite the development of either spontaneous or pharmacologically induced AV block. Tachycardias originating in the atria may be organized and repetitive resulting from either automaticity or intraatrial reentry, or may be chaotic and disorganized as is the case in AF. Therapy is directed at either moderating the ventricular response during episodes of tachycardia or suppressing the underlying atrial arrhythmia itself.

Focal arrhythmias are defined as arrhythmias originating from a point source within one of the atria with circumferential spread to encompass the rest of the atrium. Such arrhythmias display distinct P-waves separated by a clear isoelectric segment. Focal arrhythmias are commonly automatic in mechanism but in some cases may be due to microreentry involving a geographically small portion of the atrium (for example around a single pulmonary vein) followed by radial spread to the rest of the atrium. Although most commonly a single abnormal focus may be active, in the setting of severe metabolic stress, multiple foci may be active simultaneously leading to a chaotic ECG appearance with multiple distinct P-waves referred to as multifocal AT. Automatic arrhythmias tend to be episodic and unsustained,

at times recurring incessantly. Cycle length often varies within a run and between runs and with changes in autonomic tone.

Macroreentrant atrial arrhythmias are a consequence of stable reentrant circuits that encompass large portions of either atrium. All such circuits require a central obstacle and a region of slowed atrial conduction related to atrial dilatation or fibrosis. The most common of such arrhythmias is typical atrial flutter (AFL) mediated by right atrial reentry around normal anatomic obstacles. In addition to typical AFL, reentry may occur around acquired obstacles, most commonly scar resulting from prior cardiac surgery involving the atria. Reentrant arrhythmias tend to present clinically as paroxysmal sustained or persistent arrhythmias. Although they may be self-terminating and episodic, individual episodes tend to be protracted.

The final mechanism of atrial arrhythmia is AF. The modern understanding of this arrhythmia involves components of both focal automatic mechanisms and reentry. Major advances have been made in the understanding and management of this common arrhythmia in recent years and will be reviewed below.

Focal Atrial Tachycardia

Focal atrial tachycardia (AT) is commonly referred to by one of several eponyms: *focal AT*, *ectopic AT*, or *automatic AT*. All describe a characteristic clinical pattern that generally presents as runs of unifocal premature atrial contractions (PACs) lasting for seconds or minutes, usually followed by spontaneous termination and subsequent spontaneous reinitiation of additional salvos of tachycardia. Although commonly presenting as above, this mechanism can also present less commonly as a paroxysmal sustained tachycardia. When mapped in the EP laboratory, these arrhythmias are focal in origin; and although at times they are triggered by rapid pacing suggesting a triggered automatic mechanism, they appear to be automatic and not reentrant in mechanism. The ECG features are characteristic and usually permit accurate diagnosis. As the arrhythmia is focal and automatic, the morphology of the first PAC of the run is identical to the subsequent PACs. Cycle length tends to vary between and within runs, and tachycardia is unaffected by intermittent AV

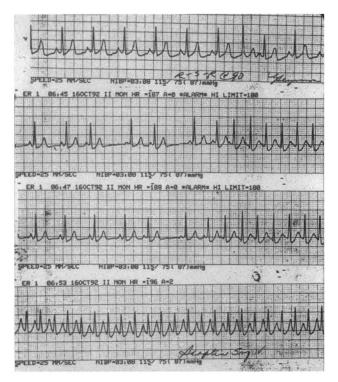

Figure 6. Focal (*eg*, automatic) AT. The tachycardia occurs in salvos with variable cycle lengths. There are frequent isolated PACs as well, and the PAC that initiates each run is the same as all the others during the run indicating a focal mechanism. Electrical cardioversion is useless for this arrhythmia as it is self reinitiating and not dependent on reentry. This arrhythmia tends to respond to nondihydropyridine calcium-channel blockers such as diltiazem or verapamil. When it is frequent and rapid like this, it can result in tachycardia-induced cardiomyopathy like AF. Frequent tachycardia like this is also straightforward to cure by ablation because its frequency makes it easy to map in the EP laboratory.

block that may occur during the runs. The same focus often fires erratically between runs, resulting in frequent atrial ectopy all morphologically identical to the P-wave observed during the runs. An example is shown in Figure 6. The arrhythmia is believed to be due to intracellular calcium overload and resultant triggered automaticity related to DADs making it responsive to calcium and β-blockers. The paroxysmal sustained form of this arrhythmia is also adenosine responsive, giving the false impression of dependence on AV conduction. The use of digoxin may exacerbate triggered causes of AT. Class Ia agents such as procainamide and class Ic agents such as flecainide and propafenone may be used in patients without structural heart disease or coronary artery disease. However, the GI side effects of procainamide and its association with drug-induced lupus limit its utility. Amiodarone can also be used in these patients

for rhythm control as well. The arrhythmia is readily amenable to catheter ablation if ectopy is frequent enough to permit mapping.

Atrial Flutter

Atrial flutter (AFL) is defined as a persistent atrial arrhythmia with an atrial rate ≥250/min. As the normal AV node cannot conduct 1:1 at these rates, this arrhythmia characteristically presents with 2:1 conduction and a ventricular response of approximately 150/min. During 2:1 conduction, the flutter waves may be very difficult to perceive, leading to diagnostic confusion. Typical AFL is the most common form of this arrhythmia and is mediated by macroreentry restricted to the right atrium. The central obstacles in this circuit consist of normal anatomic structures, accounting for its stereotyped presentation.

Typical AFL is mediated by counterclockwise reentry around the tricuspid valve as viewed from the ventricle. The valve prevents anterior collapse of the circuit, and posteriorly a long ridge in the atrial wall referred to as the *crista terminalis* forms a function line of block preventing the circuit from collapsing posteriorly. As the obstacles are already normally present, the ability for flutter to develop is due to the added presence of abnormal slowed conduction related to atrial enlargement, fibrosis, or edema, at times combined with shortened atrial refractory periods due to catecholamine stress in some clinical settings. Typical counterclockwise AFL demonstrates a deeply negative F-wave in 2, 3, and aVF, a sharply positive F-wave in V_1, and a negative F-wave in V_6. An example is shown in Figure 7. A less common reversed typical form of this arrhythmia due to clockwise reentry around the tricuspid demonstrates an ECG exactly opposite to the counterclockwise form with a strongly positive F-wave in 2, 3, and aVF, a sharply negative F-wave in V_1, and positive F-wave in V_6. In both cases, the F-waves are often difficult to perceive when presenting with 2:1 conduction. If the unusual F-wave vector is not recognized, the ECG may be misinterpreted as sinus tachycardia. Clues to the presence of AFL are persistent unexplained heart rates at approximately 150 beats/min, with only a few beats-per-minute variation over time, as well as the presence of a negative P-wave in the inferior leads, which would be

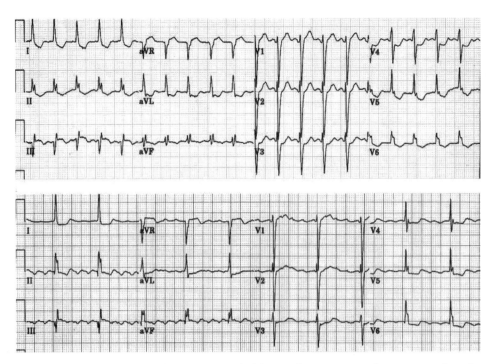

Figure 7. Typical AFL. These two ECGs are as they were recorded first in the emergency department when the patient presented with 2:1 conduction and a day later after rate control. On presentation, it was not initially suspected that this was AFL. Note that the superimposition of the T-wave with the F-waves makes it quite difficult to discern the presence of flutter. Once rate controlled, it is obvious that this is typical counterclockwise AFL with deeply negative F-waves in 2, 3, and aVF and positive F wave in V_1 and negative in V_6. This arrhythmia was confirmed to be due to typical AFL mediated by counterclockwise reentry around the tricuspid valve and readily ablated by creating a linear lesion between the tricuspid annulus and the adjacent inferior vena cava that interrupts the typical flutter circuit.

expected to be positive in sinus rhythm. The most fruitful method of diagnosis is the provocation of transient AV block either with carotid sinus massage or adenosine infusion. This will transiently expose the underlying flutter waves but will not terminate the arrhythmia. Although short-term therapy involves rate control or cardioversion if poorly tolerated, long-term rate control for this arrhythmia is difficult. Doses of drug that result in acceptable block at rest often fail to control exercise rates, and doses that result in exercise rate control often provoke bradycardia at rest. Therefore, early restoration of sinus rhythm is preferred for this arrhythmia.

AFL is a common transient arrhythmia in acute care hospital settings. The right atrial wall is thin, and pericarditis resulting from cardiac or thoracic surgery results in atrial edema and inflammation that may permit adequate slowing and promote transient AFL. Acute pulmonary decompensation may result in right-heart failure and may also promote transient AFL. In all of these settings, endogenous or pharmacologic catecholamine stimulation exacerbates the arrhythmia. Transient therapy for several weeks or a month is appropriate in these settings. When AFL occurs in the absence of an acute precipitant, long-term therapy is required. Given the difficulty achieving rate control in AFL and the need for antiarrhythmic agents with associated potential morbidity to maintain sinus rhythm, catheter ablation has become the primary means of treating this arrhythmia. Antiarrhythmic therapy for AFL is similar to that for AF and will be discussed below. Antiarrhythmic therapy should be reserved for temporary treatment of likely transient flutter or for patients who are not suitable candidates for invasive management. Catheter ablation of typical AFL is a low-risk procedure with a long-term success rate >90% in experienced centers.

Atypical AFL and Reentrant AT

In addition to typical AFL circulating around normal anatomic obstacles, the presence of atrial disease with associated fibrosis or more commonly atrial scars created at the time of cardiac surgery for either valvular or congenital heart disease may create alternative substrates for intraatrial reentry. Common to these arrhythmias is the presence of a significant region of scar with a channel of surviving myocardium either bridging the scar or between the scar and a normal anatomic obstacle. Within the channel, conduction is slow and electrocardiographically silent, resulting in an isoelectric PP interval. As the circuit differs from typical AFL, the P-wave morphology is atypical. When the rate is ≥250/min, the arrhythmia is arbitrarily classified as atypical AFL; and when <250/min, it is arbitrarily classified as AT. Like typical AFL, these arrhythmias are paroxysmal sustained or persistent arrhythmias, and when presenting with 2:1 conduction may be misdiagnosed as sinus tachycardia if the abnormal P-wave vector and fixed heart rate over time is not recognized. Therapy and prognosis are otherwise similar to typical AFL. These arrhythmias are also amenable to catheter ablation. As the circuits are unique, mapping and ablation of these arrhythmias are more complex and success rates are lower than for typical AFL. Therefore, antiarrhythmic therapy is a reasonable first option and similar to that used for AF. Ablation is used selectively in patients who are good candidates for complex ablative procedures. Like typical AFL, long-term rate control is a difficult strategy to successfully implement.

AF

AF is the most common clinically significant arrhythmia, affecting 2.2 million people in the United States. Its prevalence is from 0.4 to 1% in the general population and increases with age, reaching 8% in those >80 years old.[2] Some form of underlying cardiopulmonary disease or hypertension is present in >88% of patients. Hypertension, ischemic heart disease, heart failure, and diabetes are the most common associated conditions. Patients with AF have a higher risk of stroke, heart failure, and death. For uncertain reasons, this relative risk is greater in women than in men. However, the role of AF as an independent determinant of mortality is uncertain because it commonly coexists with other potentially important conditions. In fact, patients with truly lone AF do not have an increase in mortality, and carefully designed trials exploring the benefit of maintenance of sinus rhythm over rate control show no survival benefit to sinus rhythm. Therefore, whether AF is merely a marker for increased mortality or a mechanism remains uncertain.

Mechanisms of AF

Because of its chaotic nature, it has been difficult to study AF, and its mechanisms still remain a topic of hot debate. However, certain aspects have become clear. The initiation of spontaneous AF is a consequence of rapid electrical firing from preferential focal sites of origin. The most common site of focal origin is from left atrial muscle sleeves extending along the outer surface of the pulmonary veins.[3] When firing does not originate from a pulmonary vein, it is commonly from the left atrial tissue immediately adjacent to one of the veins, or occasionally one of the other thoracic veins such as the ostium of the superior vena cava or the ostium of the coronary sinus. Following initiation, atrial rates recorded in and around the pulmonary veins are significantly higher than other atrial sites, suggesting that activity in the region of the veins is important in perpetuating AF following initiation. These profound insights have led to highly effective techniques for the cure of AF. Ablation techniques designed to isolate these trigger sites from the atrium have success rates >70 to 80% in the cure of paroxysmal AF and somewhat lower rates in the cure of persistent AF. That ablation restricted to the region of the pulmonary veins and adjacent left atrium is curative in the majority of patients with AF implies that AF is an arrhythmia that, in most cases, is entirely contained within and maintained by the left atrium and connecting veins. Stated another way, it has become apparent that in the same way that typical AFL is the characteristic arrhythmia of the right atrium, AF is the characteristic arrhythmia of the left atrium.

Antithrombotic Therapy in AF

The overall risk of stroke in AF is 5%/yr and is associated with one in every six strokes. Multiple risk factors have been identified that predict a higher risk of stroke, including age, gender, presence of rheumatic mitral disease, prior thromboembolism or stroke, heart failure, left ventricular dysfunction, left atrial enlargement, ischemic heart disease, hypertension, and diabetes. However, these risk factors are not all independent, and the risk of stroke can be accurately estimated with only a subset of weighted factors. The CHADS$_2$ (Cardiac failure, Hypertension, Age, Diabetes, and Stroke × 2) score is a useful and well-validated clinical means of assessing stroke risk in patients with AF. The score assigns 1 point for a history of each of heart failure, hypertension, age ≥ 75 years, and diabetes, and 2 points for a history of prior stroke. A score of 0 implies a relatively low risk of 1.9%/yr, a score of 1 implies an intermediate risk of 2.8%/yr, a score of 2 implies a risk of 4.0%/yr, and a score ≥ 3 implies an annual stroke risk of > 5.9%/yr. Studies of warfarin in prevention of stroke in AF have demonstrated a significant reduction the risk of stroke, which overall including all major studies is modest at a 33% reduction. However, larger benefits were seen in studies enrolling higher-risk patients and small benefits (as little as 10%) in lower-risk patients. These studies also documented an average 1.2% rate of major hemorrhage during therapy with warfarin. Given these considerations, warfarin has been recommended in patient groups with higher annual risks of stroke and should be avoided in groups at low risk because the risk may outweigh the relatively small benefit in these low-risk groups. The current recommendations for antithrombotic therapy are contained in the American College of Cardiology/American Heart Association/European Society of Cardiology 2006 AF practice guideline,[2] and are similar to the CHADS$_2$. Moderate risk factors are defined as age ≥ 75 years, hypertension, heart failure, left ventricular ejection fraction (EF) ≤ 35, and diabetes. High risk factors are defined as previous stroke, transient ischemic attack or embolism, mitral stenosis, or presence of a prosthetic heart valve. In this scheme, patients with no risk factors should receive aspirin, 81 to 325 mg/d. Patients with only one moderate risk factor can be offered either aspirin or adjusted-dose warfarin with a target range of 2.0 to 3.0. Patients with more than one moderate risk factor or any high risk factor should be placed on adjusted-dose warfarin 2.0 to 3.0, or if a mechanical heart valve is present a target of 2.5 to 3.5. The practice guideline also recommends that patients with AFL be treated with antithrombotic therapy, as would

be the case if the arrhythmia were AF. Epidemiologic data also suggest that patients with intermittent AF have a similar risk of stroke to those with permanent AF. Therefore, the guideline suggests that these groups be treated similarly. When using warfarin it is important to target a range of 2.0 to 3.0 and attempt to remain in this range as much as possible. The risk of thromboembolism rises sharply with international normalized ratios (INRs) ≤ 1.8, so it is generally a bad strategy to target "low therapeutic" INRs in the hope of preventing bleeding. To avoid this, dosing should be targeted squarely at 2.5, which is at the middle of the therapeutic range.

Management of Anticoagulation Around Cardioversion

In the preantithrobotic era, cardioversion of AF was associated with a significant risk of thromboembolism. This typically occurred days to weeks after cardioversion and not at the moment of conversion. It is believed that the delayed presentation of thromboembolism following cardioversion is related to atrial stunning due to the period of prior AF and associated atrial remodeling. Hence, there is a time delay between restoration of electrical sinus rhythm and recovery of mechanical atrial function. The risk of thromboembolism appears to be independent of the means of cardioversion employed, whether electrical or pharmacologic. To minimize the risk of thromboembolism, it is recommended that patients with AF of > 48 h in duration undergo at least 3 weeks of therapeutic anticoagulation with a target INR between 2.0 and 3.0 prior to an additional 3 weeks of anticoagulation following successful restoration of sinus rhythm. Following this, the decision to continue anticoagulation is based on an assessment of the patient's risk for long-term thromboembolism. If the patient was receiving anticoagulation at the time of AF onset or if anticoagulation was started in the first 48 h, then it is safe to proceed with cardioversion without a 3-week run in. In addition, performance of a transesophageal echocardiography and exclusion of left atrial thrombi permit safe early cardioversion without the need for prior anticoagulation. However, in either case, anticoagulation must be continued for at least 3 weeks after conversion if the duration of AF was > 48 h before cardioversion. Finally, if the duration of AF is known to be < 48 h, the risk of thromboembolism is low and cardioversion may be safely performed without anticoagulation either before or after the procedure.

Short-term Management of AF: Rate Control

The short-term management of AF centers on the control of ventricular response, the timely restoration of sinus rhythm, and the identification of potentially reversible factors that may have precipitated the arrhythmia. AF with rapid ventricular response results in acute deterioration in stroke volume and cardiac output as well as increase in myocardial oxygen demand and the potential for coronary ischemia. Patients who are symptomatic must be controlled promptly. When pursuing rate control for acute AF of recent onset, the fastest way to achieve rate control is the restoration of sinus rhythm. Therefore, if rate control proves difficult or not well tolerated, early recourse to cardioversion should be undertaken.

Tachycardia-Induced Cardiomyopathy: In addition to the acute homodynamic consequences of rapidly conducted AF, a more subtle but important process occurs when rapid rates persist for weeks to months without control. This is the development of tachycardia-induced cardiomyopathy, which represents a true cardiomyopathy that is not simply a consequence of acute hemodynamic consequence of rapid rates. Tachycardia-induced cardiomyopathy occurs in the setting of resting rates significantly >100 beats/min. It should be suspected in a patient presenting with rapidly conducted AF, not because of the development of palpitations, but for subacute symptoms of progressive congestive heart failure occurring over many weeks or months. On evaluation, such patients will exhibit a typical dilated cardiomyopathy that is clinically indistinguishable from idiopathic dilated cardiomyopathy. However, if rate control or restoration to sinus rhythm are achieved, the cardiomyopathy will resolve over several months, often with return of normal ventricular function. When pursuing rate control, it is therefore critical to target a resting heart rate well < 100 beats/min to prevent the development of cardiomyopathy. By contrast, stress heart rates appear not to be related to the development of

cardiomyopathy, and rate control is adjusted with the intent of moderating symptoms of dyspnea and palpitations associated with high exercise rates but not for prognostic reasons.

For the short-term control of rapidly conducted AF, IV administration of a β-blocker (esmolol, metoprolol, or propranolol) or a non-dihydropyridine calcium-channel blocker (diltiazem or verapamil) is preferred. In the setting of decompensated heart failure, the use of a calcium blocker may exacerbate heart failure and should be avoided. In this setting, digoxin is a useful agent for resting rate control. Digoxin is also a useful second-line drug in addition to a β-blocker or calcium-channel blocker for resting rate control. If such therapy is ineffective or not tolerated, then IV amiodarone is a useful rate control agent, especially in the setting of congestive heart failure, and additionally may facilitate restoration of sinus rhythm. As noted above, rapidly conducted AF related to WPW can be paradoxically accelerated by calcium-channel blockers and digoxin, and these drugs should be avoided. Although in most clinical settings, any of these agents may be useful, atrial arrhythmias occurring in the ICU setting often are exacerbated by, or even primarily related to, the catecholamine stress of acute illness. If this is suspected, then withdrawal of β-adrenergic pharmacotherapy and the early use of β-blocker therapy may prove strikingly effective.

Short-term Management of AF: Restoration of Sinus Rhythm

When sinus rhythm is restored in the first 48 h of acute AF, the thromboembolic risk is low and anticoagulation is not indicated. For this reason, new-onset AF should be managed with a plan to restore sinus rhythm during this period if possible. At least half of AF episodes of new onset will terminate spontaneously in the first 24 to 48 h. Therefore, if well tolerated, it may be reasonable to wait until the next day before considering cardioversion. However if AF persists for >24 h, it is strategic to plan for either pharmacologic or electrical cardioversion before the 48-h window expires. A reasonable strategy is to pursue rate control and possibly antiarrhythmic drugs in the first 24 h, and then make the patient "nothing by mouth" and proceed with electrical cardioversion on the following day if sinus rhythm is not restored.

Pharmacologic Conversion of AF: Pharmacologic conversion of AF can be undertaken when restoration of sinus rhythm is not urgent. Several antiarrhythmic drugs have been shown to be effective in increasing the rate of early conversion of AF. Pharmacologic conversion is generally more successful with AF of recent onset than when chronic. Oral agents with efficacy in the early conversion of AF include flecainide, propafenone, and dofetilide. Oral amiodarone and sotalol have been associated with a 27% and 24% conversion rates,[4] respectively, but occurring late after 28 days of therapy. However, due to low early conversion rates, these drugs are not recommended orally for conversion. IV agents with efficacy for early conversion include ibutilide and amiodarone. Ibutilide is limited by a relatively high 4% rate of drug-induced QT prolongation and torsades de pointes VT. This risk is even higher in the setting of left ventricular dysfunction, electrolyte disturbances, or heart failure. Therefore, ibutilide should be reserved for the pharmacologic conversion of stable patients with a baseline normal QT interval. By contrast, IV amiodarone is well tolerated in unstable patients as are commonly seen in the ICU setting, and is the preferred pharmacologic agent for conversion in the critically ill.

Electrical Cardioversion of AF: Electrical cardioversion should be performed urgently in the case of severe compromise related to acute AF including angina, heart failure, hypotension, or shock. Cardioversion should also be attempted at least once electively in all cases of new-onset AF regardless of toleration. When performing electrical cardioversion, an anterior posterior patch or paddle position is more effective than the conventional anterior to lateral patch/paddle position used for ventricular defibrillation. Although low-output discharges may be effective in some patients, a strategy of starting at higher outputs decreases the number of shocks required and the average cumulative energy delivered. Therefore, an initial shock energy of at least 200 J for an older monophasic defibrillator or a minimum output of 100 J with a newer biphasic device is recommended. Following a failed initial shock, full output should be used for the next attempt. If full output shocks are ineffective, then cardioversion success can be increased by several maneuvers. Direct anterior-posterier compression over the anterior patch and timing of shock delivery to end-expiration will decrease thoracic impedance and facilitate cardioversion. Administration of an antiarrhythmic drug may also facilitate conversion. IV ibutilide significantly improves conversion success in this setting. Oral pretreatment with amiodarone, sotalol, flecainide, or propafenone may also increase defibrillation success as well as decrease the chance of relapse after successful cardioversion.

Long-term Maintenance of Sinus Rhythm

Despite the association of AF with an increase in stroke and all-cause mortality, no study to date has established a benefit to pharmacologic maintenance of sinus rhythm in terms of stroke risk or survival. This may be because AF is merely a marker and not a mechanism of stroke and mortality. It may also be a consequence of the relative inefficacy of pharmacologic therapy in the maintenance of sinus rhythm and the difficulty establishing if patients believed to be in sinus rhythm are in fact consistently in sinus rhythm in follow-up. The largest and best designed trial addressing this issue was the Atrial Fibrillation Follow-up Investigation of Rhythm Management trial,[5] which included 4,060 patients randomly assigned to a strategy of rhythm control with antiarrhythmic drugs, most commonly amiodarone, and a strategy of rate control without attempts to maintain sinus rhythm. The Atrial Fibrillation Follow-up Investigation of Rhythm Management trial demonstrated no advantage in stroke or mortality with a strategy of maintenance of sinus rhythm over rate control. Therefore, at our current state of knowledge, either strategy can be offered to patients with an expectation of similar outcomes with regard to hard end points. Usually the decision to pursue sinus rhythm involves the management of symptoms that, in selected patients, may be better addressed by maintaining sinus rhythm.

In the absence of antiarrhythmic drugs, approximately 80% of patients will relapse over the first year following cardioversion of AF. Antiarrhythmic drugs remain the primary strategy

Tachycardias: Diagnosis and Management (Roth)

for maintaining sinus rhythm following cardioversion as well as the prevention of symptomatic episodes in patients with paroxysmal AF. All antiarrhythmic drugs have the potential for proarrhythmia, the unintended precipitation of a new arrhythmic problem caused by the drug. Adverse rhythm effects of drugs may include sinus node dysfunction, heart block, promotion of drug-slowed AFL permitting rapid 1:1 conduction, and promotion of potentially lethal ventricular arrhythmias. In addition, class I drugs such as flecainide, propafenone, and disopyramide may result in significant myocardial depression and exacerbation of heart failure. The array of potential adverse effects of antiarrhythmic drugs is beyond the scope of this chapter, but certain essential concepts are important to recognize. The class I drugs such as flecainide and propafenone, which work by slowing conduction, have a high risk of ventricular proarrhythmia and potential for sudden death in the setting of heart failure, left ventricular dysfunction, and coronary artery disease. Use of these drugs is restricted to patients with preserved cardiac function and no evidence of obstructive coronary artery disease. However, in this selected group of patients with normal hearts, these drugs are exceedingly safe, well tolerated, and often effective. The conventional class III drugs, which prolong repolarization and refractoriness, including sotalol and dofetilide, are safe in the presence of coronary artery disease and in the case of dofetilide with congestive heart failure. However, these drugs may provoke torsades de pointes, even in patients with normal cardiac function, and must be used with caution. Amiodarone has a higher long-term efficacy than other drugs and a lower risk of proarrhythmia; however, long-term somatic toxicity limits the use of this drug to older patients or those with limited expected longevity or inability to safely tolerate alternate agents due to advanced cardiac disease or proarrhythmia on alternate agents. In addition to being useful agents for the prevention of AF, sotalol and amiodarone also provide substantial rate control during relapses of AF. However, rate control with other antiarrhythmic agents is not adequate to prevent rapid conduction with relapse, and some drugs may actually accelerate response at the time of relapse. Therefore, antiarrhythmic drugs other than sotalol or amiodarone

must be combined with a rate control agent such as a β-blocker or nondihydropyridine calcium-channel blocker during long-term therapy.

Catheter ablation of AF is now an important secondary strategy for maintenance of sinus rhythm. It is now routinely available in most centers performing complex ablation procedures, and success rates approaching 70 to 80% can be routinely achieved in patients with paroxysmal AF and relatively preserved cardiac function. Cure of persistent and permanent AF can also be achieved but with lower success rates, but responsiveness to previously ineffective drugs is achieved in a significant fraction of patients who are not completely cured by ablation. Finally, the older technique of AV node ablation can be used to create complete heart block, which when combined with a pacemaker permits nonpharmacologic rate control but does not prevent ongoing fibrillation within the atrium. Patients with pacemakers and prior AV node ablation will require ongoing anticoagulation because underlying AF is not prevented by simple AV node ablation. With the availability of curative AF ablation, AV node ablation has taken on a secondary role for patients who cannot tolerate a complex ablative procedure or are otherwise not good candidates for curative AF ablation.

Ventricular Arrhythmias and Sudden Cardiac Death

Cardiac death is the most common cause of death in the United States, and cardiac arrest remains the most common mechanism of cardiac death. Despite substantial advances in the early treatment of cardiac arrest, most persons who experience an out-of-hospital cardiac arrest do not survive. Those who do survive may have permanent neurologic impairment. Sustained VT and VF are the most common causes of cardiac arrest; in >90% of cases, obstructive coronary artery disease is present at autopsy.

Ventricular Ectopy and Nonsustained VT

VT is defined as three or more consecutive ventricular beats at a rate >100/min. Sustained

VT is VT that does not end without specific intervention; however, for the purposes of clinical classification, VT lasting >30 s is classified as sustained even if spontaneous termination occurs after 30 s. VT lasting three beats up to 30 s is classified as nonsustained. Nonsustained ventricular arrhythmias including premature ventricular contractions and nonsustained VT are common in the presence of left ventricular dysfunction, and nonsustained VT is associated with a higher risk of sudden death in patients with coronary artery disease and left ventricular dysfunction. Although there is a statistical association, whether such asymptomatic ventricular ectopy and nonsustained arrhythmia is causally linked to death or merely an associated finding not directly linked has been a matter of much debate. In the 1980s, attempts to systematically suppress these arrhythmias with antiarrhythmic drugs in the Cardiac Arrhythmia Suppression Trial[6] proved that the class I drugs in common use at that time, despite suppression of nonsustained tachycardia, markedly increased sudden death, and overall mortality. Subsequent studies in the 1990s testing amiodarone in the European Myocardial Infarct Amiodarone Trial[7] and the Canadian Amiodarone Myocardial Infarction Arrhythmia Trial,[8] a drug with much lower proarrhythmic potential, did not demonstrate an increase in mortality but again failed to show a significant mortality benefit despite substantial suppression of spontaneous nonsustained arrhythmias. These findings have supported the present concept that nonsustained ventricular arrhythmias are not mechanistically linked to the sustained poorly tolerated arrhythmias that eventuate in sudden death, and that asymptomatic nonsustained arrhythmias and ventricular ectopy should not be pursued as a therapeutic target in the hopes that such therapy will reduce the future risk of death.

Sustained VT and Secondary Prevention of Sudden Death

Sustained VT is associated with underlying cardiovascular pathology in >90% of cases, most commonly chronic ischemic heart disease with prior clinical or subclinical myocardial infarction (MI) with associated left ventricular dysfunction. The chance of cardiac arrest rises progressively with greater degrees of left ventricular dysfunction following MI with very low risks with EFs >40%, and a substantial precipitous rise with EFs <30 to 35%. The mechanism of sustained VT in chronic ischemic heart disease is macroreentry, similar in mechanism to that observed in the case of reentrant AT. VT in the chronic phase of ischemic heart disease is mediated by reentry through channels or sheets of surviving myocardium, especially within the partially spared border zone of a region of scar resulting from prior MI. Within these channels, conduction is abnormally slow due to poor coupling between sparse surviving myocytes, partially decoupled by interstitial fibrosis and cell loss. Tachycardia may be initiated by an ectopic beat that fails to enter one end of the channel due to unidirectional block, but enters the other end, traveling for a time within the channel then reemerging from the initially blocked end to reactivate the ventricle. Susceptibility to sustained VT increases with worsening left ventricular dysfunction and associated greater extent of scar. Such circuits may be favorably or adversely affected by antiarrhythmic drugs. As multiple functioning circuits may coexist in a single scar with multiple potential VT mechanisms, a drug may exhibit both favorable effects on one tachycardia while exacerbating alternate tachycardias.

Several trials have examined the utility of antiarrhythmic drugs, mostly amiodarone, compared with implantable cardioverter defibrillator (ICD) therapy on survival following an episode of sustained poorly tolerated VT or an episode of sudden arrhythmic death. The largest trial was the Antiarrhythmics Vs. Implantable Defibrillator trial,[9] which randomized patients with a history of poorly tolerated sustained VT or cardiac arrest between a strategy of empiric amiodarone or ICD implantation. In this trial,[9] as well as several smaller similar trials, ICD therapy was associated with a lower risk of arrhythmic and all-cause death than antiarrhythmic therapy. Therefore, for secondary prevention of cardiac arrest after an episode of sustained VT or VF in the setting of cardiac disease, ICD implantation has become the first line of therapy.

Indications for ICD Implantation for Secondary Prevention (After a First Episode of Documented or Presumed Sustained VT or VF)

Class I

1. Cardiac arrest due to VF or VT not due to a transient or reversible cause.[10]
2. Spontaneous sustained VT in association with structural heart disease.
3. Syncope of undetermined origin with clinically relevant, hemodynamically significant sustained VT, or VF induced at electrophysiologic study when drug therapy is ineffective, not tolerated, or not preferred.
4. Spontaneous sustained VT in patients without structural heart disease not amenable to other treatments.

Class IIb

1. Cardiac arrest presumed to be due to VF when electrophysiologic testing is precluded by other medical conditions.
2. Severe symptoms (*eg*, syncope) attributable to ventricular tachyarrhythmias in patients awaiting cardiac transplantation.
3. Recurrent syncope of undetermined origin in the presence of ventricular dysfunction and inducible ventricular arrhythmias at electrophysiologic study when other causes of syncope have been excluded.
4. Syncope of unexplained origin or family history of unexplained sudden cardiac death in association with typical or atypical right bundle-branch block and ST-segment elevations (Brugada syndrome).
5. Syncope in patients with advanced structural heart disease in whom thorough invasive and noninvasive investigations have failed to define a cause.

Primary Prevention of Cardiac Arrest

Patients with advanced cardiac disease, left ventricular dysfunction, and heart failure have a substantial risk of death due to both progressive heart failure and sudden death. Except in class IV (end-stage heart failure with symptoms at rest), sudden death predominates as the most common mode of death in advanced cardiac disease states. For any degree of left ventricular dysfunction, mortality rates in ischemic heart disease are higher than in nonischemic cardiomyopathy. Therefore, it has been easier to demonstrate mortality benefits with primary therapy to prevent sudden death in ischemic than nonischemic cardiomyopathy. As noted above, no form of antiarrhythmic drug, even amiodarone, has resulted in a significant mortality reduction in this population. However several ICD trials have demonstrated a significant reduction in mortality. The first such trial was the Multicenter Automatic Defibrillator Implantation Trial (MADIT),[11] which enrolled patients with prior MI, and EF ≤35%, who had frequent ventricular ectopy and inducible VT at EP testing. This study demonstrated a substantial mortality reduction with ICD therapy. The MADIT was followed by MADIT II,[12] which enrolled a simpler-to-identify population consisting of patients with simply a history of prior MI and EF ≤30% in the chronic phase. Again, a significant mortality benefit was associated with ICD therapy. Finally the recently completed Sudden Cardiac Death in Heart Failure trial[13] enrolled a broader population consisting of patients with both ischemic and nonischemic cardiomyopathy, symptomatic New York Heart Association class II or III heart failure, and EF ≤35%. Again, a survival benefit was found in patients treated with ICD when compared with conventional therapy or empiric amiodarone therapy. The degree of benefit was similar in patients with both ischemic and nonischemic cardiomyopathy, suggesting that primary prevention ICD implantation in patients with advanced nonischemic cardiomyopathy and heart failure was also appropriate. These three major trials combined with generally concordant findings in other smaller trials form the basis for the current recommendation for prophylactic primary prevention ICD implantation in patients with history of prior MI and EF ≤30% as well as patients with symptomatic heart failure of any etiology who remain New York Heart Association class II or III on optimized medical therapy and have EFs ≤35%.

Indications for ICD Implantation for Primary Prevention (in the Absence of Prior Sustained VT/VF)

Class I

Nonsustained VT in patients with coronary disease, prior MI, left ventricular dysfunction, and inducible VF or sustained VT at electrophysiologic study that is not suppressible by a class I antiarrhythmic drug.[10]

Class IIa

Patients with left ventricular EF ≤30% at least 1 month after MI and 3 months after coronary artery revascularization surgery.

Class IIb

Familial or inherited conditions with a high risk for life-threatening ventricular tachyarrhythmias such as long-QT syndrome or hypertrophic cardiomyopathy. Nonsustained VT with coronary artery disease, prior MI, left ventricular dysfunction, and inducible sustained VT or VF at electrophysiologic study.

VT and Fibrillation Without Evident Heart Disease

Although most sustained VT is related to underlying advanced structural heart disease, ventricular ectopy, nonsustained VT, at times symptomatic, and occasionally sustained VT may be seen in patients without evident underlying structural heart disease. The occurrence of VT in the absence of structural heart disease represents a heterogenous population of conditions, some benign, and some malignant. Several of the malignant conditions are familial, and therefore it is critical that they be identified to protect the welfare of the patient as well as unrecognized affected family members. It is easiest to classify such patients into three groups: idiopathic VT, right ventricular cardiomyopathy/dysplasia, and the cardiac ion-channel disorders including the long-QT syndrome.

Idiopathic VT

Right Ventricular Outflow Tract Tachycardia: Idiopathic VT typically presents in a patient with recurrent palpitations and occasionally syncope. The clinical story initially suggests SVT because the ECG is typically normal and cardiac evaluation unrevealing. However if symptoms are documented, VT is identified. The most common syndrome occurring in 75 to 90% of cases is repetitive salvos of nonsustained monomorphic VT as well as frequent unifocal premature ventricular contractions (PVCs) all with the same morphology. This arrhythmia originates in the right ventricular outflow tract (RVOT) from a focal origin usually immediately below the pulmonic valve. Ventricular ectopy is often quite frequent, and may be easily documented on 12-lead ECG in many patients. If documented, the QRS morphology has a deeply negative QRS in V_1 and strongly positive in the inferior leads, giving the beats a left bundle-branch block with inferior axis morphology (Fig 8). This arrhythmia is focal and automatic in mechanism, and its response to pacing and drugs suggests that the mechanism is likely due to triggered automaticity of the delayed afterdepolarization type. This arrhythmia is responsive to β-blockers, nondihydropyridine calcium-channel blockers such as verapamil or diltiazem, as well as transiently to adenosine infusion. It also responds to antiarrhythmic agents but, as the arrhythmia is readily cured by catheter ablation, patients who fail to respond to calcium-channel or β-blockers are commonly referred for catheter ablation. This clinical syndrome may also at times present with the same clinical pattern but with a right bundle-branch block QRS morphology and inferior axis. This arrhythmia behaves similarly to the RVOT tachycardia, but when mapped it originates in the left ventricular outflow tract instead. Although both syndromes most frequently present as repetitive bursts of nonsustained monomorphic VT, this syndrome may occasionally present as sustained monomorphic VT.

Idiopathic Left Ventricular Tachycardia: The second idiopathic VT syndrome is clinically distinct and much less common than the outflow tract tachycardias. It commonly presents as sustained monomorphic VT. This syndrome is referred to as either *idiopathic left fascicular tachycardia* or simply

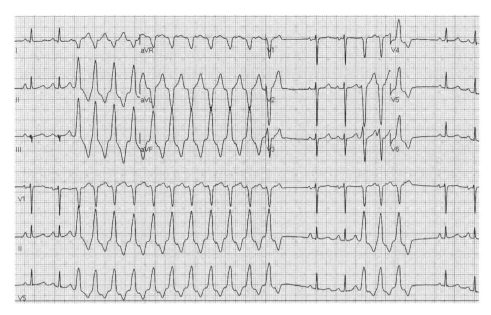

Figure 8. Idiopathic RVOT tachycardia. Note the characteristic left bundle-branch morphology and inferior right axis. This arrhythmia is automatic in mechanism and is likely similar in mechanism to focal AT. Like the focal AT shown in Figure 6, the runs have variable cycle length and occur in salvos. Like focal AT, idiopathic RVOT tachycardia responds to calcium-channel blockers and also may be helped by β-blockade. When frequent and symptomatic like this patient, most would offer ablation, and this is how this patient was treated.

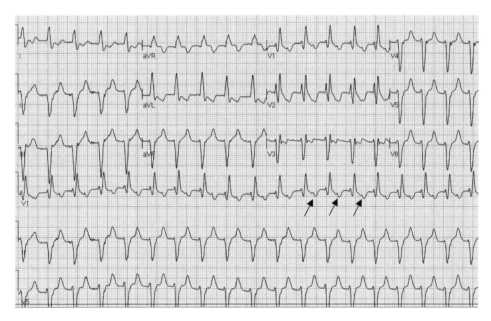

Figure 9. Idiopathic left fascicular tachycardia. This was a sustained arrhythmia in this patient, although it would tend to terminate after minutes back to sinus rhythm. Note that AV dissociation is absent during this tachycardia because there is 1:1 retrograde atrial activation (arrows). This ECG was done while the patient was already receiving β-blocker therapy, which slowed the rate of the tachycardia somewhat. This tachycardia terminated abruptly with IV diltiazem but was hard to suppress with oral medication. At EP testing, the tachycardia was mapped to the posterior apical septum in the region of the left posterior hemifascicle and ablated there.

idiopathic left ventricular tachycardia. It is a peculiar arrhythmia with a very stereotyped behavior. The arrhythmia is often well tolerated and has an ECG appearance that looks like a typical bifascicular block pattern with a right bundle-branch block and left-axis deviation (Fig 9). The arrhythmia may easily be misdiagnosed as SVT with aberrancy and if treated with a nondihydropyridine calcium-channel blocker such as diltiazem or verapamil will abruptly terminate, reinforcing the misdiagnosis. This unusual arrhythmia appears to be mediated by reentry within the left posterior

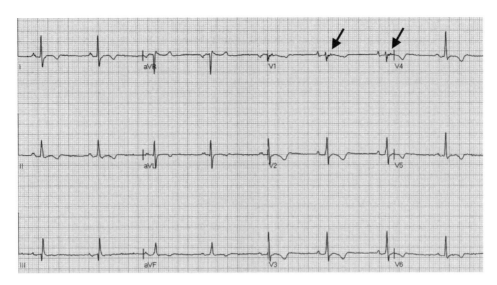

Figure 10. Arrhythmogenic right ventricular cardiomyopathy. This patient presented with sustained VT; while receiving medication for his index VT, he had another distinct sustained VT. Both had a left bundle-branch morphology and were poorly tolerated. Right ventriculography showed a dilated and aneurismal right ventricle due to fatty replacement. Note the presence of T-wave inversion beyond V_2 and a high-frequency notch in the early ST-segment following the QRS complex (arrows), which is an "epsilon wave" due to late activation of the underlying diseased right ventricle (this ECG is shown at double standard to make the epsilon wave easier to see when reproduced). This patient was orphaned, and the family history was unknown. He underwent ICD implantation.

fascicle of the left-sided conduction system, and its responsiveness to verapamil or diltiazem is surprising but characteristic. This arrhythmia, like idiopathic outflow tract tachycardia, has an excellent prognosis and may be treated medically. However, as it is often sustained, it is a common target for successful catheter ablation.

Arrhythmogenic Right Ventricular Cardiomyopathy/Dysplasia

Arrhythmogenic right ventricular cardiomyopathy (ARVC) is a familial degenerative cardiomyopathy that predominantly affects the free wall of the right ventricle. It is also referred to commonly as *arrhythmogenic right ventricular dysplasia*; however, it is now believed to be a progressive cardiomyopathy rather than a dysplastic process and *ARVC* is the preferred term. It is an important cause of unexpected sudden death in otherwise healthy persons in parts of Europe although not as frequent in the United States. Due to myocyte death/apoptosis, large portions of the right ventricular free wall may become replaced with adipose tissue leading to regional wall motion abnormalities and aneurysm formation. Although it predominantly affects the right ventricle, the left ventricle may also be

affected late in some patients. As the mechanical consequences of right ventricular dysfunction are often subclinical, this condition commonly becomes clinically apparent due to the development of ventricular arrhythmias originating in the affected portions of the right ventricle. The ventricular arrhythmias may be nonsustained or sustained and tend to exhibit a left bundle-branch block morphology consistent with a right ventricular origin. Because the right ventricle is not well imaged by routine cardiac testing, the presence of right ventricular cardiomyopathy can be easily missed; for this reason, this condition may be misdiagnosed as idiopathic RVOT VT, which is a more common condition. However, as ARVC carries a potential risk of sudden death and is commonly familial with dominant inheritance, its recognition is critical. When advanced, ARVC is associated with T-wave inversion in the anterior precordial leads, and the finding of unexplained T-wave inversion beyond V_2 is strongly suggestive. Less commonly, a late deflection at the tail of the right precordial QRS complex called an *epsilon wave* may be present and is due to late activation caused by slowed conduction in the affected right ventricle, which lies immediately under the right precordial leads (Fig 10). As the condition is a myopathic process, ventricular ectopy is often

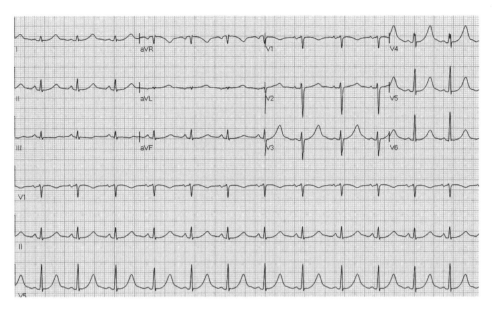

Figure 11. Familial long-QT syndrome. This 26-year-old woman presented with a cardiac arrest while at work at a manufacturing facility. She was resuscitated by bystanders and ultimately shocked out of VF by emergency medical technicians. She ultimately recovered and underwent ICD implantation. Her older sister had died suddenly 15 years earlier, but no investigation was pursued at that time. Her father also had died suddenly in his 40s, attributed to a heart attack. Genetic testing was done, and she was found to have LQT1. Her family was screened, identifying her brother and her nephew, the son of her deceased sister, as both affected but asymptomatic. A year later, this patient had a normal pregnancy. Her newborn son was found to have a QTc of 0.60 on the day of delivery. Her son, who is now 10 years old, received an ICD about a year ago; the patient is doing well but has received shocks for torsades; her brother and nephew remain asymptomatic on β-blockers 10 years later.

multiform, and this helps to distinguish it from the idiopathic arrhythmias that are focal with only a single PVC morphology. Finally, a family history of sudden death in a first-order relative should raise concern. Cardiac magnetic resonance imaging is the preferred technique to image the fatty infiltration and wall motion abnormalities in the right ventricle in ARVC. However, mild abnormalities may be seen in patients with idiopathic RVOT VT and make interpretation difficult in some patients. In the presence of sustained VT or symptoms such as syncope believed to be due to VT, ICD implantation is indicated to prevent future sudden death.

Cardiac Ion-Channel Disorders and Long-QT Syndrome

A number of familial conditions resulting in ventricular arrhythmias have been associated with point mutations in the cardiac ion channels. These conditions are often colloquially referred to as the cardiac *channelopathies*. The most important set of cardiac ion-channel disorders are the various forms of familial long-QT syndrome.

These syndromes were historically described as the *Romano-Ward syndrome*, a dominantly inherited condition associated with a long QT interval (Fig 11), recurrent syncope, and at times sudden death associated with polymorphic VT referred to as *torsades de pointes*. With modern genetic techniques, Romano-Ward syndrome has been found to be a set of long-QT syndromes due to one of several channel defects, the most common being LQT1, a defect in the KVLQT1 gene that encodes the cardiac slow potassium channel (I_{KS}); LQT2, a defect in the HERG gene that encodes a second K channel (I_{KR}); and LQT3, which is a defect in the SCN5A gene that encodes the cardiac sodium channel. Long-QT syndrome often presents with syncope as opposed to palpitations because the VT is very fast and hemodynamically ineffective. Asymptomatic patients with a long QT who have no family history of sudden death are usually followed up without treatment. If symptoms of syncope occur or there is a family history of sudden death, empiric β-blocker therapy is helpful in the most common forms (but may be harmful in the less common LQT3). If symptoms persist despite β-blocker therapy or the patient presents with resuscitated sudden death, ICD is indicated. Boys and girls have a similar rate of onset of symptoms, but in adulthood women have a higher rate of symptoms likely due to a tendency of women to have longer QT intervals than men. As this is a dominantly inherited condition, family screening is mandatory and vastly simplified by the commercial availability of genetic testing for the common forms of long-QT syndrome.

Brugada Syndrome

The Brugada syndrome was described in 1986 by Pedro and Josep Brugada when a 3-year-old boy presented with recurrent syncope and an unusual ECG. The boy's sister died at age 2 years of ventricular arrhythmias and had a similar ECG. The disorder is now known to be commonly related to distinct mutations in the sodium channel gene SCN5A, the same gene associated with LQT3. The ECG is characteristic but easily missed. The Brugada syndrome ECG is characterized by upward coved ST-segment elevation in leads V_1 to V_3 with a right bundle-branch block pattern. As the syndrome is associated with a high risk of sudden death due to polymorphic VT, is dominantly inherited, and displays otherwise normal cardiac testing and often no apparent arrhythmias between episodes, it is critical to look out for this ECG pattern in patients presenting with unexplained syncope. Unfortunately, the ECG pattern may be inconsistent from one ECG to the next. Of importance, β-blockers increase the risk of sudden death in Brugada syndrome, and many drugs with ability to block the cardiac sodium channel make this condition worse, including the class I antiarrhythmic agents as well as tricyclic antidepressants. When the diagnosis is established, and syncope is attributable to VT, or in the case of clinical ventricular tachycardia, ICD implantation is indicated because of a high risk of sudden death.

Acquired Long-QT Syndrome

Many drugs have been associated with QT prolongation and in susceptible patients with the development of torsades de points VT and at times sudden death. Table 1 gives a list of commonly associated drugs. An up-to-date database of drugs with an association with acquired long-QT

Table 1. *Drugs With a Known Risk of Torsades de Pointes**

Antiarrhythmics	Amiodarone, disopyramide, dofetilide, ibutilide, procainamide, quinidine, sotalol
Anticancer	Arsenic trioxide
Antianginal	Bepridil
Antibiotics/antiparasitics	Chloroquine, clarithromycin, erythromycin, halofantrine, pentamidine, sparfloxicin
Antipsychotics	Chlorpromazine, haloperidol, mesoridazine, pimozide, thioridazine
GI	Cisapride, domperidone, droperidol
Opiates	Levomethadyl, methadone

*Based on drug lists available from Arizona Center for Education and Research on Therapeutics.[14]

syndrome is maintained at www.qtdrugs.org, a valuable resource when evaluating a patient with unexplained QT prolongation while being treated with multiple medications. VT occurring in the drug-induced long-QT syndrome is very similar to the familial form. However some features differ. In the familial form of long-QT syndrome, VT during physical or emotional stress is common, occurring at times of elevated sinus rates. By contrast, torsades due to drug-induced long-QT syndrome tends to occur at rest during periods of low heart rates, especially following pauses often provoked by a compensatory pause from an antecedent PVC (Fig 12). Treatment involves correcting any electrolyte disturbance, and identifying and eliminating any potentially causative agents. Until the QT normalizes, treatment with IV magnesium sulfate will acutely suppress VT. As the VT is pause dependent at initiation, if VT continues to be a problem despite magnesium, VVI pacing at modest rates will prevent pauses and prevent initiation. Once torsades has developed from one drug, an effort should be made to avoid future therapy with any drug associated with this syndrome.

Summary and Conclusions

Tachyarrhythmias may be broadly classified as supraventricular arrhythmias, which are dependent on the atrium, AV node, or both; and ventricular arrhythmias, which are exclusively dependent on infranodal tissue. Supraventricular

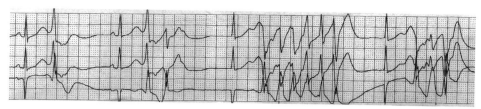

Figure 12. Torsades de pointes VT due to acquired long-QT syndrome. Note the frequent PVCs occurring on the descending limb of a very long QT interval. Note that the runs occur after pauses generated by the PVCs. Also note the very bizarre T-waves with a mountainous "giant U wave" rising off the T-waves that initiate polymorphic VT. This patient was started on amiodarone a week earlier for an unrelated arrhythmia, felt dizzy and returned to the hospital, and was readmitted. Amiodarone is the least likely of all class III drugs to cause torsades; however, it does occur occasionally. Amiodarone was stopped, and 4 days later the QT interval returned to baseline and the arrhythmias abated. This patient should never receive any drug associated with acquired QT prolongation and torsades in the future.

arrhythmias fall into two large groups: the paroxysmal SVTs, which are commonly seen in otherwise normal patients with recurrent paroxysmal sustained palpitations. More than 90% of these are due to either AV node reentry or AV reciprocating tachycardia related to an accessory pathway. The later group includes manifest WPW, in which delta waves are present and there is some potential for sudden death due to rapid conduction of AF resulting in VF and concealed WPW, in which delta waves are absent and the arrhythmia syndrome is similar to the more common AV node reentry, and sudden death is not a concern. Atrial arrhythmias may be focal or reentrant. Focal AT is usually automatic in mechanism and characterized by repeated salvos of tachycardia, often with frequent atrial ectopy between runs. Reentrant atrial arrhythmias include typical AFL, which circulates around the tricuspid valve around naturally present obstacles; AT and atypical flutters, which circulate around acquired obstacles related to atrial scar tissue and fibrosis; and finally AF, which is initiated by focal firing involving predominantly the pulmonary veins and likely maintained by chaotic left atrial reentry. The primary issues in atrial arrhythmia management are resting rate control to improve acute cardiac function and prevent the development of tachycardia-induced cardiomyopathy, restoration of sinus rhythm in selected patients, and antithrombotic therapy with aspirin or warfarin based on estimated long-term thromboembolic risk.

Ventricular arrhythmias are most commonly related to underlying structural heart disease, although an important subset occur in otherwise structurally normal hearts. In the setting of heart disease, ischemic heart disease is most commonly associated with sustained VT and sudden death. Antiarrhythmic therapy is not, based on current understanding, indicated to reduce the risk of sudden death in patients who are at high risk, including those with nonsustained arrhythmias and left ventricular dysfunction, as well as those with symptomatic sustained VT. Antiarrhythmics may have a role for symptomatic arrhythmias in low-risk patients as well as an adjunct to ICD therapy to prevent frequent ICD shocks. However the only rhythm therapy that has been shown to reduce risk of sudden death in these high-risk populations is ICD implantation. In patients with VT but a structurally normal heart, the important syndromes are idiopathic VTs, which have a generally good prognosis; occult ARVC, in which the heart is not, in fact structurally normal, but appears so unless the diagnosis is actively sought; and finally the ion-channel diseases, of which the familial long-QT syndromes are the most important clinically. The latter two syndromes are familial and have a potential for malignant arrhythmias and sudden death. Once the proband is identified, the family must also be screened. Failure to do so invites tragedy in follow-up. In managing all arrhythmias, it is the clinician's role to attempt to identify the tachycardia mechanism and the likely acute precipitants if any so they can be reversed, slow or eliminate the tachycardia to restore hemodynamic stability, and assess the likelihood for long-term recurrence and need or lack thereof for long-term management.

References

1. Delacretaz E. Supraventricular tachycardia. N Engl J Med 2006; 354:1039–1051

2. Fuster V, Rydén LE, Cannom DS, et al. ACC/AHA/ESC 2006 guidelines for the management of patients with atrial fibrillation: a report of the American College of Cardiology/American Heart Association Task Force on Practice Guidelines and the European Society of Cardiology Committee for Practice Guidelines (Writing Committee to Revise the 2001 Guidelines for the Management of Patients With Atrial Fibrillation). J Am Coll Cardiol 2006; 48:e149–e246. Available at: *http://www.acc.org/qualityandscience/clinical/guidelines/atrial_fib/pdfs/AF_Full_Text.pdf.* Accessed March 10, 2007

3. Haissaguerre M, Jais P, Shah DC, et al. Spontaneous initiation of atrial fibrillation by ectopic beats originating in the pulmonary veins. N Engl J Med 1998; 339:659–666

4. Singh BN, Singh SN, Reda DJ, et al. Amiodarone versus sotalol for atrial fibrillation (SAFE-T Trial). N Engl J Med 2005; 352:1861–1872

5. Wyse DG, Waldo AL, DiMarco JP, et al. A comparison of rate control and rhythm control in patients with atrial fibrillation. N Engl J Med 2002; 347:1825–1833

6. Echt DS, Liebson PR, Mitchell LB, et al. Mortality and morbidity in patients receiving encainide, flecainide, or placebo: the Cardiac Arrhythmia Suppression Trial. N Engl J Med 1991; 324:781–788

7. Julian DG, Camm AJ, Frangin G, et al. Randomised trial of effect of amiodarone on mortality in patients with left ventricular dysfunction after recent myocardial infarction: EMIAT. Lancet 1997; 349:667–674

8. Cairns JA, Connolly SJ, Roberts R, et al. Randomised trial of outcome after myocardial infarction in patients with frequent or repetitive ventricular premature depolarisations: CAMIAT. Canadian Amiodarone Myocardial Infarction Arrhythmia Trial Investigators. Lancet 1997; 349:675–682

9. A comparison of antiarrhythmic drug therapy with implantable defibrillators in patients resuscitated from near-fatal ventricular arrhythmias: the Antiarrhythmics Versus Implantable Defibrillators (AVID) Investigators. N Engl J Med 1997; 337:1576–1583

10. Gregoratos G, Abrams J, Epstein AE, et al. ACC/AHA/NASPE 2002 guideline update for implantation of cardiac pacemakers and antiarrhythmia devices: a report of the American College of Cardiology/American Heart Association Task Force on Practice Guidelines (ACC/AHA/NASPE Committee on Pacemaker Implantation). 2002. Available at: *http://www.acc.org/qualityandscience/clinical/guidelines/pacemaker/incorporated/index.htm.* Accessed March 10, 2007

11. Moss AJ, Hall WJ, Cannom DS, et al. Improved survival with an implanted defibrillator in patients with coronary disease at high risk for ventricular arrhythmia: Multicenter Automatic Defibrillator Implantation Trial Investigators. N Engl J Med 1996; 335:1933–1940

12. Moss AJ, Zareba W, Hall WJ, et al. Prophylactic implantation of a defibrillator in patients with myocardial infarction and reduced ejection fraction. N Engl J Med 2002; 346:877–883

13. Gust H, Bardy MD, Kerry L, et al, for the Sudden Cardiac Death in Heart Failure Trial Investigators. Amiodarone or an implantable cardioverter: defibrillator for congestive heart failure. N Engl J Med 2005; 352:225–237

14. Arizona Center for Education and Research on Therapeutics. Available at: *http://www.qtdrugs.org.* Accessed March 10, 2007

Heart Failure and Cardiac Pulmonary Edema

Steven M. Hollenberg, MD, FCCP

Objectives:

- Review the definition, demographics, and etiology of congestive heart failure diagnosis
- Understand the pathophysiology of the heart failure syndrome
- Review general treatment goals and medical therapy for heart failure, with an emphasis on acute heart failure in the ICU

Key words: aldosterone antagonism; angiotensin-converting enzyme inhibition; angiotensin receptor blockers; cardiogenic shock; congestive heart failure; remodeling; vasodilators

Definition and Epidemiology

Congestive heart failure (CHF) can be defined as the inability of the heart to provide an adequate cardiac output without invoking maladaptive compensatory mechanisms. CHF affects >5 million patients in the United States, which is an estimated 2.5% of the adult population.[1] Heart failure develops in 550,000 patients for the first time every year, and CHF results in >280,000 cardiovascular deaths and about 1.1 million hospital admissions per year in the United States. CHF is now the most common reason for hospitalization in the elderly, and annual costs are estimated at more than $33 billion.[1] The incidence of heart failure has been increasing, due not only to the aging of the population but also because improved treatment of hypertension and coronary disease is allowing patients to avoid early mortality only to have heart failure develop later.

The causes of heart failure are protean and are listed in Table 1. The predominant causes, however, are ischemia, hypertension, alcoholic cardiomyopathy, myocarditis, and idiopathic cardiomyopathy. Coronary artery disease is increasing, both as a primary cause and as a complicating factor of CHF.

Heart failure can be broken down into several different classifications, as follows: acute vs chronic; left-sided vs right-sided; and systolic vs diastolic dysfunction. It is important for the clinician to distinguish between systolic and diastolic dysfunction, as both the diagnostic workup and therapeutic sequence differ. Although CHF results most commonly from decreased systolic performance, diastolic dysfunction, which is defined clinically as cardiogenic pulmonary congestion in the presence of normal systolic performance, is becoming more common as a cause of CHF, particularly in the elderly. The estimated prevalence of diastolic heart failure is 30 to 35% overall, and >50% in patients >70 years of age.[2,3]

The severity of chronic heart failure is most commonly delineated using the classification developed by the New York Heart Association (NYHA). This classification divides patients into functional classes depending on the degree of effort needed to elicit symptoms (Table 2). More recently, stages in the evolution of heart failure have been proposed by an American College of Cardiology/American Heart Association task force to emphasize its progressive nature, and to focus on preventive measures and early intervention (Table 3). These stages have been linked to therapeutic approaches.

Pathophysiology

Heart failure is a syndrome caused not only by the low cardiac output resulting from compromised systolic performance, but also by the effects of compensatory mechanisms. Myocardial damage from any cause can produce myocardial failure. To compensate for the reduced cardiac output of a failing heart, an elevation in ventricular filling pressure occurs in an attempt to maintain output via the Frank-Starling law. These elevated diastolic filling pressures can compromise subendocardial blood flow and cause or worsen ischemia. With continued low cardiac output, additional compensatory mechanisms come into play, including sympathetic nervous system stimulation, activation of the renin-angiotensin system, and vasopressin secretion. All of these

Table 1. *Etiologies of CHF*

Ischemic
Hypertensive
Idiopathic
Valvular
Peripartum
Familial
Toxic
  Alcoholic
  Radiation
  Drug-related (anthracyclines)
  Heavy metals (cobalt, lead, or arsenic)
Metabolic/nutritional
Systemic diseases
  Hypothyroidism
  Connective tissue disease
  Diabetes
  Sarcoidosis
Infiltrative
  Amyloidosis
  Hemochromatosis
Tachycardia-induced
Autoimmune

Table 2. *NYHA Functional Classification of Heart Failure*

Class	Description
I	Symptoms of heart failure only at levels that would limit normal individuals
II	Symptoms of heart failure with ordinary exertion
III	Symptoms of heart failure on less than ordinary exertion
IV	Symptoms of heart failure at rest

Table 3. *Stages of Heart Failure*

Stage	Description
A	High risk for heart failure, without structural disease or symptoms
B	Heart disease with asymptomatic LV dysfunction
C	Prior or current symptoms of heart failure
D	Advanced heart disease and severely symptomatic or refractory heart failure

mechanisms lead to sodium and water retention and venoconstriction, increasing both preload and afterload. These increases in preload and afterload, although initially compensatory, can exacerbate the heart failure, because elevated preload increases pulmonary congestion, and elevated afterload impedes cardiac output.

Recent attention has focused on cardiac remodeling, the process by which ventricular size, shape, and function are regulated by mechanical, neurohormonal, and genetic factors, as a pathophysiologic mechanism in heart failure. Remodeling may be physiologic and adaptive during normal growth, but excessive remodeling after myocardial infarction (MI), cardiomyopathy, hypertension, or valvular heart disease can be maladaptive.[4] Early local remodeling after MI may expand the infarct zone, but late remodeling, which likely involves neurohormonal mechanisms

initiated by hemodynamic stress, involves the left ventricle (LV) globally and is associated with dilation that increases over time, distortion of ventricular shape, and hypertrophy of the walls. The failure to normalize increased wall stresses results in progressive dilatation and deterioration in contractile function. Similar processes are operative in other sorts of cardiomyopathy as well. Ventricular remodeling can be considered a primary target for treatment and a reliable surrogate for long-term outcomes.[3]

Diagnosis

The symptoms and signs of CHF relate both to low cardiac output and elevated ventricular filling pressures. Low output produces the symptoms of weakness and fatigue and an ashen appearance, sometimes with mottling. Increased left-sided filling pressures result in symptoms of pulmonary congestion such as dyspnea, cough, orthopnea, and paroxysmal nocturnal dyspnea as well as signs that may include tachycardia; pulmonary rales; a diffuse, enlarged, and laterally displaced point of maximal impulse; an S3 and S4 gallop; and a murmur of mitral regurgitation. Elevated right-sided preload can lead to symptoms such as anorexia, nausea, and abdominal pain, along with signs of systemic congestion such as jugular venous distension, a right-sided S3 gallop, a murmur of tricuspid regurgitation, hepatomegaly, ascites, and peripheral edema.

The presentation of acute heart failure and pulmonary edema can be dramatic, with the sudden onset of shortness of breath and tachypnea with use of accessory muscles. Crackles and, often, wheezing can be heard throughout the lung fields, at times obscuring some of the cardiac auscultatory findings. Hypotension and evidence of peripheral vasoconstriction and hypoperfusion may be present if cardiac output is decreased. The differential diagnosis of cardiac pulmonary edema includes other causes of acute dyspnea, such as pulmonary embolism, pneumothorax, and bronchial asthma, and causes of noncardiac pulmonary edema, such as aspiration, infection, toxins, or trauma.

The initial evaluation of the patient with pulmonary edema should include an ECG and chest radiograph. The ECG may show evidence of myocardial ischemia and can also detect arrhythmias; conduction abnormalities such as AV block and bundle branch block may be diagnosed. Q waves indicative of previous infarction or criteria diagnostic of ventricular hypertrophy may provide clues about the substrate for heart failure; atrial enlargement speaks to the chronicity of elevated filling pressures. The chest radiograph can demonstrate pulmonary vascular redistribution, with or without bilateral hazy pulmonary infiltrates, classically perihilar, as well as cardiomegaly. Pleural effusions may be identified but are neither sensitive nor specific.

Laboratory evaluation should include baseline measurement of serum electrolytes and creatinine, and blood glucose, liver function tests, and a CBC count. The measurement of plasma B-type natriuretic peptide (BNP) has been introduced[5] into the diagnostic algorithm for CHF. BNP is produced by ventricular myocytes in response to increased wall stress (ie, increased filling pressures and stretch).[5] Plasma BNP levels are increased in patients with heart failure, and the plasma concentration of BNP has been shown to correlate with NYHA functional class. The measurement of BNP has been used to distinguish between heart failure and pulmonary causes of dyspnea. In the Breathing Not Properly study of 1,586 patients presenting to the emergency department with a chief complaint of dyspnea, a plasma BNP level of >400 pg/mL accurately predicted CHF, while levels <100 pg/mL indicated noncardiac dyspnea; values between 100 and 400 pg/mL were less useful.[6] Such intermediate values may be due to CHF but may also represent preexisting LV dysfunction or right-sided heart failure. The addition of echocardiography in the acute setting may be especially valuable in patients with intermediate BNP levels.[7]

Echocardiography can provide important information about cardiac size and function, and should be performed in all patients with new-onset heart failure. Echocardiography is simple and safe, and permits the systemic interrogation of cardiac chamber size, LV and right ventricular function, valvular structure and motion, atrial size, and pericardial anatomy. Regional wall motion abnormalities are compatible with coronary heart disease but are not specific for ischemia since they are also seen in 50 to 60% of patients with idiopathic dilated cardiomyopathy. Fibrotic and thinned akinetic areas, however, indicate previous infarction. Doppler echocardiography can be used to evaluate the severity of mitral and tricuspid regurgitation, and the tricuspid regurgitation velocity can be used to estimate pulmonary artery pressure. In addition, Doppler echocardiography is increasingly used in the diagnosis of diastolic dysfunction.[8]

Therapy

Treatment Goals

The goals of CHF therapy are to control symptoms, improve exercise tolerance, prolong life, and, where possible, correct the underlying cause. Different therapies can have disparate effects on these goals.

Therapeutic agents can be viewed in the light of the pathophysiologic mechanisms of CHF development. Traditionally, these have been considered in hemodynamic terms. Fluid restriction and diuretic and venodilator agents decrease cardiac preload. Angiotensin-converting enzyme (ACE) inhibitors, angiotensin receptor blockers (ARBs), and aldosterone antagonists counteract the activation of the renin-angiotensin-aldosterone system and reduce afterload as well. Arterial dilators can also reduce afterload. Inotropic agents can improve cardiac pump function and increase output. More recently, the effects of therapy on counterproductive neurohormonal activation have received attention. β-blockers can counteract sympathetic activation and are being used more commonly in heart failure management. The most current approaches, however, take into account the effects of different therapies on ventricular remodeling. Agents used for therapy that have been shown to have a beneficial effect on remodeling, such as ACE inhibitors, ARBs, aldosterone antagonists, and β-blockers, reduce

Table 4. *Remodeling and Survival by Drug Class**

Established Therapy	Remodeling Effects	Survival Effects
ACE-I	Benefit	Benefit
ARB	Benefit (+ACE better)	Benefit (+ACE better)
Aldosterone antagonists	Benefit	Benefit
β-blocker	Benefit	Benefit
Diuretic	No benefit	No benefit
Digoxin	No benefit	No benefit
Other therapies		
Endothelin antagonists	No benefit	No benefit
TNF-α	No benefit	No benefit
Inotropes	Adverse	Adverse

*TNF = tumor necrosis factor.

Table 5. *Precipitating Causes of CHF*

Myocardial ischemia or infarction
Excess salt or fluid intake
Noncompliance or inadequate drug regimen
Renal failure
Arrhythmias
Anemia
Infection
Fever
Thyrotoxicosis
Pregnancy
Pulmonary embolism

mortality and are effective across the whole spectrum of heart failure severity (Table 4). Mechanical approaches to remodeling, most notably cardiac resynchronization therapy (CRT), also appear to be effective.

General Measures

The first order of business in the therapy for patients with new or decompensated CHF is to address the precipitating causes, the most prominent of which are listed in Table 5. Bypass surgery or percutaneous intervention for cardiac ischemia can improve both symptoms and ventricular performance. Registry data consistently support the notion that in the presence of significant amounts of ischemic yet viable myocardium, revascularization confers a survival benefit.[9] For patients with arrhythmias, either cardioversion or rate control can produce marked improvement.

Patients with acute heart failure should be put on bed rest (which by itself can produce a diuresis), with sodium restriction to <2 g per day and fluid restriction in severe cases. Attention should be paid to prophylaxis for deep venous thrombosis.

Pharmacologic Therapy

Diuretics

Diuretics cause renal sodium and water loss, decreasing preload, and thus pulmonary and systemic congestion. For inpatient treatment of decompensated heart failure, loop diuretics such as furosemide are usually chosen initially because of their rapid onset, and are administered in IV bolus doses. When used for patients who present with pulmonary edema, most of the rapid effect of furosemide is attributable to venodilation.

If there is no response to a bolus dose of a loop diuretic, the dose is titrated to achieve the desired effect, usually by doubling the dose. Loop diuretics enter the glomerulus primarily by tubular secretion into the proximal tubule and so exhibit a threshold effect. Once the effective dose has been determined, the degree of diuresis is usually adjusted by changing the frequency of diuretic administration. If intermittent bolus doses of loop diuretics are ineffective or are poorly tolerated due to large fluid shifts and consequent hypotension, continuous infusion may be preferable.[10] Alternatively, another diuretic with a different mechanism of action, such as metolazone or chlorothiazide, may be added.

The use of diuretics can lead to significant hypokalemia or hypomagnesemia, which can predispose the patient to arrhythmias. The careful addition of a potassium-sparing diuretic can be considered in some settings.

Nitrates

Nitrates are still the first-line agents for the symptomatic relief of angina pectoris and in cases when MI is complicated by CHF. Given the high incidence of coronary artery disease in patients with CHF, the use of nitrates to reduce preload is often desirable. In patients with severely decompensated CHF, therapy with IV nitroglycerin is preferred because of the questionable absorption of oral and transdermal preparations and for the

Heart Failure and Cardiac Pulmonary Edema (Hollenberg)

ease of titration. IV nitroglycerin should be started at 5 µg/min and increased in increments of 5 µg/min every 3 to 5 min as needed for symptomatic relief. The major adverse effects of nitrates are hypotension and headache.

Long-term therapy with oral nitrates alone does not impact ventricular remodeling and, thus, in the absence of ongoing ischemia, is not usually a first-line choice. When combined with hydralazine, however, salutary effects on outcome have been demonstrated, first in the V-Heft,[11] and more recently in the A-HeFT trial.[12] These trials are described below in the "Hydralazine" subsection.

ACE Inhibitors

ACE inhibitors inhibit the conversion of angiotensin I to angiotensin II and also inhibit the breakdown of bradykinin. Both of these actions produce vasodilation, the latter through bradykinin-induced nitric oxide production, but the increased inhibition of ventricular remodeling seen with ACE inhibitors compared to that seen with other vasodilators speaks to the potential for involvement of other mechanisms. Local renin-angiotensin systems, both intracardiac and intravascular, contribute to myocardial hypertrophy and remodeling, and their inhibition by ACE inhibitors may explain part of their beneficial effects.[13] ACE inhibitors also modulate sympathetic nervous system activity, and increased nitric oxide production may exert direct beneficial effects on cardiac myocytes.

ACE inhibitors improve hemodynamics, functional capacity, and survival in patients across the spectrum of severity of chronic CHF and also after MI. The CONSENSUS group[14] compared therapy with enalapril to placebo in 253 patients with advanced heart failure (NYHA class III or IV) and showed a 40% reduction in 6-month mortality; this benefit was sustained, with a risk reduction averaged over the 10-year duration of the trial of 30%. The SOLVD treatment trial[15] compared therapy with enalapril to placebo in 2,569 patients with symptomatic heart failure (NYHA class II to III) and showed a 16% mortality reduction. Moreover, therapy with ACE inhibitors also prevented the development of CHF in patients

with asymptomatic LV dysfunction in the SOLVD prevention trial.[16]

ACE inhibitors also improve the outcome in patients with asymptomatic LV dysfunction or overt heart failure after an acute MI. In the Survival and Ventricular Enlargement Trial (or SAVE) trial,[17] 2,231 asymptomatic patients with an ejection fraction (EF) of <40% were randomly assigned to receive either captopril or placebo. Captopril therapy decreased mortality by 19% at 42 months, and also decreased hospitalization for heart failure and, interestingly, recurrent MI.[17] The latter effect may have been due to an improvement in endothelial function. The Acute Infarction Ramipril Efficacy (or AIRE) trial[18] compared therapy with ramipril to placebo in 2,006 patients with clinical heart failure and showed a 27% reduction in mortality at 15 months. The survival benefit was maintained in the long term in both trials.

Patients should be started on therapy with low doses and titrated upward to the range demonstrated to be beneficial in clinical trials (*ie*, captopril, 50 mg three times daily, enalapril, 20 mg twice daily, or lisinopril, 40 mg once daily). The side effects of ACE inhibitors include cough, renal failure (usually occurring in the setting of renal artery stenosis), hyperkalemia, and angioedema.

ARBs

An alternative approach to inhibiting the effects of angiotensin II is the use of agents that block the angiotensin II receptor (*ie*, ARBs). Since these agents do not increase bradykinin levels, the incidence of some side effects, such as cough and angioedema, is greatly reduced. The hemodynamic effects of ARBs have been shown in a number of trials to be similar to those of ACE inhibitors. Trials comparing ACE inhibitors to ARBs in patients with heart failure have suggested similar mortality reductions.[19] Nonetheless, the number of heart failure patients treated with ARBs and followed up for mortality is still relatively small compared to those treated with ACE inhibitors, and so therapy with ARBs is usually reserved for patients who cannot tolerate ACE inhibitors; however, ARBs are a good alternative.

The recognition that angiotensin II is produced by pathways other than ACEs has provided a rationale for using ACE inhibitors and ARBs in combination therapy. This approach was tested in the 2001 V-Heft,[20] in which valsartan or placebo was added to usual therapy in patients with heart failure. Although mortality was unchanged, a combined end point of mortality and hospital admission for CHF was reduced with valsartan therapy. A subset analysis of this trial yielded the provocative finding that although valsartan therapy improved mortality in patients who were receiving ACE inhibitors but not β-blockers, and also those receiving β-blockers but not ACE inhibitors, when valsartan was added as triple therapy on top of both ACE inhibitors and β-blockers mortality was increased.[20] Other trials, however, have not shown adverse effects of triple combination therapy. In the VALIANT trial,[21] which compared therapy with valsartan, captopril, and the combination of the two agents in patients with acute MI and CHF, an adverse effect of the combination of ARBs, ACE inhibitors, and β-blockers was not seen. Increased mortality was also not observed when the ARB candesartan was added to therapy with ACE inhibitors and β-blockers in heart failure patients in the CHARM-Added trial.[22]

Aldosterone Antagonists

Although aldosterone is predominantly known for its role in the regulation of renal sodium and potassium excretion, its neurohumoral effects are gaining increasing recognition. Aldosterone inhibition impacts ventricular remodeling as well. The RALES trial[23] randomized 1,653 patients with class III and IV heart failure to receive spironolactone or placebo, and found a reduction in the 24-month mortality rate from 46 to 35% (relative risk, 30%; p <0.001). Hyperkalemia was uncommon, and the main side effect was gynecomastia. The recently reported EPHESUS trial[23a] randomized 6,632 patients with LV dysfunction after MI to receive eplerenone or placebo, and found a 15% reduction in mortality (relative risk, 0.85; 95% confidence interval, 0.75 to 0.96; p <0.01). In this trial, hyperkalemia was noted in 5.5% of the eplerenone group compared to 3.9% of the placebo group (p <0.01), but, interestingly, the incidence of hypokalemia was reduced from 13.1 to 8.4%.

It should be noted that the doses of aldosterone antagonists used in these heart failure trials were well below those used for diuresis. Nonetheless, careful attention to serum potassium levels is warranted when using these agents for any indication.

β-Blockers

Symptomatic heart failure results in the activation of neurohumoral mechanisms, including the sympathetic nervous system, which initially support the performance of the failing heart. Long-term activation of the sympathetic nervous system, however, exerts deleterious effects. Circulating catecholamine levels correlate with survival in these patients.[24] Sympathetic activation can increase ventricular volumes and pressure by causing peripheral vasoconstriction and impairing sodium excretion by the kidneys, and can also provoke arrhythmias. The long-term stimulation of β-receptors reduces the responsiveness to β-adrenergic agonists due to the down-regulation and desensitization of the β-receptor and its coupled signaling pathways; β-blockade can up-regulate adrenergic receptor density, restoring inotropic and chronotropic responsiveness.[25] Catecholamines induce oxidative stress in cardiac myocytes, potentially leading to programmed cell death, which is a process that is counteracted by β-blockers.[26] β-blockers also reduce the circulating level of vasoconstrictors and mitigate their effects, decreasing afterload. Perhaps most importantly, catecholamines promote deleterious ventricular remodeling, and β-blockers can decrease LV end-systolic and end-diastolic volume.[25] Thus, although it is perhaps counterintuitive on hemodynamic grounds, there is now compelling evidence that β-blockers are beneficial not only for patients with acute MI complicated by heart failure but also with chronic heart failure from all causes.[25]

β-blockers have now been evaluated in >10,000 patients with heart failure and systolic dysfunction. This collective experience indicates that long-term treatment with β-blockers can relieve symptoms, improve ventricular performance, and reduce both mortality and the need for hospitalization. The following three different agents have been shown to decrease mortality in patients with

NYHA class II and III heart failure: metoprolol XL[27]; bisoprolol[28]; and carvedilol.[29] Studies[30] with carvedilol have suggested that the benefits extend to patients with class IV heart failure. These benefits of β-blockers are seen in patients with or without coronary artery disease and in patients with or without diabetes, and are also observed in patients who are already receiving ACE inhibitors.

The initiation of therapy with β-blockers, however, can be problematic during the acute phase of heart failure, as they can depress contractility. When administered for the treatment of heart failure indications *per se*, β-blockers should be introduced when the patient is in a well-compensated and euvolemic state, typically in the ambulatory setting and at low doses. Patients who experience an exacerbation of heart failure while receiving maintenance β-blocker therapy, particularly at a higher dose, present a previously rare dilemma that is becoming more common. No controlled observations are available to guide therapy, so current practice remains largely at the discretion of individual clinicians. Discontinuing therapy with β-blockers, or decreasing their dose, may expose myocardial β-receptors to endogenous catecholamines and may result in a brief increase in contractility. On the other hand, the slow titration of β-blockers will need to begin anew after the resolution of acute CHF. It is usually best to attempt to resolve acute episodes of heart failure by diuresis and the adjustment of other medications while holding β-blocker doses constant, and to halve the dose if heart failure persists.

Hydralazine

Hydralazine reduces afterload by directly relaxing smooth muscle. Its effects are almost exclusively confined to the arterial bed. In healthy subjects, the hypotensive actions of hydralazine provoke a marked reflex tachycardia, but this response is often blunted in patients with heart failure.

Hydralazine therapy is effective in increasing cardiac output in patients with heart failure. Therapy with hydralazine in combination with oral nitrates was the first therapy shown to improve mortality in CHF patients, reducing mortality in patients with class III and IV heart failure in the V-Heft trial.[11] Enalapril was shown to be superior to this combination.[31] In addition, oral hydralazine must be administered four times a day, and prolonged administration is attended by the development of a lupus-like syndrome in up to 20% of patients; so hydralazine has usually been reserved for ACE-intolerant patients.

In 2004, a fixed dose of both isosorbide dinitrate and hydralazine administered twice daily was tested in black patients with class III and IV heart failure, a subgroup that was previously noted to have a favorable response to this therapy and that may not respond as well to ACE inhibition.[12] Therapy with hydralazine and nitrates improved mortality, hospitalization for heart failure, and quality of life.[12]

Nesiritide

Nesiritide is a recombinant form of human BNP. Assays of circulating BNP levels have been used in the diagnosis of heart failure and have some prognostic value, but the therapeutic use of BNP differs. When infused IV, nesiritide is a balanced arterial and venous vasodilator that may also have a modest natriuretic effect.

In patients with heart failure, IV nesiritide has been shown to increase stroke volume and cardiac output and to decrease right atrial and pulmonary capillary wedge pressure.[32] Its effects, compared to those of IV nitroglycerin, in patients with acute heart failure were tested in the randomized VMAC trial.[33] In this trial, 489 patients, including 246 who underwent pulmonary artery catheterization, were randomly assigned to receive nesiritide, IV nitroglycerin, or placebo for 3 h. After this initial placebo-controlled period, the placebo-treated patients were randomly reassigned to receive either nesiritide or IV nitroglycerin, and all patients were observed for 24 h (*ie*, the active-treatment phase).[33] Therapy with nesiritide decreased the mean PCWP significantly more than therapy with either IV nitroglycerin or placebo at 3 h (5.8 vs 3.8 and 2.0 mm Hg, respectively) and significantly more than therapy with nitroglycerin at 24 h (8.2 vs 6.3 mm Hg, respectively). Symptoms of dyspnea were decreased and global clinical status was improved with nesiritide therapy compared with placebo, but there was no significant difference in these parameters when compared to therapy with IV nitroglycerin. There was no significant difference in 30-day rehospitalization rate or the 6-month mortality rate.[33]

Nesiritide is given as an initial IV bolus of 2 μg/kg, followed by a continuous infusion of 0.01 μg/kg/min; the dose can be increased every 3 h by 0.005 μg/kg/min up to a maximum of 0.03 μg/kg/min. Hypotension is the most common side effect.

Although nesiritide has natriuretic properties, it has not been shown to improve either the glomerular filtration rate or renal plasma flow.[34] In addition, metaanalyses of data from the VMAC trial[33] and other trials have suggested that nesiritide may worsen renal function[35] and decrease survival at 30 days compared to conventional therapies.[36] The degree to which these issues are applicable for use in patients with acute heart failure and hemodynamic decompensation is controversial, but the potential adverse effect on long-term outcome is a significant concern, the resolution of which awaits the completion of appropriately powered prospective clinical trials.

Digoxin

Digitalis, which has been used to treat heart failure for >200 years, works by inhibiting Na-K-dependent adenosine triphosphatase activity, causing intracellular sodium accumulation and increasing intracellular calcium via the sodium-calcium exchange system. Digoxin improves myocardial contractility and increases cardiac output, but its inotropic effects are mild in comparison to those of catecholamines. The effect of digoxin on patient survival was definitively addressed in the Digoxin Investigators' Group (or DIG) trial,[37] a study of 6,800 patients with symptomatic CHF and systolic dysfunction. There was no difference in survival between the digoxin and placebo groups, but survival did significantly decrease during hospitalization for heart failure patients.[37] Thus, apart from its use as an antiarrhythmic agent, digoxin is recommended for therapy in patients with systolic dysfunction and symptomatic heart failure despite therapy with diuretics, ACE inhibitors, and β-blockers.

Inotropic Agents

In severe decompensated heart failure, inotropic support may be initiated. Dobutamine is a selective β₁-adrenergic receptor agonist that can improve myocardial contractility and increase cardiac output. Dobutamine is the initial inotropic agent of choice in patients with decompensated acute heart failure and adequate systolic BP. Dobutamine has a rapid onset of action and a plasma half-life of 2 to 3 min; infusion is usually initiated at 5 μg/kg/min and then titrated. Tolerance of the effects of dobutamine may develop after 48 to 72 h, possibly due to the down-regulation of adrenergic receptors. Dobutamine has the potential to exacerbate hypotension in some patients and can precipitate tachyarrhythmias.

Milrinone is a phosphodiesterase inhibitor with both positive inotropic and vasodilatory actions. Because milrinone does not stimulate adrenergic receptors directly, it may be effective when added to therapy with catecholamines or when β-adrenergic receptors have been down-regulated. Compared to catecholamines, phosphodiesterase inhibitors have fewer chronotropic and arrhythmogenic effects.

Although they clearly are useful in improving hemodynamics in the acute setting, controversy has arisen regarding the use of inotropic agents (other than digoxin) as outpatient maintenance therapy for chronic heart failure. Concerns have included exacerbation of arrhythmic complications, either by induction of myocardial ischemia or by independent pathways, and the perpetuation of neurohumoral activation that might accelerate the progression of myocardial damage. Milrinone has been examined in a prospective manner in the OPTIME-CHF trial[38] in order to determine whether its use could reduce hospitalization time following an exacerbation of acute heart failure. Although these observations did not demonstrate any advantage for patients who were treated with milrinone, patients whom the investigators felt "needed" acute inotropic support were not included in the trial, thereby biasing the enrollment toward a less severely afflicted cohort.[38] Therefore, the utilization of such agents today remains at the discretion of the clinician. The proof that these agents have beneficial effects on hard clinical end points remains elusive, but their hemodynamic effects are attractive for treating decompensated patients.

Inotropic infusions need to be titrated carefully in patients with ischemic heart disease to maximize coronary perfusion pressure with the least possible increase in myocardial oxygen demand. Invasive hemodynamic monitoring can be extremely useful for the optimization of therapy in these unstable patients, because clinical estimates of filling pressure can be unreliable, and because changes in myocardial performance and compliance and therapeutic interventions can change cardiac output and filling pressures precipitously. The optimization of filling pressures and serial measurements of cardiac output (and other parameters, such as mixed venous oxygen saturation) allow for the titration of inotropes and vasopressors to the minimum dosage required to achieve the chosen therapeutic goals, thus minimizing the increases in myocardial oxygen demand and arrhythmogenic potential.

Arrhythmias

Arrhythmias are common in patients with heart failure. Nonsustained ventricular tachycardia may occur in as many as 50% of patients, and complex ventricular depolarizations in as many as 80%. Forty to 50% of deaths are sudden, and many of these deaths are attributable to arrhythmias.

The mortality benefits of some of the standard therapies for heart failure, particularly β-blockers, may be attributable in part to antiarrhythmic properties. Specific antiarrhythmic agents, however, have not proven to be very effective for the prevention of sudden death in patients with heart failure,[39] and so attention has focused on identifying patients who would benefit from the placement of an implantable cardiac defibrillator (ICD).

The insertion of ICDs as secondary prevention in survivors of sudden cardiac death or patients with hemodynamically significant sustained ventricular tachycardias has been well demonstrated to improve survival in clinical trials.[39] Virtually all of the patients enrolled in the study had LV dysfunction, and about half had clinical heart failure.

ICDs are effective as primary prevention in selected heart failure patients as well. The MADIT I trial[40] and MUSST[41] showed a mortality benefit

with ICD therapy in patients with LV dysfunction (EF, <35 to 40%) and nonsustained VT in whom sustained VT was inducible in an electrophysiologic study.[40,41] The MADIT II trial[42] showed a mortality benefit with ICD therapy in a trial in which the entry criterion was simply an EF of <30%. Most of the patients in these trials had ischemic cardiomyopathy. More recently, the SCD-HeFT[43] compared ICD implantation to amiodarone therapy in patients with heart failure due either to ischemic or nonischemic cardiomyopathy (EF, <35%) and found a mortality benefit with ICD in both groups.

Cardiac Resynchronization

Left bundle branch block or other conduction system abnormalities can cause dyssynchronous ventricular contraction. Such dyssynchrony causes abnormal septal motion, decreasing contractile performance and myocardial efficiency, reduces diastolic filling times, and can increase the duration and degree of mitral regurgitation. The goal of CRT is to pace the LV and right ventricle to restore physiologic atrioventricular timing and contraction synchrony. This is accomplished by placing the standard leads in the right atrium and right ventricle and also by placing a special lead through the coronary sinus to enable pacing of the lateral aspect of the LV.

CRT, by optimizing the coordination of contraction, improves LV contractile function, stroke volume, and cardiac output, with decreased pulmonary capillary wedge pressures. This improved performance is associated with either no increase in myocardial oxygen consumption or a decrease, thus increasing myocardial efficiency. Most importantly, biventricular pacing is associated with reverse ventricular remodeling. In the MIRACLE trial,[44] biventricular pacing produced significant decreases in LV end-systolic and end-diastolic dimensions, a significant reduction in mitral regurgitation jet area, and a reduction in LV mass, all of which are signs of reverse remodeling. Cardiac resynchronization also improved exercise capacity, functional class, and quality of life in this trial.[44]

Studies of outcomes after CRT are beginning to emerge.[44] The COMPANION trial[45] compared optimal medical therapy to CRT with and without an ICD in 1,520 patients with NYHA class III to IV heart failure and an LV EF of <35%. The primary end point, a combination of all-cause mortality and hospitalization, was reduced in both the CRT-alone arm and the CRT-plus-ICD arm compared to medical therapy.[45] The reduction in the secondary end point of all-cause mortality alone was significant only in the CRT-plus-ICD arm compared to medical therapy. In the recently reported Cardiac Resynchronization-Heart Failure (or CARE-HF) trial,[46] cardiac resynchronization reduced the interventricular mechanical delay, ventricular volume, and mitral regurgitation, increased EF, improved symptoms and quality of life, and reduced both death and the combined end point of death and hospitalization compared to medical therapy.

References

1. Rosamond W, Flegal K, Friday G, et al. Heart disease and stroke statistics: 2007 update; a report from the American Heart Association Statistics Committee and Stroke Statistics Subcommittee. Circulation 2007; 115:e69–e171

2. Zile MR, Brutsaert DL. New concepts in diastolic dysfunction and diastolic heart failure: part I. Diagnosis, prognosis, and measurements of diastolic function. Part II: causal mechanisms and treatment. Circulation 2002; 105:1387–1393, 1503–1508

3. Zile MR, Brutsaert DL. New concepts in diastolic dysfunction and diastolic heart failure: part II. Causal mechanisms and treatment. Circulation 2002; 105:1503–1508

4. Sutton MG, Sharpe N. Left ventricular remodeling after myocardial infarction: pathophysiology and therapy. Circulation 2000; 101:2981–2988

5. de Denus S, Pharand C, Williamson DR. Brain natriuretic peptide in the management of heart failure: the versatile neurohormone. Chest 2004; 125:652–668

6. Maisel AS, Krishnaswamy P, Nowak RM, et al. Rapid measurement of B-type natriuretic peptide in the emergency diagnosis of heart failure. N Engl J Med 2002; 347:161–167

7. Logeart D, Saudubray C, Beyne P, et al. Comparative value of Doppler echocardiography and B-type natriuretic peptide assay in the etiologic diagnosis of acute dyspnea. J Am Coll Cardiol 2002; 40:1794–1800

8. Oh JK, Hatle L, Tajik AJ, et al. Diastolic heart failure can be diagnosed by comprehensive two-dimensional and Doppler echocardiography. J Am Coll Cardiol 2006; 47:500–506

9. CASS Principal Investigators. A randomized trial of coronary artery bypass surgery: survival of patients with a low ejection fraction. N Engl J Med 1985; 312:1665–1671

10. Dormans TP, van Meyel JJ, Gerlag PG, et al. Diuretic efficacy of high dose furosemide in severe heart failure: bolus injection versus continuous infusion. J Am Coll Cardiol 1996; 28:376–382

11. Cohn JN, Archibald DG, Ziesche S, et al. Effect of vasodilator therapy on mortality in chronic congestive heart failure: results of a Veterans Administration cooperative study. N Engl J Med 1986; 314:1547–1552

12. Taylor AL, Ziesche S, Yancy C, et al. Combination of isosorbide dinitrate and hydralazine in blacks with heart failure. N Engl J Med 2004; 351: 2049–2057

13. Dzau VJ, Bernstein K, Celermajer D, et al. The relevance of tissue angiotensin-converting enzyme: manifestations in mechanistic and endpoint data. Am J Cardiol 2001; 88:1L–20L

14. CONSENSUS Trial Study Group. Effects of enalapril on mortality in severe congestive heart failure: results of the Cooperative North Scandanavian Enalapril Survival Study (CONSENSUS). N Engl J Med 1987; 316:1429–1435

15. SOLVD Investigators. Effect of enalapril on survival in patients with reduced left ventricular ejection fractions and congestive heart failure. N Engl J Med 1991; 325:293–302

16. SOLVD Investigators. Effect of enalapril on mortality and the development of heart failure in asymptomatic patients with reduced left ventricular ejection fractions. N Engl J Med 1992; 327: 685–691

17. Pfeffer MA, Braunwald E, Moye LA, et al. Effect of captopril on mortality and morbidity in patients with left ventricular dysfunction after myocardial infarction: results of the Survival and Ventricular Enlargement Trial. N Engl J Med 1992; 327: 669–677

18. Acute Infarction Ramipril Efficacy (AIRE) Study Investigators. Effect of ramipril on mortality and morbidity of survivors of acute myocardial infarction with clinical evidence of heart failure. Lancet 1993; 342:821–828

19. Pitt B, Poole-Wilson PA, Segal R, et al. Effect of losartan compared with captopril on mortality in patients with symptomatic heart failure: randomised trial; the Losartan Heart Failure Survival Study ELITE II. Lancet 2000; 355:1582–1587

20. Cohn JN, Tognoni G. A randomized trial of the angiotensin-receptor blocker valsartan in chronic heart failure. N Engl J Med 2001; 345:1667–1675

21. Pfeffer MA, McMurray JJ, Velazquez EJ, et al. Valsartan, captopril, or both in myocardial infarction complicated by heart failure, left ventricular dysfunction, or both. N Engl J Med 2003; 349:1893–1906

22. McMurray JJ, Ostergren J, Swedberg K, et al. Effects of candesartan in patients with chronic heart failure and reduced left-ventricular systolic function taking angiotensin-converting-enzyme inhibitors: the CHARM-Added trial. Lancet 2003; 362:767–771

23. Pitt B, Zannad F, Remme WJ, et al. The effect of spironolactone on morbidity and mortality in patients with severe heart failure. N Engl J Med 1999; 341:709–717

23a. Pitt B, Remme W, Zannad F, et al. Eplerenone, a selective aldosterone blocker, in patients with left ventricular dysfunction after myocardial infarction. N Engl J Med 2003; 348:1309–1321

24. Cohn JN, Levine TB, Olivari MT, et al. Plasma norepinephrine as a guide to prognosis in patients with chronic congestive heart failure. N Engl J Med 1984; 311:819–823

25. Hunt SA, Abraham WT, Chin MH, et al. ACC/AHA 2005 guideline update for the diagnosis and management of chronic heart failure in the adult: summary article. J Am Coll Cardiol 2005; 46:1116–1143

26. Lohse MJ, Engelhardt S, Eschenhagen T. What is the role of β-adrenergic signaling in heart failure? Circ Res 2003; 93:896–906

27. Metoprolol CR/XL Randomised Intervention Trial in Congestive Heart Failure Investigators. Effect of metoprolol CR/XL in chronic heart failure: Metoprolol CR/XL Randomised Intervention Trial in Congestive Heart Failure (MERIT-HF). Lancet 1999; 353:2001–2007

28. CIBIS-II Investigators. The Cardiac Insufficiency Bisoprolol Study II (CIBIS-II): a randomised trial. Lancet 1999; 353:9–13

29. Packer M, Coats AJ, Fowler MB, et al. Effect of carvedilol on survival in severe chronic heart failure. N Engl J Med 2001; 344:1651–1658

30. Krum H, Roecker EB, Mohacsi P, et al. Effects of initiating carvedilol in patients with severe chronic heart failure: results from the COPERNICUS Study. JAMA 2003; 289:712–718

31. Cohn JN, Johnson G, Ziesche S, et al. A comparison of enalapril with hydralazine-isosorbide dinitrate in the treatment of chronic congestive heart failure. N Engl J Med 1991; 325:303–310

32. Colucci WS, Elkayam U, Horton DP, et al. Intravenous nesiritide, a natriuretic peptide, in the treatment of decompensated congestive heart failure: Nesiritide Study Group. N Engl J Med 2000; 343:246–253

33. VMAC Investigators. Intravenous nesiritide vs nitroglycerin for treatment of decompensated congestive heart failure: a randomized controlled trial. JAMA 2002; 287:1531–1540

34. Wang DJ, Dowling TC, Meadows D, et al. Nesiritide does not improve renal function in patients with chronic heart failure and worsening serum creatinine. Circulation 2004; 110:1620–1625

35. Sackner-Bernstein JD, Skopicki HA, Aaronson KD. Risk of worsening renal function with nesiritide in patients with acutely decompensated heart failure. Circulation 2005; 111:1487–1491

36. Sackner-Bernstein JD, Kowalski M, Fox M, et al. Short-term risk of death after treatment with nesiritide for decompensated heart failure: a pooled analysis of randomized controlled trials. JAMA 2005; 293:1900–1905

37. Digitalis Investigation Group. The effect of digoxin on mortality and morbidity in patients with heart failure. N Engl J Med 1997; 336:525–533

38. Cuffe MS, Califf RM, Adams KF Jr, et al. Short-term intravenous milrinone for acute exacerbation of chronic heart failure: a randomized controlled trial. JAMA 2002; 287:1541–1547

39. Antiarrhythmics Versus Implantable Defibrillators (AVID) Investigators. A comparison of antiarrhythmic-drug therapy with implantable defibrillators in patients resuscitated from near-fatal ventricular arrhythmias: the Antiarrhythmics Versus Implantable Defibrillators (AVID) Investigators. N Engl J Med 1997; 337:1576–1583

40. Moss AJ, Hall WJ, Cannom DS, et al. Improved survival with an implanted defibrillator in patients with coronary disease at high risk for ventricular arrhythmia. N Engl J Med 1996; 335:1933–1940

41. Buxton AE, Lee KL, Fisher JD, et al. A randomized study of the prevention of sudden death in

patients with coronary artery disease: Multicenter Unsustained Tachycardia Trial Investigators. N Engl J Med 1999; 341:1882–1890

42. Moss AJ, Zareba W, Hall WJ, et al. Prophylactic implantation of a defibrillator in patients with myocardial infarction and reduced ejection fraction. N Engl J Med 2002; 346:877–883

43. Bardy GH, Lee KL, Mark DB, et al. Amiodarone or an implantable cardioverter-defibrillator for congestive heart failure. N Engl J Med 2005; 352: 225–237

44. Abraham WT, Fisher WG, Smith AL, et al. Cardiac resynchronization in chronic heart failure. N Engl J Med 2002; 346:1845–1853

45. Bristow MR, Saxon LA, Boehmer J, et al. Cardiac-resynchronization therapy with or without an implantable defibrillator in advanced chronic heart failure. N Engl J Med 2004; 350:2140–2150

46. Cleland JG, Daubert JC, Erdmann E, et al. The effect of cardiac resynchronization on morbidity and mortality in heart failure. N Engl J Med 2005; 352:1539–1549

Acute Coronary Syndromes

Steven M. Hollenberg, MD, FCCP

Objectives:

- Review the diagnosis of myocardial infarction, with emphasis on diagnostic pitfalls
- Understand indications, contraindications, and use of thrombolytic therapy
- Understand the role of cardiac catheterization, angioplasty, and surgical revascularization
- Review adjunctive medical therapy of acute myocardial infarction
- Review complications of acute myocardial infarction

Key words: antiplatelet agents; antithrombotic agents; complications; fibrinolytic therapy; myocardial infarction; non-ST elevation; percutaneous coronary intervention; ST elevation

Acute Coronary Syndromes

Terminology

Acute coronary syndromes (ACSs) describe the spectrum of disease in patients who present with any constellation of clinical symptoms that are compatible with acute myocardial ischemia. ACSs comprise a family of disorders that share similar pathogenic mechanisms and represent different points along a common continuum. These syndromes are caused by recent thrombus formation on preexisting coronary artery plaque leading to impaired myocardial oxygen supply. In this sense, they differ from stable angina, which is usually precipitated by increased myocardial oxygen demand (*eg*, exertion, fever, or tachycardia) with background coronary artery narrowing (*ie*, limitation of the oxygen supply).

ACSs have traditionally been classified into Q-wave myocardial infarction (MI), non-Q-wave MI (NQMI), and unstable angina. More recently, the classification has shifted and is now based on the initial ECG findings. Patients are divided into the following three groups: patients with ST-elevation MI (STEMI); patients without ST elevation but with enzyme evidence of myocardial damage (*ie*, non-STEMI [NSTEMI]); and patients with unstable angina. Classification according to the presenting ECG findings coincides with current treatment strategies, since patients presenting with ST elevation benefit from immediate reperfusion and should be treated with thrombolytic therapy or urgent revascularization, whereas fibrinolytic agents are not effective treatment in patients with other acute coronary syndromes. The discussion in this chapter will follow this schematization.

Pathophysiology

The common link among the various ACSs is the rupture of a vulnerable, but previously quiescent, coronary atherosclerotic plaque.[1] The exposure of plaque contents to the circulating blood pool triggers the release of vasoactive amines, and the activation of platelets and the coagulation cascade. The extent of the resultant platelet aggregation, thrombosis, vasoconstriction, and microembolization dictates the clinical manifestations of the syndrome. The relative fibrin and platelet contents of these lesions vary, with unstable angina/NSTEMI more often associated with platelet-rich lesions and STEMI more often associated with fibrin-rich clots, although it should be noted that all lesions contain some degree of both components.[2] These observations form the scientific rationale for the use of fibrinolytic agents in the treatment of STEMI and the use of platelet inhibitors in the treatment of unstable angina/NSTEMI.

Diagnosis

Signs and Symptoms

Patients with myocardial ischemia can present with chest pain or pressure, shortness of breath, palpitations, syncope, or sudden death. The pain of MI is typically severe, constant, and retrosternal. The pain commonly spreads across the chest and may radiate to the throat or jaw, or down the arms. Its duration is most often >20 min. Diaphoresis, nausea, pallor, and anxiety are often present. Prodromal symptoms of myocardial ischemia occur in 20 to 60% of patients in the days preceding the infarction. The pain of unstable angina may be similar, although it is often milder.

Although these are the classic signs of infarction, it is important to recognize that the pain of MI may sometimes be atypical in terms of location or perception. It may be epigastric; confined to the jaw, arms, wrists, or interscapular region; or perceived as burning or pressure.

The physical examination can be insensitive and nonspecific, but is useful in diagnosing specific complications and in excluding alternative diagnoses, both cardiovascular (such as aortic dissection or pericarditis) and noncardiac. Distended jugular veins signal right ventricular diastolic pressure elevation, and the appearance of pulmonary crackles (in the absence of pulmonary disease) indicates elevated left ventricular filling pressures. Left ventricular failure is suggested by the presence of basal crackles, tachycardia, and tachypnea, and an S3 gallop, which usually indicates a large infarction with extensive muscle damage. A systolic murmur of mitral regurgitation may be present due to papillary muscle dysfunction or left ventricular dilation. A pansystolic murmur may also result from an acute ventricular septal defect due to septal rupture.

The ECG

The ECG abnormalities in myocardial ischemia depend on the extent and nature of coronary stenosis and the presence of collateral flow, but the pattern of ECG changes generally gives a guide to the area and extent of the infarction (Table 1).

The number of leads involved broadly reflects the extent of myocardium involved.

With total acute occlusion of a coronary artery, the first demonstrable ECG changes are peaked T-wave changes in the leads, reflecting the anatomic area of the myocardium that is in jeopardy. As total occlusion continues, there is elevation of the ST segments in the same leads. With continued occlusion, there is an evolution of ECG abnormalities, with biphasic and then inverted T waves. If enough myocardium is infarcted, Q waves, which represent unopposed initial depolarization forces away from the mass of the infarcted myocardium, may appear. At times, the diminution of R-wave voltage in the affected area may be the only ECG evidence for the presence of permanent myocardial damage. Right ventricle infarction may be detected by ST elevation in recordings from the right precordial leads, particularly the V4R.[3]

The clinician must also be careful not to be fooled by ECG "imposters" of acute infarction, which include pericarditis, J-point elevation, Wolff-Parkinson-White syndrome, and hypertrophic cardiomyopathy. In patients with pericarditis, ST segments may be elevated, but the elevation will be diffuse, and the morphology of the ST segments in patients with pericarditis tends to be concave upward while that of ischemia is convex. Pericarditis may also be distinguished from infarction by the presence of PR-segment depression in the inferior leads (and also by PR-segment elevation in lead aVR).[4]

Cardiac Biomarkers

Measurement of enzymes released into the serum from necrotic myocardial cells after

Table 1. *Localization of MI by ECG**

Area of Infarction	ECG Leads	Infarct-Related Artery
Inferior	II, III, aVF	RCA or posterolateral branch of Cx
Anterior	V2, V3, V4	LAD or diagonal branch of LAD
Lateral	I, aVL, V5, V6	Cx
True posterior	Tall R wave in V1	Posterolateral branch of Cx or posterior descending branch of RCA
Septal	V1-V3	LAD or diagonal branch of LAD
Anterolateral	I, aVL, V2-V6	Proximal LAD
Inferolateral	II, III, aVF, I, aVL, V5, V6	Proximal Cx or large RCA in right dominant system
Right ventricular	V3R, V4R	RCA

*RCA = right coronary artery; LAD = left anterior descending coronary artery; Cx = circumflex coronary artery.

Acute Coronary Syndromes (Hollenberg)

infarction can aid in the diagnosis of MI.[5] The classic biochemical marker of acute MI is the elevation of the CPK-MB isoenzyme, which begins to appear in the plasma 4 to 8 h after the onset of infarction, peaks at 12 to 24 h after the onset of infarction, and returns to baseline at 2 to 4 days after the onset of infarction. To be diagnostic for MI, the total plasma CPK value must exceed the upper limit of normal, and the MB fraction must exceed a certain value (usually >5%, but it depends on the CPK-MB assay used).

A newer serologic test for the detection of myocardial damage employs the measurement of cardiac troponins.[5] Troponin T and troponin I are constituents of the contractile protein apparatus of the cardiac muscle, and are more specific than the conventional CPK-MB assays for the detection of myocardial damage. Their use is becoming more widespread and has superceded the use of CPK-MB assays in most settings.[6] Troponins are also more sensitive for the detection of myocardial damage, and troponin elevation in patients without ST elevation (or in fact, without elevation of CPK-MB) identifies a subpopulation of patients who are at increased risk for complications. Rapid point-of-care troponin assays, which have become available in the past few years, have further extended the clinical utility of this marker. Troponins may not be elevated until 6 h after an acute event, and so critical therapeutic interventions should not be delayed pending assay results. Once elevated, troponin levels can remain high for days to weeks, limiting their utility to detect late reinfarction.

STEMI

Symptoms suggestive of MI are usually similar to those of ordinary angina but are greater in intensity and duration. Nausea, vomiting, and diaphoresis may be prominent features, and stupor and malaise attributable to low cardiac output may occur. Compromised left ventricular function may result in pulmonary edema with the development of pulmonary bibasilar crackles and jugular venous distention; a fourth heart sound can be present with small infarctions or even mild ischemia, but a third heart sound is usually indicative of more extensive damage.

Patients presenting with suspected myocardial ischemia should undergo a rapid evaluation, and should be treated with oxygen, sublingual nitroglycerin (unless systolic pressure is <90 mm Hg), adequate analgesia, and aspirin, 160 to 325 mg orally.[7] Narcotics, the salutary effects of which have been known for decades and must not be underestimated, should be used to relieve pain and also to reduce anxiety. It is also important to provide reassurance to the patient. A 12-lead ECG should be performed and interpreted expeditiously.

ST-segment elevation of at least 1 mV in two or more contiguous ECG leads provides strong evidence of thrombotic coronary occlusion, and the patient should be considered for immediate reperfusion therapy. The diagnosis of STEMI can be limited in the presence of preexisting left bundle-branch block (LBBB) or a permanent pacemaker. Nonetheless, a new LBBB with a compatible clinical presentation should be treated as acute MI and treated accordingly. Indeed, recent data suggest that patients with STEMI and new LBBB may stand to gain greater benefit from reperfusion strategies than those patients with ST elevation and preserved ventricular conduction.

Fibrinolytic Therapy

Early reperfusion of an occluded coronary artery is indicated for all eligible candidates. Overwhelming evidence from multiple clinical trials has demonstrated the ability of fibrinolytic agents administered early in the course of an acute MI to reduce infarct size, preserve left ventricular function, and reduce short-term and long-term mortality.[8,9] Patients treated early derive the most benefit. Indications and contraindications for fibrinolytic therapy are listed in Table 2. Because of the small, but nonetheless significant, risk of a bleeding complication, most notably intracranial hemorrhage, the selection of patients with acute MI for the administration of a fibrinolytic agent should be undertaken with prudence and caution. Some patients may be better treated with emergent coronary angiography with percutaneous coronary intervention (PCI) as clinically indicated. In contrast to the treatment of STEMI, fibrinolytic agents have shown no benefit when used for the treatment of unstable angina/NSTEMI,[10] and there is currently no role for their use in treating these latter syndromes.

Table 2. *Indications for and Contraindications to Thrombolytic Therapy in Patients With Acute MI*

Indications
  Symptoms consistent with acute MI
  ECG showing 1-mm (0.1 mV) ST elevation in at least two
    contiguous leads or new left bundle-branch block
  Presentation within 12 h of symptom onset
  Absence of contraindications
Contraindications
  Absolute
    Active internal bleeding
    Intracranial neoplasm, aneurysm, or A-V malformation
    Stroke or neurosurgery within 6 wk
    Trauma or major surgery within 2 wk that could be
      a potential source of serious rebleeding
    Aortic dissection
  Relative
  Prolonged (>10 min) or clearly traumatic
    cardiopulmonary resuscitation*
  Noncompressible vascular punctures
  Severe uncontrolled hypertension (>200/110 mm Hg)*
  Trauma or major surgery within 6 wk (but >2 wk)
  Preexisting coagulopathy or current use of anticoagulants
    with INR >2–3
  Active peptic ulcer
  Infective endocarditis
  Pregnancy
  Chronic severe hypertension

*Could be an absolute contraindication in low-risk patients with MI.

Fibrinolytic Agents

Streptokinase (SK) is a single-chain protein produced by α-hemolytic streptococci. SK is given as a 1.5 million-unit IV infusion over 1 h, which produces a systemic lytic state for about 24 h. Hypotension with infusion usually responds to the administration of fluids and a decreased infusion rate, but allergic reactions are possible. Hemorrhagic complications are the most feared side effect, with a rate of intracranial hemorrhage of approximately 0.5%. SK produces coronary arterial patency approximately 50 to 60% of the time and has been shown to decrease mortality by 18% compared to placebo.[8]

Tissue plasminogen activator (t-PA) is a recombinant protein that is more fibrin-selective than SK and produces a higher early coronary patency rate (70 to 80%). In the large (41,021 patients) Global Utilization of Streptokinase and Tissue Plasminogen Activator for Occluded Coronary Arteries (GUSTO) trial, t-PA demonstrated a small but significant survival benefit compared to SK in patients with STEMI (absolute

reduction, 1.1%; relative reduction, 15%).[11] The GUSTO angiographic substudy showed that the difference in patency rates explains the difference in clinical efficacy between these two agents.[12] t-PA is usually given in an accelerated regimen consisting of a 15-mg bolus, 0.75 mg/kg (up to 50 mg) IV over the initial 30 min, and 0.5 mg/kg (up to 35 mg) over the next 60 min. Allergic reactions do not occur because t-PA is not antigenic, but the rate of intracranial hemorrhage may be slightly higher than that with SK (approximately 0.7%).

Reteplase (r-PA) is a deletion mutant of t-PA with an extended half-life, and is given as two 10-mg boluses 30 min apart. r-PA was originally evaluated in angiographic trials, which demonstrated improved coronary flow at 90 min compared to t-PA, but subsequent trials showed similar 30-day mortality rates.[13] Why enhanced patency attained with r-PA therapy did not translate into lower mortality is uncertain.

Tenecteplase (TNK-tPA) is a genetically engineered t-PA mutant with amino acid substitutions that result in prolonged half-life, resistance to plasminogen-activator inhibitor-1, and increased fibrin specificity. TNK-tPA is given as a single bolus, adjusted for weight. A single bolus of TNK-tPA has been shown to produce coronary flow rates identical to those seen with accelerated t-PA, with equivalent 30-day mortality and bleeding rates.[14] Based on these results, therapy with single-bolus TNK-tPA is an acceptable alternative to t-PA that can be given as a single bolus.

Because these newer agents, in general, have equivalent efficacy and side-effect profiles, currently have no additional cost compared to t-PA, and are simpler to administer, they have gained popularity. The ideal thrombolytic agent has not yet been developed. Newer recombinant agents with greater fibrin specificity, slower clearance from the circulation, and more resistance to plasma protease inhibitors are being studied.

Primary PCI in Acute MI

As many as one half to two thirds of patients presenting with acute MI may be ineligible for thrombolytic therapy, and these patients should be considered for primary PCI. The major advantages of therapy with primary PCI over thrombolytic therapy include a higher rate of normal flow (thrombolysis in myocardial infarction [TIMI] grade 3), a lower risk of intracranial hemorrhage, and the ability to stratify risk based on the severity and distribution of coronary artery disease. Data from several randomized trials[15] have suggested that PCI is preferable to thrombolytic therapy for acute MI patients at higher risk, including those patients who are >75 years old, those with anterior infarctions, and those with hemodynamic instability. The largest of these trials is the GUSTO-IIb Angioplasty Substudy, which randomized 1,138 patients. At 30 days, there was a clinical benefit in the combined primary end points of death, nonfatal reinfarction, and nonfatal disabling stroke in the patients treated with percutaneous coronary angioplasty (PTCA) compared to those treated with t-PA, but there was no difference in the "hard" end points of death and MI at 30 days.[16]

It should be noted that these trials were performed in institutions in which a team skilled in primary angioplasty for acute MI was immediately available, with standby surgical backup, allowing for prompt reperfusion of the infarct-related artery. More important than the method of revascularization is the time to revascularization, and that this is achieved in the most efficient and expeditious manner possible.[17] Procedural volume is important as well.[18] A metaanalysis[15,19] from 2003 comparing direct PTCA therapy with thrombolytic therapy found lower rates of mortality and reinfarction among those patients receiving direct PTCA. Thus, direct angioplasty, if performed in a timely manner (ideally within 60 min) by highly experienced personnel, may be the preferred method of revascularization since it offers more complete revascularization with improved restoration of normal coronary blood flow and detailed information about coronary anatomy.

Historically, it has been thought that when the performance of PCI requires a substantial time delay, thrombolytic therapy may be preferable. Recently reported studies comparing in-house thrombolysis to hospital transfer for PCI have challenged this notion, however. In the PRAGUE-2 study,[20] there was no difference in mortality between patients treated within 3 h with either thrombolysis using SK or off-site

Table 3. *Situations in Which Primary Angioplasty Is Preferred in Acute MI**

Situations in which PTCA is clearly preferable to therapy with thrombolytic agents
    Contraindications to thrombolytic therapy
    Cardiogenic shock
    Patients in whom uncertain diagnosis prompted cardiac catheterization, which revealed coronary occlusion
Situations in which PTCA may be preferable to thrombolytic agents
    Elderly patients (>75 yr)
    Hemodynamic instability
    Patients with prior CABG
    Large anterior infarction
    Patients with a prior MI

*CABG =coronary artery bypass grafting.

PCI. Interestingly, in patients treated between 3 and 12 h, transfer for PCI conferred a significant mortality benefit despite adding to the time to treatment.[20] Similar results were found in the DANAMI-2 study,[21] in which referral for primary PCI reduced the occurrence of a composite end point of death, reinfarction, or stroke, compared with thrombolysis using t-PA. While these data are intriguing, the importance of procedural volume and experience has been underscored by retrospective studies suggesting that in the community setting (as opposed to PCI performed as part of a controlled clinical trial), mortality rates after MI with routine primary PCI and thrombolytic therapy are currently equivalent. More controversial is the issue of performing PCI at centers without onsite surgical backup. While emerging data suggest that this practice is not only feasible but also safe,[22] further large-scale investigations will be necessary to clarify this issue.

There are certain subpopulations in which primary PCI is preferred. In patients who do not respond to thrombolytic therapy, salvage PTCA is indicated; although the initial success rate is lower than that of primary angioplasty, reocclusion is more common, and mortality is higher.[23] Emergent cardiac catheterization is also preferred in patients with cardiogenic shock. Other indications are listed in Table 3.

There is no convincing evidence to support empirical delayed PTCA in patients without evidence of recurrent or provocable ischemia after thrombolytic therapy. The TIMI IIB trial[24] and other studies have suggested that a strategy of "watchful waiting" allows for the identification of patients who will benefit from revascularization.

Adjunctive Therapies in STEMI

Antiplatelet Agents

Aspirin has been shown to reduce mortality in patients with acute infarction to the same degree as thrombolytic therapy, and its effects are additive to thrombolytic agents.[25] In addition, aspirin reduces the risk of reinfarction. Unless contraindicated, all patients with a suspected ACS (ie, STEMI, NSTEMI, or unstable angina) should be given aspirin as soon as possible.

The efficacy of the addition of clopidogrel to aspirin for therapy in STEMI patients was recently shown in the Clopidogrel and Metoprolol Myocardial Infarction Trial (or COMMIT) trial.[26] In 45,852 STEMI patients (half of whom received fibrinolytic therapy), the addition of clopidogrel to the treatment regimen reduced both total mortality and the composite end point of death, reinfarction, or stroke; there was no significant excess risk of bleeding in this study.[26]

Heparin

The administration of full-dose heparin after thrombolytic therapy with t-PA is essential to diminish reocclusion after successful reperfusion.[8,25] Dosing should be adjusted to weight, with a bolus of 60 U/kg up to a maximum of 4,000 U and an initial infusion rate of 12 U/kg/h up to a maximum of 1,000 U/h, with adjustment to keep the partial thromboplastin time between 50 and 70 s. Therapy with heparin should be continued for 24 to 48 h.

Therapy with enoxaparin was compared to therapy with unfractionated heparin in the EXTRACT-TIMI 25 trial,[27] which randomized 20,506 patients with STEMI for treatment with fibrinolytic therapy, using death or MI at 30 days as the primary end point. This combined end point was significantly reduced with therapy with enoxaparin (although mortality was unchanged) at the cost of a small but significant increase in major bleeding.[27] The composite of death, reinfarction, or nonfatal intracranial hemorrhage (termed the net clinical benefit) was also reduced with enoxaparin therapy, suggesting that low-molecular-weight heparin (LMWH) is an attractive agent for therapy in patients receiving fibrinolysis for STEMI.

Nitrates

Nitrates have a number of beneficial effects in the treatment of acute MI. They reduce myocardial oxygen demand by decreasing preload and afterload, and may also improve the myocardial oxygen supply by increasing subendocardial perfusion and collateral blood flow to the ischemic region. Occasionally, patients with ST elevation due to occlusive coronary artery spasm may have dramatic resolution of ischemia with the use of nitrates. In addition to their hemodynamic effects, nitrates also reduce platelet aggregation. Despite these benefits, the Gruppo Italiano per lo Studio Della Streptochinasi Nell'Infarto Miocardico (or GISSI)-3 trial[28] and the International Study of Infarct Survival (or ISIS)-4 trial[29] failed to show a significant reduction in mortality from routine short-term and long-term nitrate therapy. Nonetheless, nitrates are still first-line agents for the symptomatic relief of angina pectoris and when MI is complicated by congestive heart failure.

ß-Blockers

β-blockers are beneficial both in the early management of MI and as long-term therapy. In the prethrombolytic era, early therapy with IV atenolol was shown to significantly reduce reinfarction, cardiac arrest, cardiac rupture, and death.[30] In conjunction with thrombolytic therapy with t-PA, immediate β-blockade with metoprolol resulted in a significant reduction in recurrent ischemia and reinfarction, although mortality was not decreased.[24] These findings were confirmed in a very large (45,852 patient) trial[31] randomizing patients with STEMI to metoprolol (IV and then oral) or placebo (n = 22,923). Although the risk of reinfarction or ventricular fibrillation was significantly decreased, mortality was unchanged.[31] Further analysis showed that an excess of cardiogenic shock in the metoprolol group, particularly in patients presenting with Killip class III heart failure (as heart failure on presentation was not an exclusion criterion).[31]

These findings suggest that IV β-blockade should be considered for all patients with STEMI who have continued ischemic discomfort, particularly those with hypertension, but should be avoided in patients with moderate or severe heart failure, hypotension, severe bradycardia or heart block, and severe bronchospastic disease.

Oral β-blockade has been clearly demonstrated to decrease mortality after acute MI[9,32,33] and should be initiated in all patients who can tolerate it, even if they have not been treated with IV β-blockers. Diabetes mellitus is not a contraindication.

Lipid-Lowering Agents

Extensive epidemiologic, laboratory, and clinical evidence links cholesterol and coronary artery disease.[34] Impressive results have been achieved using hydroxymethylglutaryl-coenzyme A (HMG-CoA) reductase inhibitors (statins) in patients with documented coronary artery disease[35] in the 4S trial, and also in patients after MI,[35-37] as well as in the CARE study[36] and the Long-Term Intervention with Pravastatin in Ischaemic Disease (or LIPID) trial.[37] More recent studies[38] have suggested that therapy with statins should be started in the hospital, as the benefits can be demonstrated early, perhaps as a result of the antiinflammatory effects of statins.

The 2004 PROVE-IT trial[39] showed that the reduction of low-density lipoprotein (LDL) cholesterol to a mean concentration of 62 mg/dL with atorvastatin was associated with improved outcomes compared to therapy with pravastatin at a dose that achieved a mean LDL concentration of 95 mg/dL. Although current guidelines[40] suggest an LDL concentration goal of 70 to 100 mg/dL, newer recommendations are likely to be even more aggressive. Maximum benefit may require the management of other lipid abnormalities (ie, elevated triglycerides and low high-density lipoprotein cholesterol concentrations) and the treatment of other atherogenic risk factors.

Angiotensin-Converting Enzyme Inhibitors

Therapy with angiotensin-converting enzyme (ACE) inhibitors is clearly beneficial in patients with congestive heart failure. ACE inhibitors were shown to decrease mortality in the SAVE trial,[41] in which patients with left ventricular dysfunction (ejection fraction, <40%) after an MI had a 21% improvement in survival after treatment with the ACE inhibitor captopril. A smaller but still significant reduction in mortality was seen when all patients were treated with captopril in the ISIS-4 study.[29] The mechanisms responsible for the benefits of therapy with ACE inhibitors probably include limitation in the progressive left ventricular dysfunction and enlargement (remodeling) that often occur after infarction, but a reduction in ischemic events was seen as well.

Therapy with ACE inhibitors should be started early, preferably within the first 24 h after the MI. Immediate IV ACE inhibition with enalaprilat has not been shown to be beneficial.[42] Patients should be started on low doses of oral agents (captopril, 6.25 mg three times daily) and rapidly increased to the dosage range that has been demonstrated to be beneficial in clinical trials (captopril, 50 mg three times daily; enalapril, 10 to 20 mg twice daily; lisinopril, 10 to 20 mg once daily; or ramipril, 10 mg once daily).

Calcium Channel Blockers

Randomized clinical trials have not demonstrated that the routine use of calcium channel blockers improves survival after MI. In fact, metaanalyses have suggested[43] that high doses of the short-acting dihydropyridine nifedipine increase mortality in patients with MI. Calcium channel blockers may be useful in the treatment of patients whose postinfarction course is complicated by recurrent angina, because these agents not only reduce myocardial oxygen demand but inhibit coronary vasoconstriction. Diltiazem is the only calcium channel blocker that has been proven to have tangible benefits, reducing reinfarction and recurrent ischemia in patients with NQMIs who do not have evidence of congestive heart failure.[44] The adverse effects of calcium-channel blockers include bradycardia, atrioventricular block, and exacerbation of heart failure

For hemodynamically stable patients, diltiazem can be given orally, starting at 60 to 90 mg every 6 to 8 h. In patients with severe left ventricular dysfunction, long-acting dihydropyridine agents without prominent negative inotropic effects, such as amlodipine, nicardipine, or the

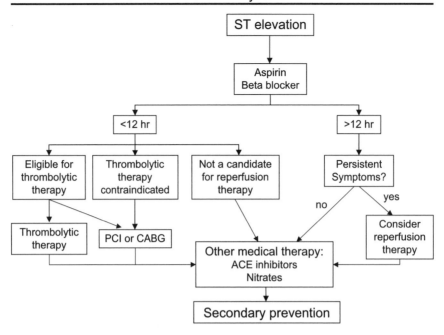

Figure 1. Possible treatment algorithm for patients presenting with STEMI.

long-acting preparation of nifedipine, may be preferable; increased mortality with these agents has not been demonstrated.

Antiarrhythmic Therapy

A major purpose for admitting MI patients to the ICU is to monitor for and prevent malignant arrhythmias. Ventricular extrasystoles are common after MI and are a manifestation of electrical instability of periinfarct areas. The incidence of sustained ventricular tachycardia or fibrillation is highest in the first 3 to 4 h, but these arrhythmias may occur at any time. Malignant ventricular arrhythmias may be heralded by frequent complex ectopy but may occur suddenly without these preceding "warning" arrhythmias.

Although lidocaine increases the frequency of premature ventricular contractions and of early ventricular fibrillation, overall mortality is not decreased. In fact, metaanalyses[45] of pooled data have demonstrated increased mortality from the routine use of lidocaine. Therefore, the routine prophylactic administration of lidocaine is no longer recommended.

Nonetheless, lidocaine infusion may be useful after an episode of sustained ventricular tachycardia or ventricular fibrillation, and could be considered in patients with nonsustained

ventricular tachycardia. Toxic manifestations primarily involve the CNS, and can include confusion, lethargy, slurred speech, and seizures

Therapy with IV amiodarone is an alternative to therapy with lidocaine for ventricular arrhythmias. Amiodarone is given as a 150-mg IV bolus infused over 10 min, followed by infusion of 1 mg/min for 6 h, then 0.5 mg/min for 18 h.

Perhaps the most important point in the prevention and management of arrhythmias after acute MI is correcting hypoxemia, and maintaining normal serum potassium and magnesium levels. The serum levels of electrolytes should be monitored closely, particularly after diuretic therapy. Magnesium depletion is also a frequently overlooked cause of persistent ectopy, and serum magnesium levels, even within normal limits, may not reflect myocardial concentrations. The routine administration of magnesium has not been shown to reduce mortality after acute MI,[29] but the empiric IV administration of 2 g of magnesium in patients with early ventricular ectopy is probably a good idea. A potential treatment algorithm for treating patients with STEMI is shown in Figure 1.

NSTEMI

The key to the initial management of patients with ACSs who present without ST elevation is risk stratification. The overall risk of a patient is related to both the severity of the preexisting heart disease and the degree of plaque instability. Risk stratification is an ongoing process, which begins with hospital admission and continues through hospital discharge. The risk of progression to acute MI or death in patients with ACSs is dependent on clinical factors such as age, presentation with heart failure, and ST-segment depression seen on the ECG.[46] Conversely, a normal ECG finding confers an excellent short-term prognosis. Biochemical markers of cardiac injury, in particular elevated levels of troponin, are associated with an increased risk of cardiac events and a higher 30-day mortality rate.[47] Conversely, low levels are associated with low event rates, although the absence of troponin elevation does not guarantee a good prognosis and is not a substitute for good clinical judgment.

Antiplatelet Therapy

As previously noted, aspirin is a mainstay of therapy for ACSs. Both the Veterans Administration Cooperative Study Group[48] and the Canadian Multicenter Trial[49] showed that aspirin reduces the risk of death or MI by approximately 50% in patients with unstable angina or NQMI. Aspirin also reduces the number of events after the resolution of an ACS and should be continued indefinitely.

Clopidogrel, a thienopyridine that inhibits adenosine diphosphate-induced platelet activation, is more potent than aspirin and can be used in its place if necessary. Clopidogrel is used in combination with aspirin when intracoronary stents are placed. Clopidogrel added to aspirin significantly reduced the risk of MI, stroke, or cardiovascular death in 12,562 patients with unstable angina in the randomized CURE trial,[50] both in patients managed invasively with stents and those managed medically. It should be noted that this benefit came with a 1% absolute increase in major, non-life-threatening bleeds as well as a 2.8% absolute increase in major/life-threatening bleeds associated with coronary artery bypass grafting (CABG) within 5 days.[50] These data have raised concerns about administering clopidogrel prior to having information about the coronary anatomy.

Anticoagulant Therapy

Heparin is an important component of primary therapy for patients with unstable coronary syndromes without ST elevation. When added to therapy with aspirin, heparin has been shown to reduce refractory angina and the development of MI,[51] and a metaanalysis[52] of the available data has indicated that the addition of heparin to therapy reduces the composite end point of death or MI.

Heparin, however, can be difficult to administer, because the anticoagulant effect is unpredictable in individual patients; this is due to heparin binding to heparin-binding proteins, to endothelial cells and other cells, and heparin inhibition by several factors released by activated platelets. Therefore, the activated partial thromboplastin time must be monitored closely. The potential for heparin-associated thrombocytopenia is also a safety concern.

LMWHs, which are obtained by the depolymerization of standard heparin and the selection of fractions with lower molecular weight, have several advantages. Because they bind less avidly to heparin-binding proteins, there is less variability in the anticoagulant response and a more predictable dose-response curve, obviating the need to monitor activated partial thromboplastin time. The incidence of thrombocytopenia is lower (but not absent, and patients with heparin-induced thrombocytopenia with antiheparin antibodies cannot be switched to LMWH). Finally, LMWHs have longer half-lives and can be given by subcutaneous injection.

The beneficial effects of LMWH therapy in patients with unstable coronary syndromes were documented in the ESSENCE trial[53] and the TIMI IIB trial,[54] which showed that the LMWH enoxaparin reduced the combined end point of death, MI, or recurrent ischemia compared to unfractionated heparin. In these early trials, most of the patients were managed conservatively. In the SYNERGY trial,[55] which was performed in high-risk patients, most of whom were treated invasively, no difference was found in efficacy between enoxaparin and unfractionated heparin, with a slightly higher major bleeding rate with enoxaparin. Specific considerations with the use of LMWH include decreased clearance in renal insufficiency and the lack of a readily available test to measure the anticoagulant effect.

Recently, fondaparinux, a pentasaccharide that inhibits factor Xa, was tested in patients with non-ST-elevation ACSs. The OASIS-5 trial[56] compared fondaparinux to enoxaparin in 20,078 patients with ACSs (most of whom were treated conservatively), with death, MI, or refractory ischemia at 9 days as the primary outcome. This outcome was equivalent, satisfying noninferiority for fondaparinux, and major bleeding was lower in the fondaparinux group.[56] A secondary end point, mortality at 30 days, was significantly reduced with fondaparinux therapy.[56]

These studies suggest that alternatives to therapy with unfractionated heparin are safe and effective. Further testing of their effects when combined with an invasive strategy will clarify their appropriate role.

Glycoprotein IIb/IIIa Antagonists

Given the central role of platelet activation and aggregation in the pathophysiology of unstable coronary syndromes, attention has focused on platelet glycoprotein IIb/IIIa antagonists, which inhibit the final common pathway of platelet aggregation.[57] The following three agents are currently available: abciximab, a chimeric murine-human monoclonal antibody Fab fragment; eptifibatide, a small-molecule cyclic heptapeptide; and tirofiban, a small-molecule, synthetic, nonpeptide agent. The benefits of therapy with glycoprotein IIb/IIIa inhibitors as adjunctive treatment in patients undergoing PCI have been substantial and consistently observed.[57] Abciximab has been most extensively studied, but a benefit for eptifibatide has also been demonstrated.

In patients with ACSs, the evidence supporting the efficacy of therapy with glycoprotein IIb/IIIa inhibitors is somewhat less impressive. Taken together, the major trials[58-61] show a small but significant reduction in composite end points (ie, death and MI, with refractory ischemia in some patients). Additional analysis suggests that glycoprotein IIb/IIIa inhibition is most effective in high-risk patients, those with either

ECG changes or elevated troponin levels.[57] The benefits appear to accrue primarily to patients undergoing PCI, which may not be entirely surprising.

Interventional Management

Cardiac catheterization may be undertaken in patients presenting with symptoms suggestive of unstable coronary syndromes for one of the following reasons: to assist with risk stratification; as a prelude to revascularization; and to exclude significant epicardial coronary stenosis as a cause of symptoms when the diagnosis is uncertain.

An early invasive approach has now been compared to a conservative approach in several prospective studies. The results of two earlier trials, the TIMI IIIb study[10] and the VANQWISH trial,[62] both of which were performed before use of coronary stenting and platelet glycoprotein IIb/IIIa inhibitors was widespread, were negative. More recently, several trials, including a substudy of the FRagmin and Fast Revascularisation during InStability in Coronary artery disease (or FRISC) II study,[63] the TACTICS TIMI-18 study,[64] and the RITA-3 study[65] found a significant reduction in the combined end point of death, MI, or recurrent angina with invasive management. The most recent comparison, the ICTUS study,[66] found no difference in a composite end point of death, MI, or rehospitalization for angina at 1 year between a group assigned to early invasive management and another assigned to selectively invasive management. As > 40% of patients in the selectively invasive group were revascularized in the first month, this trial likely argues not so much against an early invasive strategy as for the selection of those patients who are most likely to benefit. Alternatively (or in parallel), improved adjunctive antiplatelet, antithrombin, and lipid-lowering therapy may have narrowed the difference between strategies.

Risk stratification is the key to managing patients with NSTEMI ACSs. One possible algorithm for managing patients with NSTEMI is shown in Figure 2. An initial strategy of medical management with attempts at stabilization is warranted in patients with lower risk, but

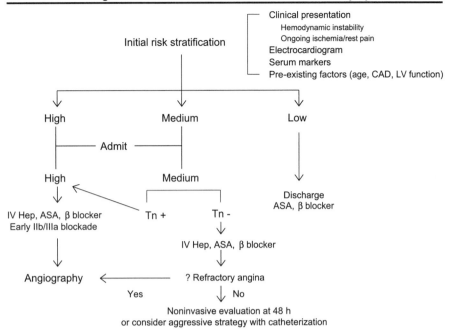

Figure 2. Possible treatment algorithm for patients with non-ST-elevation ACSs. Hep = heparin; ASA = aspirin; Tn = troponin.

patients at higher risk should be considered for cardiac catheterization. Pharmacologic and mechanical strategies are intertwined because the selection of patients for early revascularization will influence the choice of antiplatelet and anticoagulant medication. When good clinical judgment is employed, early coronary angiography in selected patients with ACSs can lead to better management and lower morbidity and mortality.

Complications of Acute MI

Postinfarction Ischemia

Ischemia after MI can be due to mechanical problems that increase myocardial oxygen demand and to extracardiac factors, such as hypertension, anemia, hypotension, or hypermetabolic states, but it usually results from decreased myocardial oxygen supply due to coronary reocclusion or spasm. Immediate management includes therapy with aspirin, β-blockers, IV nitroglycerin, heparin, the consideration of calcium-channel blockers, and diagnostic coronary angiography.

Post-infarction angina is an indication for revascularization. PTCA can be performed if the culprit lesion is suitable. CABG should be considered for patients with left main artery disease and three-vessel disease, and in those patients who are unsuitable to undergo PTCA. If the angina cannot be controlled medically or is accompanied by hemodynamic instability, an intraaortic balloon pump should be inserted.

Ventricular Free-Wall Rupture

Ventricular free-wall rupture typically occurs during the first week after MI. The classic patient is elderly, female, and hypertensive. The early use of thrombolytic therapy reduces the incidence of cardiac rupture, but late use may actually increase the risk.[67] Free-wall rupture presents as a catastrophic event with shock and electromechanical dissociation. Salvage is possible with prompt recognition, pericardiocentesis to relieve acute tamponade, and thoracotomy for repair.[68] Emergent echocardiography or pulmonary artery catheterization can help to make the diagnosis.

Ventricular Septal Rupture

Septal rupture presents as severe heart failure or cardiogenic shock, with a pansystolic murmur and parasternal thrill. The hallmark finding is a left-to-right intracardiac shunt (ie, a "step-up" in oxygen saturation from the right atrium to the right ventricle), but the diagnosis is most easily made with echocardiography.

The rapid institution of intraaortic balloon pumping and supportive pharmacologic measures is necessary. Operative repair is the only viable option for long-term survival. The timing of surgery has been controversial, but most authorities now suggest[69,70] that repair should be undertaken early, within 48 h of the rupture.

Acute Mitral Regurgitation

Ischemic mitral regurgitation is usually associated with inferior MI and ischemia or with infarction of the posterior papillary muscle, although anterior papillary muscle rupture can also occur. Papillary muscle rupture typically occurs 2 to 7 days after an acute MI, and presents dramatically with pulmonary edema, hypotension, and cardiogenic shock. When a papillary muscle ruptures, the murmur of acute mitral regurgitation may be limited to early systole because of the rapid equalization of pressures in the left atrium and left ventricle. More importantly, the murmur may be soft or inaudible, especially when cardiac output is low.[71]

Echocardiography is extremely useful in the differential diagnosis, which includes free-wall rupture, ventricular septal rupture, and infarct extension with pump failure. Hemodynamic monitoring with pulmonary artery catheterization may also be helpful. Management includes afterload reduction with nitroprusside and intraaortic balloon pumping as temporizing measures. Inotropic or vasopressor therapy may also be needed to support cardiac output and BP. Definitive therapy, however, is surgical valve repair or replacement, which should be undertaken as soon as possible since clinical deterioration can be sudden.[71,72]

Right Ventricular Infarction

Right ventricular infarction occurs in up to 30% of patients with inferior infarction and is clinically significant in 10% of patients.[73] The combination of a clear chest radiograph with jugular venous distention in a patient with an inferior wall MI should lead to the suspicion of a coexisting right ventricular infarction. The diagnosis is substantiated by the demonstration of ST segment elevation in the right precordial leads (ie, V3R to V5R) or by characteristic hemodynamic findings on right heart catheterization (ie, elevated right atrial and right ventricular end-diastolic pressures with normal to low pulmonary artery occlusion pressure and low cardiac output). Echocardiography can demonstrate depressed right ventricular contractility.[74] Patients with cardiogenic shock due to right ventricular infarction have a better prognosis than those with left-sided pump failure.[73] This may be due in part to the fact that right ventricular function tends to return to normal over time with supportive therapy,[75] although such therapy may need to be prolonged.

In patients with right ventricular infarction, right ventricular preload should be maintained with fluid administration. In some cases, however, fluid resuscitation may increase pulmonary capillary occlusion pressure but may not increase cardiac output, and overdilation of the right ventricle can compromise left ventricular filling and cardiac output.[75] Inotropic therapy with dobutamine may be more effective in increasing cardiac output in some patients, and monitoring with serial echocardiograms may also be useful to detect right ventricular overdistention.[75] The maintenance of atrioventricular synchrony is also important in these patients to optimize right ventricular filling.[74] For patients with continued hemodynamic instability, intraaortic balloon pumping may be useful, particularly because elevated right ventricular pressures and volumes increase wall stress and oxygen consumption, and decrease right coronary perfusion pressure, exacerbating right ventricular ischemia.

Reperfusion of the occluded coronary artery is also crucial. A study[76] using direct angioplasty demonstrated that the restoration of normal flow resulted in dramatic recovery of right ventricular function and a mortality rate of only 2%, whereas unsuccessful reperfusion was associated with persistent hemodynamic compromise and a mortality rate of 58%.

References

1. Libby P. Current concepts of the pathogenesis of the acute coronary syndromes. Circulation 2001; 104:365–372

2. Ambrose JA, Martinez EE. A new paradigm for plaque stabilization. Circulation 2002; 105: 2000–2004

3. Croft CH, Nicod P, Corbett JR, et al. Detection of acute right ventricular infarction by right precordial electrocardiography. Am J Cardiol 1982; 50: 421–427

4. Lange RA, Hillis LD. Clinical practice. Acute pericarditis. N Engl J Med 2004; 357:2195–2202

5. Jaffe AS, Babuin L, Apple FS. Biomarkers in acute cardiac disease: the present and the future. J Am Coll Cardiol 2006; 48:1–11

6. Jaffe AS, Ravkilde J, Roberts R, et al. It's time for a change to a troponin standard. Circulation 2000; 102:1216–1220

7. Antman EM, Anbe DT, Armstrong PW, et al. ACC/AHA guidelines for the management of patients with ST-elevation myocardial infarction: executive summary; a report of the American College of Cardiology/American Heart Association Task Force on Practice Guidelines. Circulation 2004; 110: 588–636

8. Gruppo Italiano per lo Studio Della Streptochinasi Nell'Infarto Miocardico (GISSI). Effectiveness of intravenous thrombolytic treatment in acute myocardial infarction. Lancet 1986; 2:397–402

9. International Study Group. In-hospital mortality and clinical course of 20,891 patients with suspected acute myocardial infarction randomised between alteplase and streptokinase with or without heparin. Lancet 1990; 336:71–75

10. TIMI Investigators. Effects of tissue plasminogen activator and a comparison of early invasive and conservative strategies in unstable angina and non-Q-wave myocardial infarction: results of the TIMI IIIB Trial. Circulation 1994; 89:1545–1556

11. GUSTO Investigators. An international randomized trial comparing four thrombolytic strategies for acute myocardial infarction. N Engl J Med 1993; 329:673–682

12. GUSTO Angiographic Investigators. The effects of tissue plasminogen activator, streptokinase, or both on coronary-artery patency, ventricular function, and survival after acute myocardial infarction. N Engl J Med 1993; 329:1615–1622

13. Global Use of Strategies to Open Occluded Coronary Arteries (GUSTO III) Investigators. A comparison of reteplase with alteplase for acute myocardial infarction. N Engl J Med 1997; 337: 1118–1123

14. ASSENT-2 Investigators. Single-bolus tenecteplase compared with front-loaded alteplase in acute myocardial infarction: the ASSENT-2 double-blind randomised trial. Lancet 1999; 354:716–722

15. Grines C, Patel A, Zijlstra F, et al. Primary coronary angioplasty compared with intravenous thrombolytic therapy for acute myocardial infarction: six-month follow up and analysis of individual patient data from randomized trials. Am Heart J 2003; 145:47–57

16. GUSTO IIb Investigators. A comparison of recombinant hirudin with heparin for the treatment of acute coronary syndromes. N Engl J Med 1996; 335:775–782

17. Cannon CP, Gibson CM, Lambrew CT, et al. Relationship of symptom-onset-to-balloon time and door-to-balloon time with mortality in patients undergoing angioplasty for acute myocardial infarction. JAMA 2000; 283:2941–2947

18. Canto JG, Every NR, Magid DJ, et al. The volume of primary angioplasty procedures and survival after acute myocardial infarction: National Registry of Myocardial Infarction 2 Investigators. N Engl J Med 2000; 342:1573–1580

19. Keeley EC, Boura JA, Grines CL. Primary angioplasty versus intravenous thrombolytic therapy for acute myocardial infarction: a quantitative review of 23 randomised trials. Lancet 2003; 361:13–20

20. Widimsky P, Budesinsky T, Vorac D, et al. Long distance transport for primary angioplasty vs immediate thrombolysis in acute myocardial infarction: final results of the randomized national multicentre trial; PRAGUE-2. Eur Heart J 2003; 24:94–104

21. Andersen HR, Nielsen TT, Rasmussen K, et al. A comparison of coronary angioplasty with fibrinolytic therapy in acute myocardial infarction. N Engl J Med 2003; 349:733–742

22. Aversano T, Aversano LT, Passamani E, et al. Thrombolytic therapy vs primary percutaneous coronary intervention for myocardial infarction in patients presenting to hospitals without on-site cardiac surgery: a randomized controlled trial. JAMA 2002; 287:1943–1951

23. Gershlick AH, Stephens-Lloyd A, Hughes S, et al. Rescue angioplasty after failed thrombolytic therapy

for acute myocardial infarction. N Engl J Med 2005; 353:2758–2768

24. TIMI Study Group. Comparison of invasive and conservative strategies after treatment with intravenous tissue plasminogen activator in acute myocardial infarction: Results of the Thrombolysis in Myocardial Infarction (TIMI) phase II trial. N Engl J Med 1989; 320:618–627

25. ISIS-2 Collaborative Group. Randomised trial of intravenous streptokinase, oral aspirin, both, or neither among 17 187 cases of suspected acute myocardial infarction: ISIS-2. Lancet 1988; 2:349–360

26. Chen ZM, Jiang LX, Chen YP, et al. Addition of clopidogrel to aspirin in 45,852 patients with acute myocardial infarction: randomised placebo-controlled trial. Lancet 2005; 366:1607–1621

27. Antman EM, Morrow DA, McCabe CH, et al. Enoxaparin versus unfractionated heparin with fibrinolysis for ST-elevation myocardial infarction. N Engl J Med 2006; 354:1477–1488

28. Gruppo Italiano per lo Studio della Strepto chinasi nell'Infarto Miocardico (GISSI). GISSI-3: effects of lisinopril and transdermal glyceryl trinitrate singly and together on 6-week mortality and ventricular function after acute myocardial infarction. Lancet 1994; 343:1115–1122

29. ISIS-4 (Fourth International Study of Infarct Survival) Study Group. ISIS-4: a randomised factorial trial assessing early oral captopril, oral mononitrate, and intravenous magnesium sulphate in 58,050 patients with suspected acute myocardial infarction. Lancet 1995; 345:669–685

30. First International Study of Infarct Survival Collaborative Group. Randomised trial of intravenous atenolol among 16,027 cases of suspected acute myocardial infarction: ISIS-1. Lancet 1986; 2: 57–66

31. Chen ZM, Pan HC, Chen YP, et al. Early intravenous then oral metoprolol in 45,852 patients with acute myocardial infarction: randomised placebo-controlled trial. Lancet 2005; 366:1622–1632

32. MIAMI Trial Research Group. Metoprolol in acute myocardial infarction (MIAMI): a randomised placebo-controlled international trial. Eur Heart J 1985; 6:199–226

33. Dargie HJ. Effect of carvedilol on outcome after myocardial infarction in patients with left-ventricular dysfunction: the CAPRICORN randomised trial. Lancet 2001; 357:1385–1390

34. Lipid Research Clinics Program. The lipid research clinics coronary primary prevention trial results: I. Reduction in incidence of coronary heart disease. JAMA 1984; 251:351–364

35. Scandinavian Simvastatin Survival Study Group. Randomised trial of cholesterol lowering in 4444 patients with coronary heart disease: the Scandinavian Simvastatin Survival Study (4S). Lancet 1994; 344:1383–1389

36. Sacks FM, Pfeffer MA, Moye LA, et al. The effect of pravastatin on coronary events after myocardial infarction in patients with average cholesterol levels. N Engl J Med 1996; 335:1001–1009

37. Long-Term Intervention with Pravastatin in Ischaemic Disease (LIPID) Study Group. Prevention of cardiovascular events and death with pravastatin in patients with coronary heart disease and a broad range of initial cholesterol levels. N Engl J Med 1998; 339:1349–1357

38. Schwartz GG, Olsson AG, Ezekowitz MD, et al. Effects of atorvastatin on early recurrent ischemic events in acute coronary syndromes: the MIRACL study: a randomized controlled trial. JAMA 2001; 285:1711–1718

39. Cannon CP, Braunwald E, McCabe CH, et al. Intensive versus moderate lipid lowering with statins after acute coronary syndromes. N Engl J Med 2004; 350:1495–1504

40. Gibbons RJ, Abrams J, Chatterjee K, et al. ACC/AHA 2002 guideline update for the management of patients with chronic stable angina: summary article; a report of the American College of Cardiology/American Heart Association Task Force on Practice Guidelines (Committee on the Management of Patients With Chronic Stable Angina). Circulation 2003; 107:149–158

41. Pfeffer MA, Braunwald E, Moye LA, et al. Effect of captopril on mortality and morbidity in patients with left ventricular dysfunction after myocardial infarction: results of the Survival and Ventricular Enlargement Trial. N Engl J Med 1992; 327: 669–677

42. Swedberg K, Held P, Kjekshus J, et al. Effects of the early administration of enalapril on mortality in patients with acute myocardial infarction: results of the Cooperative New Scandinavian Enalapril Survival Study II (CONSENSUS II). N Engl J Med 1992; 327:678–384

43. Furberg CD, Psaty BM, Meyer JV. Nifedipine: dose-related increase in mortality in patients

with coronary heart disease. Circulation 1995; 92: 1326–1331

44. Gibson RS, Boden WE, Theroux P, et al. Diltiazem and reinfarction in patients with non-Q-wave myocardial infarction. N Engl J Med 1986; 315:423–429

45. MacMahon S, Collins R, Peto R, et al. Effects of prophylactic lidocaine in suspected acute myocardial infarction: an overview of results from the randomized, controlled trials. JAMA 1988; 260: 1910–1916

46. Braunwald E, Antman EM, Beasley JW, et al. ACC/AHA guidelines for the management of patients with unstable angina and non-ST-segment elevation myocardial infarction: executive summary and recommendations; a report of the American College of Cardiology/American Heart Association task force on practice guidelines (committee on the management of patients with unstable angina). Circulation 2000; 102:1193–1209

47. Ohman EM, Armstrong PW, Christenson RH, et al. Cardiac troponin T levels for risk stratification in acute myocardial ischemia. N Engl J Med 1996; 335:133–1341

48. Lewis HD Jr., Davis JW, Archibald DG, et al. Protective effects of aspirin against acute myocardial infarction and death in men with unstable angina: results of a Veterans Administration cooperative study. N Engl J Med 1983; 309:396–403

49. Cairns JA, Gent M, Singer J, et al. Aspirin, sulfinpyrazone, or both in unstable angina: results of a Canadian multicenter trial. N Engl J Med 1985; 313:1369–1375

50. Yusuf S, Zhao F, Mehta SR, et al. Effects of clopidogrel in addition to aspirin in patients with acute coronary syndromes without ST-segment elevation. N Engl J Med 2001; 345:494–502

51. Theroux P, Ouimet H, McCans J, et al. Aspirin, heparin, or both to treat acute unstable angina. N Engl J Med 1988; 319:1105–1111

52. Oler A, Whooley MA, Oler J, et al. Adding heparin to aspirin reduces the incidence of myocardial infarction and death in patients with unstable angina: a meta-analysis. JAMA 1996; 276:811–815

53. Antman EM, Cohen M, Radley D, et al. Assessment of the treatment effect of enoxaparin for unstable angina/non-Q-wave myocardial infarction: TIMI 11B-ESSENCE meta-analysis. Circulation 1999; 100:1602–1608

54. Antman EM, McCabe CH, Gurfinkel EP, et al. Enoxaparin prevents death and cardiac ischemic events in unstable angina/non-Q-wave myocardial infarction: results of the Thrombolysis in Myocardial Infarction (TIMI) 11B trial. Circulation 1999; 100:1593–1601

55. Ferguson JJ, Califf RM, Antman EM, et al. Enoxaparin vs unfractionated heparin in high-risk patients with non-ST-segment elevation acute coronary syndromes managed with an intended early invasive strategy: primary results of the SYNERGY randomized trial. JAMA 2004; 292:45–54

56. Yusuf S, Mehta SR, Chrolavicius S, et al. Comparison of fondaparinux and enoxaparin in acute coronary syndromes. N Engl J Med 2006; 354: 1464–1476

57. Chew DP, Moliterno DJ. A critical appraisal of platelet glycoprotein IIb/IIIa inhibition. J Am Coll Cardiol 2000; 36:2028–2035

58. Platelet Receptor Inhibition in Ischemic Syndrome Management in Patients Limited by Unstable Signs and Symptoms (PRISM-PLUS) Study Investigators. Inhibition of the platelet glycoprotein IIb/IIIa receptor with tirofiban in unstable angina and non-Q-wave myocardial infarction. N Engl J Med 1998; 338:1488–1497

59. Platelet Receptor Inhibition in Ischemic Syndrome Management (PRISM) Study Investigators. A comparison of aspirin plus tirofiban with aspirin plus heparin for unstable angina. N Engl J Med 1998; 338:1498–1505

60. PURSUIT Trial Investigators. Inhibition of platelet glycoprotein IIb/IIIa with eptifibatide in patients with acute coronary syndromes. N Engl J Med 1998; 339:436–443

61. Simoons ML. Effect of glycoprotein IIb/IIIa receptor blocker abciximab on outcome in patients with acute coronary syndromes without early coronary revascularisation: the GUSTO IV-ACS randomised trial. Lancet 2001; 357:1915–1924

62. Boden WE, O'Rourke RA, Crawford MH, et al. Outcomes in patients with acute non-Q-wave myocardial infarction randomly assigned to an invasive as compared with a conservative management strategy. N Engl J Med 1998; 338: 1785–1792

63. FRagmin and Fast Revascularisation during Instability in Coronary artery disease Investigators. Invasive compared with non-invasive treatment in unstable coronary- artery disease: FRISC II prospective randomised multicentre study. Lancet 1999; 354:708–715

64. Cannon CP, Weintraub WS, Demopoulos LA, et al. Comparison of early invasive and conservative strategies in patients with unstable coronary syndromes treated with the glycoprotein IIb/IIIa inhibitor tirofiban. N Engl J Med 2001; 344:1879–1887

65. Fox KA, Poole-Wilson P, Clayton TC, et al. 5-year outcome of an interventional strategy in non-ST-elevation acute coronary syndrome: the British Heart Foundation RITA 3 randomised trial. Lancet 2005; 366:914–920

66. de Winter RJ, Windhausen F, Cornel JH, et al. Early invasive versus selectively invasive management for acute coronary syndromes. N Engl J Med 2005; 353:1095–1104

67. Bueno H, Martinez-Selles M, Perez-David E, et al. Effect of thrombolytic therapy on the risk of cardiac rupture and mortality in older patients with first acute myocardial infarction. Eur Heart J 2005; 26:1705–1711

68. Reardon MJ, Carr CL, Diamond A, et al. Ischemic left ventricular free wall rupture: prediction, diagnosis, and treatment. Ann Thorac Surg 1997; 64:1509–1513

69. Killen DA, Piehler JM, Borkon AM, et al. Early repair of postinfarction ventricular septal rupture. Ann Thorac Surg 1997; 63:138–142

70. Chaux A, Blanche C, Matloff JM, et al. Postinfarction ventricular septal defect. Semin Thorac Cardiovasc Surg 1998; 10:93–99

71. Khan SS, Gray RJ. Valvular emergencies. Cardiol Clin 1991; 9:689–709

72. Bolooki H. Emergency cardiac procedures in patients in cardiogenic shock due to complications of coronary artery disease. Circulation 1989; 79: I137–I148

73. Zehender M, Kasper W, Kauder E, et al. Right ventricular infarction as an independent predictor of prognosis after acute inferior myocardial infarction. N Engl J Med 1993; 328:981–988

74. Nedeljkovic ZS, Ryan TJ. Right ventricular infarction. In: Hollenberg SM, Bates ER, eds. Cardiogenic shock. Armonk, NY: Futura Publishing Company, 2002; 161–186

75. Dell'Italia LJ, Starling MR, Blumhardt R, et al. Comparative effects of volume loading, dobutamine, and nitroprusside in patients with predominant right ventricular infarction. Circulation 1985; 72:1327–1335

76. Bowers TR, O'Neill WW, Grines C, et al. Effect of reperfusion on biventricular function and survival after right ventricular infarction. N Engl J Med 1998; 338:933–940

Shock

John P. Kress, MD, FCCP

Objectives:

- Describe the clinical evaluation of patients with shock
- Describe the different types of shock
- Describe resuscitation of shock
- Describe new therapies for septic shock
- Describe vasoactive drugs used for treatment of shock

Key words: left ventricular failure; right ventricular failure; sepsis; shock; vasopressors

Shock is a common condition necessitating admission of the patient to the ICU or occurring in the course of critical care. This chapter discusses the pathophysiology of various shock states, followed by recommendations for the diagnosis and treatment of each category of shock. Last, a brief review of commonly used vasoactive agents is presented.

Shock Defined

Shock is defined by the presence of multisystem end-organ hypoperfusion. Clinical indicators include reduced mean BP, tachycardia, tachypnea, cool skin and extremities, acute altered mental status, and oliguria. Hypotension is usually, though not always, present. The end result of multiorgan hypoperfusion is tissue hypoxia, which is often clinically seen as lactic acidosis.

Clinical Evaluation of Patients in Shock

Most patients who present with shock are hypotensive. Since the mean BP is the product of the cardiac output (CO) and the systemic vascular resistance (SVR), reductions in BP can be categorized by decreased CO and/or decreased SVR. Accordingly, the initial evaluation of a hypotensive patient should evaluate the adequacy of the CO. Clinical evidence of diminished CO includes a narrow pulse pressure (a surrogate marker for stroke volume) and cool extremities with delayed capillary refill. Signs of increased CO include a widened pulse pressure (particularly with a reduced diastolic pressure), warm extremities with bounding pulses and rapid capillary refill. If a hypotensive patient has clinical signs of increased CO, one can infer that the reduced BP is a result of decreased SVR.

In hypotensive patients with clinical evidence of reduced CO, an assessment of intravascular and cardiac volume status is appropriate. A hypotensive patient with decreased intravascular and cardiac volume status may have a history suggesting hemorrhage or other volume losses (eg, vomiting, diarrhea, and polyuria). The jugular venous pulse is often reduced in such a patient. A hypotensive patient with an increased intravascular and cardiac volume status may have S3 and/or S4 gallops, increased jugular venous pressure (JVP), extremity edema, and crackles on lung auscultation. The chest radiograph may show cardiomegaly, congestion of the vascular pedicle,[1] Kerley B lines, and pulmonary edema. Chest pain and ECG changes consistent with ischemia may also be noted.

In hypotensive patients with clinical evidence of increased CO, a search for the causes of decreased SVR is appropriate. The most common cause of high-CO hypotension is sepsis. Accordingly, one should search for signs of the systemic inflammatory response syndrome (SIRS), which include abnormalities in temperature ($\geq38°C$ or $\leq36°C$), heart rate (≥90 beats/min), respiratory rate (≥20 breaths/min), and WBC count ($\geq12,000$ or $\leq4,000$ cells/μL or ≥10 bands).[2] A person with SIRS and a presumed or confirmed infectious process fulfills the criteria for sepsis. A person with sepsis and one or more organ failures fulfills the criteria for severe sepsis. Other causes of high-CO hypotension include the following: liver failure; severe pancreatitis; burns and other trauma that elicit SIRS; anaphylaxis; thyrotoxicosis; and peripheral arteriovenous shunts.

In summary, the three most common categories of shock include cardiogenic, hypovolemic, and high CO with decreased SVR. Certainly, these categories may overlap and occur simultaneously (*eg*, hypovolemic and septic shock, or septic and cardiogenic shock).

The initial assessment of a patient in shock as outlined above should take only a few minutes. It is important that aggressive, early resuscitation is instituted based on the initial assessment, particularly since there are data suggesting that the early resuscitation of shock (both septic and cardiogenic) may improve survival.[3,4] If the initial bedside assessment yields equivocal or confounding data, more objective assessments such as echocardiography and/or central venous or pulmonary artery catheterization may be useful. The goal of early resuscitation is to reestablish adequate perfusion to prevent or minimize end-organ injury.

During the initial resuscitation of patients in shock, the principles of advanced cardiac life support should be followed. Since patients in shock may be obtunded and unable to protect the airway, an early assessment of the patient's airway is mandatory during resuscitation from shock. Early intubation and mechanical ventilation are often required. The reasons for the institution of endotracheal intubation and mechanical ventilation include acute hypoxemic respiratory failure as well as ventilatory failure. Acute hypoxemic respiratory failure may occur in cardiogenic shock (pulmonary edema) as well as septic shock (pneumonia or ARDS). Ventilatory failure often occurs as a result of an increased load on the respiratory system. This load may present in the form of acute metabolic acidosis (often lactic acidosis) or decreased compliance of the lungs as a result of pulmonary edema. Inadequate perfusion to respiratory muscles in the setting of shock may be another reason for early intubation and mechanical ventilation. Normally, the respiratory muscles receive a very small percentage of the CO.[5] However, in patients who are in shock with respiratory distress for the reasons listed above, the percentage of CO dedicated to respiratory muscles may increase $\geq$10-fold.[6,7] Mechanical ventilation may relieve the patient of the work of breathing and permit the redistribution of a limited CO to other vital organs. Such patients often demonstrate signs of respiratory muscle fatigue, including the following: inability to speak full sentences; accessory respiratory muscle use; paradoxical abdominal muscle activity; extreme tachypnea

(>40 breaths/min); and decreasing respiratory rate despite an increasing drive to breathe.

Endotracheal intubation and mechanical ventilation with sedation, and, if necessary, muscle paralysis will decrease oxygen demand of the respiratory muscles allowing improved oxygen delivery to other hypoperfused tissue beds.[8] Patients in shock should be intubated before other procedures are performed, since attention to the airway and breathing may wane during such procedures.

Resuscitation

Resuscitation should focus on improving end-organ perfusion, not simply raising the BP. Accordingly, a patient with a reduced CO by clinical assessment with a decreased intravascular and cardiac volume status should receive aggressive IV resuscitation. The question of which type of IV fluid to use is controversial,[9,10] although data[10] from 2004 suggest that colloid (albumin) is not better than crystalloid, and indeed may be associated with increased morbidity and mortality. Though one study[11] reported improved outcomes in trauma patients whose volume resuscitation was delayed until definite surgical repair (average time to operation, approximately 2 h), aggressive volume resuscitation in patients with reduced intravascular and cardiac volume status is merited in virtually all patients except for torso trauma patients, who can undergo surgical repair quickly. The early administration of vasoactive drugs in hypovolemic patients in order to increase BP is not recommended. This practice may impair the assessment of the patient's circulatory status and potentially delay definitive treatment. The transfusion of packed RBCs to anemic patients in order to improve oxygen delivery is physiologically rational; however, some data[12] have suggested that, as long as hemoglobin levels remain >7 g/dL, this practice may not improve outcomes and perhaps may even worsen outcomes in select subgroups of patients. Certainly, a conservative transfusion strategy does not apply to hemorrhaging hypovolemic patients who are in shock. Blood products should be administered through a blood warmer to minimize hypothermia and subsequent disturbances in coagulation. In summary, it is important to remember that oxygen delivery is the product of CO, the oxygen-carrying capacity of the blood, and arterial oxygen saturation. Each of these components must be considered and optimized when addressing the resuscitation of patients who are in shock.

Early reassessment of the patient with purported hypovolemic shock after the initial resuscitation is extremely important. Concrete end points such as increased BP and pulse pressure, improved capillary refill, urine output, and mental status should be sought. The absence of a response suggests that the volume challenge may not be adequate. Careful and repeated searches for signs of volume overload (ie, increased JVP, new gallop or extra heart sounds, and pulmonary edema) should be performed while the resuscitation is ongoing.

If the patient remains in shock despite adequate volume resuscitation, support with vasoactive drugs is appropriate. Occasionally, vasoactive drugs must be started "prematurely" when volume resuscitation needs are large. When severe hypotension and hypovolemia are present, this approach is occasionally needed to "buy time" while volume resuscitation is ongoing. This strategy is only rarely necessary and should only be instituted temporarily until volume resuscitation is accomplished. It is important to remember that vasoactive drugs may obscure hypovolemic shock by raising BP despite a low CO state.

Once intravascular volume has been restored, patients who remain in shock may benefit from therapy with vasoactive drugs. These drugs should be titrated to end-organ perfusion, rather than to an arbitrary BP value. Accordingly, mental status, urine output, lactic acidosis, capillary refill and skin temperature, and venous oxygen saturation are reasonable end points to target in these patients. If evidence of hypoperfusion persists, one should consider inadequate volume resuscitation, impaired CO, inadequate hemoglobin concentration, and/or inadequate oxygen saturation as likely explanations. If the objective information obtained by physical examination is unclear or ambiguous, additional information obtained via invasive monitoring (ie, central venous pressure, pulmonary artery catheterization, or echocardiography) may be useful. Echocardiography is a useful adjunct or even replacement to invasive pressure measurements and can be used to distinguish poor ventricular pumping function

from hypovolemia; a good study can exclude or confirm tamponade, pulmonary hypertension, or significant valve dysfunction, all of which influence therapy and may supplement or replace the more invasive right heart catheterization. These topics are covered separately in another chapter in the syllabus.

Cardiogenic Shock

The model of the heart as a pump is useful in considering cardiogenic shock. By definition, pump failure is seen when CO is inappropriately low despite adequate input in the form of venous return (determined by right atrial pressure). The specific cause of decreased pump function must be considered. Left ventricular (LV) and/or right ventricular (RV) dysfunction may occur due to decreased systolic contractility, impaired diastolic relaxation, increases in afterload, valvular dysfunction, or abnormal heart rate and rhythm.

LV Failure

Systolic Dysfunction: This is the classic example of cardiogenic shock. When LV systolic function is impaired, the most common reason is acute coronary ischemia. The result is a reduction of CO relative to the increases in preload. Attempted compensation for this impaired pump function occurs via the Frank-Starling mechanism as well as by fluid retention by the kidneys and by increased venous tone mediated by the sympathetic nervous system. Patients present with reduced CO and a resulting increased oxygen extraction ratio by the peripheral tissues. The low mixed venous oxygen saturation may exacerbate hypoxemia, especially in patients with pulmonary edema and intrapulmonary shunt physiology. As mentioned above, acute myocardial infarction or ischemia is the most common cause of LV failure leading to shock. Cardiogenic shock is reported to complicate up to 10% of acute myocardial infarctions.[13] Some evidence[4] supports the use of early aggressive revascularization using angioplasty or coronary artery bypass grafting in patients with cardiogenic shock. A survival benefit was seen in patients subjected to this strategy compared to the medical management of cardiogenic shock, including those patients to whom thrombolytic therapy was administered. The treatment of cardiogenic shock due to systolic dysfunction includes the judicious administration of intravenous crystalloid if hypovolemia is present. A more precise characterization of the circulation can be obtained with the use of pulmonary artery catheterization and/or echocardiography, topics that are discussed in more detail in another chapter of the syllabus. Inotropic support includes the use of agents such as dobutamine, milrinone, or levosimendan. Intraaortic balloon counterpulsation may be used to support the circulation as a bridge to coronary artery revascularization.

Diastolic Dysfunction: Increased LV diastolic chamber stiffness and impaired LV filling occur most commonly as a result of myocardial ischemia, although LV hypertrophy and restrictive myocardial diseases may also contribute. Patients usually present with increased cardiac filling pressures despite a small LV end-diastolic volume, as documented by echocardiography (usually best seen in the short-axis view at the level of the papillary muscles). Aside from the management of acute ischemia, this condition may be difficult to treat. Volume administration can be tried, but many times there are only further increases in diastolic pressure with little change in diastolic volume. Therapy with inotropic agents are usually ineffective. The aggressive management of tachycardia with volume administration and the cautious use of negative chronotropic agents is a rational approach to therapy. Since very little ventricular filling occurs late in diastole in these patients, a very low heart rate (*eg*, sinus bradycardia) may be detrimental. Often, the careful titration of chronotropic agents to achieve the "optimal" heart rate that maximizes CO is necessary. The maintenance of a normal sinus rhythm is important to maximize ventricular filling.

Valvular Dysfunction: The management of valvular disease contributing to cardiogenic shock is guided by interventions to counter the specific pathophysiology. Accordingly, aortic stenosis is managed by efforts to decrease heart rate while maintaining sinus rhythm. Preload should be maintained, and afterload must not be reduced, since there is a fixed afterload imposed by the aortic stenosis, which may not tolerate further reductions in afterload via arteriolar dilation. Surgical evaluation or palliative valvuloplasty are other important considerations in patients with cardiogenic shock complicated by aortic stenosis. Cardiogenic shock due to aortic insufficiency may present acutely and may require urgent surgical repair. Medical management includes the use of chronotropic agents to decrease regurgitant filling time and afterload-reducing agents to facilitate forward flow. Mitral regurgitation may occur acutely as a result of ischemic injury to papillary muscles. Medical management includes attempts to establish and maintain sinus rhythm, as well as afterload reduction to decrease the percentage of regurgitant blood flow. This may be accomplished with medications such as nitroprusside or intraaortic balloon counterpulsation as a bridge to mitral valve repair or replacement. Mitral stenosis contributing to cardiogenic shock is managed by negative chronotropic agents, which seek to maximize diastolic filling time across the stenotic valve. Last, hypertrophic cardiomyopathy may contribute to cardiogenic shock. This lesion is managed by the maintenance of preload with volume administration and therapy with negative inotropic and chronotropic agents, which serve to decrease the obstruction of the LV outflow tract during systole. Rarely, acute obstruction of the mitral valve by left atrial thrombus or myxoma may also result in cardiogenic shock. These conditions generally require acute surgical interventions.

Cardiac Arrhythmias: Dysrhythmias may exacerbate shock in critically ill patients. A detailed discussion on the management of dysrhythmias is beyond the scope of this chapter, and the reader is referred to other chapters of the syllabus for further discussion of this topic.

RV Failure

RV failure resulting in cardiogenic shock is typically associated with increased right atrial pressure and reduced CO.[14] Although the most common reason for RV failure is concomitant LV failure, this section will discuss the management of isolated RV failure. RV infarction may result in RV failure, usually accompanied by inferior myocardial infarction. Elevated JVP in the presence of clear lungs is the classic physical finding seen in patients with acute RV infarction. It is important to distinguish RV infarction from cardiac tamponade. Echocardiography may be helpful in making this distinction. Therapy includes careful volume administration to maintain preload; however, volume overload is common with RV failure, and RV dilation may increase tricuspid regurgitation, leading to worsening hepatic and renal congestion. Therapy with dobutamine may be used to increase RV inotropy,[15] and therapy with norepinephrine may improve RV endocardial perfusion.

RV failure as a result of increases in right heart afterload may be due to pulmonary embolism, ARDS, and other causes of alveolar hypoxia, hypercapnia, and metabolic acidosis. Management is focused on treating the underlying physiologic derangement, with circulatory support again centered around inotropic agents as well as norepinephrine.[16,17] Norepinephrine is more effective at improving RV function and RV coronary perfusion pressure than phenylephrine.[18] The treatment of RV failure is complicated, since volume administration may result in worsening RV function by causing mechanical overstretch and/or by reflex mechanisms that depress contractility.[19] However, some investigators[20] have found volume administration to result in favorable hemodynamics in patients with acute RV failure due to increased RV afterload. Optimal management is often facilitated by echocardiographic or pulmonary artery catheter-directed therapy. Thrombolytic therapy for acute pulmonary embolism complicated by cardiogenic shock has been shown to improve survival[21] and is currently accepted as a recommended strategy.[22] Hypoxic pulmonary vasoconstriction may be reduced by improving alveolar and mixed venous oxygenation with the administration of supplemental oxygen. More aggressive correction of hypercapnia and acidemia may be necessary in patients with acute right heart syndromes. Pulmonary vasodilator therapy (eg, inhaled nitric oxide and prostaglandin E1) may be considered, although outcome benefits in the acute setting are largely lacking. Recently, levosimendan (the first of a new class of drugs known as *calcium sensitizers*) has become available. Levosimendan is discussed in more detail in the section on "Vasoactive Agents."

Pericardial Tamponade and Other Syndromes Causing External Compression of the Heart

Cardiac tamponade impairs diastolic filling, resulting in shock. The diagnosis is established by the presence of elevated jugular venous pulse with Kussmaul sign and pulsus paradoxus. Pulmonary artery catheterization may reveal a decreased CO with equalization of right atrial, left atrial (ie, pulmonary capillary wedge pressure), and RV diastolic pressures. Echocardiography reveals pericardial fluid with diastolic collapse of the atria and RV, and right-to-left septal shift during inspiration. Other causes of external cardiac compression include tension pneumothorax, elevated intraabdominal pressure (eg, tense ascites), so-called *abdominal tamponade*, large pleural effusions, and pneumopericardium. Treatment is focused at the underlying cause and includes pericardial drainage with a catheter or surgical "window" in the case of pericardial tamponade. In unstable patients, blind drainage of the pericardial sac with a needle may be necessary. Medical management of the circulatory pathophysiology of tamponade includes the use of aggressive volume administration as well as inotropic and chronotropic support to increase heart rate and thus maintain forward flow.

Decreased Venous Return

Hypovolemia is the most common cause of shock due to decreased venous return. The venous circuit has tremendous capacitance potential, and venoconstriction in response to hypovolemia can compensate for the initial decreases in intravascular volume. Orthostatic changes in BP and heart rate may be seen early in patients in hypovolemic shock.[20] At a level of approximately 40% loss of intravascular volume, venoconstriction driven by the sympathetic nervous system can no longer maintain mean arterial BP.

In patients with hypovolemic shock, tissue injury (especially gut ischemia) and the resulting systemic inflammation may lead to ongoing shock despite the replacement of volume losses.[21] This is particularly relevant if resuscitation is delayed and underscores the importance of early aggressive resuscitation in patients with hypovolemic shock. The phenomenon of systemic inflammation as it pertains to shock will be discussed in more detail in the section on "Septic Shock."

Other causes of shock due to decreased venous return include severe neurologic damage or drug exposure resulting in hypotension due to a loss of venous tone. The prototypical example of loss of venous tone due to drug exposure is anaphylaxis. This unregulated immunologically mediated release of histamine can result in profound shock requiring aggressive catecholamine support (epinephrine is the drug of choice). Septic shock is a common cause of shock due to decreased venous tone and is discussed separately in the next section. All of these processes result in decreased venous tone and impaired venous return, resulting in decreased CO and BP. The obstruction of veins due to compression (eg, pregnancy or intraabdominal tumor), thrombus formation, or tumor invasion increases the resistance to venous return and may occasionally result in shock.

The principal therapy of hypovolemic shock and other forms of shock due to decreased venous return is aggressive volume resuscitation while attempting to reverse the underlying problem driving the pathophysiology. This has been described in more detail above. In patients with hemorrhagic shock, resuscitation with packed RBCs should be performed through a blood warmer. The optimal hemoglobin concentration is controversial, and transfusion should be paced by the extent of ongoing blood loss. After large-volume RBC transfusions, dilutional thrombocytopenia and reduction in clotting factors should be anticipated, sought out, and corrected with platelet and plasma product transfusions, as directed by the findings of a platelet count and coagulation assays.

High-CO Hypotension

Septic Shock

Septic shock is the most extreme presentation of a spectrum of pathophysiologic responses to an infectious insult. Sepsis is defined by the presence of SIRS in the presence of known or suspected infection.[2] Severe sepsis occurs when patients with sepsis accrue one or more organ failures. Septic shock is seen in patients with severe sepsis who manifest shock, as described above. Any

infectious organism may result in sepsis and septic shock, including all bacteria, fungi, viruses, and parasites. As noted above, patients typically present with evidence of high CO (assuming hypovolemia has been resuscitated). These patients have a widened pulse pressure, warm extremities, brisk capillary refill, and a reduced diastolic and mean BP. A subgroup of patients with septic shock may present with depressed cardiac function. Circulating myocardial depressant factors have been identified in some septic patients,[23–25] but the reason that only a small subgroup of patients manifest cardiac depression is not well understood.

Sepsis is a significant problem in the care of critically ill patients. It is the leading cause of death in noncoronary ICUs in the United States.[26] Current estimates suggest that >750,000 patients are affected each year,[27] and these numbers are expected to increase in the coming years as the population continues to age and a greater percentage of people who are vulnerable to infection seek medical care.

Decades of research have focused on modifying the pathophysiologic responses of the body to severe infection. For many years, an unregulated proinflammatory state was thought to be the driving force behind severe sepsis and septic shock. Numerous trials[28] attempting to block a particular inflammatory pathway were conducted without any survival benefits noted. More recently, the pathophysiology behind severe sepsis has become better understood. Currently, the pathophysiology of severe sepsis is thought to be driven by unregulated inflammation (via cytokines such as interleukin 6 and tumor necrosis factor) coupled to a hypercoagulable state favoring microvascular coagulation and impaired fibrinolysis. Such unregulated microvascular coagulation is thought to lead to impaired tissue perfusion and to predispose patients to the multiple organ dysfunction syndrome that is commonly observed in patients with severe sepsis.[29] Therapy with activated protein C has a salutary impact on all three pathophysiologic derangements noted in patients with severe sepsis. A survival benefit has been reported[30] in patients with severe sepsis who were treated with recombinant activated protein C. This study was the first ever to demonstrate a survival benefit from a therapy directed at modifying the underlying pathophysiology of severe sepsis. Because of its anticoagulant properties, there was a small but significant increase in bleeding complications associated with activated protein C.

The mainstay of therapy for septic shock is aggressive supportive care. This includes early identification of the source of infection with eradication by surgical or percutaneous drainage, if possible. More than 80% of patients with severe sepsis will require ventilatory support for respiratory failure, which should be instituted early for the reasons outlined earlier in this chapter. Circulatory failure is supported with aggressive volume administration to correct any component of hypovolemia. Objective monitoring using central venous catheterization, pulmonary artery catheterization, and echocardiography should be used early to guide therapy. Vasoactive support is directed by the underlying circulatory derangement. The optimal extent of volume resuscitation is controversial. Some clinicians favor aggressive volume administration, while others favor the earlier use of vasoactive drugs (ie, keeping patients "dry"). Trials are ongoing to attempt to better answer this difficult question. The early institution of broad-spectrum antibiotic therapy focused on potential pathogens has been shown to improve survival.[31,32] Acute renal failure in patients with septic shock carries a poor prognosis. Some more recent studies[33] in the literature supports the use of an aggressive approach to renal replacement therapy, with a survival benefit demonstrated with daily hemodialysis compared to alternate-day hemodialysis. The use of low-dose dopamine as a renal protective strategy has been found[34] to be of no benefit in preventing acute tubular necrosis in patients with SIRS and acute renal insufficiency. Other therapeutic interventions in patients with severe sepsis await further evaluation. Early trials evaluating the utility of high-dose corticosteroids in patients with septic shock have failed to demonstrate a survival benefit.[35, 36] Corticosteroid therapy remains controversial, and further studies are needed before it can be recommended for widespread use. Some data[37] suggest that the response to an adrenocorticotropic hormone (ACTH) stimulation test may have important prognostic implications. Furthermore, a 2002 multicenter trial[38] found that a combination of low-dose hydrocortisone and fludrocortisone improved survival in patients with septic shock who had relative adrenal insufficiency.

Other Types of Shock

Adrenal insufficiency is often viewed as a rare occurrence in critically patients. However, one study[39] has reported a 54% incidence of blunted adrenal response to ACTH in patients with septic shock. This number may be a generous estimate since the parameters for defining adrenal insufficiency have not been universally agreed on[39]; nevertheless, adrenal insufficiency may not be as rare as previously thought. It is reasonable to consider testing all patients who present with septic or other occult reasons for shock with an ACTH stimulation test. Conventionally, this test is performed in the morning with a baseline cortisol level drawn and then 250 μg of ACTH administered IV. Thirty-minute and 60-min cortisol levels are then drawn. A level of >20 μg/dL is viewed as an appropriate response. If adrenal insufficiency is suspected, dexamethasone (which does not cross-react with the cortisol laboratory assay) should be administered while the ACTH stimulation test is being performed.

Neurogenic shock typically occurs as a result of severe injury to the CNS. The loss of sympathetic tone results in venodilation and venous blood pooling. The mainstays of therapy include volume repletion and vasoactive support with drugs that have venoconstricting properties.

Severe hypothyroidism or hyperthyroidism may result in shock. Myxedema presenting as shock should be treated with the administration of IV thyroid hormone. One should watch carefully for myocardial ischemia and/or infarction, which may complicate aggressive thyroid replacement. Thyroid storm requires urgent therapy with Lugol solution, propylthiouracil, steroids, propranolol, fluid resuscitation, and the identification of the precipitating cause. Pheochromocytoma often presents with a paradoxical hypertension despite a state of shock and impaired tissue perfusion. Intravascular volume depletion is masked by extreme venoconstriction from therapy with endogenous catecholamines in patients with pheochromocytoma. The increase in afterload caused by endogenous catecholamines may also precipitate a shock-like state. Treatment includes aggressive volume replacement as well as α-adrenergic and β-adrenergic blockades. A search for the location of the pheochromocytoma with subsequent surgical removal is indicated.

Vasoactive Agents

The choice of vasoactive medications should be based on the underlying pathophysiology of the circulation as gleaned by the physical examination and supplemented by more sophisticated measurements. It is sobering to realize that despite the widespread use of these agents for many decades, there are no outcome studies to guide clinicians with regard to the use of a particular agent in the management of shock.

Dobutamine

Dobutamine is a powerful inotrope, which stimulates both β_1 and β_2 receptors. The end result is typically an increase in CO with diminished SVR. This reduction in afterload may benefit patients with LV systolic dysfunction.

Milrinone

Milrinone is an inotropic agent that induces a positive inotropic state via phosphodiesterase inhibition. It has potent vasodilating properties that decrease both systemic and pulmonary vascular resistance. One study[42] of patients with acute exacerbations of congestive heart failure did not demonstrate a benefit with regard to the number of days hospitalized for cardiovascular causes, the in-hospital mortality rate, the 60-day mortality rate, or the composite incidence of death or hospital readmission. Rather, hypotension and new atrial arrhythmias were found to occur more frequently in patients who received milrinone compared to placebo.[40]

Levosimendan

Levosimendan is the first clinically available agent from a new class of drugs known as *calcium sensitizers*. Calcium sensitizers improve myocardial contractility without significantly increasing intracellular calcium levels. Levosimendan increases the sensitivity of the cardiac myofilaments to calcium during systole, which increases the force and rate of contraction. It appears to enhance CO without increasing myocardial oxygen consumption. These drugs may improve diastolic relaxation or at least are neutral with regard to diastolic function.[41,42] Levosimendan causes the dilation of systemic, pulmonary, and coronary arteries.[43,44] Studies have shown levosimendan to be superior to placebo and dobutamine in patients with chronic congestive heart failure.[45,46] Preliminary studies have suggested that levosimendan may improve RV mechanical efficiency.[42] The role of levosimendan in the management of shock or RV failure has not been studied extensively.

Dopamine

Dopamine is purported to have varying physiologic effects at different doses. Classically, "low-dose" dopamine (1 to 3 μg/kg/min) is thought to stimulate dopaminergic receptors and to increase renal and mesenteric blood flow. This notion has been disproven, however.[34,47] Indeed, there is evidence that dopamine may impair mesenteric perfusion to a greater degree than norepinephrine.[48] Because data are accumulating that report the ill effects of dopamine in patients with shock, this agent has fallen out of favor in the view of many clinicians, with other agents such as norepinephrine being more widely used (see next section).[49]

Norepinephrine

Norepinephrine stimulates β_1 receptors as well as α receptors. Data are now accumulating that suggest that norepinephrine may be a preferred drug in the treatment of septic shock and other vasodilatory types of shock. It appears to have a lesser propensity to cause renal injury[50] and provides a more reliable increase in BP compared to dopamine.[51] A prospective observational cohort study[52] found a significant reduction in mortality when compared to therapy with dopamine and/or epinephrine in patients with septic shock.

Phenylephrine

Phenylephrine is a pure α_1-agonist, which results in venous and arteriolar constriction. It often elicits a reflex bradycardia that is mediated via baroreceptors. This may prove useful in patients with tachydysrhythmias accompanied by hypotension. In a prospective observational study[53] of patients with septic shock, phenylephrine was found to increase BP, SVR, and cardiac index when added to low-dose dopamine or dobutamine after volume resuscitation. There is a theoretical concern that α-agonism may precipitate myocardial ischemia, though there are few objective data to support or refute this concern.

Epinephrine

Epinephrine has both β-agonist as well as α-agonist properties. It has potent inotropic as well as vasoconstricting properties. It appears to have a higher propensity toward precipitating mesenteric ischemia,[54] a property that limits its utility as a first-line agent for the management of shock, regardless of the underlying etiology.

Vasopressin

The use of vasopressin as a vasoactive agent has increased tremendously in the last few years. Patients who present with septic shock or late-phase hemorrhagic shock have been shown to have a relative deficiency of vasopressin. A 2001 study[55] found that patients with septic shock demonstrate an increase in BP and urine output without evidence of impaired cardiac, mesenteric, or skin perfusion when treated with "low-dose" (ie, 40 mU/min) vasopressin. The exact role of vasopressin in the treatment of patients who are in various shock states requires further investigation.

References

1. Ely EW, Smith AC, Chiles C, et al. Radiologic determination of intravascular volume status using portable, digital chest radiography: a prospective investigation in 100 patients. Crit Care Med 2001; 29:1502–1512

2. Bone RC, Balk RA, Cerra FB, et al. Definitions for sepsis and organ failure and guidelines for the use of innovative therapies in sepsis: the ACCP/SCCM Consensus Conference Committee; American College of Chest Physicians/Society of Critical Care Medicine. Chest 1992; 101:1644–1655

3. Rivers E, Nguyen B, Havstad S, et al. Early goal directed therapy in the treatment of severe sepsis and septic shock. N Engl J Med 2001; 345:1368–1377

4. Hochman JS, Sleeper LA, Webb JG, et al. Early revascularization in acute myocardial infarction complicated by cardiogenic shock: SHOCK Investigators; should we emergently revascularize occluded coronaries for cardiogenic shock. N Engl J Med 1999; 341:625–634

5. Rochester DF, Pradel-Guena M. Measurement of diaphragmatic blood flow in dogs from xenon 133 clearance. J Appl Physiol 1973; 34:68–74

6. Hussain SNA, Roussos C. Distribution of respiratory muscle and organ blood flow during endotoxic shock in dogs. J Appl Physiol 1985; 59:1802–1808

7. Robertson CH Jr, Foster GH, Johnson RL Jr. The relationship of respiratory failure to the oxygen consumption of, lactate production by, and distribution of blood flow among respiratory muscles during increasing inspiratory resistance. J Clin Invest 1977; 59:31–42

8. Hall JB, Wood LDH. Liberation of the patient from mechanical ventilation. JAMA 1987; 257:1621-1628

9. Cochrane Injuries Group Albumin Reviewers. Human albumin administration in critically ill patients: systematic review of randomised controlled trials. BMJ 1998; 317:235–240

10. Finfer S, Bellomo R, Boyce N, et al. A comparison of albumin and saline for fluid resuscitation in the intensive care unit. N Engl J Med 2004; 350:2247–2256

11. Bickell WH, Wall MJ Jr, Pepe PE, et al. Immediate versus delayed fluid resuscitation for hypotensive patients with penetrating torso injuries. N Engl J Med 1994; 331:1105–1109

12. Hebert PC, Wells G, Blajchman MA, et al. A multicenter, randomized, controlled clinical trial of transfusion requirements in critical care: Transfusion Requirements in Critical Care Investigators, Canadian Critical Care Trials Group. N Engl J Med 1999; 340:409–417

13. Goldberg RJ, Gore JM, Alpert JS, et al. Cardiogenic shock after acute myocardial infarction: incidence and mortality from a community-wide perspective, 1975 to 1988. N Engl J Med 1991; 325:1117–1122

14. Mebazaa A, Karpati P, Renaud E, et al. Acute right ventricular failure: from pathophysiology to new treatments. Intensive Care Med 2004; 30:185–196

15. Dell'Italia LJ, Starling MR, Blumhardt R, et al. Comparative effects of volume loading, dobutamine and nitroprusside in patients with predominant right ventricular infarction. Circulation 1985; 72:1327–1335

16. Hirsch LJ, Rooney MW, Wat SS, et al. Norepinephrine and phenylephrine effects on right ventricular function in experimental canine pulmonary embolism. Chest 1991; 100:796–801

17. Layish DT, Tapson VF. Pharmacologic hemodynamic support in massive pulmonary embolism. Chest 1997; 111:218–224

18. Hirsch LJ, Rooney MW, Wat SS, et al. Norepinephrine and phenylephrine effects on right ventricular function in experimental canine pulmonary embolism. Chest 1991; 100:796–801

19. Ghignone M, Girling L, Prewitt RM. Volume expansion versus norepinephrine in treatment of a low cardiac output complicating an acute increase in right ventricular afterload in dogs. Anesthesiology 1984; 60:132–135

20. Mathru M, Venus B, Smith R, et al. Treatment of low cardiac output complicating acute pulmonary hypertension in normovolemic goats. Crit Care Med 1986; 14:120–124

21. Jerjes-Sanchez C, Ramirez-Rivera A, Gareia M de L, et al. Streptokinase and heparin versus heparin alone in massive pulmonary embolism: a randomized controlled trial. J Thromb Thrombolysis 1995; 2:227–229

22. Arcasoy SM, Kreit JW. Thrombolytic therapy of pulmonary embolism: a comprehensive review of current evidence. Chest 1999; 115:1695–1707

23. Parker MM, Shelhamer JH, Bacharach SL, et al. Profound but reversible myocardial depression in patients with septic shock. Ann Intern Med 1984; 100:483–490

24. Schremmer B, Dhainault J. Heart failure in septic shock: effects of inotropic support. Crit Care Med 1990; 18:S49–S55

25. Parrillo JE, Burch C, Shelhamer JH, et al. A circulating myocardial depressant substance in humans with septic shock. J Clin Invest 1985; 76:1539–1553

26. Sands KE, Bates DW, Lanken PN, et al. Epidemiology of sepsis syndrome in eight academic medical centers. JAMA 1997; 278:234–240

27. Angus DC, Linde-Zwirble WT, Lidicker J, et al. Epidemiology of severe sepsis in the United States: analysis of incidence, outcome, and associated costs of care. Crit Care Med 2001; 29:1303–1310

28. Bone RC. Why sepsis trials fail. JAMA 1996; 276:565–566

29. Kidokoro A, Iba T, Fukunaga M, et al. Alterations in coagulation and fibrinolysis during sepsis. Shock 1996; 5:223–228

30. Bernard GR, Vincent JL, Laterre PF. Recombinant human protein C Worldwide Evaluation in Severe Sepsis (PROWESS) study group: efficacy and safety of recombinant human activated protein C for severe sepsis. N Engl J Med 2001; 344:699–709

31. Ibrahim EH, Sherman G, Ward S, et al. The influence of inadequate antimicrobial treatment of bloodstream infections on patient outcomes in the ICU setting. Chest 2000; 118:146–155

32. Kollef MH, Sherman G, Ward S, et al. Inadequate antimicrobial treatment of infections: a risk factor for hospital mortality among critically ill patients. Chest 1999; 115:462–474

33. Schiffl H, Lang SM, Fischer R. Daily hemodialysis and the outcome of acute renal failure. N Engl J Med 2002; 346:305–310

34. Bellomo R, Chapman M, Finfer S, et al. Low-dose dopamine in patients with early renal dysfunction: a placebo-controlled randomised trial: Australian and New Zealand Intensive Care Society (ANZICS) Clinical Trials Group. Lancet 2000; 356:2139–2143

35. Bone RC, Fisher CJ, Clemmer TP, et al. A controlled clinical trial of high-dose methylprednisolone in the treatment of severe sepsis and septic shock. N Engl J Med 1987; 317:653–658

36. Veterans Administration Systemic Sepsis Cooperative Study Group. Effect of high-dose glucocorticoid therapy on mortality in patients with clinical signs of systemic sepsis. N Engl J Med 1987; 317:659–665

37. Annane D, Sebille V, Troche G, et al. A 3-level prognostic classification in septic shock based on cortisol levels and cortisol response to corticotropin. JAMA 2000; 283:1038–1045

38. Annane D, Sebille V, Charpentier C, et al. Effect of treatment with low doses of hydrocortisone and fludrocortisone on mortality in patients with septic shock. JAMA 2002; 288:862–871

39. Zaloga GP. Sepsis-induced adrenal deficiency syndrome. Crit Care Med 2001; 29:688–690

40. Cuffe MS, Califf RM, Adams KF, et al. Short-term intravenous milrinone for acute exacerbation of chronic heart failure: a randomized controlled trial. JAMA 2002; 287:1541–1547

41. Haikala H, Nissinen E, Etemadzadeh E, et al. Troponin C-mediated calcium sensitization induced by levosimendan does not impair relaxation. J Cardiovasc Pharmacol 1995; 25:794–801

42. Ukkonen H, Saraste M, Akkila J, et al. Myocardial efficiency during levosimendan infusion in congestive heart failure. Clin Pharmacol Ther 2000; 68:522–531

43. Yokoshiki H, Katsube Y, Sunagawa M, et al. Levosimendan, a novel calcium sensitizer, activates the glibenclamide-sensitive K^+ channel in rat arterial myocytes. Eur J Pharmacol 1997; 333:249–259

44. Slawsky MT, Colucci WS, Gottlieb SS. Acute hemodynamic and clinical effects of levosimendan in patients with severe heart failure. Circulation 2000; 102:2222–2227

45. Follath F, Cleland JG, Just H, et al. Efficacy and safety of intravenous levosimendan compared with dobutamine in severe low-output heart failure (the LIDO study): a randomised double-blind trial. Lancet 2002; 20:196–202

46. Moiseyev VS, Poder P, Andrejevs N, et al. Safety and efficacy of a novel calcium sensitizer, levosimendan, in patients with left ventricular failure due to an acute myocardial infarction: a randomized, placebo-controlled, double-blind study (RUSSLAN). Eur Heart J 2002; 23:1422–1432

47. Hannemann L, Reinhart K, Grenzer O, et al. Comparison of dopamine to dobutamine and norepinephrine for oxygen delivery and uptake in septic shock. Crit Care Med 1995; 23:1962–1970

48. Marik PE, Mohedin M. The contrasting effects of dopamine and norepinephrine on systemic and splanchnic oxygen utilization in hyperdynamic sepsis. JAMA 1994; 272:1354–1357

49. Nasraway SA. Norepinephrine: no more "leave 'em dead"? Crit Care Med 2000; 28:3096–3098

50. Desjars P, Pinaud M, Bugnon D, et al. Norepinephrine therapy has no deleterious renal effects in human septic shock. Crit Care Med 1989; 17:426–429

51. Martin C, Papazian L, Perrin G, et al. Norepinephrine or dopamine for the treatment of hyperdynamic septic shock? Chest 1993; 103:1826–1831

52. Martin C, Viviand X, Leone M, Thirion X. Effect of norepinephrine on the outcome of septic shock. Crit Care Med 2000; 28:2758–2765

53. Gregory JS, Bonfiglio MF, Dasta JF, et al. Experience with phenylephrine as a component of the pharmacologic support of septic shock. Crit Care Med 1991; 19:1395–1400

54. Levy B, Bollaert PE, Charpentier C, et al. Comparison of norepinephrine and dobutamine to epinephrine for hemodynamics, lactate metabolism, and gastric tonometric variables in septic shock: a prospective, randomized study. Intensive Care Med 1997; 23:282–287

55. Tsuneyoshi I, Yamada H, Kakihana Y, et al. Hemodynamic and metabolic effects of low-dose vasopressin infusions in vasodilatory septic shock. Crit Care Med 2001; 29:487–493

Notes

Mechanical Ventilation

Gregory A. Schmidt, MD, FCCP

Objectives:

- Provide a rationale for distinguishing two aspects of mechanical ventilation: oxygen and ventilation
- Review new evidence regarding the role of positive end-expiratory pressure in the treatment of patients with acute lung injury (ALI)/ARDS
- Describe the role of pressure and flow waveforms in determining respiratory mechanics
- Recommend disease-specific ventilator strategies aimed at reducing the adverse consequences of mechanical ventilation
- Review new information regarding lung-protective ventilation and effective strategies in patients with ALI and ARDS
- Address the role of noninvasive ventilation
- Discuss the complications of mechanical ventilation

Key words: acute lung injury; ARDS; assist-control ventilation; COPD; inverse ratio ventilation; lung-protective ventilation; mechanical ventilation; noninvasive ventilation; pressure control; pressure support; status asthmaticus; synchronized intermittent mandatory ventilation; tidal volume; ventilator-induced lung injury

This chapter offers an approach in which two aspects of mechanical ventilation, oxygenation (largely determined by fraction of inspired oxygen [F_{IO_2}] and positive end-expiratory pressure [PEEP]) and ventilation (depending mostly on mode, rate, and tidal volume [V_T] or set inspiratory pressure [Pinsp]) are considered separately. Then, the ventilator is used as a probe of the patient's respiratory system mechanical derangements, and ventilator settings are tailored to the patient's mechanical and gas exchange abnormalities. This facilitates early stabilization of the patient on the ventilator in such a way as to optimize carbon dioxide removal and oxygen delivery within the limits of abnormal neuromuscular function, lung mechanics, and gas exchange. The impact of new information regarding ventilator-induced lung injury (VILI) on current practice will be covered, as well as the potential roles of high-frequency ventilation (HFV), prone positioning, and recruitment maneuvers.

The fundamental purpose of mechanical ventilation is to assist in the elimination of carbon dioxide and the uptake of adequate oxygen while the patient is unable to do so or should not be allowed to do so. Such patients fall into the following two main groups: (1) patients in whom full rest of the respiratory muscles is indicated (*eg*, during shock; severe, acute pulmonary derangement; or deep sedation or anesthesia); and (2) patients in whom some degree of respiratory muscle use is desired (*eg*, to strengthen or improve the coordination of the respiratory muscles, to assess the ability of the patient to sustain the work of breathing, or to begin spontaneous ventilation). It is important for the intensivist to be explicit about whether the respiratory muscles should be rested or exercised because the details of ventilation (*ie*, mode and settings) usually follow logically from this fundamental point. For example, in a patient who is in profound shock, the ventilator should be set to fully take over the work of breathing (*eg*, using volume assist-control ventilation [ACV] mode) while the flow and pressure waveforms are examined to determine whether this goal has been met.

Using the Ventilator To Control Oxygenation

The ventilator settings most concerned with oxygenation are the F_{IO_2} and PEEP. Generally, mode, V_T, rate, and other settings have only very modest effects on Pao_2. For example, in the ARDS Network V_T trial, use of the 6 vs 12 mL/kg predicted body weight was associated with a small but real decrement in the Pao_2/F_{IO_2} ratio (156 vs 178, respectively).[1]

Oxygen is clearly toxic in high concentrations, likely due to the effects of reactive oxygen species on many biological systems. The threshold for toxicity is uncertain, especially in the injured lung. Generally, an F_{IO_2} of <0.6 is considered nontoxic, while higher fractions are avoided when possible. There is some experimental evidence that the injured lung may be more resistant to oxygen-induced injury. Given the uncertainties in this area, most clinicians strive to limit exposure to concentrations in excess of 0.6 to less than 24 h, using PEEP, diuresis, positional maneuvers, or inhaled vasodilators.

Evidence arose >30 years ago that PEEP could protect the injured lung. Repeated recruitment and derecruitment was postulated to amplify lung injury. By keeping some portion of the lung open at end-expiration, PEEP was postulated to reduce this aspect of VILI. In a clinical study performed more than a decade ago, Amato and colleagues[2] used a higher than usual level of PEEP (set 2 cm H_2O above the Pinsp at which the slope of the volume-pressure relationship steepened), combined with low Vts, in an "open-lung approach," which improved outcomes in ARDS patients. The two individual components of this ventilatory approach (ie, lower VT and higher PEEP) were investigated subsequently by the ARDS Network in separate trials. The beneficial effect of low VT was confirmed in the ARMA trial.[1] The role of PEEP was clarified subsequently in the ALVEOLI study.[3] In this study, various combinations of FIO_2 and PEEP were allowed, so that in one group the PEEP was set higher than in the other (13.2 vs 8.3 cm H_2O on average, respectively). There was no significant difference in outcome, suggesting that the lower PEEP was sufficient to adequately protect the lung or that PEEP is simply not important in the treatment of VILI.

Given these findings, PEEP should be set using the ARDS Network table of FIO_2 and PEEP, or, similarly, the "least PEEP" approach, in which PEEP is set at the lowest value that allows adequate saturation of hemoglobin (arterial oxygen saturation, >0.87) on a nontoxic FIO_2, should be used. Some lung lesions are not responsive to PEEP (some lesions may even be worsened by increasing PEEP), so the effect of PEEP should always be judged before further adjustments are made. When PEEP is ineffective and oxyhemoglobin saturation is unacceptable, additional approaches such as prone positioning may be useful. By recruiting lung, PEEP raises the pleural pressure, a feature that could have hemodynamic consequences. Most often, however, the effects are modest, probably because if the lung gets very much bigger with PEEP (lots of recruitment), not

much PEEP is needed. Another concern regarding PEEP has been the potential to cause pneumothorax. However, Palv is determined largely by VT, not PEEP. The current use of lung-protective VTs, combined with the regular assessment of plateau airway pressure (Pplat) [see section on "Modes of Mechanical Ventilation"], makes this effect of PEEP of little consequence.

Using the Ventilator To Effect Carbon Dioxide Elimination

The $PaCO_2$ depends on total body carbon dioxide production and alveolar ventilation. The ventilator can be used to set minute ventilation, the sum of alveolar ventilation and dead space ventilation. Various ventilatory modes control minute ventilation by delivering a VT (either directly, as in volume-preset modes, or indirectly, as in pressure-preset modes).

Modes of Mechanical Ventilation

Technologic innovations have provided a plethora of differing modes by which a patient can be mechanically ventilated.[4] Various modes have been developed with the hope of improving gas exchange, patient comfort, or speed of return to spontaneous ventilation. Aside from minor subtleties, however, nearly all modes allow full rest of the patient, on the one hand, or substantial exercise on the other. Thus, in the great majority of patients, the choice of mode is merely a matter of patient or physician preference. Noninvasive ventilation (NIV) should be considered before intubation and ventilation in many patients who are hemodynamically stable and do not require an artificial airway, especially those with acute-on-chronic respiratory failure, postoperative respiratory failure, cardiogenic pulmonary edema, or acute respiratory failure complicating severe immunosuppression.

During volume-preset ventilation (and assuming a passive patient), the Pplat is determined by the VT and the static compliance of the respiratory system (Crs):

$$Pplat = VT/Crs + PEEP$$

where PEEP also includes auto-PEEP.

On the other hand, in pressure-preset modes a fixed Pinsp is applied to the respiratory system, whatever the resulting VT. However, the VT is predictable (again, assuming a passive patient) when the Crs is known:

$$VT = (Pinsp - PEEP) \times Crs$$

assuming time for equilibration between Pinsp and Palv. Thus, a patient with a Crs of 50 mL/cm H_2O ventilated on ACV at a VT of 500 mL with no PEEP (or auto-PEEP) will have a Pplat of about 10 cm H_2O, while the same patient ventilated on pressure-control ventilation (PCV) mode at 10 cm H_2O will have a VT of about 500 mL. Thus, while physicians' comfort level with volume-preset and pressure-preset modes may be very different, the modes can be similar as they are tied to each other through the patient's Crs.

A potential advantage of pressure-preset ventilation is greater physician control over the peak airway opening pressure (Ppeak) [since Ppeak = Pinsp] and the peak Palv, which could lessen the incidence of VILI. However, this same reduction in volutrauma risk should be attainable during volume-preset ventilation if a VT appropriate to the lung derangement is chosen. Indeed, the ARDS Network ARMA trial, which demonstrated a mortality reduction in the low-VT group, used ACV and a VT of 6 mL/kg predicted body weight. Pressure-preset modes could make such a lung-protection strategy easier to carry out by dispensing with the need to repeatedly determine Pplat and periodically adjust the VT. During the use of pressure-preset modes, the patient also has greater control over inspiratory flow rate, and therefore potentially increased comfort. Several features of pressure-preset modes have raised concern that lung protection cannot be assured. Most importantly, a safe level of maximal Palv is not known. Moreover, unless the patient is fully passive, the transpulmonary pressure cannot be controlled using pressure-preset modes and is not even known. A final limitation is that pressure-preset modes do not allow ready determination of the respiratory system mechanical properties.

In the following descriptions, each mode is first illustrated for a passive patient, such as following muscle paralysis, then for the more common situation in which the patient plays an active role in ventilation. On some ventilators, VT can be selected by the physician or respiratory therapist, while on others a minute ventilation and respiratory rate (f) are chosen, secondarily determining the VT. Similarly, on some machines an inspiratory flow rate is selected, while on others flow depends on the ratio of inspiratory time (TI) to total respiratory cycle time and f, or an inspiratory/expiratory (I:E) ratio and f.

Conventional Modes of Ventilation

Volume ACV

Volume ACV was found to be the most commonly used mode in an international survey of mechanical ventilation. Among its advantages are that it was the mode used in the ARMA trial demonstrating reduced mortality in patients with acute lung injury (ALI) and ARDS, and that respiratory mechanics can be measured readily.

Passive Patient: The set parameters of the ACV mode are the inspiratory flow rate, f, and VT. The ventilator delivers f equal breaths per minute, each of the set VT. VT and flow determine the TI, expiratory time (TE), and the I:E ratio. Pplat is related to VT, the compliance of the respiratory system, and PEEP, while the difference between Ppeak and Pplat includes contributions from flow and inspiratory resistance.

Active Patient: The patient has the ability to trigger extra breaths by exerting an inspiratory effort exceeding the preset trigger sensitivity, each at the set VT and flow, and to thereby change TI, TE, and I:E ratio, and to potentially create or increase auto-PEEP. Typically, each patient will display a preferred rate for a given VT and will trigger all breaths when the controlled ventilator f is set a few breaths per minute below the patient's rate; in this way, the control rate serves as an adequate support should the patient stop initiating breaths. When high inspiratory effort continues during the ventilator-delivered breath, the patient may trigger a second, superimposed ("stacked") breath (rarely a third as well). Patient effort can be increased (if the goal is to exercise the patient) by increasing the magnitude of the trigger or by lowering VT (which increases the rate of assisting). Lowering f at the same VT generally has no effect on work of breathing when the patient is initiating all breaths.

Synchronized Intermittent Mandatory Ventilation

In the passive patient, synchronized intermittent mandatory ventilation (SIMV) cannot be distinguished from controlled ventilation in the ACV mode. Ventilation is determined by the mandatory f and V_T. However, if the patient is not truly passive, he may perform respiratory work during the mandatory breaths. More to the point of the SIMV mode, the patient can trigger additional breaths by lowering the airway opening pressure (Pao) below the trigger threshold. If this triggering effort comes in a brief, defined interval before the next mandatory breath is due, the ventilator will deliver the mandatory breath ahead of schedule in order to synchronize with the patient's inspiratory effort. If a breath is initiated outside of the synchronization window, V_T, flow, and I:E ratio are determined by patient effort and respiratory system mechanics, not by ventilator settings. The spontaneous breaths tend to be of small volume and are highly variable from breath to breath. The SIMV mode has historically been used to gradually augment the patient's work of breathing by lowering the mandatory breath f, but SIMV has been shown to prolong weaning.[5,6] Although this mode continues to be used widely, there is little rationale for it, and the use of SIMV is falling out of favor.

PCV

In the passive patient, ventilation is determined by f, the Pinsp increment (ie, Pinsp − PEEP), I:E ratio, and the time constant of the patient's respiratory system. In patients without severe obstruction (ie, the time constant not elevated) given a sufficiently long T_I, there is equilibration between the ventilator-determined Pinsp and alveolar pressure (Palv) so that inspiratory flow ceases. In this situation, V_T is highly predictable, based on Pinsp (= Palv), and the mechanical properties of the respiratory system (Crs). In the presence of severe obstruction or if the T_I is too short to allow equilibration between ventilator and alveoli, V_T will fall below that predicted based on Pinsp and Crs. It is typically the case during PCV that alveolar and ventilator pressures do not equilibrate either at end-inspiration or at end-expiration.

Thus, the maximal inspiratory Palv is generally less than the set Pinsp on the ventilator and the end-expiratory pressure exceeds the set expiratory pressure (ie, there is auto-PEEP).

The active patient can trigger additional breaths by reducing the Pao below the triggering threshold, raising the I:E ratio. The inspiratory reduction in pleural pressure combines with the ventilator Pinsp to augment the transpulmonary pressure and the V_T. This point has led many intensivists to be skeptical regarding the ability of PCV to assure lung-protective V_Ts in patients with ALI and ARDS. Because T_I is generally set by the physician, care must be taken to discern the patient's neural T_I (from the waveform display) and adjust the ventilator accordingly; otherwise, additional sedation might be necessary.

Pressure-Support Ventilation

The patient must trigger the ventilator in order to activate this mode, so pressure support is not applied to passive patients. Ventilation is determined by Pinsp, patient-determined f, patient effort, and the respiratory mechanics. Once a breath is triggered, the ventilator attempts to maintain Pao at the physician-determined Pinsp, using whatever flow is necessary to achieve this. Eventually, flow begins to fall as a result of either the cessation of the patient's inspiratory effort or the increasing elastic recoil of the respiratory system as V_T rises. The ventilator will maintain a constant Pinsp until inspiratory flow falls by an arbitrary amount (eg, to 25% of initial flow) or below an absolute flow rate. Since patients' respiratory system time constants vary widely (so that the time for flow to fall to 25% varies widely), many patients have to work actively to turn off the Pinsp, raising the work of breathing. Some ventilators allow the intensivist to adjust the threshold for turning off the expiratory flow, allowing the ventilator to be tailored to the respiratory mechanics. Especially in patients with exacerbations of COPD, a threshold well >50% is often necessary to minimize this unintended expiratory work. During pressure-support ventilation (PSV), the work of breathing can be increased by lowering Pinsp or making the trigger less sensitive, and can inadvertently increase if respiratory system mechanics change, despite no change in ventilator settings. Respiratory system mechanical parameters cannot be determined readily on this mode because the ventilator and patient contributions to VT and flow are not represented by Pao; accordingly, these important measurements of Pplat, Ppeak – Pplat, and auto-PEEP are measured during a brief, daily switch from PSV to volume-preset ventilation. A potential advantage of PSV is improved patient comfort and, for patients with very high drive, reduced work of breathing compared with volume-preset modes.

Mixed Modes

Some ventilators allow combinations of modes, most commonly SIMV plus PSV. There is little reason to use such a hybrid mode, although some physicians use the SIMV as a means to add sighs to PSV, an option that is not otherwise generally available. Because SIMV plus PSV guarantees some backup minute ventilation (which PSV does not), this mode combination may have value in occasional patients who are at high risk for abrupt deterioration in central drive.

Dual-Control Modes

The sophisticated microprocessors included with modern ventilators allow remarkably complex modes of ventilation. These modes typically try to meld the best features of the volume-preset and pressure-preset modes. Some cause a switch of modes between breaths (eg, pressure-regulated volume control [PRVC]; volume support ventilation [VSV]) or within a breath (eg, volume-assured pressure support). In general, these modes are complex, and their effects may vary greatly depending on the details of the patient's effort. None have been shown to be safer or more useful than more conventional modes. The greatest problem with such newer modes is that they are very complex, the algorithm describing their function is not usually understood by practitioners, and they change during a breath, or from breath to breath, depending on patient effort, sometimes in ways that can provoke unanticipated effects.

PRVC

This is a pressure-preset mode with a set TI (ie, it is time cycled) in which the ventilator compares the VT with a physician-set VT and automatically and gradually adjusts the Pinsp of subsequent breaths in order to deliver the desired VT. A downside of PRVC is that as patient effort increases, the ventilator reduces support. Proponents of PRVC argue that this mode provides the benefits of pressure-preset modes, while at the same time guaranteeing VT. Whether this guarantee makes the mode better or worse for the patient is debated.

VSV

VSV is a pressure-preset mode in which Pinsp is automatically varied to gradually bring VT in line with the desired VT over several breaths; it differs from PRVC in that the TI is not set but, rather, depends on patient effort, as in PSV. It is unknown whether this mode speeds or impedes weaning.

Volume-Assured Pressure Support

This mode begins as PSV, but, if a desired VT is not met, the ventilator switches to ACV within the same breath in order to guarantee VT. As with many dual-control modes, the physician delegates decision making to the ventilator. Complex adjustments and their potentially detrimental effects on the patient may come into play at any time of day or night, depending on changes in the mechanical properties of the respiratory system or changes in the patient's level of consciousness, comfort, or neuromuscular competence.

Choosing Mode and Settings

If full rest of the respiratory muscles is desired, it is incumbent on the physician to assure that this is indeed achieved. Although some patients are fully passive while being ventilated (eg, patients with deep sedation or therapeutic paralysis, some forms of coma, metabolic alkalosis, or sleep-disordered breathing), most patients will make active respiratory efforts, even on volume ACV, at times performing extraordinary amounts of work. Unintended patient effort can be difficult to recognize but, aside from obvious patient effort, may be signaled by an inspiratory fall in intrathoracic pressure (as noted on a central venous or pulmonary artery pressure tracing, or with an esophageal balloon) or by triggering of the ventilator. Recognizing patient effort has been greatly aided by the provision of real-time displays of flow and pressure waveforms. Using waveforms, it is easiest to gather information regarding the patient-ventilator interaction when patients are ventilated with a volume-preset mode (ie, ACV or SIMV). Still, some useful information can be gleaned from waveforms during pressure-preset ventilation (ie, PSV and PCV).

The first step is to seek signs of inspiratory effort in the pressure tracing. In volume-preset modes, the signs of persistent effort include the presence of triggering, concavity during inspiration, and a variable Ppeak. When the goal of ventilation is to rest the respiratory muscles, ventilator adjustments, psychological measures, and pharmacologic sedation all may be effective. Ventilator strategies to reduce the patient's work of breathing include increasing the minute ventilation to reduce Pco_2 (although this may run counter to other goals of ventilation, especially in patients with ARDS or severe obstruction), increasing the inspiratory flow rate, and changing the mode to pressure-preset ventilation (ie, PSV or PCV). Only rarely is therapeutic paralysis required to achieve ventilatory goals.

The next step is to determine whether the patient has significant airflow obstruction. This can be inferred by inserting a brief end-inspiratory pause, then determining the difference between Ppeak and Pplat. Alternatively, one can examine the expiratory flow waveform, seeking low-flow and prolonged expiration, signs that are present regardless of the mode of ventilation (eg, ACV, SIMV, PSV, or PCV). Bronchodilator therapy can be assessed by noting whether expiratory flow increases, the TE shortens, or there is a reduction in Ppeak, Pplat, or auto-PEEP.

Finally, one should ensure that the patient and ventilator are synchronized (ie, that each attempt by the patient to trigger the ventilator generates a breath). The most common situation in which the patient fails to trigger breaths occurs in patients with severe obstruction when auto-PEEP is present. This is recognized at the bedside when the patient makes obvious efforts that fail to produce a breath. Using waveforms, these ineffective efforts cause a temporary slowing of expiratory flow, sometimes halting it completely.

Triggered Sensitivity

In the ACV, SIMV, and pressure-support modes, the patient must lower the Pao below a preset threshold in order to "trigger" the ventilator. In most situations, this is straightforward. The more negative the sensitivity, the greater the effort demanded of the patient. This can be used intentionally to increase the work of breathing when the goal is to strengthen the inspiratory muscles. When auto-PEEP is present, however, the patient must lower Palv by the auto-PEEP amount in order to have any impact on Pao, then lower it further by the trigger amount to initiate a breath. This can dramatically increase the required effort for breath initiation.

Flow-triggering systems (or *flow-by* systems) have been used to further reduce the work of triggering the ventilator. In contrast to the usual approach in which the patient must open a demand valve in order to receive ventilatory assistance, continuous-flow systems maintain a continuous high flow, then further augment flow when the patient initiates a breath. These systems can reduce the work of breathing slightly below that present when using conventional demand valves, but do not solve the problem of triggering when auto-PEEP is present.

Unconventional Ventilatory Modes

Inverse-Ratio Ventilation

Inverse-ratio ventilation (IRV) is defined as a mode in which the I:E ratio is >1. There are two general ways to apply IRV, as follows: pressure-controlled IRV (PC-IRV), in which a preset airway pressure is delivered for a fixed period of time at an I:E ratio >1; or volume-controlled IRV (VC-IRV), in which a VT is delivered at a slow (or decelerating) inspiratory flow rate (or an end-inspiratory pause is inserted) to yield an I:E >1. For PC-IRV, the physician must specify the inspiratory airway pressure, f, and I:E ratio, while VT and flow profile are determined by respiratory system impedance, as discussed for PCV above. Commonly, the initial Pinsp is 20 to 40 cm H_2O (or 10 to 30 cm H_2O above the PEEP), f is 20 breaths/min, and the I:E is 2:1 to 4:1. For VC-IRV, the operator selects a VT, f, flow (typically a low value), flow profile, and, possibly, an end-inspiratory pause. The chosen values result in an I:E ratio >1:1 and as high as 5:1.

Compared with conventional modes of ventilation, lung oxygen exchange is often improved with IRV, owing to increased mean Palv and volume consequent to the longer time above functional residual capacity, or due to the creation of auto-PEEP. It is remotely possible that IRV causes better ventilation of lung units with long time constants, but these are so short in healthy lungs (and shorter in patients with acute hypoxemic respiratory failure) that such redistribution is unlikely to occur with slower flow, and could not reduce shunt even if it did. Because auto-PEEP is a common consequence of IRV, serial determination of its magnitude is essential for the safe use of this mode. Both PC-IRV and VC-IRV generally require heavy sedation of the patient with or without muscle paralysis.

Airway Pressure-Release Ventilation

Airway pressure-release ventilation consists of continuous positive airway pressure, which is intermittently released to allow a brief expiratory interval. Conceptually, this mode is PC-IRV during which the patient is allowed to initiate spontaneous breaths. An advantage over IRV is that patients are more comfortable, requiring less sedation. It is not known whether airway pressure-release ventilation can deliver lung-protective ventilation, so this mode is not a good choice in patients with ALI or ARDS. Whether this mode provides any benefit over modern low-VT ventilation remains to be shown.

Proportional-Assist Ventilation

Proportional-assist ventilation is intended only for spontaneously breathing patients. The goal of this novel mode is to attempt to normalize the relationship between patient effort and the resulting ventilatory consequences.[7] The ventilator adjusts Pinsp in proportion to patient effort both throughout any given breath and from breath to breath. This allows the patient to modulate his breathing pattern and total ventilation. This is implemented by monitoring the instantaneous flow and volume of gas from the ventilator to the patient and varying the Pinsp as follows:

$$Pinsp = f1 \times V + f2 \times Flow$$

where V is volume, and f1 and f2 are selectable functions of volume (elastic assist) and flow (resistive assist), values that can be estimated from the patient's respiratory mechanics. The potential advantages of this method are greater patient comfort, lower Ppeak, and enhancement of the patient's reflex and behavioral respiratory control mechanisms.

HFV

Several modes of ventilation have in common the use of VT smaller than the dead space volume.[8] Gas exchange does not occur through convection as during conventional ventilation, but through bulk flow, Taylor diffusion, molecular diffusion, nonconvective mixing, and possibly other mechanisms. These modes include high-frequency oscillatory ventilation and high-frequency jet ventilation. The theoretical benefits of HFV include a lower risk of barotrauma as a result of smaller tidal excursions, improved gas exchange through a more uniform distribution of ventilation, and improved healing of bronchopleural fistulas. HFV is attractive as a lung-protective mode, since the lung is kept open, yet barely tidally distended. A substantial risk is that dynamic hyperinflation is the rule and Palv is greatly underestimated by monitoring pressure at the airway opening. HFV holds promise as the natural extension of lowering the VT as a means to prevent volutrauma, and there is renewed interest in this old technique. In a controlled trial[9] in patients with ARDS, HFV showed no advantage in terms of gas exchange or of short-term or long-term mortality, but did appear to be safe, at least during the performance of a clinical trial. A nonsignificant trend toward a short-term mortality benefit for HFV has been interpreted as a reason to pursue additional clinical studies. It is worth mentioning, however, that the control arm ventilation strategy was not lung-protective, potentially biasing the study in favor of HFV.

NIV

Mechanical ventilation for acute respiratory failure carries a high morbidity and mortality due, in part, to violation of the glottis by the endotracheal tube. In patients with acute-on-chronic respiratory failure, numerous studies have demonstrated that NIV effectively relieves symptoms, improves gas exchange, reduces the work of breathing, lessens complications, shortens the ICU length of stay, and improves survival.[10,11]

Nasal, oronasal, and full facial masks, as well as full-head helmets have been used successfully. Nasal masks are especially difficult to use in edentulous patients who are unable to control mouth leak. Careful attention to mask leaks and adjusting air flow and pressure-support levels are important considerations. Inflatable cuffs, nasal bridge protection, and the availability of a range of mask sizes to ensure proper fit can minimize mask complications. I find it useful to initiate ventilation by briefly holding the mask (already connected to the ventilator) onto the patient's face, rather than first strapping the mask on and then initiating ventilatory assistance. Sedative medications are occasionally appropriate and can improve tolerance of NIV, but carry some risk of respiratory depression and aspiration.

Patient-ventilator asynchrony (PVA) describes patient breathing efforts that are not coupled to machine output. During NIV, two mechanisms of PVA are common. The first is the failure of the patient to sufficiently lower the proximal airway pressure (ie, mask pressure) due to the presence of auto-PEEP. As during invasive ventilation, counterbalancing the auto-PEEP with externally applied PEEP provides a means by which to lower the work of triggering. The second common mechanism for PVA is the failure of the ventilator to detect end-inspiration because the patient's subsiding effort is cloaked by a mask leak. Most pressure-support ventilators terminate inspiration when inspiratory flow falls to a preset threshold, often at an arbitrary low value of flow or at a fixed percentage of the peak inspiratory flow. Mask leaks prevent the flow from falling to this threshold, so the ventilator fails to switch off the Pinsp even while the patient is making active expiratory efforts. This serves to increase patient discomfort and the work of breathing. Ventilators designed for NIV are very "leak tolerant" as are some newer ICU ventilators that have been redesigned with NIV in mind. Using other methods for terminating inspiration, such as time-cycled PSV or volume ACV, can minimize this problem.

Either conventional ICU ventilators or one of many portable bilevel pressure-targeted ventilators, which were initially designed for home ventilation, can be used. The limitations of portable pressure-targeted ventilators include the lack of waveform displays, the inability to deliver a high F_{IO_2} (greater than approximately 40%; some new machines allow an F_{IO_2} as high as 1.0), and the potential for the rebreathing of exhaled gas. Whether volume-preset ventilation (eg, ACV) or pressure-preset ventilation is superior for NIV remains under debate, but nearly all practitioners now use a pressure-support mode. Both modes have been used successfully, but direct comparisons between modes are few.

I believe the following points will minimize the chances that NIV will fail:

1. Develop an individual and institutional commitment to NIV.
2. Select patients carefully, excluding those with hemodynamic instability, inadequate airway protective reflexes, or little prospect of improvement within the next several days.
3. Have available a selection of masks to increase the probability of a good fit.
4. Use the pressure-support mode, beginning with modest settings, such as a PEEP of 3 cm H_2O, a PSV of 8 cm H_2O, and the most sensitive trigger, periodically removing the mask to allow the patient to sense its effect.
5. Education, reassurance, and modest sedation (when required) may improve tolerance to the mask and ventilator.
6. Increase the PEEP to ease the work of triggering with a goal of (typically) 4 to 6 cm H_2O; raise the level of PSV until the patient's breathing subjectively improves, the VT is sufficient, and the rate begins to fall, with a goal of 10 to 15 cm H_2O.
7. Detect and correct mask leaks by repositioning, achieving a better fit, changing the type of mask, removing nasogastric tubes (gastric decompression is not recommended during NIV), or adjusting the ventilator to reduce peak airway pressure.
8. Pay particular attention in the first hour to patient-ventilator synchrony, using waveform displays as a guide.

Management of the Patient

Initial Ventilator Settings

Initial ventilator settings depend on the goals of ventilation (*eg*, full respiratory muscle rest vs partial exercise), the patient's respiratory system mechanics, and minute ventilation needs. Although each critically ill patient presents myriad challenges, it is possible to identify the following five subsets of ventilated patients: (1) the patient with normal lung mechanics and gas exchange; (2) the patient with severe airflow obstruction; (3) the patient with acute-on-chronic respiratory failure; (4) the patient with acute hypoxemic respiratory failure; and (5) the patient with restrictive lung or chest wall disease.[12]

In all patients, the initial FIO_2 should usually be 0.5 to 1.0 to assure adequate oxygenation, although it can usually be lowered within minutes when guided by pulse oximetry and, in the appropriate setting, applying PEEP. In the first minutes following the institution of mechanical ventilation, the physician should remain alert for several common problems. These include, most notably, airway malposition, aspiration, and hypotension. Positive-pressure ventilation may reduce venous return and so cardiac output, especially in patients with a low mean systemic pressure (*eg*, hypovolemia, venodilating drugs, decreased sympathetic tone from sedating drugs, or neuromuscular disease) or a very high ventilation-related pleural pressure (*eg*, chest wall restriction, large amounts of PEEP, or obstruction causing auto-PEEP). If hypotension occurs, intravascular volume should be rapidly expanded while steps are taken to lower the pleural pressure (*eg*, smaller VT or less minute ventilation).

The Patient With Normal Respiratory Mechanics and Gas Exchange

Patients with normal lung mechanics and gas exchange can require mechanical ventilation for several of the following reasons: (1) because of the loss of central drive to breathe (*eg*, drug overdose or structural injury to the brainstem); (2) because of neuromuscular weakness (*eg*, high cervical cord injury, acute idiopathic myelitis, or myasthenia gravis); (3) as an adjunctive therapy in

the treatment of shock; or (4) in order to achieve hyperventilation (*eg*, in the treatment of elevated intracranial pressure following head trauma). Following intubation, initial ventilator orders should be an FIO_2 of 0.5 to 1.0, a VT of 8 to 15 mL/kg, a respiratory rate of 8 to 12 breaths/min, and an inspiratory flow rate of 40 to 60 L/min. Alternatively, if the patient has sufficient drive and is not profoundly weak, PSV can be used. The level of pressure support is adjusted (usually to the range of 10 to 20 cm H_2O above PEEP) to bring the f down into the low 20 breaths/min, usually corresponding to a VT of approximately 400 mL. If gas exchange is entirely normal, the FIO_2 can likely be lowered further based on pulse oximetry or arterial blood gas determinations. In patients who do not have acute lung injury but are at risk of it developing, it may be prudent to use a low VT since there is some evidence that mechanical ventilation at VTs of roughly 11 mL/kg predicted body weight can induce lung injury.[13]

Soon after the initiation of ventilation, airway pressure and flow waveforms should be inspected for evidence of patient-ventilator dyssynchrony or undesired patient effort. If the goal of ventilation is full rest, the patient's respiratory drive can often be suppressed by increasing the inspiratory flow rate, f, or VT; of course, the latter two changes may induce respiratory alkalemia. If such adjustments do not diminish breathing effort (despite normal blood gas levels) to an undetectable level, sedation may be necessary. If this does not abolish inspiratory efforts and full rest is essential (as in patients who in shock), muscle paralysis should be considered. A small amount of PEEP (5 to 7.5 cm H_2O) is used to prevent atelectasis.

Patients With Severe Airflow Obstruction

Severe obstruction is seen most commonly in patients with status asthmaticus, but also rarely in those with inhalation injury or central airway lesions, such as a tumor or a foreign body, that are not bypassed with the endotracheal tube. Some of these patients may benefit from NIV, but most will require invasive ventilation. These patients are usually extremely anxious and distressed. Deep sedation should be provided in such instances, supplemented in some patients by therapeutic paralysis. These interventions help to reduce oxygen consumption (and hence carbon dioxide production) to lower airway pressures and to reduce the risk of self-extubation.

Because the gas exchange abnormalities of airflow obstruction are largely limited to ventilation-perfusion mismatch, an FIO_2 of 0.5 suffices in the vast majority of patients. Ventilation should be initiated using the ACV mode (or SIMV mode), the VT should be small (5 to 7 mL/kg), and the f should be 12 to 15 breaths/min. A peak flow of 60 L/min is recommended; higher flow rates do little to increase TE. For example, if the VT is 500 mL/kg, the f is 15 breaths/min, and the flow is 60 L/min, the TE is 3.5 s. Raising flow (dramatically) to 120 L/min increases the TE to only 3.75 s, which is a trivial improvement. In contrast, a small reduction in f to 14 breaths/min increases the TE to 3.8 s. This example serves to emphasize not only the relative lack of benefit of raising the flow rate but also the importance of minimizing minute ventilation when the goal is to reduce auto-PEEP. Some patients who remain agitated during ACV can be made more comfortable by using PSV mode (or PCV mode) with a total Pinsp of approximately 30 cm H_2O. Finally, if the patient is triggering the ventilator, some PEEP should be added to reduce the work of triggering.[14] Although this occasionally compounds the dynamic hyperinflation, potentially compromising cardiac output, usually auto-PEEP increases little as long as PEEP is not set higher than about 85% of the auto-PEEP. The goals are (1) to minimize alveolar overdistention (Pplat, <30 cm H_2O) and (2) to minimize dynamic hyperinflation (auto-PEEP, <15 cm H_2O; or end-inspiratory lung volume, <20 mL/kg), a strategy that largely prevents barotrauma.[15,16] Reducing minute ventilation to achieve these goals generally causes the PCO_2 to rise to >40 mm Hg, and often to ≥70 mm Hg. Although this requires sedation, such permissive hypercapnia is tolerated quite well, except in patients with increased intracranial pressure, and perhaps in those with ventricular dysfunction or critical pulmonary hypertension.[17]

Patients With Acute-on-Chronic Respiratory Failure

Acute-on-chronic respiratory failure is a term that is used to describe the exacerbations of chronic ventilatory failure, often requiring ICU admission, usually occurring in patients with COPD. Unlike patients with status asthmaticus, patients in this population tend to have relatively smaller increases in inspiratory resistance, their expiratory flow limitation arising largely from the loss of elastic recoil. As a consequence, in the patient with COPD and minimally reversible airway disease, peak airway pressures on the ventilator tend not to be extraordinarily high, yet auto-PEEP and its consequences are common. At the time of intubation, hypoperfusion is common, as manifested by tachycardia and relative hypotension, and typically responds to briefly ceasing ventilation combined with fluid loading.

Because the majority of these patients receive ventilation after days to weeks of progressive deterioration, the goal is to rest the patient (and respiratory muscles) for 24 to 48 h. Also, because the patient typically has an underlying compensated respiratory acidosis, excessive ventilation risks severe respiratory alkalosis and, over time, bicarbonate wasting by the kidney. Many such patients can be ventilated effectively with NIV, as described above. For those patients who require intubation, the goals of rest and appropriate hypoventilation can usually be achieved with initial ventilator settings of a VT of 5 to 7 mL/kg and an f of 20 to 24 breaths/min, with ACV mode set on minimal sensitivity. Because gas exchange abnormalities are primarily those of ventilation-perfusion mismatch, supplemental oxygenation with FIO_2 in the range of 0.4 should achieve >90% saturation of arterial hemoglobin.

The majority of patients with COPD will appear exhausted at the time when mechanical support is instituted and will sleep with minimal sedation. To the extent that muscle fatigue has played a role in a patient's functional decline, rest and sleep are desirable. Two days of such rest presumably will restore biochemical and functional changes associated with muscle fatigue, but 24 h may not be sufficient. Small numbers of patients will have difficulty resting while receiving ventilation, continuing to demonstrate a high work of breathing. An examination of airway pressure and flow waveforms can be very helpful in identifying this extra work of breathing and in suggesting strategies for improving the ventilator settings. In many patients, this is the result of auto-PEEP-induced triggering difficulty. Adding extrinsic PEEP to nearly counterbalance the auto-PEEP dramatically improves the patient's comfort.

Patients With Acute Hypoxemic Respiratory Failure

Acute hypoxemic respiratory failure is caused by alveolar filling with blood, pus, or edema, the end results of which are impaired lung mechanics and gas exchange. The gas exchange impairment results from intrapulmonary shunt that is largely refractory to oxygen therapy. In ARDS, the significantly reduced functional residual capacity arising from alveolar flooding and collapse leaves many fewer alveoli to accept the VT, making the lung appear stiff and dramatically increasing the work of breathing. The lung of the ARDS patient should be viewed as a small lung, however, rather than a stiff lung. In line with this current conception of ARDS, it is now clearly established that excessive distention of the lung of the ARDS patient compounds lung injury and may induce systemic inflammation.[1,18] Ventilatory strategies have evolved markedly in the past decade, changing clinical practice and generating tremendous excitement.

The goals of ventilation are to reduce shunt, avoid toxic concentrations of oxygen, and choose ventilator settings that do not amplify lung damage. The initial FIO_2 should be 1.0 in view of the typically extreme hypoxemia. PEEP therapy is indicated in patients with diffuse lung lesions but may not be helpful in patients with focal infiltrates, such as occurs with lobar pneumonia. In patients with ARDS, PEEP should be instituted immediately, then rapidly adjusted to the lowest PEEP necessary to produce an arterial saturation of 90% on an FIO_2 no higher than 0.6 (ie, the "least-PEEP approach"). Recruitment maneuvers have generally applied a sustained inflation pressure while the patient is therapeutically paralyzed. For example, continuous positive airway pressure of 40 cm H_2O for 40 s has often been chosen. Although these maneuvers have shown some ability to transiently raise the PO_2, they have not been shown to change clinically meaningful outcomes. The VT should be 6 mL/kg while receiving ACV; a higher VT is associated with higher mortality. Potentially, PCV could be used as well, but the parameters that assure lung-protective

ventilation are not known. In either mode, the f should be set at 24 to 36 breaths/min. An occasional consequence of lung-protective ventilation is hypercapnia. This approach of preferring hypercapnia to alveolar overdistention, termed *permissive hypercapnia*, is very well tolerated.

The Patient With Restriction of the Lungs or Chest Wall

A small VT (5 to 7 mL/kg) and rapid breathing rate (18 to 24 breaths/min) are especially important in order to minimize the hemodynamic consequences of positive-pressure ventilation and to reduce the likelihood of barotrauma. The FIO_2 is usually determined by the degree of alveolar filling or collapse, if any. When the restrictive abnormality involves the chest wall (including the abdomen), the large ventilation-induced rise in pleural pressure has the potential to compromise cardiac output. This in turn will lower the mixed venous PO_2 and, in the setting of ventilation-perfusion mismatch or shunt, the PaO_2 as well. If the physician responds to this falling PaO_2 by augmenting PEEP or increasing the minute ventilation, further circulatory compromise ensues. A potentially catastrophic cycle of worsening gas exchange, increasing ventilator settings, and progressive shock is begun. This circumstance must be recognized because the treatment is to reduce dead space (*eg*, by lowering minute ventilation or correcting hypovolemia).

The Airway During Split-Lung Ventilation

The lungs may be separated for purposes of differential ventilation in two major ways: (1) blocking the bronchus of a lobe or whole lung while ventilating with a standard endotracheal tube, or (2) passing a double-lumen tube (DLT). A number of different devices have been used to obstruct a bronchus, but experience is greatest with the Fogarty embolectomy catheter. DLTs carry the advantages of allowing each lung to be ventilated, collapsed, reexpanded, or inspected independently.

Split-lung ventilation is only rarely useful in the critical care unit, but occasionally its benefits are dramatic. Large bronchopleural fistulas severely compromise ventilation and may not respond to HFV. A DLT will maintain ventilation of the healthy lung while facilitating closure of the bronchopleural fistula. During massive hemoptysis, lung separation may be life-saving by minimizing blood aspiration, maintaining airway patency, and tamponading the bleeding site while awaiting definitive therapy. Finally, patients with focal causes of acute hypoxemic respiratory failure, such as lobar pneumonia or acute total atelectasis, may benefit from differential ventilation and the application of PEEP.

Annotated References

1. The Acute Respiratory Distress Syndrome Network. Ventilation with lower tidal volumes as compared with traditional tidal volumes for acute lung injury and the acute respiratory distress syndrome. N Engl J Med 2000; 342:1301–1308
Signal study establishing that VT is an important determinant of outcome in patients with acute lung injury and ARDS.

2. Amato MBP, Barbas CSV, Medeiros DM, et al. Effect of a protective-ventilation strategy on mortality in the acute respiratory distress syndrome. N Engl J Med 1998; 338:347–354
Fifty-three subjects with early acute lung injury were ventilated with a "conventional" versus "lung-protective" approach, where the lung-protective strategy involved both lower tidal volumes and higher PEEPs than the conventional approach. The protective approach improved 28-day survival, weaning from ventilation, and the incidence of barotrauma. This key study indicated that the details of ventilating acute lung injury patients affected outcome but raised questions as to which component or components of the "protective" strategy led to the benefit.

3. The National Heart, Lung, and Blood Institute ARDS Clinical Trials Network. Higher versus lower positive end-expiratory pressures in patients with the acute respiratory distress syndrome. N Engl J Med 2004; 351:327–336
This study sought to compare higher versus lower PEEP in 549 subjects with acute lung injury who were receiving a lung-protective tidal volume of 6 mL/kg predicted body weight. Outcomes were similar regardless of the level of PEEP.

4. Slutsky A. Mechanical ventilation. Chest 1993; 104:1833–1859
A comprehensive review of many aspects of mechanical ventilation.

5. Brochard L, Rauss A, Benito S, et al. Comparison of three methods of gradual withdrawal from ventilatory support during weaning from mechanical ventilation. Am J Respir Crit Care Med 1994; 150:896–903
One of two large multicenter trials comparing weaning modes. SIMV was clearly shown to be inferior.

6. Esteban A, Alía I, Gordo F, et al. Extubation outcome after spontaneous breathing trials with T-tube or pressure support ventilation. Am J Respir Crit Care Med 1997; 156:459–465
The other major weaning trial.

7. Younes M, Puddy A, Roberts D, et al. Proportional assist ventilation: results of an initial clinical trial. Am Rev Respir Dis 1992; 145:121–129
A mode that adjusts pressure to meet patient demand.

8. Drazen JM, Kamm RD, Slutsky AS, et al. High-frequency ventilation. Physiol Rev 1984; 64:505–543
Description of ventilation using VTs less than the dead space volume.

9. Derdak S, Mehta S, Stewart TE, et al. High-frequency oscillatory ventilation for acute respiratory distress syndrome in adults: a randomized, controlled trial. Am J Respir Crit Care Med 2002; 166:801–808
Randomized trial showing that HFV can be performed safely, but failing to demonstrate any significant clinical benefits compared with PCV in patients with ARDS.

10. Brochard L, Mancebo J, Wysocki M, et al. Noninvasive ventilation for acute exacerbations of chronic obstructive pulmonary disease. N Engl J Med 1995; 333:817–822
The first trial to show convincingly the benefits of NIV.

11. Kramer N, Meyer TJ, Meharg J, et al. Randomized, prospective trial of noninvasive positive pressure ventilation in acute respiratory failure. Am J Respir Crit Care Med 1995; 151:1799–1806
This trial confirmed the trial of Brochard et al.[10]

12. Schmidt GA, Hall JB. Management of the ventilated patient. In: Hall JB, Schmidt GA, Wood LDH, eds. Principles of critical care. 2nd ed. New York, NY: McGraw-Hill, 1998
Describes ventilation based on individual patient physiology.

13. Gajic O, Dara SI, Mendez JL, et al. Ventilator-associated lung injury in patients without acute lung injury at the onset of mechanical ventilation. Crit Care Med 2004; 32:1817–1824

    This retrospective study found an association between the initial V_T and subsequent development of acute lung injury, suggesting that V_Ts of 11 mL/kg may be injurious even before lung injury is established.

14. Ranieri VM, Giuliani R, Cinnella G, et al. Physiologic effects of positive end-expiratory pressure in patients with chronic obstructive pulmonary disease during acute ventilatory failure and controlled mechanical ventilation. Am Rev Respir Dis 1993; 147:5–13

    Demonstrates the impact of externally applied PEEP in patients receiving auto-PEEP, showing reduced work of breathing.

15. Tuxen DV, Lane S. The effects of ventilatory pattern on hyperinflation, airway pressures, and circulation in mechanical ventilation of patients with severe air-flow obstruction. Am Rev Respir Dis 1987; 136:872–879

    This key article demonstrated the link between minute ventilation and potentially detrimental consequences, such as barotraumas and hypotension.

16. Tuxen DV, Williams TJ, Scheinkestel CD, et al. Use of a measurement of pulmonary hyperinflation to control the level of mechanical ventilation in patients with acute severe asthma. Am Rev Respir Dis 1992; 146:1136–1142

    Demonstrated improved outcome by limiting minute ventilation.

17. Feihl F, Perret C. Permissive hypercapnia: how permissive should we be? Am J Respir Crit Care Med 1994; 150:1722–1737

    A comprehensive review of the risks and benefits of hypercapnic ventilation.

18. Ranieri VM, Suter PM, Tortoella C, et al. Effects of mechanical ventilation on inflammatory mediators in patients with acute respiratory distress syndrome: a randomized controlled trial. JAMA 1999; 282:54–61

    Demonstrated that large V_Ts elaborate potentially damaging cytokine levels in patients.

Notes

Hypertensive Emergencies and Urgencies

R. Phillip Dellinger, MD, FCCP

Objectives:

- Identify acute end-organ dysfunction due to hypertension
- Recognize the importance of lowering BP in a timely but finite manner
- Match appropriate drugs for the treatment of hypertensive emergencies/urgencies based on patient characteristics
- Appreciate the potential toxicities and side effects of the drug chosen

Key words: hypertensive emergency; hypertensive encephalopathy; hypotensive urgency; postoperative hypertension

Severe hypertension with acute organ dysfunction is a reason for admission to the ICU, and uncontrolled hypertension may complicate ICU stay for those patients admitted for other reasons. *Hypertensive emergency* is defined as a severe elevation in BP that is associated with acute end-organ damage. These conditions require immediate control of BP to ameliorate organ injury. IV medications are required, and invasive monitoring and ICU admission are typical. The organ systems that are most frequently involved include the CNS, the cardiovascular system, and the kidneys. Both the absolute level of BP and the time to reach that level are important in the development of organ injury. Therefore, acute end-organ injury may occur at different blood values in different patients. Defining hypertensive emergency based on acute end-organ damage is more appropriate than using specified numbers for systolic or diastolic BP. Hypertensive urgencies identify patients who are at risk for organ dysfunction due to hypertension; based on clinical assessment, the lowering of BP needs to be immediate or may be accomplished over hours based on the assessment of risk.

Identification of End-Organ Damage

Most patients with hypertensive emergencies will have a history of poorly controlled essential hypertension. Secondary hypertension (*eg*, renal artery stenosis) should, however, be considered. Symptoms and physical examination findings are important clues to trigger a search for acute organ dysfunction in hypertensive patients. Headache, confusion, or seizures may indicate hypertensive encephalopathy. Chest pain may signify aortic dissection or myocardial ischemia. A physical examination of the chest may reveal rales associated with hypertension-induced pulmonary edema, a murmur of aortic insufficiency associated with proximal aortic dissection, or extremity pulse deficits related to aortic dissection. Pertinent laboratory tests performed in the evaluation of patients with known or suspected hypertensive emergencies or urgencies include a urine analysis in search of glomerulonephritis as a secondary cause of hypertension or creatinine measurement as a marker of hypertension-induced acute renal dysfunction (when the baseline value is known). An ECG may reveal myocardial ischemia exacerbated by hypertension, and a chest radiograph may offer clues to aortic dissection (*eg*, widened mediastinum) or hypertension-induced pulmonary edema.

Hypertensive Encephalopathy

A 52-year-old man presented with generalized seizures and a BP of 244/160 mm Hg. The patient received lorazepam IV with the cessation of seizures. He was intubated and mechanically ventilated. A fundus examination revealed papilledema, supporting the diagnosis of hypertensive encephalopathy.

Clinical manifestations of a hypertensive encephalopathy-induced increase in intracranial pressure include headache, nausea, vomiting, confusion, lethargy, generalized seizures, and coma. A differential diagnosis of hypertensive encephalopathy includes severe hypertension in association with subarachnoid hemorrhage or stroke. A CT scan may be required to assure the absence of these entities.

General Principles of IV Drug Therapy for Hypertensive Emergencies

In hypertensive encephalopathy, as well as in most hypertensive emergencies and urgencies, the initial BP therapeutic target is to decrease the mean arterial pressure by 15 to 25%. In patients with chronic hypertension, the cerebral blood flow autoregulation curve is shifted to the right. In the normotensive patient, cerebral blood flow is auto-regulated such that cerebral blood flow remains constant between mean arterial pressures of 50 and 150 mm Hg (Fig 1). In chronically hypertensive patients, this autoregulation shifts to the right, and the regulation of cerebral blood flow occurs at a much higher pressure range. Overzealous lowering of the mean arterial pressure in patients with severe hypertension to even high normal BPs may drop the BP to a level that is below the lower range of autoregulation and decrease cerebral blood flow. This may be particularly problematic in patients with underlying cerebral vascular disease, producing iatrogenic strokes.

In patients with hypertensive encephalopathy, as in those with other causes of hypertensive emergencies, the ideal drug is an IV vasodilator with quick onset of action and quick offset of action. Drugs that offer these traits include nitroprusside, nicardipine, fenoldopam, and nitroglycerin.

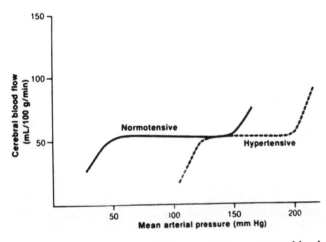

Figure 1. Cerebral autoregulation maintains constant blood flow (in the absence of acute brain injury) between approximately 50 and 150 mm Hg mean arterial pressure. With chronic sustained elevations in blood pressure the autoregulation curve shifts to the right and puts the patient at risk for cerebral hypoperfusion and stroke when blood pressure is aggressively lowered, even when the value is within normal range.

Therapy with sodium nitroprusside, long a staple drug in the treatment of hypertensive emergencies, is begun with an initial infusion of 0.5 to 1.0 µg/kg/min with a maximum dosage of 10 µg/kg/min for 10 min or a maximum sustained dose of 3 µg/kg/min. Cyanide and thiocyanate toxicity are potential problems with nitroprusside infusion. This rarely occurs with recommended infusion rates occurring over ≤48 h of therapy. Even in patients with anuric renal failure, therapy with nitroprusside, used at recommended doses during the initial stabilization of BP, is safe. Nitroprusside is nonenzymatically converted to cyanide in the blood, and cyanide is converted to thiocyanate in the liver. Thiocyanate is excreted by the kidney. Patients with liver disease are at an increased risk of cyanide toxicity, and patients with kidney disease are at an increased risk of thiocyanate and cyanide toxicity. In patients without renal dysfunction, thiocyanate levels can be followed as a marker for the risk of cyanide and thiocyanate toxicity. An arterial line is advised for the administration of nitroprusside due to the sudden drops in BP that may occur with the titration of nitroprusside.

IV nicardipine is an effective, titratable continuous-infusion calcium-channel blocker that is used for the treatment of hypertensive emergencies/urgencies. It has a rapid onset and intermediate half-life, and is an arterial vasodilator that is associated with increased cardiac index. Unlike other calcium-channel blockers, it is unlikely to produce negative inotropic effects. Infusion is begun at 5 mg/h and is increased by 2.5 mg/h every 10 min to a maximum rate of 15 mg/h.

IV labetalol is a reliable drug for the treatment of hypertensive encephalopathy as well as other etiologies of hypertensive emergencies. The onset of action of labetalol is 2 to 5 min with peak hypotensive effect occurring at 5 to 10 min and an effect lasting up to 4 h. Its combined α/β effect typically produces a significant lowering of peripheral vascular resistance with a minimal decrease in heart rate and a minimal change in cardiac output. Drug loading is accomplished with incremental dosing (an IV bolus of 20 to 80 mg every 10 to 15 min, depending on the response). Loading by continuous infusion at 0.5 to 2 mg/min is also possible. Unlike nitroprusside, labetalol may be utilized in most patients without arterial line placement. Although maintenance continuous infusions have been successfully utilized, labetalol was primarily developed for the initial control of BP through loading followed by conversion to labetalol administered orally or other alternative antihypertension therapies. Labetalol should not be used in patients with second-degree heart block or greater, patients with asthma, or patients with signifi cant systolic cardiac dysfunction.

Fenoldopam is a drug with a very similar pharmacodynamic profile as nitroprusside. As a selective dopamine-1 receptor agonist, it has been demonstrated to increase renal blood flow, although clinical studies have not been able to demonstrate a renal clinical outcome benefit compared to that with nitroprusside. Administration is begun at 0.03 to 0.10 µg/kg/min and titrated in increments of 0.05 to 0.1 µg/kg no more frequently than every 15 min. The use of fenoldopam is safer than nitroprusside in patients with moderate-to-severe renal dysfunction (fenoldopam carries no risk for cyanide toxicity) but is more expensive.

Nitroglycerin is a direct-acting vasodilator and, unlike nitroprusside, which is a balanced arteriolar IV acting drug, has predominately venous capacitance effects. It also has the potential to redistribute coronary artery blood flow to benefit the ischemic myocardium. Primary consideration for the use of nitroglycerin should be in hypertensive emergencies/urgencies associated with congestive heart failure, coronary artery disease, postcoronary artery bypass surgery, or increased left ventricular (LV) filling pressures. It is particularly useful in patients with active myocardial ischemia, high LV filling pressures, and mild-to-moderate hypertension.

Hypertension Associated With Cardiac Dysfunction

Hypertensive Crisis With High-Pressure Pulmonary Edema

Clinical features of a severe hypertension-induced rise in LV end-diastolic pressure with associated high pulmonary capillary pressure and pulmonary edema include severe hypoxemia, CO_2 retention, pink frothy sputum, and pulmonary edema seen on a chest radiograph. The typical patient will have chronic LV hypertrophy with

diastolic function and normal or increased ejection fraction. Initial therapy targets any intervention that lowers the LV end-diastolic pressure. This includes an increase in venous capacitance, a decrease in arteriolar resistance, and increasing compliance (softening) of the LV. Diuresis is an effective therapy, although studies have demonstrated that most patients with this diagnosis do not have increased intravascular blood volume; therefore, vasodilatation is the most effective therapy. The use of diuretics, although effective in abating pulmonary edema, may leave the patient's intravascular volume depleted with prerenal azotemia. Since diastolic function is often present, therapy with β-blockers is also very effective. Labetalol may also be useful as a combination α/β-blocker. Acute ischemia, associated with hypertension, may occur during weaning from mechanical ventilation, and also may produce an increase in BP, an associated rise in LV end-diastolic pressure, and pulmonary edema as a cause of weaning failure. This presentation is likely to be more insidious than the presentation of the patient presenting to the emergency department with acute hypertension-induced pulmonary edema, since lower ranges of BP elevation may be present with a contribution of myocardial ischemia-induced wall stiffness playing a prominent role in the rise in pulmonary capillary pressure.

Hypertension and Systolic Dysfunction

Enalaprilat is an IV drug with a potential to treat hypertension and to improve cardiac function. It is an afterload reducer with an onset of action of 15 min and a duration of action of 12 h. The dose is 0.625 to 5 mg administered as a single bolus every 6 h. It may be chosen to treat mild-to-moderate hypertension in patients with congestive heart failure due to systolic dysfunction or in patients with an activation of the renin-angiotensin system such as scleroderma kidney. It is not usually a "go-to" drug to treat severe life-threatening hypertension. The potential disadvantages of enalaprilat include idiopathic angioedema. It should not be used in patients with bilateral renovascular disease or in pregnant women in the second or third trimester. When used on an ongoing basis in the ICU, creatinine levels should be followed and therapy should be discontinued if the creatinine level begins to rise. Therapy with enalaprilat can, however, be instituted in patients with stable elevated creatinine levels.

Hypertension With Acute CNS Events

An increase in BP is thought to be a normal physiologic response to acute CNS strokes, including bland stroke, hemorrhagic stroke, intracranial hemorrhage, and subarachnoid hemorrhage. The optimum method to be used for the management of BP following cerebral vascular accidents remains controversial. Hypertension is common after both ischemic and hemorrhagic strokes, and at least some component of the rise is thought to be a body-compensatory mechanism. However, extreme elevations in BP are associated with poor outcomes after both ischemic and hemorrhagic cerebrovascular accidents and are thought to play a role in this bad outcome. Concerns of severe elevations in BP after stroke include reinfarction, cerebral edema, increased hemorrhage size, and

hemorrhagic transformation. Cerebral edema is problematic in light of a dysfunctional ability to autoregulate cerebral blood flow following a stroke. It is a double-edged sword, however, as neurologic deterioration may occur in this circumstance with aggressive pharmacologic lowering of BP. In general, withholding therapy for hypertension in the acute phase of ischemic strokes is the recommendation, unless thrombolysis is planned, acute end-organ damage is occurring, or arbitrary selected limits for systolic BP are present.

Although increased BP is considered to put the patient at risk for increased edema in areas of injury as well as to increase the chance of bleeding or rebleeding, equally important in these patients are watershed areas of brain penumbra that are at risk for further ischemic injury, which might benefit from higher BP-induced collateral flow. There is general agreement that in an unclipped subarachnoid hemorrhage BP should be normalized, and once the aneurysm is clipped that very high BPs may be tolerated as there is no significant risk

Table 1. *Approach to Arterial Hypertension in Acute Ischemic Stroke*

Indication that patient is eligible for treatment with intravenous rtPA or other acute reperfusion intervention
    Blood pressure level
        Systolic >185 mm Hg or diastolic >110 mm Hg
            Labetalol 10–20 mg IV over 1–2 min, may repeat ×1;
            or Nitropaste 1–2 inches;
            or
            Nicardipine infusion, 5 mg/h, titrate up by 2.5 mg/h at 5- to 15-min intervals, maximum dose 15 mg/h; when desired blood pressure attained, reduce to 3 mg/h
        If blood pressure does not decline and remains >185/110 mm Hg, do not administer rtPA
Management of blood pressure during and after treatment with rtPA or other acute reperfusion intervention
    Monitor blood pressure every 15 min during treatment and then for another 2 h, then every 30 min for 6 h, and then every hour for 16 h
    Blood pressure level
        Systolic 180–230 mm Hg or diastolic 105–120 mm Hg
            Labetalol 10 mg IV over 1–2 min, may repeat every 10–20 min, maximum dose of 300 mg;
            or
            Labetalol 10 mg IV followed by an infusion at 2–8 mg/min
        Systolic >230 mm Hg or diastolic 121–140 mm Hg
            Labetalol 10 mg IV over 1–2 min, may repeat every 10–20 min, maximum dose of 300 mg;
            or
            Labetalol 10 mg IV followed by an infusion at 2–8 mg/min;
            or
            Nicardipine infusion, 5 mg/h, titrate up to desired effect by increasing 2.5 mg/h every 5 min to maximun of 15 mg/h
        If blood pressure not controlled, consider sodium nitroprusside

*Reprinted with permission from Adams H, del Zoppo G, Alberts MJ, et al. Stroke 2007; 38:1655–1711

Hypertensive Emergencies and Urgencies (Dellinger)

of rebleeding, and hypertension may be protective against a postbleed vasospasm.

Less hypertension is tolerated when thrombolysis is planned. The current recommendation is to administer thrombolytic therapy with a systolic BP of ≤185 mm Hg and a diastolic BP of ≤110 mm Hg (Table 1).

In patients who experience intracerebral hemorrhage, the penumbra issues are very important. The degree of BP rise likely is associated with a risk for rebleeding, but it is also likely that a higher BP better maintains perfusion of the risk area surrounding the stroke. The lowering of BP by 15% likely does not put the penumbra at risk after intracerebral hemorrhage and may decrease the risk of bleeding. Recommended drugs include labetalol, nicardipine, and nitroprusside. Maintaining systolic pressure ≤ 180 seems reasonable.

Severe Hypertension-Induced Renal Dysfunction

A patient may present with severe hypertension and acute deterioration in renal function. Drugs that may be particularly suited to the treatment of this group of patients include labetalol and hydralazine, where a greater preservation of renal blood flow may occur. Dialysis is the treatment of choice for severe hypertension (and associated hypoxemia), primarily driven by volume overload.

Postoperative Hypertension

Hypertension-induced postoperative complications include arrhythmias, myocardial ischemia/infarction, stroke, and wound hemorrhage. Indications for the treatment of postoperative hypertension have been arbitrarily defined as a systolic BP of > 190 mm Hg or a diastolic BP of >100 mg on two consecutive readings. A history of hypertension, high body mass index, age, and the grade of the surgical stress are risk factors for postoperative hypertension. It is important to evaluate for possible causes of hypertension that are secondary to pain, hypercarbia, hypoxemia, or urinary retention.

A wide variety of drugs may by used to manage postoperative hypertension depending on particular patient characteristics. These include nitroprusside, nicardipine, hydralazine, labetalol, esmolol, and fenoldopam.

Esmolol is a cardioselective β-adrenergic blocker with quick onset of action (peak effects within 5 to 15 min) and a short half-life (9 to 10 min). Esmolol is rapidly metabolized by RBCs and does not depend on renal or hepatic function. Esmolol may be administered by IV bolus or by continuous infusion. Continuous infusion is usually initiated following a loading dose. It is a good fit for patients with tachycardia, hypertension, and good systolic function. Either esmolol or intermittent bolus metoprolol may offer an advantage to postoperative patients with hypertension, tachycardia, and good systolic function. These drugs should be used with caution in patients with obstructive airways disease and avoided in patients with asthma. When a β-blocker is used in the treatment of patients with potential side effects of β-blockade, esmolol is preferred over intermittent metoprolol. Table 2 contrasts esmolol with two other choices of IV antihypertensive agents.

Aortic Dissection

Aortic dissection is caused by a tear in the intima of the aorta that is propagated by the aortic pulse wave. The aortic pulse wave, or "shearing force," depends on a combination of myocardial contractility, heart rate, and BP. The risk factors for aortic dissection include advanced atherosclerosis, connective tissue diseases, and aortic coarctation. Dissections involving the area proximal to the left subclavian artery are considered to be type A, and when this area is not involved are considered to be type B (ie, involving the descending aorta only). Chest pain is the typical presenting symptom, and the classic chest radiographic finding is a widened mediastinum. Diagnosis is made either with a contrast-enhanced CT scan or transesophageal echocardiography. Dissection is usually diagnosed utilizing CT scanning with and without contrast enhancement, which demonstrates a grayish/whitish false lumen predominately filled with a clot alongside a bright-white, dye-filled true aortic channel. Dissecting thoracic aortic aneurysms involving the arch and descending aorta that do not interfere with major vessel outflow are typically managed medically with BP control. Aneurysms involving the ascending aorta or are comprimizing organ blood flow are typically surgically treated.

Table 2. *Contrasting Effects of Nicardipine, Esmolol, and Labetalol**

	Nicardipine	Esmolol	Labetalol
Administration	Continuous infusion	Continuous infusion	Bolus continuous infusion
Onset	Rapid	Rapid	Rapid
Offset	Rapid	Rapid	Slower
HR	Minimal increase	Decreased	Minimal decrease
SVR	Decreased	0	Decreased
Cardiac output	Increased	Decreased	No change
Myocardial O$_2$ balance	Positive	Positive	Positive

*HR, heart rate; SVR, systemic vascular resistance.

Aneurysms of the ascending aorta may dissect proximally, producing a murmur of aortic insufficiency or acute pericardial tamponade. Distal migration may produce an obstruction of the major vascular outflow vessels or a rupture into the thorax. Occasionally, a leak may occur into the thorax, which is diagnosed in time to allow life-saving surgery. The propagating force for a dissection is the change in blood pressure over the shearing force. This shearing force is minimized by a combination therapy of keeping the heart rate normal, normalizing BP, and decreasing inotropy. Dissection of the aorta is another circumstance (unclipped aneurysm was discussed earlier) in which the immediate normalization of BP is indicated.

Severe Hypertension in Pregnancy

Hypertension is responsible for 18% of maternal deaths in the United States. Hypertension of pregnancy is defined as a systolic BP of ≥ 140 mm Hg or a diastolic BP of ≥90 mm Hg. Preeclampsia is defined by new-onset hypertension accompanied by proteinuria and edema. Eclampsia is defined as the development of seizures or coma in a preeclamptic patient. The treatment of severe preeclampsia and eclampsia includes delivery of the fetus combined with therapy with magnesium sulfate for the prevention and treatment of seizures and BP control. The typical recommendation is to reduce diastolic BP to 110 mm Hg or mean arterial pressure by 20%. In addition to magnesium, hydralazine has traditionally been the drug of choice in the treatment of these patients. Potential problems include tachycardia and side effects that mimic the symptoms of eclampsia (eg, nausea, vomiting, headaches, and anxiety). Excessive hypotension can be dangerous to both mother and fetus. Hydralazine is a direct arteriolar vasodilator with an onset of action in 15 to 30 min and a duration of effect of 2 to 4 h. It is also advocated as a drug of particular benefit in patients with eclampsia. It is associated with reflex tachycardia, and its use should be avoided in patients with dissecting aortic aneurysm and acute myocardial ischemia. Although hydralazine has historically been recommended as the antihypertensive agent of choice, recent data have suggested that labetalol and nifedipine may be more viable options.

Catecholamine-Associated Hypertensive Crisis

Catecholamine-induced hypertensive crisis may be associated with consumption of sympathomimetic agents such as amphetamines, or certain diet pills, decongestants such as ephedrine and other agents (alkaloids). A rapid surge in catecholamines resulting in hypertension may also accompany withdrawal from β-blocker or α-blocker agents. In this circumstance, reinitiation of the drug may be sufficient to treat the elevated BP. Rare causes of catecholamine-associated hypertensive crisis include pheochromocytoma, autonomic dysfunction (Guillain-Barré syndrome), and tyramine ingestion in the presence of monoamine oxidase inhibitor therapy. In general, the use of β-blocker therapy alone as the initial therapy should be avoided because of the possibility of the loss of β-adrenergically mediated vasodilation leading to an unopposed α effect. Pheochromocytoma, which is more likely to be encountered on board examinations as opposed to in real life, is a rare tumor producing a catecholamine-excess state with the potential for severe hypertension accompanied by headache, palpitations, diaphoresis, abdominal pain, and anxiety. The drug of choice for therapy is phentolamine.

Annotated Bibliography

Adams HP, del Zoppo G, Alberts MJ, et al. Guidelines for the early management of adults with ischemic stroke. Stroke 2007; 38:1655–1711
Current AHA American Stroke (ASA) Association recommendations.

Aggarwal M, Khan IA. Hypertensive crisis: hypertensive emergencies and urgencies. Cardiol Clin 2006; 24:135–146
General review of hypertensive emergencies and urgencies.

Broderick J, Connolly S, Feldmann E, et al. Guidelines for the management of spontaneous intracerebral hemorrhage in adults. Stroke 2008; 38:2001–2023
Current recommendations for management in intracerebral hemorrhage.

Elliott WJ. Clinical features in the management of selected hypertensive emergencies. Prog Cardiovasc Dis 2006; 48:316–325
Review and update targets selected end-organ dysfunction scenarios.

Elliott WJ. Clinical features in the management of selected hypertensive emergencies. Prog Cardiovasc Dis 2006; 48:316–325
A cardiologists' perspective on hypertensive emergencies.

Feldstein C. Management of hypertensive crises. Am J Ther 2007; 14:135–139
Renew presenting a logical approach to specific organ dysfunctions and causes of hypertensive crises.

Flanigan JS, Vitberg D. Hypertensive emergency and severe hypertension: What to treat, who to treat, and how to treat. Med Clin North Am 2006; 90:439–451
Concise management-based format.

Goldberg ME, Weaver FA. Strategies for managing perioperative hypertension. Crit Care Clin 2007; 23:7–21
Covers issues related to intravenous option only and co-morbidities to prevent operation specific complications (wound hemorrhage) and not operation specific complications.

Haas CE, LeBlanc JM. Acute postoperative hypertension: a review of therapeutic options. Am J Health Syst Pharm 2004; 61:1661–1675
This is a clinical pharmacology-related review that includes both narrative and tabular summaries of drug treatment options for postoperative hypertension.

Haas AR, Marik PE. Current diagnosis and management of hypertensive emergency. Semin Dial 2006; 19:502–512
Covers both diagnostic approach as well as medical intervention.

Ince H, Nienaber CA. Diagnosis and management of patients with aortic dissection. Heart 2007; 93: 266–270
This is a concise but informative review of both pathophysiology and treatment of aortic dissection.

Khoynezhad A, Plestis KA. Managing emergency hypertension in aortic dissection and aortic aneurysm surgery. J Card Surg 2006; 21(suppl):S3–S7

McCoy S, Baldwin K. Pharmacotherapeutic options for the treatment of preeclampsia. Am J Health Syst Pharm 2009; 66:337–344
Up to date review of the changes that have occurred over the last 5 years about this important topic.
This review includes perioperative and operative management.

Perez MI, Musini VM. Pharmacological interventions for hypertensive emergencies: a Cochrane systematic review. J Hum Hypertens 2008; 22:596–607
The Cochrane methodology applied to interventions to control blood pressure in the presence of organ dysfunction.

Powers WJ, Zazulia AR, Videen TO, et al. Autoregulation of cerebral blood flow surrounding cute (6 to 22 hours) intracerebral hemorrhage. Neurology 2001; 57:18–24
This article discusses issues related to autoregulation of cerebral blood flow, its preservation or lack of preservation, and how that influences perihemorrhagic blood flow in small-sized to medium-sized acute intracranial hemorrhages.

Rosei EA, Salvetti M, Farsang C. Treatment of hypertensive urgencies and emergencies. Blood Press 2006; 15:255–256
General review of hypotensive urgencies and emergencies across all settings.

Rosei EA, Salvetti M, Farsang C. Treatment of hypertensive urgencies and emergencies. Blood Press 2006; 15:255–256
Another good general review.

Slama M, Modeliar SS. Hypertension in the intensive care unit. Curr Opin Cardiol 2006; 21:279–287
Review specifically targeting ICU presentations and treatment.

Varon J. Treatment of acute severe hypertension: current and newer agents. Drugs 2008; 68:283–297
Good general view of both established and more recent agents for treatment of severe hypertension.

Varon J, Marik PE. Clinical review: the management of hypertensive crises. Crit Care 2003; 7:374–384
This article reviews the initial therapeutic approach to hypertensive emergencies and the most commonly used medical therapies.

Vidaeff AC, Carroll MA, Ramin SM. Acute hypertensive emergencies in pregnancy. Crit Care Med 2005; 33(suppl):S307–S312
Covers predisposition and management.

Notes

Critical Illness in Pregnancy

Mary E. Strek, MD, FCCP

Objectives:

- Understand the normal physiologic changes of pregnancy
- Review the causes and management of respiratory disorders in pregnancy
- Understand the diagnosis and treatment of venous thromboembolism in pregnancy
- Review the causes, diagnosis, and treatment of cardiovascular disorders of pregnancy including preeclampsia

Key words: critical illness; preeclampsia; pregnancy; venous thromboembolism

The development of critical illness during pregnancy is a rare but potentially devastating occurrence because two lives are affected. Understanding the normal maternal physiologic adaptation to pregnancy is essential to the accurate diagnosis and treatment of critical illness in the gravid patient. Awareness of the determinants of oxygen delivery to the fetoplacental unit is important to maintain fetal viability. Critical illnesses in pregnancy may result from worsening of an underlying cardiac or pulmonary disease or the onset of a unique pregnancy-related illness. The need for intensive care in pregnancy ranges from 1 to 9 in 1,000 gestations with a mortality of 12 to 20%.[1] In the United States, the overall pregnancy-related mortality from 1991 to 1999 was 11.8 deaths per 100,000 live births.[2] During this period, the leading causes of death were embolism, hemorrhage, and pregnancy-induced hypertension.

This chapter will review the normal physiology of pregnancy as well as the diagnosis and treatment of disorders of the respiratory and circulatory systems that account for the vast majority of admissions to the ICU during pregnancy. Asthma, venous thromboembolism (VTE), and preeclampsia are especially important topics that will be covered in detail. Assessment, monitoring, and treatment of the gravid patient in the ICU must take into account both maternal and fetal well-being and require a multidisciplinary approach to care.

Physiology of Pregnancy

Adaptive changes occur in the maternal respiratory system, circulation, gastrointestinal system, and kidneys to meet the increased metabolic demands of the mother, fetus, and placenta.[1,3,4] Knowledge of the normal changes in these organ systems is essential to distinguish between expected adaptive and pathologic findings so that early recognition and treatment of critical illness during pregnancy is possible.

Adaptation of the Respiratory System

Oxygen consumption increases 20 to 35% in normal pregnancy; during labor, there is a further increase.[5] This occurs to meet fetal and placental needs as well as maternal increases in cardiac output and work of breathing. The increased oxygen consumption and associated increase in carbon dioxide production requires an increase in minute ventilation that begins in the first trimester and peaks at 20 to 40% above baseline at term. Alveolar ventilation is increased above the level needed to eliminate carbon dioxide, and Pco_2 falls to 27 to 32 mm Hg throughout pregnancy. The augmented alveolar ventilation is attributed to respiratory stimulation due to increased levels of progesterone and results from a 30 to 35% increase in tidal volume (from 450 to 600 mL) while respiratory rate is unchanged to mildly increased (Table 1). Renal compensation results in a maternal pH that is only slightly alkalemic, in the range of 7.40 to 7.45, with serum bicarbonate decreasing to 18 to 21 mEq/L (Table 2).

Maternal Pao_2 is increased throughout pregnancy by virtue of augmented minute ventilation, but this increase does not significantly increase oxygen delivery. Mild hypoxemia and an increased alveolar-to-arterial oxygen gradient may occur in the supine position as pregnancy progresses. This results from ventilation-perfusion mismatch from airway narrowing or closure in gravid

Table 1. *Respiratory Changes in Pregnancy*

Parameters*	Direction
Oxygen consumption	Increases
Respiratory rate	Unchanged
V_T	Increases
Total lung capacity	Unchanged
FRC	Decreases
FVC	Unchanged
FEV_1	Unchanged

*FRC = functional residual capacity.

individuals during normal tidal breathing (Table 2). When possible, arterial blood gas samples should be obtained in the seated position to avoid the mild positional hypoxemia of pregnancy.

Functional residual capacity decreases progressively 10 to 25% at term as a result of increased abdominal pressure from the enlarged uterus, which results in diaphragmatic elevation and decreased chest wall compliance (Table 1). Expiratory reserve volume and residual volume are decreased during the second half of pregnancy. Total lung capacity decreases minimally because the function of the diaphragm and thoracic muscles is unimpaired, and widening of the thoracic cage results in an increased inspiratory capacity. FVC remains unchanged during pregnancy. Diffusing capacity is unchanged or mildly increased early in pregnancy and then decreases to normal or just below normal after the first trimester. The decreased functional residual capacity, when combined with the increased oxygen consumption in pregnancy, makes the pregnant woman and fetus more vulnerable to hypoxia in the event of hypoventilation or apnea. This is an important consideration during endotracheal intubation.

Despite increases in levels of many hormones known to affect smooth muscle, the function of large airways does not appear to be altered in

pregnancy. FEV_1, the ratio of FEV_1 to FVC, and specific airways conductance are unchanged during pregnancy. The fact that flow-volume loops are also unaffected by pregnancy is further evidence of normal airway function. Lung compliance also is unchanged.

Adaptation of the Circulation

During pregnancy, numerous circulatory adjustments occur that ensure adequate oxygen delivery to the fetus.[3,5] Maternal blood volume increases early, reaching a level 40% above baseline by the 30th week. The increased number of erythrocytes and even greater increase in plasma volume result in a mild dilutional anemia, with a decrease in hematocrit of approximately 12%. The increase in blood volume is greater with multiple births. Parallel decreases in colloid osmotic pressure and serum albumin concentration from 4.0 to 3.4 g/dL occur. Mild peripheral edema is noted in 50 to 80% of normal pregnancies.

The increase in maternal blood volume contributes to a 30 to 50% increase in cardiac output, most of which occurs in the first trimester and continues throughout gestation (Table 3). The augmented cardiac output results from an increase in heart rate and stroke volume, with heart rate reaching a maximum of 15 to 20 beats/min above resting nonpregnant levels by weeks 32 to 36. The increase in stroke volume is due to an increase in preload caused by augmented blood volume and a decrease in afterload from a 20 to 30% fall in systemic vascular resistance (SVR). The fall in SVR is attributed both to arteriovenous shunting through the low-resistance uteroplacental bed and hormonally mediated vasodilation. Left ventricular end-diastolic pressure remains normal, but left ventricular wall thickness and mass increase. There is no increase in ejection fraction as calculated from echocardiography.

Table 2. *Typical Arterial Blood Gas Values**

Variables	Pao_2, mm Hg	$Paco_2$, mm Hg	pH	Alveolar-Arterial Pressure Gradient, mm Hg
Nonpregnant	98	40	7.40	2
Term pregnancy, seated	101	28	7.45	14
Term pregnancy, supine	95	28	7.45	20

*To convert millimeters of mercury to kilopascals, multiply the value by 0.1333.

Critical Illness in Pregnancy (Strek)

Table 3. *Circulatory Changes in Pregnancy*

Parameters	Direction	Percentage	Time Course
Heart rate	Increases	10–30	Peak at 32 wk
BP	Decreases	10–20	Nadir at 28 wk
Cardiac output	Increases	30–50	Peak at 25–32 wk
Stroke volume	Increases		First trimester
SVR	Decreases	20–30	
Pulmonary vascular resistance	Decreases	20–30	

During the course of pregnancy, cardiac output becomes more dependent on body position because the gravid uterus can cause significant obstruction of the inferior vena cava with reduced venous return. This effect is most notable in the third trimester. Vena caval obstruction is maximal in the supine position and much less pronounced in the left lateral decubitus position. During labor, uterine contraction can increase cardiac output 10 to 15% over resting pregnant levels by increasing blood return from the contracting uterus. This effect on cardiac output, however, may be tempered by blood loss during delivery.

Blood pressure decreases early in pregnancy from peripheral vasodilation. Peak decreases in systolic and diastolic pressures average 5 to 9 mm Hg and 6 to 17 mm Hg, respectively, and occur at 16 to 28 weeks. Blood pressure then increases gradually, returning to baseline shortly after delivery. Diastolic pressures of 75 mm Hg in the second trimester and 85 mm Hg in the third trimester should be considered the upper limits of normal.

Normal adaptation of the circulatory system to pregnancy results in a physiologic third heart sound in the majority of pregnant patients. The chest radiograph reveals an enlarged cardiac silhouette. Right ventricular, pulmonary artery, and pulmonary capillary wedge pressures (PCWPs) are unchanged from prepartum values in the healthy pregnant woman.

Renal and GI Adaptation

Renal blood flow increases greatly during pregnancy.[1] The glomerular filtration rate rises early in pregnancy to 50% above baseline at 12 to 16 weeks and remains increased throughout pregnancy. During pregnancy, serum creatinine is somewhat lower than baseline (0.5 to 0.7 mg/dL); therefore, creatinine levels that would be normal in a nonpregnant patient can indicate renal dysfunction in pregnancy.

Lower esophageal sphincter tone decreases during the first trimester of pregnancy and remains low until near term, perhaps as a result of increased plasma progesterone levels.[1] The gravid uterus displaces the stomach, further reducing the effectiveness of the gastroesophageal sphincter. Basal gastric acid secretion and pH remain unchanged during pregnancy. Labor and narcotic analgesics given during labor delay gastric-emptying time, significantly increasing the risk of aspiration.

Fetal Oxygen Delivery

Oxygen delivery to the fetal tissues depends on the oxygen content of uterine artery blood, as determined by maternal Po_2, hemoglobin concentration and saturation, and uterine artery blood flow.[3] The anemia of pregnancy reduces the oxygen content significantly; therefore, the critically ill gravid patient is more dependent than the nonpregnant individual on cardiac output to maintain oxygen delivery. Should maternal cardiac output fall, uterine artery blood flow and fetal oxygen delivery decrease.

Numerous factors affect uterine artery blood flow. The uterine vasculature is maximally dilated under normal conditions and therefore unable to adapt to stress by increasing flow through local vascular adjustment. Fetal oxygen delivery can be decreased by uterine artery vasoconstriction. Exogenous or endogenous sympathetic stimulation and maternal hypotension elicit uterine artery vasoconstriction. In addition, maternal alkalosis may cause uteroplacental vasoconstriction with decreased uteroplacental perfusion and fetal hypoxia.

Despite a low umbilical vein Po_2 of 30 to 40 mm Hg and fetal Pao_2 of 20 to 25 mm Hg at baseline, compensatory mechanisms maintain fetal oxygen delivery. At all levels of Po_2, fetal hemoglobin has a higher affinity for oxygen than maternal hemoglobin, being 80 to 90% saturated at a Po_2 of 30 to 35 mm Hg. In addition, the fetus has a high hemoglobin concentration (15 g/dL) and a high systemic cardiac output, with both left and right ventricles delivering blood to the systemic circulation. Protective responses to hypoxic stress include a shift to anaerobic metabolism; redirection of the fetal cardiac output to the brain, heart, and adrenal glands; and decreased oxygen consumption.

In summary, during pregnancy, oxygen delivery to maternal and fetoplacental tissue beds is highly dependent on adequate blood flow and maternal oxygen content. Maternal oxygen consumption increases progressively during gestation and rises further in labor. The fetoplacental unit is unable to increase oxygen delivery by local vascular adjustment. The fetus, however, is protected from hypoxic insult by the avidity of fetal hemoglobin for oxygen relative to maternal hemoglobin, the high fetal hemoglobin content and cardiac output, and the autoregulatory responses of the fetal circulation to hypoxic insult. An understanding of these physiologic concepts suggests some general principles for management of the critically ill gravid patient (Table 4). Obstetrical consultation and assessment of fetal well-being by monitoring fetal heart rate is essential.

US Food and Drug Administration Drug Classification

When prescribing medications for pregnant patients with critical illness, it is important to be aware of the US Food and Drug Administration safety ratings for medication use in pregnancy. Category A drugs are those in which adequate, well-controlled studies in pregnant women have not demonstrated a risk to the fetus. Category B drugs are those with no evidence of fetal risk in humans (if animal studies demonstrate risk, human findings do not, or if human studies are not adequate, animal findings are negative). Category C agents are those in which risk cannot

be ruled out but potential benefits may outweigh risk (human studies are lacking and animal studies are either positive for fetal risk or lacking). Category D includes agents with evidence of fetal risk by virtue of investigation or postmarketing human data (in critical illness, potential benefits may outweigh risks). Category X includes drugs contraindicated in pregnancy.

Respiratory Disorders of Pregnancy

This section focuses on the diagnosis and management of respiratory disorders in the gravid patient.[5,6] Asthma is the most common disease to complicate pregnancy, affecting 4 to 8% of all gravidas. Venous thromboembolic disease is the major cause of maternal mortality in the United States. ARDS is infrequent but has a high mortality. Tocolytic-induced pulmonary edema has a much better outcome. The institution of mechanical ventilation in the pregnant patient requires careful attention to the special needs of both mother and fetus.

Asthma

Acute asthma requiring a visit to the emergency department or hospitalization may occur in about 10% of pregnant women cared for by an asthma specialist.[7] In an individual patient, the course of asthma during pregnancy is variable. In approximately one-third of pregnant asthmatic women, asthma does not change; in one-third it improves; and in one-third it worsens. Patients with more severe asthma are more likely to experience worsening asthma during pregnancy. Asthma typically worsens during the second and third trimesters, with improvement during the last month of pregnancy. Adverse maternal outcomes in pregnant woman with asthma have been noted, including preterm labor, preeclampsia, and

Table 4. *General Principles of Management in Critical Illness in Pregnancy*

Echocardiogram to assess maternal cardiac function due to high flow state of pregnancy
Oxygen delivery to fetus is maximized by adequate maternal circulation, left lateral decubitus position, and supplemental oxygen
Early elective intubation and mechanical ventilation for respiratory failure
Continuous monitoring of fetal heart rate to assess fetal well-being
Delivery of the fetus may be in the best interest of mother and fetus if the fetus is beyond the age of viability

cesarean delivery. Adverse fetal outcomes include preterm birth and infants small for gestational age. Studies show that active treatment of the gravid patient to control asthma improves both maternal and fetal outcomes.

The management of the pregnant patient with status asthmaticus is similar to that of the nonpregnant patient, with a few exceptions.[7,8] Mild hypoxemia should be treated aggressively because it may be detrimental to the fetus. An arterial blood gas with a $Paco_2$ of >35 mm Hg during status asthmaticus may be a sign of impending ventilatory failure, given the baseline respiratory alkalosis in normal pregnancy. Indications for mechanical ventilation include (1) hypercapnia, (2) altered consciousness, (3) maternal exhaustion, and (4) fetal distress. Cesarean section in refractory cases has been successful and should be considered when fetal viability is likely. The specifics of mechanical ventilation will be discussed later.

Most asthma medications are safe for use during pregnancy. Inhaled albuterol should be administered every 20 min or continuously and may be mixed with ipratropium bromide. Use of parenteral β-agonists is limited to the rare situations in which inhaled agents have been ineffective. Because epinephrine causes vasoconstriction of the uteroplacental circulation in animal studies, parenteral terbutaline is preferred but may inhibit labor and cause pulmonary edema if administered near term. Systemic corticosteroids are given for acute asthma exacerbations. An IV infusion of magnesium sulfate can be considered for its potential bronchodilator effect in refractory cases as long as the patient is monitored carefully for respiratory depression. Heliox, a low-density mixture of helium and oxygen, may decrease the work of breathing and preclude intubation and mechanical ventilation when administered to patients in status asthmaticus. Guidelines for managing asthma in pregnancy have been updated and are readily available online.[8]

VTE

Pulmonary embolism (PE) is the leading cause of pregnancy-related death in the United States.[2] The risk of VTE is increased fourfold during pregnancy. Hypercoagulability, venous stasis, and endothelial damage to pelvic vessels during delivery or cesarean section all occur in normal pregnancy; thus, all pregnant women are at increased risk of VTE. Known risk factors include age >35 years, cesarean section, obesity, heart disease, lupus, diabetes, sickle cell disease, black race, smoking, and multiple pregnancies.[9] Thrombophilia increases the risk even further and is noted in approximately 50% of woman with VTE during pregnancy. Deep venous thrombosis (DVT) and subsequent PE occurs in all three trimesters and the postpartum period. More cases of DVT in pregnancy are ileofemoral and more likely to embolize than in the nonpregnant individual. There is a 70 to 90% incidence of left leg DVT, thought to be due to stasis in the left iliac vein caused by increased compression where it is crossed by the right iliac artery as the gravid uterus enlarges.

Diagnosis and treatment of both DVT and PE are more complicated in pregnancy (Table 5). The diagnosis of VTE requires a high index of suspicion because dyspnea, tachycardia, and mild lower-extremity edema are often noted in normal pregnancy. Pregnant women occasionally

Table 5. *Challenging Problems in Management of Pregnant Patients vs Nonpregnant Patients With VTE*

Nonpregnant	Pregnant
1. Hypercoagulable states less common	1. Underlie 50% of cases of VTE in pregnancy
2. Negative d-dimer result helpful	2. Helpful if compression ultrasonography findings are normal
3. Compression ultrasonography of legs helpful	3. Less accurate for isolated calf and iliac vein thrombosis
4. CT angiography safe	4. CT angiography safe for fetus, increases future risk maternal breast cancer
5. Thrombolytic therapy an option	5. Riskier and contraindicated at term
6. Inferior vena cava filter below renal veins	6. Inferior vena cava filter placed suprarenally
7. Partial thromboplastin time monitoring	7. Antifactor Xa (heparin level) may be preferable
8. Warfarin long term	8. Crosses placenta and contraindicated

present with lower abdominal pain, fever, and an elevated WBC count mimicking acute appendicitis. It is important to remember that patients may be without symptoms and have a normal physical examination, so a high clinical suspicion must be maintained.

If DVT or PE is suspected, treatment with low-molecular-weight heparin (LMWH) should be begun while diagnostic testing is pursued.[9] Compression ultrasonography is the diagnostic test of choice, although it is less accurate for isolated calf and iliac vein thrombosis. A positive study is considered sufficient to justify treatment, and anticoagulation is begun. In patients suspected of having DVT who have negative compression ultrasonography results, a negative d-dimer test result with a highly specific assay in the first and second trimester makes DVT unlikely. Because the d-dimer increases as pregnancy progresses, a positive d-dimer test requires further imaging with magnetic resonance direct thrombus imaging, which has a high sensitivity for iliac vein thrombosis and is not harmful to the fetus, or repeat compression ultrasonography in 5 to 7 days.

In a pregnant woman with suspected PE, with negative-compression ultrasonography of the legs, a normal perfusion lung scan rules out PE and avoids the extra radiation exposure from the ventilation scan. If the lung scan finding is abnormal, a ventilation scan is performed and anticoagulation is begun for a high-probability study. In patients with asthma or an abnormal chest radiograph, CT pulmonary angiography is performed rather than a ventilation-perfusion lung scan, with the advantage of providing additional imaging of the chest. Radiation exposure to the fetus from either test is low and within the amount considered safe in pregnancy. Ventilation-perfusion lung scanning, compared with CT angiography, slightly increases the risk of childhood cancer in the offspring but has a lower risk of maternal breast cancer. Echocardiography may be useful to document right-sided clot or right-heart strain. It is important to make a definitive diagnosis, and the clinical presentation alone cannot be relied on to diagnose or exclude VTE.

Once a diagnosis of either DVT or PE is made, anticoagulation with heparin is begun. This is the treatment of choice because heparin does not cross the placenta. Adjusted-dose subcutaneous

LMWH or IV adjusted-dose unfractionated heparin is recommended for treatment of acute VTE.[10] Subcutaneous heparin should be continued throughout the duration of pregnancy, with anticoagulation continued for at least 6 weeks postpartum. Current guidelines favor LMWH because of the decreased risk of bleeding and heparin-related thrombocytopenia and osteoporosis with these agents.[10] The half-life of LMWH is shorter in pregnancy so twice-daily dosing may be preferable, especially during the initial treatment phase. As the pregnancy progresses, the potential volume of distribution for LMWH changes, so the dose may be adjusted based on increased weight or periodic antifactor Xa LMWH levels performed 4 to 6 h after injection with dose adjustments to achieve an antifactor Xa level of 0.6 to 1.0 U/mL. The current guidelines suggest that the decision to make dose adjustments and monitor heparin levels should be based on the clinician's judgment and experience. For patients with heparin-induced thrombocytopenia, danaparoid (a low-molecular-weight heparinoid) or fondaparinux (a synthetic pentasaccharide and direct inhibitor of factor Xa) may be given.[9,10] Warfarin crosses the placenta and is absolutely contraindicated (category X) because of the high incidence of embryopathy in the first trimester, small incidence of fetal central nervous system abnormalities throughout pregnancy, and possible fetal hemorrhage.

Life-threatening VTE should prompt consideration of thrombolytic therapy. Thrombolysis can be performed safely in pregnancy, although there is the potential risk of maternal or fetal hemorrhage and fetal loss. Recombinant tissue plasminogen activator does not cross the placenta and is the preferred thrombolytic agent.

Amniotic Fluid Embolism

Amniotic fluid embolism is a rare occurrence but is estimated to account for 10% of maternal deaths.[11,12] Previously the mortality rate has been reported to be 80 to 90%, but more recent series suggest it is much lower (25%). Most survivors develop permanent neurologic deficits from cerebral hypoxia.

Risk factors may include advanced maternal age, multiparity, turbulent labor, and trauma. Although most cases occur during labor and delivery or immediately postpartum, amniotic fluid embolism occurs up to 48 h after delivery and during first- and second-trimester abortions.

The classic presentation is the abrupt onset of severe dyspnea, tachypnea, and hypoxemia in association with cardiovascular collapse and altered mental status. Disseminated intravascular coagulation (DIC) is common. Entry of amniotic fluid and fetal products into the maternal circulation may result in an inflammatory cascade or "anaphylactoid syndrome of pregnancy." Vasoconstriction of the pulmonary vasculature is thought to cause hypoxia and right-heart failure followed by left-heart failure with shock and pulmonary edema. The third phase involves neurologic impairment with seizures and coma. Cytologic examination of pulmonary artery catheter blood may show fetal squamous cells and lanugo hairs but is not sufficient to make the diagnosis because small numbers of fetal squamous cells have been observed in patients without clinical evidence of amniotic fluid embolism.

Treatment is supportive and aimed at ensuring adequate oxygenation, stabilizing the circulation, and controlling bleeding. After administration of 100% oxygen, intubation, mechanical ventilation, and positive end-expiratory pressure (PEEP) often are required. Fluid resuscitation and vasopressors may reverse hypotension. Once DIC is established, factor replacement and fresh-frozen plasma are given based on laboratory findings and bleeding. IV corticosteroid therapy, plasma exchange transfusion, continuous hemofiltration, and inhaled nitric oxide are some of the treatments described to be of benefit in small case reports.

Venous Air Embolism

Venous air embolism may occur during normal labor or delivery, abortions, orogenital sex, central venous access, and surgical procedures, especially cesarean delivery.[13] Symptoms include chest pain, dyspnea, dizziness, tachypnea, tachycardia, and diaphoresis. Sudden hypotension is usually followed by respiratory arrest. A "mill-wheel murmur" or bubbling sound is occasionally heard over the precordium. Right-heart strain, ischemia, and arrhythmias have been noted on the ECG. ARDS may develop in patients who survive the initial cardiopulmonary collapse.

When venous air embolism is suspected, the patient should be placed immediately in the left lateral decubitus position and Trendelenburg to direct the air embolus away from the right ventricular outflow tract. The patient should be given 100% oxygen in an effort to decrease the size of the embolus by removing nitrogen. Hyperbaric therapy may benefit patients with paradoxic cerebral embolism.

Tocolytic Therapy

Pulmonary edema associated with β-adrenergic agents that are administered to inhibit preterm labor is seen in up to 9% of women receiving these drugs.[3,13] Most of the reported cases have resulted from use of IV β-mimetics such as ritodrine, terbutaline, isoxuprine, and salbutamol. There is an increased incidence in women with multiple gestations, concurrent infection, and those receiving corticosteroid therapy. Most women have intact membranes at the time of presentation. Pulmonary edema typically develops during tocolytic therapy or within 24 h after the discontinuation of these drugs. When pulmonary edema develops postpartum, the vast majority of cases are encountered within 12 h of delivery.

Most patients complain of chest discomfort and dyspnea, they manifest tachypnea and tachycardia with crackles on lung auscultation, and have pulmonary edema on chest radiography. A positive fluid balance is often noted in the hours to days preceding the onset of symptoms. The history and clinical findings should help in distinguishing this disorder from acute thromboembolic disease, acid aspiration, and amniotic fluid embolism.

The course of this disease is usually benign, and invasive hemodynamic monitoring is usually not required. Treatment consists of discontinuation of tocolytic therapy, oxygen administration, and diuresis. Response is usually rapid, with resolution of tachypnea and hypoxemia often occurring within hours.

Aspiration

Aspiration is an uncommon but well-described and ominous complication of the peripartum period.[13] Factors that increase the risk of aspiration in the pregnant woman include the increased intragastric pressure that results from external compression by the enlarged uterus, relaxation of the lower esophageal sphincter resulting from use of progesterone, delayed gastric emptying during labor, and depressed mental status and vocal cord closure from analgesia. Injury due to aspiration of gastric contents is related to the volume of aspirated material, its acidity, the presence of particulate material, the bacterial burden of the aspirated material, and host resistance to subsequent infection. The early injury is a chemical pneumonitis followed by the development of ARDS. A late complication of aspiration is the evolution to bacterial pneumonia.

Prevention of this dread complication should be the primary goal of all physicians assessing and managing the patient's airway. Once aspiration has occurred, treatment is supportive and is similar to that for the nonpregnant individual. Antibiotics should be given only if bacterial pneumonia develops.

Pneumonia

Pneumonia during pregnancy most often occurs from community-acquired bacterial organisms, with asthma and anemia increasing the risk.[14,15] An increased incidence of influenza pneumonia was noted among pregnant patients during the 1918 and 1957 influenza pandemics, with death from fulminant influenza pneumonia, rather than secondary bacterial infection, as is usually the case in the nonpregnant population. Pregnant women may have more frequent influenza-related morbidity. Primary infection with varicella-zoster virus progresses to pneumonia more often in adults than in children. Coccidioidomycosis is the fungal infection associated with increased risk of dissemination during pregnancy, especially if it is contracted in the third trimester. With appropriate chemotherapy, the prognosis for pregnant women with tuberculosis is excellent. Obstetric complications of pneumonia include preterm labor, preterm delivery, and fetal mortality. Respiratory failure requiring mechanical ventilation and maternal mortality also occur.

In the pregnant woman, HIV infection is complicated by the risk of perinatal transmission to the fetus, preterm delivery, and opportunistic infection, especially pneumonia. Testing for HIV infection and antiretroviral therapy to prevent vertical transmission are standard of care in the pregnant patient. Pneumocystis pneumonia (PCP) may complicate pregnancy and be especially virulent. It is the most common cause of AIDS-related death in pregnant women in the United States, with respiratory failure requiring mechanical ventilation occurring in 59% of patients and a mortality rate of 50%. Fetal mortality is also high and may be worse if PCP occurs during the first or second trimester. The clinical presentation is not altered by pregnancy.

The choice of antibacterial agents should take into account potential fetal toxicity. Penicillins, cephalosporins, and azithromycin are safe. Tetracycline and chloramphenicol are contraindicated, and sulfa-containing regimens should be avoided near term except for the treatment of PCP. Drugs used to treat influenza (oseltamivir, zanamivir, amantadine, and rimantadine) are category C. Recommendations have been made to use them in patients who contract influenza in the third trimester and in patients with cardiopulmonary disease. Favorable results have been obtained using acyclovir to treat pregnant women with varicella pneumonia, especially when used early. No teratogenic effects have been noted in animal studies of acyclovir. Amphotericin B should be used to treat disseminated coccidioidal infections in pregnancy. Some azole antifungal agents are category D and are known teratogens in animals. They should not be used in pregnancy. No adverse effects on the fetus have been reported for amphotericin. Active tuberculosis during pregnancy is treated with isoniazid, rifampin, and ethambutol plus pyridoxine until drug susceptibility testing is complete. These medications cross the placenta, but are not teratogenic. Streptomycin is the only antituberculosis drug with documented harmful effects on the human fetus, and should not be used in pregnancy. PCP is treated with trimethoprim-sulfamethoxazole, which results in an improved outcome compared with other therapies. Its use near term can increase the risk of fetal kernicterus. Corticosteroids are added if clinically indicated, as for the nonpregnant patient.

ARDS

Many of the respiratory disorders previously discussed can cause acute lung injury and ARDS during pregnancy (Table 6). In addition, pregnancy-specific causes such as placental abruption, chorioamnionitis, endometritis, septic abortion, and eclampsia as well as the more typical causes of ARDS such as sepsis, transfusion, and trauma may occur.[13] Acute lung injury is more likely to result in pulmonary edema given the increased plasma volume and decreased plasma oncotic pressure noted in pregnancy. Fetal distress and premature labor are common. The management of ARDS is directed at treatment of the underlying cause, supportive care, and close monitoring of the fetus. Intubation and mechanical ventilation are usually necessary.

Mechanical Ventilation

The indications for intubation and mechanical ventilation are not significantly changed by pregnancy, although it is important that intubation occur in an early and elective fashion.[13,16] Several difficulties in airway management should be anticipated (Table 7). Pharyngeal, laryngeal, and vocal cord edema are common, and the highly vascular upper airway may bleed from even minor intubation-related trauma. Relatively small endotracheal tubes (6 to 7 mm in diameter)

Table 6. *Causes of ARDS in Pregnancy*

Sepsis (chorioamnionitis, endometritis, septic abortion)
Pneumonia
Aspiration
Trauma
Preeclampsia
Obstetric hemorrhage
Amniotic fluid embolism
Venous air embolism
Obstetric hemorrhage and transfusions

Table 7. *Problems With Airway Management*

Upper airway edema
Diminished airway caliber
Propensity for bleeding
Increased risk of aspiration

may be necessary, and nasotracheal intubation is best avoided. There is an increased risk of aspiration during pregnancy because of delayed gastric emptying, increased intra-abdominal pressure from compression by the gravid uterus, and diminished competence of the gastroesophageal sphincter. Use of cricoid pressure to minimize the risk of pulmonary aspiration is recommended. Control of the airway should be achieved by a skilled individual. Noninvasive mask ventilation for acute respiratory failure has not been studied in pregnancy. In the awake patient needing temporary ventilatory assistance, noninvasive positive pressure ventilation is a reasonable first step but the patient must be monitored closely. Theoretical limitations include pregnancy-related upper airway edema and increased risk of aspiration.

Initial ventilator settings should aim for eucapnia (Pco_2 of 27 to 34 mm Hg). Respiratory alkalosis should be avoided because animal models suggest that hyperventilation can reduce fetal oxygenation by decreasing uteroplacental blood flow. In the asthmatic patient, the use of a lower tidal volume (V_T) and respiratory rate minimizes the adverse effects of intrinsic PEEP.

The patient with ARDS should be ventilated with a small V_T (4 to 6 mL/kg) and a high respiratory rate (24 to 30 breaths/min) to avoid ventilator-induced lung injury. The safety of permissive hypercapnia in pregnancy has not been studied but in the few case reports of lung-protective ventilation in pregnancy, no adverse effects were noted when Pco_2 was maintained at ≤ 50 mm Hg. Ventilatory changes associated with fetal distress by fetal heart rate monitoring should be avoided. During the third trimester of pregnancy, chest wall stiffness from the gravid uterus may cause high airway pressures unrelated to lung stiffness or overdistention. In summary, continuous fetal heart rate monitoring, a low V_T ventilation strategy, avoiding rapid rises in $Paco_2$, and allowing plateau airway pressures to be slightly higher than normal are recommended in these patients.

When ARDS is present requiring high levels of oxygen, sufficient PEEP should be used to correct arterial hypoxemia at a nontoxic fraction of inspired oxygen (< 0.6). In the pregnant patient, the aim is to keep the $Pao_2 > 70$ mm Hg or oxygen saturation $> 95\%$, values higher than that used in the nonpregnant patient, to prevent fetal distress. To minimize the decrease in venous return that occurs with positive pressure ventilation, it is important that the pregnant patient be managed in a lateral position whenever possible.

In patients with ARDS requiring high levels of PEEP, and in patients with hemodynamic instability, muscle relaxation and sedation may decrease oxygen consumption. Nondepolarizing neuromuscular blocking agents, including cisatracurium, pancuronium, vecuronium, and atracurium, produce no adverse fetal effects with short-term use. Of these, cisatracurium is preferred because it does not depend on renal or hepatic function for elimination. Benzodiazepines may increase the risk of cleft palate when used early in pregnancy. Narcotic analgesics such as morphine sulfate and fentanyl may be used safely during pregnancy. These agents all cross the placenta; therefore, if administered near the time of delivery, immediate intubation of the neonate may be required.

Circulatory Disorders of Pregnancy

In pregnancy, circulatory impairment may be life-threatening because mother and fetus depend on cardiac output for oxygen delivery. Common causes of hypoperfusion include hemorrhage, cardiac dysfunction, trauma, and sepsis. Preeclampsia is a vascular disorder unique to pregnancy that is associated with maternal hypertension.

The initial approach to the critically ill hypoperfused gravida is to distinguish between low-flow states, caused by inadequate circulating volume, cardiac dysfunction, or trauma, and high-flow states such as septic shock, while keeping in mind the physiologic alterations of pregnancy. Most often the state of perfusion can be determined by bedside assessment. Left and right ventricular hemodynamics assessed by echocardiography correlated with pulmonary artery catheter pressures in a heterogenous group of critically ill obstetric patients, suggest echocardiography may be an alternative to invasive monitoring. Right-heart catheterization has not been shown to improve mortality in nonobstetric critical illness. When this procedure is necessary, a subclavian or internal jugular approach is recommended. Femoral vein catheterization is relatively contraindicated because of obstruction of the vena cava

by the uterus and the possible need for emergent delivery. In the healthy pregnant woman, right ventricular, pulmonary artery, and PCWPs are unchanged from prepartum values. Cardiac output is increased, and SVR and pulmonary vascular resistance are decreased during pregnancy.

Should cardiac arrest occur, certain modifications to resuscitation algorithms are required.[17,18] The best hope of fetal survival is maternal survival. To prevent the gravid uterus from limiting the effectiveness of chest compressions, the patient should be placed 15 to 30° from the left lateral position by use of a wedge under the right hip or by pulling the gravid uterus manually to the side. Chest compressions should be performed higher on the sternum to adjust for the elevation of the diaphragm and abdominal contents caused by the gravid uterus. Fetal or uterine monitors should be removed prior to delivering shocks. The femoral vein should not be used for venous access because drugs administered through these sites may not reach the maternal heart. An emergency hysterotomy may save the life of both the mother and the fetus if gestational age is >24 weeks. Should resuscitation be unsuccessful, the best survival rate for infants occurs when delivery is no more than 5 min after the mother's heart stops beating.

Hemorrhagic Shock

The common causes of hemorrhagic shock in pregnancy are listed in Table 8. Hemorrhage in pregnancy can be massive and swift, necessitating immediate intervention. It is the second most common cause of maternal death and a common reason for admission to the ICU. Antepartum hemorrhage is most often caused by premature separation of the normal placental attachment site (placental abruption), disruption of an abnormal placental attachment (placenta previa), and spontaneous uterine rupture.[3,5]

Placental abruption occurs in patients with hypertension, high parity, cigarette or cocaine use, and previous abruption. The severity of maternal blood loss is correlated with the extent and duration of abruption and fetal demise. Blood loss averages 2 to 3 L when abruption results in fetal death, and much of this may remain concealed within the uterus. Maternal complications include

Table 8. *Etiology of Hemorrhagic Shock in Pregnancy*

Early	Late (Third Trimester)	Postpartum
Trauma	Trauma	Uterine atony
Ectopic or abdominal pregnancy	Placenta previa or abruption	Surgical trauma
Abortion	Uterine rupture	Uterine inversion
DIC	DIC	DIC
Hydatidiform mole	Marginal sinus rupture	Retained placenta

acute renal failure and DIC. Patients may initially present with painful vaginal bleeding and be misdiagnosed as having premature labor. The diagnosis is made using clinical information and ultrasound.

Placenta previa infrequently causes massive hemorrhage because ultrasound examination during pregnancy leads to identification prior to delivery. Nonetheless, if vaginal examination results in disruption of the placenta over the cervical os, or if trophoblastic tissue invades the myometrium (placenta previa et accreta), the patient is at risk for massive hemorrhage at delivery. Fetal mortality is low.

Uterine rupture typically occurs spontaneously in the multipara with protracted labor. Other risk factors include prior cesarean section, operative (assisted) vaginal delivery, and use of uterotonic agents. In overt rupture, peritoneal signs may be observed. Substantial blood loss can occur in the absence of significant physical findings.

Common causes of postpartum hemorrhage include uterine atony, surgical obstetric trauma, uterine inversion, retained placental tissue, and coagulopathies due to DIC. Uterine atony occurs after prolonged labor, overdistention of the uterus from multiple gestation or hydramnios, abruptio placentae, oxytocin administration, or cesarean section, or as a result of retained intrauterine contents or chorioamnionitis. Hemorrhage from surgical obstetric trauma may be due to cervical or vaginal lacerations or uterine incision for cesarean section.

Trauma is a leading cause of nonobstetric maternal mortality. Hypoperfusion and shock may occur as a result of injury from motor vehicle accidents, falls, and assaults. The gravid woman is at greater risk of hemorrhage after trauma, as blood flow to the entire pelvis is increased. Some injuries are unique to pregnancy, including amniotic membrane rupture, placental abruption, uterine rupture, premature labor, and fetal trauma. Rapid deceleration injury can cause placental abruption as a result of deformation of the elastic uterus around the less elastic placenta. In most cases, vaginal bleeding will be present when abruption has occurred. The cephalad displacement of abdominal contents in pregnancy increases the risk of visceral injury from penetrating trauma of the upper abdomen, including splenic rupture. The urinary bladder is a target for injury because it is displaced into the abdominal cavity beyond 12 weeks of gestation.

Patients at increased risk of bleeding should be identified early so that IV access and blood typing can be done.[19] The physiologic changes of pregnancy make evaluation and treatment of the gravid patient more difficult. Borderline tachycardia and supine hypotension may be caused by pregnancy itself, and thus vital signs may not indicate significant blood loss. When hypovolemia is clinically evident in gravid patients, it signifies enormous blood loss because of the expanded blood volume associated with pregnancy. The initial management of the patient is similar to that of the nonpregnant patient, and two or three large-bore ($\geq$ 16-gauge) venous catheters should be inserted. Immediate volume replacement with crystalloid is instituted until blood is available, along with supplemental oxygen. The patient should be placed in the left lateral decubitus position. Fetal monitoring is important because fetal distress in the setting of obstetric hemorrhage indicates hemodynamic compromise.

If shock is not immediately reversed by volume resuscitation or is accompanied by respiratory dysfunction, elective intubation and mechanical ventilation are indicated. Blood replacement with packed red blood cells should begin immediately. Massive obstetric hemorrhage is a setting in which initial resuscitation may require the use of unmatched type-specific blood until more complete cross-matching can be accomplished. Because critical illness in pregnancy is frequently associated with DIC, massive bleeding should prompt an evaluation for a coagulopathy.

Measurement of factor VIII levels is inexpensive and can be accomplished more quickly than a full DIC screen. Massive blood loss can result in a dilutional coagulopathy with secondary thrombocytopenia, which needs to be corrected.

Uterine atony is treated with uterine massage, draining the bladder, and IV oxytocin. Oxytocin can cause hyponatremia by virtue of its antidiuretic effect. Alternatively, prostaglandin analogs such as carboprost tromethamine can be used to improve uterine contraction and decrease bleeding. Side effects include hypertension, bronchoconstriction, and intrapulmonary shunt with arterial oxygen desaturation. Ergot preparations such as methylergonovine have been associated with cerebral hemorrhage and are contraindicated if the patient is hypertensive. Recombinant factor VIIa has been used successfully in the management of severe obstetric hemorrhage and is thought to be most effective when used early.[20] Thrombotic complications are a rarely reported side effect of this medication. Ultrasonography is used to diagnose retained intrauterine products of conception that require curettage. Balloon tamponade, compression sutures, and uterine artery embolization may control hemorrhage in many cases. Surgical exploration to repair lacerations, ligate the uterine artery, or remove the uterus may be necessary when these measures fail.

Cardiogenic Shock

Shock from cardiac dysfunction is most often caused by congestive heart failure due to preexisting myocardial or valvular heart disease or to a cardiomyopathy arising *de novo*. Heart disease during pregnancy is uncommon but increases the likelihood of maternal and fetal morbidity and mortality. Prior subclinical heart disease may manifest itself for the first time during pregnancy owing to the physiologic changes of pregnancy previously described.

Patients with Eisenmenger syndrome, cyanotic congenital heart disease, or pulmonary hypertension have a mortality rate of up to 40% during pregnancy. Predictors of maternal cardiac complications include prior cardiac events, New York Heart Association class III or IV or cyanosis, aortic or mitral stenosis, and left ventricular systolic dysfunction. Neonatal complications are associated with poor functional class or cyanosis, left-heart obstruction, anticoagulation, smoking, and multiple gestations. In 1 of every 1,300 to 4,000 deliveries, peripartum cardiomyopathy presents in the last month of pregnancy or the first 6 months after parturition.[21] Risk factors include race, older age, twin gestations, multiparity, anemia, preeclampsia, and postpartum hypertension. Bacterial endocarditis has been reported, particularly in patients with a history of IV drug use. Myocardial infarction is uncommon but should be considered in the hypoperfused patient with chest pain. There is an increased incidence of aortic dissection during pregnancy, perhaps related to the increased shear stress on the aorta associated with pregnancy. Aortic dissection presents most commonly during the third trimester, often as a tearing interscapular pain. Pulse asymmetry or aortic insufficiency may be noted on examination.

It is essential to identify the exact cause of the underlying cardiac dysfunction and hypoperfusion. The chest radiograph may suggest the diagnosis; mediastinal widening is often noted in patients with aortic dissection. Echocardiography can help determine the volume status and detect valvular abnormalities, myocardial dysfunction, or ischemia. Transesophageal echocardiography and MRI are the most sensitive and specific tests for detecting aortic dissection, although CT scan of the chest is often done first given its ready availability. Once the cause of cardiac dysfunction is determined, the initial management should focus on volume status, and hypovolemia should be excluded. Vasoactive drugs are reserved for situations in which hypovolemia has been corrected and maternal perfusion remains inadequate. If cardiogenic shock persists despite an adequate preload, dobutamine is the drug of choice. When cardiogenic shock is complicated by pulmonary edema, parenteral furosemide should be given.

When cardiogenic shock persists despite inotropic drug support, afterload reduction with nicardipine should be considered. IV sodium nitroprusside or nitroglycerin is a second-line agent, and the dose and duration of therapy should be minimized. Oral agents, such as hydralazine or labetalol, should be substituted as soon as possible to avoid nitroprusside toxicity. Angiotensin-converting enzyme inhibitors are absolutely contraindicated during pregnancy because they cause fetal growth retardation, oligohydramnios, congenital malformations, and anuric renal failure in human neonates exposed *in utero*, as well as neonatal death.

Labor and delivery is an especially dangerous time for women with cardiac disease. The optimal method of delivery is an assisted vaginal delivery in the left lateral decubitus position. Epidural anesthesia will ameliorate tachycardia in response to pain, and its vasodilatory actions may be of benefit in patients with congestive heart failure. Because decreased SVR may lead to further decompensation in patients with aortic stenosis, hypertrophic cardiomyopathy, or pulmonary hypertension, general anesthesia may be preferred in these patients. Cesarean section should be reserved for patients with obstetric complications or fetal distress, although with improved surgical techniques and close hemodynamic monitoring, cesarean sections are safer than in the past. Invasive monitoring or echocardiography may be required to follow shifts in volume status that occur from the tremendous "autotransfusions" produced by each uterine contraction during labor and the blood loss that occurs with delivery.

Septic Shock

The diagnosis of sepsis in the febrile gravid patient can be obscured by the normal hemodynamic changes of pregnancy (*ie*, increased cardiac output, decreased SVR). An awareness of the usual settings and patients at risk will increase the chance of recognizing this life-threatening state.[22,23] Animal data suggest that pregnancy may cause increased vulnerability to the systemic effects of bacteremia and endotoxemia. In addition, pregnant patients have an increased susceptibility to infection with *Listeria monocytogenes* and disseminated herpesvirus and coccidioidomycosis infections, perhaps owing to a decreased cell-mediated immune response during pregnancy.

The common causes of sepsis in pregnancy include septic abortions, antepartum pyelonephritis, chorioamnionitis, and postpartum infections (Table 9). Chorioamnionitis or intra-amniotic infection occurs most commonly after prolonged rupture of membranes or prolonged labor or after invasive procedures such as amniocentesis

Table 9. *Bacterial Infections Associated With Sepsis in Pregnancy and Postpartum**

Obstetric
   Postpartum endometritis
   Chorioamnionitis (intra-amniotic infection)
   Septic abortion
   Septic pelvic thrombophlebitis
   Antepartum pyelonephritis
Nonobstetric
   Appendicitis
   Cholecystitis
   Pyelonephritis
   Pneumonia
Invasive procedures
   Abdominal wall or perineal incisions (necrotizing fasciitis)
   Amniocentesis/chorionic villus sampling (septic abortion)
   Infected cerclage (chorioamnionitis)

*Reprinted with permission from Fein AM, Duvivier R. Sepsis in pregnancy. Clin Chest Med 1992; 13:709

or cervical cerclage, but occasionally reflects hematogenous spread from maternal bacteremia. Patients present with fever, maternal and fetal tachycardia, uterine tenderness, and foul-smelling amniotic fluid.

Sepsis in obstetric patients occurs postpartum following cesarean section, prolonged rupture of membranes, or prior instrumentation of the genitourinary tract. Infection at the placental site results in endometritis. Patients with endometritis may present with fever, abdominal pain and tenderness, and purulent lochia. Episiotomy sites and cesarean section incisions are less common sources of postpartum infection. Life-threatening wound infection with group A streptococci results in necrotizing fasciitis, and Clostridium spp may cause gas gangrene of the uterus. A wide range of Gram-positive, Gram-negative, and anaerobic organisms must be considered. Rarely, toxic streptococcal syndrome may occur as a result of infection with pyrogenic exotoxin A-producing group A streptococci in patients with necrotizing fasciitis or may unexpectedly follow an uncomplicated pregnancy and delivery. Toxic shock syndrome may also result from infection with *Clostridium sordellii*, with recent reports of this occurring after medical abortion with oral agents.

The hemodynamic profile in septic shock is similar to that of the nonpregnant septic patient. Although evidence of myocardial depression is often present, the predominant abnormality is high-output hypotension with a decreased SVR. Complications of sepsis in pregnancy include ARDS and DIC.

The septic gravid patient requires thorough culturing and evaluation of pelvic sites. Empiric antibiotic therapy to cover polymicrobial infection involving Gram-positive, Gram-negative, and anaerobic organisms is administered until specific cultures are available. Reasonable regimens include clindamycin and a third-generation cephalosporin; in certain patients, it is necessary to expand the initial regimen to a semisynthetic penicillin, an aminoglycoside, or another broad-spectrum agent. It is best to avoid aminoglycosides in patients with sepsis antepartum because these agents can be ototoxic and nephrotoxic to the fetus. Chorioamnionitis associated with sepsis requires delivery of the fetus. Postpartum deterioration in septic patients receiving antibiotics suggests a localized abscess, a resistant organism, or septic pelvic thrombophlebitis. Surgical drainage of appropriate pelvic and abdominal sources, with possible hysterectomy, may be required, particularly in patients with myometrial microabscesses or gas gangrene from clostridial species.

Early goal-directed therapy improves survival in the non-pregnant population. Goals include fluid to achieve a central venous pressure >8 to 12 mm Hg, the use of vasoactive agents to achieve a mean arterial pressure >65 to 90 mm Hg, and packed RBCs and inotropes to increase central venous oxygen saturation of >70%.[24] Recommended vasoactive drugs are ephedrine and dopamine, with dobutamine the inotrope of choice.[25] When necessary, norepinephrine may be used, but epinephrine should be avoided. Close fetal monitoring is required as dopamine and norepinephrine can decrease uterine blood flow. The role of vasopressin in the pregnant patient with septic shock remains undefined, but institution of an infusion at 10 to 40 milliunits per hour is reasonable in refractory shock. Mechanical ventilatory support should be instituted if needed.

As in the nonpregnant septic patient, corticosteroids are given if adrenal insufficiency is documented. The corticotropin stimulation test may be difficult to interpret in the pregnant woman because baseline cortisol may be elevated in pregnancy and stimulation tests have not been studied in this population. Recombinant protein C has not been systematically evaluated in pregnant patients, and it is impossible to make informed commentary on its risk/benefit profile in this setting. The essentials of treatment are early appropriate antibiotics, identification and control of the source of infection with surgical treatment if necessary, and meticulous supportive care.

Preeclampsia

Preeclampsia is a disorder unique to pregnancy that accounts for a substantial proportion of obstetric ICU admissions.[3,5] It complicates 5 to 10% of all pregnancies, causing 10 to 15% of maternal deaths.[2] It occurs most often in nulliparous women after the 20th week of gestation, typically near term, and may even occur postpartum. Although the exact pathogenesis is not known, it may begin with placental hypoperfusion from abnormally formed uteroplacental spiral arteries.[26] Excess production of placenta-derived vascular endothelial growth factor receptor, known as soluble fms-like tyrosine kinase 1, neutralizes the proangiogenic actions of vascular endothelial growth factor and placental growth factor, leading to maternal endothelial dysfunction.[27] Ultimately, an exaggerated inflammatory response, endothelial damage, vasoconstriction, and microthrombi affect multiple organ systems. Cardiac output and plasma volume are decreased, and SVR is increased. Right-heart catheterization reveals low normal right atrial pressure and PCWP. Cardiac output may be low, normal, or high.

Clinically, preeclampsia is characterized by hypertension, proteinuria, and generalized edema; however, these features may be mild and may not occur simultaneously, making the diagnosis of early disease difficult in many cases. An increased ratio of serum soluble fms-like tyrosine kinase 1 to placental growth factor is thought to show promise as a biomarker for preeclampsia. Risk factors for the development of preeclampsia, besides the primigravid state, include preexisting and gestational hypertension, maternal or paternal family history of preeclampsia, preexisting renal disease, diabetes mellitus, multiple gestation, body mass index >35, maternal age >40 years, and antiphospholipid antibody syndrome.[28] Preeclampsia may progress without warning to a convulsive and potentially lethal phase, termed *eclampsia*. An especially fulminant complication of preeclampsia is the HELLP (hemolysis, elevated liver enzymes, low platelets) syndrome. Maternal and fetal morbidity and mortality are significant if eclampsia or the HELLP syndrome develops or if preeclampsia develops prior to 34 weeks of gestation.

Maternal complications of severe preeclampsia include seizures (eclampsia), cerebral hemorrhage or edema, renal dysfunction, pulmonary edema, placental abruption with DIC, the HELLP syndrome, and hepatic infarction, failure, subcapsular hemorrhage, or rupture. Although the risks of eclampsia are higher when these markers of disease severity are present, in one large clinical series 20% of eclamptic patients had a diastolic BP <90 mm Hg or no proteinuria prior to experiencing convulsions. Renal dysfunction may result from intravascular volume depletion, renal ischemia, and glomerular disease characterized by swollen glomerular endothelial cells known as *glomeruloendotheliosis*. Acute renal failure is rare and most often seen in patients with the HELLP syndrome. Pulmonary edema most commonly occurs after parturition. In a subgroup of patients who are obese and chronically hypertensive with secondary left ventricular hypertrophy, antepartum pulmonary edema may develop. The increased intravascular volume of pregnancy and the hemodynamic derangements of preeclampsia cause diastolic dysfunction with an elevated PCWP and pulmonary edema in these patients.

The HELLP syndrome is characterized by multiorgan dysfunction arising from dysfunction with secondary fibrin deposition and organ hypoperfusion.[29] A microangiopathic hemolytic anemia and consumptive coagulopathy develop. The liver involvement is characterized by periportal or focal parenchymal necrosis with elevated liver function tests. Intrahepatic hemorrhage or subcapsular hematoma occurs in 2% of patients and may progress to hepatic rupture.

The HELLP syndrome occurs in 4 to 20% of patients with preeclampsia. Patients are more often preterm than those with uncomplicated eclampsia. In up to 30% of patients, the HELLP syndrome develops after parturition; it has been reported up to 7 days postpartum. Presenting symptoms are usually nonspecific, the most common being malaise, epigastric or right upper quadrant pain, nausea, vomiting, and edema. Patients less frequently present with jaundice, GI bleeding, or hematuria. Complications include acute renal failure, ARDS, hemorrhage, hypoglycemia, hyponatremia, and nephrogenic diabetes insipidus. Maternal mortality ranges from 0 to 24%, with higher perinatal mortality (8 to 60%).

Laboratory values that suggest the HELLP syndrome include (1) hemolysis on peripheral smear, (2) bilirubin ≥ 1.2 mg/dL or lactate dehydrogenase ≥ 600 U/L, (3) increased liver enzyme levels, and (4) a platelet count of $< 100,000/\mu L$. Isolated thrombocytopenia that progresses may be one of the first clues to the diagnosis.

The principles of management of preeclampsia include early diagnosis, close medical observation, and timely delivery. Delivery is curative in most cases. The differential diagnosis of preeclampsia includes thrombotic thrombocytopenic purpura (TTP), hemolytic uremic syndrome (HUS), acute fatty liver of pregnancy, and idiopathic postpartum renal failure. Once the diagnosis is made, further management is based on an evaluation of the mother and fetus. The presence of symptoms and proteinuria increases the risk of placental abruption and eclampsia. These patients and those with disease progression should be hospitalized and observed closely. In patients who have mild preeclampsia at term and have a favorable cervix, labor should be induced. Based on a number of clinical trials, there is no clear benefit to antihypertensive drug treatment in women with mild gestational hypertension or preeclampsia.

Immediate delivery is appropriate when there are signs of impending eclampsia, multiorgan involvement, or fetal distress, and in patients who are >34 weeks pregnant. Early in gestation, conservative management with close monitoring to improve neonatal survival and morbidity may be appropriate in selected cases at tertiary perinatal centers. The objective of antihypertensive therapy is to prevent cerebral complications such as encephalopathy and hemorrhage.[30] A sustained diastolic BP >110 mm Hg should be treated to keep the mean arterial pressure from 105 to 126 mm Hg and the diastolic pressure from 90 to 105 mm Hg. Although hydralazine has been the traditional treatment, IV labetalol is now favored in the

ICU. A loading dose of labetalol, 20 mg, is recommended, followed by either repeated incremental doses of 20 to 80 mg at 20- to 30-min intervals or an infusion starting at 1 to 2 mg/min and titrated up until the target BP is achieved. Nicardipine may be an acceptable alternative. Because calcium-channel blockers may be potentiated by magnesium infusion, care should be taken to avoid hypotension when the two medications are used together. Acute nicardipine infusion can induce severe maternal tachycardia. Nitroprusside is relatively contraindicated, and angiotensin-converting enzyme inhibitors are absolutely contraindicated in pregnancy. Diuretics should be used with caution because they may aggravate the reduction in intravascular volume that is often seen in preeclampsia. Antihypertensive therapy has no effect on the progression of preeclampsia and does not prevent complications such as HELLP.

Magnesium sulfate prophylaxis has been shown to be better than placebo, phenytoin, or nimodipine in the prevention of eclampsia.[31] In a recent large study, magnesium sulfate was superior to both phenytoin and diazepam for the treatment and prevention of recurrent convulsions in women with eclampsia.[32] Magnesium sulfate should be administered to all women with either preeclampsia or eclampsia and for a minimum of 24 h postpartum (Table 10). Aspirin has no role in the treatment of preeclampsia.

The preeclamptic patient with oliguria may benefit from judicious volume loading. Patients with delayed postpartum resolution of the HELLP syndrome with persistent thrombocytopenia, hemolysis, or organ dysfunction may benefit from plasmapheresis with fresh-frozen plasma. These patients may actually have TTP or HUS,

which can be difficult to distinguish from the HELLP syndrome. In two studies, administration of corticosteroids resulted in improved maternal platelet counts and liver function test results and in a trend toward better fetal outcome. No significant effect in delaying delivery was noted. Management of intrahepatic hemorrhage with subcapsular hematoma includes administration of blood products, delivery, and control of liver hemorrhage. Embolization of the hepatic artery is often successful, but evacuation of the hematoma and packing of the liver may be required.

Other Disorders of Pregnancy

Acute Renal Failure

The incidence of acute renal failure associated with pregnancy is from 0.02 to 0.05%.[33] Acute renal failure may complicate preeclampsia, the HELLP syndrome, and acute fatty liver of pregnancy. Acute tubular necrosis may occur from hemorrhage or sepsis. Acute cortical necrosis is associated with placental abruption, septic abortion, prolonged intrauterine retention of a dead fetus, hemorrhage, and amniotic fluid embolism. Acute oliguric renal failure necessitating dialysis typically results. Arteriography may demonstrate loss of the cortical circulation, and renal biopsy can confirm the diagnosis. Although renal function often improves, end-stage renal failure is the eventual outcome. Idiopathic postpartum acute renal failure is an unusual complication of pregnancy and may occur days to weeks after a normal pregnancy and delivery. The etiology is unknown. The disorder may be a variant of HUS or TTP because it is clinically and pathologically

Table 10. *Magnesium Dosing in Severe Preeclampsia/Eclampsia*

Variables	Normal Renal Function	Renal Insufficiency, Creatinine > 1.0 mL/dL
Initial	6 g IV over 15–20 min	4–6 g IV over 15–20 min
Maintenance	2 g/h infusion	1 g/h infusion
Serum levels	4.8–8.4 mg/dL	Monitor every 6 h
Monitor	Patellar reflex present	Patellar reflex present
	Respiratory rate > 12 breaths/min	Respiratory rate > 12 breaths/min
	Urine output > 100 mL / 4 h	Urine output > 100 mL / 4 h
Adverse effects	Hypotension/asystole	Hypotension/asystole
	Respiratory depression	Respiratory depression
Drug interactions	Calcium-channel blockers may enhance adverse/toxic effects	Calcium-channel blockers may enhance adverse/toxic effects

Critical Illness in Pregnancy (Strek)

similar to these entities, although without hemolysis or thrombocytopenia, and many patients respond to treatment with prednisone administration and plasmapheresis. In general, the treatment of acute renal failure in pregnancy is similar to that in the nonpregnant patient, with supportive care and dialysis as necessary. Renal dysfunction associated with preeclampsia and the HELLP syndrome should respond to delivery of the fetus, while TTP and HUS require plasmapheresis with fresh-frozen plasma.

Acute Liver Failure

Acute liver failure is an uncommon complication of pregnancy. In pregnancy, *de novo* liver function test abnormalities are uncommon and occur in < 5% of pregnancies in the United States. Serum alkaline phosphatase increases during the first 7 months of pregnancy, peaking at two to four times normal at term. Serum albumin concentrations decrease in pregnancy. Levels of serum aminotransferases and bilirubin are unchanged in normal pregnancy.

Liver failure rarely complicates preeclampsia and the HELLP syndrome; subcapsular hematoma and rupture are more common complications.[34] Acute fatty liver of pregnancy is estimated to occur in 1 of 13,000 deliveries. Risk factors include male fetus, multiple gestations, and a first pregnancy. Mean onset is at 36 weeks of gestation, although the disorder can be seen as early as 26 weeks and postpartum. Patients present with headache, nausea and vomiting, right upper quadrant or epigastric pain, malaise, and anorexia. The onset of acute fatty liver of pregnancy may be similar to the onset of preeclampsia with peripheral edema, hypertension, and proteinuria. Jaundice may follow 1 to 2 weeks later. Cholestasis with mild-to-moderate elevations in serum aminotransferases is the rule. Ultrasound may show increased echogenicity. CT abdominal scans are more sensitive and may demonstrate decreased attenuation, although this imaging exposes the fetus to significant radiation. Liver biopsy is sometimes necessary to make the diagnosis but must be undertaken with caution because these patients often have a coagulopathy. The biopsy is characterized by microvesicular fatty infiltration detected only on frozen sections. Acute fatty liver of pregnancy progresses to fulminant hepatic failure complicated by encephalopathy, renal failure, pancreatitis, hemorrhage, DIC, seizures, coma, and death. Because deterioration may occur rapidly, expectant management is generally not advised. The treatment is delivery of the fetus. Jaundice, liver dysfunction, and DIC may worsen for a few days after delivery but then should improve. Maternal and fetal mortality has improved with early delivery and is < 20%. Full maternal recovery is to be expected. Because long-chain 3-hydroxyacyl-coenzyme dehydrogenase deficiency in the fetus has been reported to be associated with acute fatty liver of pregnancy in women in a recent study, infants may have hypoglycemia, hypotonia, acute or chronic skeletal and cardiac muscle dysfunction, and sudden infant death syndrome.

References

1. Naylor DF, Olson MM. Critical care obstetrics and gynecology. Crit Care Clin 2003; 19:127–149
2. Chang J, Elam-Evans LD, Berg CJ, et al. Pregnancy-related mortality surveillance—United States, 1991-1999. MMWR Surveill Summ 2003; 52:1–8
3. Lapinsky SE, Kruczynski K, Slutsky AS. Critical care in the pregnant patient. Am J Respir Crit Care Med 1995; 152:427–455
4. Rizk NW, Kalassian KG, Gilligan T, et al. Obstetric complications in pulmonary and critical care medicine. Chest 1996; 110:791–809
5. Strek ME, O'Connor M, Hall JB, et al. Critical illness in pregnancy. In: JB Hall, GA Schmidt, LD Wood, eds. Principles of critical care. 3rd ed. New York, NY: McGraw-Hill, 2005; 1593–1614
6. Pereira A, Kreiger BP. Pulmonary complications of pregnancy. Clin Chest Med 2004; 25:299–310
7. Hanania NA, Belfort MA. Acute asthma in pregnancy. Crit Care Med 2005; 33:S319–S324
8. National Asthma Education and Prevention Program. Working Group Report on managing asthma during pregnancy: recommendations for pharmacologic treatment. Bethesda, MD: National Institutes of Health, 2004; 2-11; publication 05–5246
9. Marik PE and Plante LA. Venouos thromboembolic disease and pregnancy. N Engl J Med 2008; 359:2025–2033
10. Bates SM, Greer IA, Pabinger I, et al. Venous thromboembolism, thrombophilia, antithrombotic therapy, and pregnancy. Chest 2008; 133:844S–886S

11. Aurangzeb I, George L, Raoof S. Amniotic fluid embolism. Crit Care Clin 2004; 20:643–650

12. Moore J, Baldisseri MR. Amniotic fluid embolism. Crit Care Med 2005; 33:S279–S285

13. Bandi VD, Munnur U, Matthay MA. Acute lung injury and acute respiratory distress syndrome in pregnancy. Crit Care Clin 2004; 20:577–607

14. Ramsey PS, Ramin KD. Pneumonia in pregnancy. Obstet Gyncol Clin North Am 2001; 28:553–569

15. Goodnight WH, Soper DE. Pneumonia in pregnancy. Crit Care Med 2005; 33:S390–S397

16. Cole DE, Taylor TL McCullough DM, et al. Acute respiratory distress syndrome in pregnancy. Crit Care Med 2005; 33:S269–S278

17. Cardiac arrest associated with pregnancy. Circulation 2005; 112:150–153

18. Mallampalli A, Guy E. Cardiac arrest in pregnancy and somatic support after brain death. Crit Care Med 2005; 33:S325–S331

19. Roberts WE. Emergent obstetric management of post-partum hemorrhage. Obstet Gynecol Clin North Am 1995; 22:283–302

20. Franchini M, Franchini M, Bergamini V, et al. A critical review on the use of recombinant factor VIIa in life-threatening obstetric postpartum hemorrhage. Semin Thromb Hemost 2008; 34:104–112

21. Murali S, Baldisseri MR. Peripartum cardiomyopathy. Crit Care Med 2005; 33:S340–S346

22. Fein AM, Duvivier R. Sepsis in pregnancy. Clin Chest Med 1992; 13:709–722

23. Fernandez-Perez ER, Salman S, Pendem S, et al. Sepsis during pregnancy. Crit Care Med 2005; 33:286–293

24. Guinn DA, Abel DE, Tomlinson MW. Early goal directed therapy for sepsis during pregnancy. Obstet Gynecol Clin North Am 2007; 34:459–479

25. Ko R, Mazur JE, Pastis NJ, et al. Common problems in critically ill obstetric patients, with an emphasis on pharmacotherapy. Am J Med Sci 2008; 335: 65–70

26. Roberts JM, Gammill HS. Preeclampsia. Hypertension 2005; 46:1243–1249

27. Carty DM, Delles C, Dominiczak AF. Novel biomarkers for predicting preeclampsia. Trends Cardiovasc Med 2008; 18:186–194

28. Duckitt K, Harrington D. Risk factors for pre-eclampsia at antenatal booking: systematic review of controlled studies. BMJ 2005; 330:565–567

29. Gilson G, Golden P, Izquierdo L, et al. Pregnancy-associated hemolysis, elevated liver functions, low platelets (HELLP) syndrome: an obstetric disease in the intensive care unit. J Intensive Care Med 1996; 11:173–178

30. Vigil-DeGracia P, Lasso M, Ruiz E, et al. Severe hypertension in pregnancy: hydralazine or labetalol a randomized clinical trial. Eur J Obstet Gynecol Reprod Biol 2006; 128:157–162

31. The Magpie Trial Collaborative Group. Do women with pre-eclampsia, and their babies, benefit from magnesium sulphate? The Magpie Trial: a randomized placebo-controlled trial. Lancet 2002; 359:1877–1890

32. Eclampsia Trial Collaborative Group. Which anticonvulsant for women with eclampsia: evidence from the Collaborative Eclampsia Trial. Lancet 1995; 345:1455–1463

33. Gammill HS, Jeyabalan A. Acute renal failure in pregnancy. Crit Care Med 2005; 33:S372–S384

34. Guntupalli SK, Steingrub J. Hepatic disease and pregnancy: an overview of diagnosis and management. Crit Care Med 2005; 33:S332–S339

Venous Thromboembolic Disease

R. Phillip Dellinger, MD, FCCP

Objectives:

- Recognize the risk factors for pulmonary embolism (PE)
- Appreciate the typical clinical presentations of PE
- Choose rationally among perfusion lung scanning, leg ultrasound, CT scanning, and d-dimer assay in the diagnostic approach to PE
- Understand the place of anticoagulation, inferior vena cava filter placement, and thrombolytic therapy in the management of PE

Key words: anticoagulation; compression ultrasound; deep-vein thrombosis; pulmonary embolism; thromboembolism; thrombolytic therapy; perfusion lung scanning

---

Risk Factors

Major risk factors for pulmonary thromboemboli are processes that predispose a patient to the development of deep-vein thrombosis (DVT) [ie, any cause of venous stasis, such as venous valvular insufficiency, right-sided heart failure, the postoperative period, and prolonged bed rest, or immobilization] (Table 1). Abdominal operations requiring general anesthesia >30 min place the patient at risk for venous thromboembolism (VTE). Orthopedic surgery of the lower extremity has long been recognized as one of the greatest risk factors for VTE. DVT develops in >50% of patients who do not receive prophylactic therapy while undergoing elective total hip replacement and knee replacement surgery. Over 90% of proximal thrombi occur in hip replacement patients on the operated side. Since the first controlled trials demonstrating a reduced rate of pulmonary embolism (PE) mortality with anticoagulant prophylaxis were performed in this high-risk group, patients with fractures of the pelvis, hip, or femur are of significant historical relevance.

Trauma to the extremities, advanced malignancy (increasingly recognized as a major risk factor), pregnancy, the postpartum state, and, to a lesser degree, birth control pills (current formulations have lower estrogen content) are significant risk factors. Long-distance air travel has also been linked to PE. There is an estimated 40% risk of VTE and a 5% incidence of PE in patients with traumatic spinal cord injury and associated paralysis of lower extremities. The period of greatest risk is during the first 2 weeks after the initial injury; death occurs rarely in PE patients after 3 months.

The frequency of VTE increases exponentially between the ages of 20 and 80 years. Although an age of >40 years has often been used as a break point for age-related increase in VTE, increasing age increases risk beginning with adulthood and continues to increase after the age of 40 years, nearly doubling with each decade. One study demonstrated a 23% incidence of PE in 175,730 tertiary-care hospital admissions with linear relation to age. The incidence in women was higher in individuals ≥50 years old but not in those <50 years old (Stein et al, 1999). In patients with a history of thromboembolic disease who undergo hospitalization, there is nearly an eightfold increase in acute thromboembolism compared with patients without such a history, therefore making acute thromboembolism one of the more important risk factors for VTE.

Patients with a history of VTE who undergo major surgery, periods of immobility, or who are hospitalized for serious medical illnesses must be aggressively targeted for prophylaxis therapy. Although precise estimates of risk increase in malignancy are difficult to ascertain, advanced cancer is associated with a high risk of VTE.

With other risk factors considered equal, surgery for malignant disease results in a twofold to threefold increase in thromboembolism compared with surgery for nonmalignant conditions. Hypercoagulable states secondary to deficiencies of antithrombin, protein C, or protein S, as well as the presence of anticardiolipin antibody, lupus anticoagulant, prothrombin G20210A mutation, or factor V Leiden mutation are predisposing factors for thromboembolic disease.

Table 1. *Risk Factors for Pulmonary Emboli*

Right-sided heart failure
Postoperative period
Prolonged bed rest
Travel "economy class syndrome"
Trauma
Advanced malignancy
Pregnancy
Postpartum state
Birth control pills
Previous DVT
Hypercoagulable states

Hypercoagulable states include the following: (1) antiphospholipid syndrome (lupus anticoagulant, anticardiolipin antibody; (2) factor V mutation; (3) prothrombin G20210A mutation; (4) hyperhomocysteinemia; and (5) deficiencies (antithrombin, protein C, protein S). Screening for select hypercoagulable states is appropriate in patients with no obvious risk factors who acquire PE. This screening is most appropriate for the three coagulopathies that can be easily accurately measured accurately in the presence of acute clot burden/anticoagulation and have therapeutic implications: factor V Leiden (most common hypercoagulable state and would warrant more aggressive prophylaxis), anticardiolipin antibody or lupus anticoagulant (dictates more aggressive warfarin therapy), and hyperhomocysteinemia (may benefit from treatment with B vitamins). Although most pulmonary emboli come from deep veins of the lower extremities, clinically significant emboli also occur from other sites of venous thrombosis including the iliac veins, pelvic veins and, less frequently, the inferior vena cava (IVC). Central venous catheters are risk factors for superior vena cava/axillary/subclavian vein thrombosis, as well as femoral vein thrombosis.

Clinical Findings

The clinical diagnosis of PE is difficult. Clinical acumen falters due to both sensitivity and specificity problems. The most common symptoms/signs of dyspnea, tachypnea, and tachycardia are seen with a myriad of other disorders. Tachypnea and tachycardia may be transient. The physical examination is not typically helpful in considering PE, with the exception of the

presence of findings to support acute increases of right-sided pressure such as a new right-axis deviation or new right bundle-branch block, widely split-second heart sound, murmur of tricuspid regurgitation, or an accentuated pulmonary closure sound. Examination of the lower extremity is unreliable for predicting the presence or absence of DVT. Nevertheless, new findings supportive of acute deep-vein obstruction, particularly unilateral leg swelling in the setting of pulmonary symptoms compatible with thromboembolism, should strengthen the possibility of PE.

Pulmonary infarction is the classic presentation of PE and is characterized by a pulmonary infiltrate that is often peripheral and wedge shaped (Hampton hump), pleuritic chest pain, hemoptysis and, not infrequently, a bloody pleural effusion. These findings represent the "textbook" version of PE that is taught to medical students but seen in only 10% of pulmonary emboli. Pulmonary infarction is rare due to three sources of oxygen and two sources of nutrient supply to the lung: the bronchial and pulmonary arteries and the airways. In addition, back-perfusion from the pulmonary venous system may also be a potential source of oxygen and nutrient supply. Pulmonary infarction is more likely to occur in the face of preexisting compromise of nutrient or oxygen supply, such as in intrinsic lung disease or in the presence of reduced cardiac output.

A more frequent presentation of PE is acute onset of shortness of breath or hypoxemia in the absence of pulmonary infarction, with or without chest pain (often pleuritic when present). Radiographic infiltrates may or may not be present. Chest radiographic findings of PE include the following: atelectasis and parenchymal densities; enlarged right descending pulmonary artery; decreased pulmonary vascularity; wedge-shaped infiltrate; cardiomegaly; and may be normal (up to 25%)

Less frequent, but more lethal, is acute massive PE characterized by a large thromboembolus lodging in the proximal pulmonary circulation resulting in hypotension and possible syncope. Chest pain may be present and is probably due to right ventricular (RV) or left ventricular (LV) myocardial ischemia. Infiltrates are usually absent in massive PE unless the embolus has fragmented and moved peripherally. Acute pulmonary hypertension with

Table 2. *Distribution of Temperature in PE*

Temperature, °F	No. (%)
<99.9	268 (86)
100.0–100.9	24 (8)
101.0–101.9	14 (5)
102.0–102.9	3 (1)
103.0–103.9	1 (<1)
>104.0	1 (<1)

central dilated pulmonary arteries may also be present (Westermark sign). Hypoxemia is almost always present, although hypotension is usually the primary clinical concern.

Fever (temperature ≥100.0°F) has been demonstrated to be present in 14% of angiographically documented PE with no other cause of fever (Stein et al, Chest 2000). Only 2 of 228 patients had temperatures ≥103.0°F (Table 2). Leukocytosis may or may not be present.

Tachycardia and nonspecific ST-T changes are the most common ECG findings in PE. In massive PE, right-heart strain may be indicated by P-wave pulmonale, $S_1Q_3T_3$ pattern, right-axis deviation, or right bundle-branch block. Chest radiographic abnormalities due to PE include pulmonary infiltrate, pleural effusion, elevated hemidiaphragm, and atelectasis. A pleural-based, wedge-shaped infiltrate called a Hampton hump may be seen in some cases of pulmonary infarction. An unremarkable chest radiograph with significant hypoxemia and no obvious cause, such as asthma or exacerbation of COPD, should also raise the concern for PE. Patients who acquire PE in the ICU typically have abnormal chest radiographic findings due to preexisting pulmonary disease. One study found cardiomegaly to be the most common chest radiographic abnormality.

Analysis of pleural fluid in a patient suspected of having PE is useful only to confirm other diagnoses. There are no pathognomonic pleural effusion findings with PE; the effusion may be a transudate or exudate; it may or may not be bloody. A bloody pleural effusion that accompanies PE usually implies pulmonary infarction. Other potential etiologies of bloody pleural effusions include malignancy and trauma.

Echocardiography may be helpful in delineating other etiologies of clinical findings, such as myocardial ischemia or pericardial tamponade.

However, findings such as acute RV dilation and hypokinesis, tricuspid regurgitation, pulmonary hypertension estimated from tricuspid regurgitation jet, pulmonary artery dilation, loss of respiratory variation in IVC diameter, interventricular septum bulge into the left ventricle, and reduced diastolic-shaped LV size may support the diagnosis of PE but are not specific enough to establish the diagnosis. A distinct radiograph pattern has recently been noted in patients with large PE in which regional RV dysfunction is noted but the apex is spared. (McConnell, Am J Cardiol) Clinically significant PE may also occur in the absence of any abnormal RV findings on echocardiography. Rarely, a clot may be visualized in the right heart and thus allows a specific diagnosis.

Recent (nonlatex agglutination) assays are clinically useful in the evaluation for possible PE since a nonelevated d-dimer makes PE unlikely. A d-dimer measured by enzyme-linked immunosorbent assay (ELISA) was noted to be normal in ≤10% of angiographically documented PE in one study (Quinn et al). An elevated d-dimer, however, may be seen in many circumstances other than PE (recent surgery, malignancy, total bilirubin >2 mg/dL, sepsis, late pregnancy, trauma, advanced age). The traditional ELISA assay typically requires 24 h for results. Newer, second-generation tests, including rapid ELISA, may offer reliable and rapid bedside testing. The d-dimer assay may be particularly important in the emergency department, in low pretest clinical suspicion scenarios, and in combination with other studies in the inpatient population. A fall in end-tidal CO_2 may also be useful in raising the clinical suspicion of PE, while a decrease in $Paco_2$ may be a marker of success of thrombolytic therapy in patients with PE.

Respiratory alkalosis is a common finding in the tachypneic patient with PE. With massive pulmonary embolus, respiratory acidosis may be present due to increased dead space. Although a room air Pao_2 >80 mm Hg (>10.7 kPa) or a normal alveolar-arterial gradient makes the diagnosis of PE less likely, neither can be relied on to exclude PE. Patients with PE may have a normal alveolar-arterial gradient. This finding is more likely to occur in the presence of previous normal cardiopulmonary status. Hypoxemia and an increase in alveolar-arterial gradient may also be transient.

Forty-two patients in the Prospective Investigation of Pulmonary Embolism Diagnosis (PIOPED) trial had suspected PE, no prior cardiopulmonary disease, and fulfilled all of the following criteria: Pao_2 >80 mm Hg (>10.7 kPa), $Paco_2$ >35 mm Hg (>4.7 kPa), and normal alveolar-arterial gradient. Sixteen patients (38%) had angiographically documented PE. In patients who had prior cardiopulmonary disease and who met all three criteria mentioned above, 14% had PE. Therefore, normal arterial blood gases, in general, and in patients with no prior history of cardiopulmonary disease, in particular, do not allow discontinuation of the pursuit of PE.

Nonmassive PE produces hypoxemia by release of bronchoconstrictors, production of atelectasis (surfactant depletion over hours), and perhaps reperfusion injury to the endothelial-epithelial barrier. Massive PE is almost always associated with hypoxemia and frequently with CO_2 retention. In addition to the same causes of hypoxemia as related above for nonmassive PE, the amputation of pulmonary vascular bed in massive PE produces both a large increase in dead space (as a cause of increased $Paco_2$) and a large amount of blood flow diverted to noninvolved areas of the lung, causing low ventilation/perfusion ratio due to overperfusion with resultant hypoxemia.

Other potential causes of hypoxemia in massive PE include low mixed venous oxygen due to low cardiac output, as well as the potential for opening of a probe-patent foramen ovale due to high right-sided pressures. A probe-patent foramen ovale is present in a small but significant percentage of the general population. In the presence of very high right-heart pressures, this right-to-left shunt produces hypoxemia unresponsive to oxygen therapy and also places the patient at risk for embolic cerebral vascular events.

Diagnosis

The treatment of PE or DVT is essentially the same as in patients with suspected PE; therefore, either diagnosis is sufficient for decision making.

CT

CT angiography (CTA; spiral [helical] or electron beam) is of significant value in detecting pulmonary emboli. In patients other than those with pretest high clinical suspicion (80 to 99%), a negative spiral CT result makes pulmonary emboli very unlikely when using the most recent CT imaging with digital reconstruction and a welltrained reader. It typically allows diagnosis and treatment. The same is true for a positive result, with the exception of those patients with low pretest clinical suspicion (0 to 20%).

The specificity of CT for the diagnosis of PE has traditionally been better than sensitivity, although the latter has improved with newer generation scanners (multidetector/digital reconstruction). It must also be remembered that a CTA may allow identification of other pulmonary processes as the cause of clinical findings.

The PIOPED II trial was designed to study the ability of the CTA to predict presence or absence of PE. All patients being evaluated for possible PE underwent a ventilation/perfusion scan, leg ultrasound, and a CTA that was not used to make or exclude the diagnosis of PE and was read blinded to the following: (1) other test results, and (2) pretest assessment of likelihood of PE. PE was considered present in the presence of a high- probability ventilation/perfusion scan or a positive leg ultrasound. PE was considered absent in the presence of a normal perfusion scan. All other subjects received digital subtraction angiography for definitive diagnosis of presence or absence of PE. Sensitivity and specificity were ascertained. Pretest probability of PE was ascertained for all subjects. Positive and negative predictive values of CTA referenced to pretest clinical probability are shown (Table 3). It is apparent that, like perfusion scanning, CTA looses diagnostic yield in circumstances of extreme discordance (high clinical probability/negative CTA and low clinical probability/positive CTA).

One sensitivity issue with the CTA diagnosis of PE is the decreased ability to detect vessels beyond the segmental arteries. This may be of less clinical relevance, however, since the natural history of pulmonary emboli limited to subsegmental arteries is usually a benign course, especially in patients with self-limited risk factors. Withholding anticoagulant therapy in patients with a 380 Venous Thromboembolic Disease (Dellinger) negative CT scan coupled with a negative ultrasonographic study of the legs is a safe strategy, except in those patients who present with a high pretest clinical probability of embolism.

Table 3. *PIOPED II Results**

Variables	Clinical Suspicion of PE		
	High	Moderate	Low
True-positive CT (positive predictive value), %	96	92	58
True-negative CT (negative predictive value), %	60	89	96

*CT sensitivity, 83%; specificity, 96%.

Perfusion Lung Scanning

Perfusion lung scanning (usually done in combination with ventilation scanning) is typically classified into high probability, intermediate probability, low probability, and normal. Probability of PE increases with size of perfusion defect, number of moderate-to-large size defects, and perfusion defects that are significantly larger than ventilation defects or present in the absence of ventilation defects. Although ventilation scanning is usually performed in combination with perfusion scanning to quantify ventilation defects, chest radiographs can be used in place of ventilation scanning in patients without chronic pulmonary disease or acute bronchospasm. The chance of a perfusion defect being due to PE increases with increasing number and size of defects, lower-lobe distribution, matching of vascular tree distribution, and defect larger than any ventilation defects that may accompany the perfusion defect by chest radiograph or ventilation scanning (so-called "mismatched defect"). Using these characteristics, perfusion scans are classified as normal, low, or intermediate probability scans. The PIOPED study is the most frequently utilized reference for assessing utility of perfusion scanning in the diagnosis of PE.

The PIOPED I study supported the following findings: (1) normal lung scans make PE very unlikely; (2) reliability of a high-probability scan increases with (a) the degree of clinical suspicion using history, physical examination, and clinical information; (b) no underlying cardiopulmonary disease; and (c) no history of pulmonary emboli; (3) a minority of patients have high-probability perfusion scans; (4) a low-probability scan does not exclude PE; (5) a clinical impression of low likelihood of PE when combined with a low-probability scan increases the predictive value of the low-probability scan; (6) intermediate-probability scans cannot be used for definitive decision making; (7) the great majority of patients with suspected PE cannot have PE excluded with perfusion scanning; (8) it is best to call low- and intermediate-probability scans "nondiagnostic," with the classification system then becoming high probability, nondiagnostic, and normal.

Nondiagnostic scans require additional testing because they do not allow a decision as to the presence or absence of PE. In anticipation of a later question of failure of heparin therapy, a baseline perfusion scan should be considered even when the clinical diagnosis of PE is made by other methods. This will allow repeat scanning for the presence or absence of additional perfusion defects if new symptoms develop or symptoms continue.

Lower-Extremity Ultrasound

Compression ultrasound (CUS) combines Doppler venous flow detection with venous imaging and has become the imaging procedure of choice for DVT in most medical centers in the United States. The diagnostic utility of CUS is related to imaging of a venous filling defect that persists with compression of the lesion. Impressive sensitivity and specificity for proximal vein thrombosis are usually obtained with this technique in patients with leg symptoms. This technique does not detect isolated thrombosis in the iliac veins or the superficial femoral veins within the adductor canal. It is, however, unlikely that these areas will be involved unless thrombus is also present in the more readily imageable popliteal and deep femoral system.

Diagnosis of calf vein thrombosis is more challenging because these veins are smaller, have slower flow, and have more anatomic variability. CUS may also diagnose other etiologies of clinical findings such as Baker cyst, hematoma, lymphadenopathy, and abscess. CUS cannot be performed if the leg is cast. CUS may also be limited by pain and edema.

Diagnosis of DVT by CUS allows treatment because treatments for PE and DVT are essentially the same. Absence of DVT by CUS, in combination with low-probability perfusion scan or failure to detect PE on helical CT and the absence of high clinical suspicion, usually allows withholding treatment. One concern with regard to this approach, however, is that the sensitivity of CUS is significantly diminished in high-risk patients without leg symptoms or signs.

Clinically evident pulmonary emboli are even more unlikely in the presence of serial negative noninvasive leg studies (typically repeated one to three times over a period of 3 to 14 days) and if negative further enhance clinical acumen. A negative leg ultrasound in a patient with an intermediate-probability scan usually implies the need for a spiral CT or pulmonary angiography.

Diagnosis of PE With Pulmonary Angiography

Pulmonary angiography remains the "gold standard" for diagnosis of PE, and morbidity and mortality rates are low and usually acceptable. Angiography is considered positive when a persistent filling defect or cut-off sign is noted. Risk is increased if angiography is followed by thrombolytic therapy. The risk of pulmonary angiography to the patient is usually greater from anticoagulation in the absence of PE or failure to treat PE that is present. The death rate from pulmonary angiogram in the PIOPED I study was 0.5%, with a low incidence (0.8%) of major nonfatal complications (respiratory failure, renal failure or hematoma necessitating transfusion). Major nonfatal complications were four times more likely to occur in ICU patients.

Despite early studies that suggested a higher incidence of mortality due to pulmonary angiography in patients with high pulmonary artery pressures, this was not found to be true in the PIOPED I study. Pulmonary angiography done within 1 week of acute symptoms should reliably detect pulmonary emboli even in the presence of anticoagulation. In patients with angiographically proven PE, perfusion defects persist for at least 7 days without resolution, and in the majority for 14 days. This is an important consideration since patients may be referred to a tertiary-care center with uncertain diagnosis of PE, having received therapy for a considerable period of time.

Diagnosis of PE in Pregnancy

The pursuit of diagnosis of PE in pregnant women is challenging. Ventilation/perfusion scanning is low risk. In pregnant patients with negative leg ultrasound findings, identifying the location of perfusion defects on an indeterminant diagnosis perfusion scan and following with selective pulmonary angiography targeting those defects is likely the best approach because it potentially minimizes dye load if PE is present. Warfarin is an absolute contraindication in the first trimester and a relative contraindication in the second and third trimesters. Long-term heparin administration in the pregnant woman is a significant risk for osteoporosis.

Treatment

Anticoagulation

Heparin therapy is discontinued after a minimum of 4 to 5 days of therapy, at least 48 h of warfarin therapy, and a warfarin-induced prolongation of international normalized ratio for prothrombin time >2.0. For patients with antiphospholipid syndrome, this target is typically higher (>2.5). The activated partial thromboplastin time (aPTT) should be maintained at 1.5 to 2 times control with heparin therapy. Although subtherapeutic aPTT is strongly correlated with thromboembolic recurrence, a supratherapeutic aPTT does not appear to correlate with important bleeding complications. Instead, bleeding complications correlate with concurrent illness such as renal disease, heavy ethanol consumption, aspirin use, and peptic ulcer disease.

Based on this information, targeting an aPTT of 2.0 times normal rather than 1.5 times normal may be ideal. Adequate heparinization prevents additional clot formation, but the body's own fibrinolytic system must clear the clot that is already present so that patients who are hemodynamically unstable or who have poor cardiopulmonary reserve may remain at risk during early anticoagulation therapy. In patients without a contraindication for anticoagulation, heparin therapy should be instituted as soon as thromboembolic disease is considered. A loading dose of 5,000 to 10,000 U of heparin is indicated for PE.

Failure to achieve adequate heparinization in the first 24 h of treatment has been demonstrated to increase the risk of recurrent emboli. Additionally, less heparin is typically required to maintain adequate anticoagulation after the first low-molecular-weight heparin (LMWH) is an effective subcutaneous therapy for DVT and PE. It is at least as effective as standard heparin therapy in inpatient nonmassive PE and may be cost efficacious. An advantage of LMWH over unfractionated heparin is a decreased incidence of heparin-induced thrombocytopenia. A disadvantage in the critically ill patient, for whom invasive procedures may be required, is that the longer half-life may be problematic. Decreased administration costs and no need for monitoring coagulation in most patients may make LMWH cost efficacious in the appropriate patient group. Thrombocytopenia is uncommon enough that no more than one platelet count is recommended during a treatment period of 5 to 7 days. If therapy is prolonged >7 days, subsequent platelet counts should be done. LMWH does not prolong the aPTT. Anti-factor Xa levels reflect LMWH activity but are not routinely necessary in most treated patients. LMWH dose adjustment is required in patients with renal insufficiency (creatinine clearance of 30 mL/min) in very large persons (>150 kg) or very small persons (<50 kg). Anti-factor Xa levels may be needed to optimize dosing if LMWH is used in these groups. When bleeding occurs after recent administration of LMWH, protamine is recommended for reversal, but the degree of effectiveness in this circumstance is difficult to judge.

It is important to remember that warfarin therapy is contraindicated in pregnancy and anticoagulation should be maintained with heparin. In addition, heparin dosage requirements are increased in pregnancy. Decreases in platelet count (heparin-induced thrombocytopenia [HIT]) may occur with heparin therapy. A nonimmunologically mediated decrease in heparin (HIT-1) may occur, and is usually mild without dramatic drops in platelet count, occurs early in treatment, and does not usually require discontinuation of

heparin. A more dramatic and clinically significant decrease in platelet count (HIT-2) may rarely occur in heparin therapy (days 3 to 4 or earlier with previous heparin exposure), is immunologically mediated, and does require immediate discontinuation of heparin therapy. Arterial thrombosis (white clot) and worsening vs thrombosis may be a part of this more severe syndrome. When the platelet count falls precipitously or in a sustained fashion and HIT-2 is suspected, heparin therapy should be stopped. The addition of a direct thrombin inhibitor at this time to prevent or treat heparin-induced thrombosis is indicated. When the platelet count falls to <100,000/μL, heparin therapy should be stopped. There is a chance for cross-reactivity with LMWH, and that is not advisable as a therapeutic option. Therefore, although LMWH might be chosen as a better option than unfractionated heparin in patients with thrombocytopenia at baseline, once thrombocytopenia occurs on unfractionated heparin, switching to LMWH is not a good option. With HIT-2, warfarin should not be instituted for 2 days because of the possibility of increased clot formation. Since 4 to 5 days may be required to achieve anticoagulation with warfarin in that circumstance, a direct thrombin inhibitor or a heparinoid is recommended to protect in the interim.

Thrombolytic Therapy

Indications for thrombolytic therapy are controversial because thrombolytic therapy has not been proven to alter clinical end points, such as mortality rates in randomized clinical trials. Thrombolytic therapy followed by heparin has, however, been shown to provide more rapid improvement in RV function than heparin alone; therefore, its utility in the face of hemodynamic instability is assumed. Although rarely encountered, persistent hypoxemia despite maximum oxygen supplementation is also an accepted indication.

Streptokinase and recombinant plasminogen activator (rTPA) are both thrombolytic agents for consideration of treatment of PE, although rTPA is almost exclusively used in the United States. Traditional absolute contraindications for thrombolytic therapy are active internal bleeding, recent acute cerebrovascular event (2 months), or recent cerebrovascular procedure (2 months). One report noted, however, the successful use of urokinase thrombolytic therapy of PE in nine neurosurgical patients (mean, 19 days after surgery) with no intracranial hemorrhage (one subgaleal hematoma). Intracranial bleeding, a primary concern, occurs in 1 to 2% of patients with PE who are treated with thrombolytic therapy. Retroperitoneal hemorrhage can also be life threatening, and most frequently occurs as a sequela of previous femoral vein access for pulmonary angiography or other associated femoral lines. Relative contraindications to thrombolytic therapy include any history of cerebrovascular event; a <10-day postpartum period; recent organ biopsy or puncture of a noncompressible vessel; recent serious internal trauma; surgery within the last 7 days; uncontrolled coagulation defects; pregnancy; cardiopulmonary resuscitation with rib fracture; thoracentesis; paracentesis; lumbar puncture; and any other conditions that place the patient at risk for bleeding. In general, angiographic or CTA documentation of PE should be obtained before thrombolytic therapy. Occasionally, thrombolytic therapy may be considered in hemodynamically unstable patients with a high-probability perfusion scan who cannot be moved to receive additional testing. Bedside echocardiography, if immediately available, offers support for diagnosis in this circumstance. When neither angiography, CTA, or perfusion scanning are possible, the patient is at risk for death, and the clinical scenario is strongly suggestive, echocardiography supporting PE should be adequate for initiating therapy. No coagulation tests are typically necessary during thrombolysis. Blood samples should be limited during the thrombolytic agent infusion period. Heparin should not be administered during thrombolysis, but heparin therapy should be resumed without a bolus when the aPTT is 1.5 to 2 times control. If bleeding should occur during thrombolytic therapy, drug should be discontinued (half-life is short). If bleeding should persist, cryoprecipitate infusion or fresh-frozen plasma should be considered.

Although no study has demonstrated thrombolytic therapy-induced improvement in survival or decrease in recurrent thromboembolic events, its use is advocated by some in the presence of large clot burden or especially with echocardiographic evidence of acute RV dilation. This latter argument is based on the fact that RV dysfunction strongly correlates with mortality in patients with PE. Those who argue against thrombolytic use in this circumstance point to the low mortality rate once PE is diagnosed in the presence of RV dysfunction, the absence of studies demonstrating clinical outcome benefit in this group, and the low but potentially catastrophic incidence of intracranial hemorrhage with thrombolytic therapy. One study evaluated 200 consecutive patients with documented PE (diagnosis made by high-probability perfusion scan spiral CT, or angiography) who had echocardiography to document the presence or absence of acute RV dysfunction. Of the 65 normotensive patients with acute RV dysfunction (31% of patients), PE-related shock developed in 6 patients after admission and 3 died. A contrasting study comes to an opposite opinion. Using a retrospective cohort analysis of two matched groups of 64 patients, the study concluded that although thrombolytic therapy improved lung scan more rapidly, there were no differences in recurrences or death rate from PE except increased death rate from bleeding. Another study showed that although thrombolytic therapy of acute RV dysfunction in the absence of hemodynamic instability did not decrease mortality, it did decrease escalation of therapy (institution of vasopressor therapy, intubation/mechanical ventilation, and secondary thrombolysis).

The management of free-floating RV thrombi remains controversial. Echocardiography usually demonstrates evidence of RV overload (>90%), paradoxical interventricular septal motion (75%), and pulmonary hypertension (86%). The clots are usually worm-like, mortality rate is high (45%), and thrombolytic therapy, if not contraindicated, is recommended as the treatment of choice by some investigators. Infusion of a thrombolytic agent directly onto a pulmonary thrombus via the pulmonary artery has never been shown to be superior to infusion of the agent through a peripheral vein. There are some data in the radiology literature that suggest this approach is useful for DVT. The use of thrombolytic agents in PE remains controversial. The American College of Chest Physicians (ACCP) consensus statement on thromboembolism states that the use of thrombolytic agents continues to be highly individualized, and clinicians should have latitude in their use. They are, however, recommended in general for hemodynamic instability and massive ileofemoral thrombosis.

In the United States, the most frequently used thrombolytic agent for the treatment of PE is rTPA. Food and Drug Administration-approved dosing is 100 mg over 2 h. In the patient with massive PE in whom death appears imminent without thrombolytic intervention, more rapid administration may be appropriate. One proposed alternative that seems reasonable in that circumstance is 40 mg over minutes followed by 60 mg over the remainder of the 2-h period. Empiric thrombolytic therapy might be considered in hospitalized patients with sudden unexpected arrest who are at risk for PE and in whom there is no obvious alternative diagnosis. Based on autopsy series, it is estimated that up to 70% of sudden unanticipated in-hospital arrests are due to either PE or acute myocardial infarction, with both diagnoses amenable to treatment with thrombolytic therapy. If the decision is made to administer thrombolytic therapy in this circumstance, the timing and dosing are less clear and best left to the bedside clinician. Timing considerations vary from too early (patient was going to be successfully resuscitated without thrombolytic therapy) to too late (missed opportunity for thrombolytic therapy to make a difference). Dosing considerations for initial front loading vary from 60 to 100% of standard infusion dose as bolus.

IVC Filter

Traditional indications for IVC filter placement include contraindication to anticoagulation, onset of bleeding with anticoagulation, and failure of anticoagulation to abate thromboembolic events. Other indications for filter placement include hemodynamically unstable patients who will not be given thrombolytic therapy and patients with HIT as a bridge to warfarin therapy. Direct thrombin inhibitors, if available, are less invasive and more appropriate alternatives in this situation. The empiric use of IVC filter in patients with a large clot burden or poor cardiopulmonary reserve is more controversial. Filter placement may also be considered in patients with high risk for DVT and relative or absolute contraindications for anticoagulation prophylaxis of DVT. The decision to anticoagulate patients who have had an IVC filter placed is controversial, but the use of anticoagulation may prevent further clot formation and increase the patency rate of the filter over time and, therefore, facilitate venous drainage. Patency can be maintained, however, without concomitant heparin therapy. Documentation of DVT disease is usually required before placement of an IVC filter. This is usually accomplished at the time of filter placement using dye venogram. A filter may also benefit patients at high risk for chronic anticoagulation, such as poorly compliant patients or patients at risk for falls. Complications of filter placement include vessel injury at the time of insertion, subsequent venous thrombosis at the insertion site, filter migration and embolization into the heart, filter erosion through the IVC, and IVC obstruction. There are good data to indicate that one tradeoff of IVC filter ability to decrease PE is subsequent development of femoral vein thrombosis at the site of insertion. Retrievable filters are now available and offer utility in patients who have short-term need for filter and who are expected to return to an active lifestyle. The filter should be removed within several months.

PE-Induced Tissue Hypoperfusion

The right ventricle cannot increase stroke volume in response to sudden increases in afterload. Instead, the right ventricle dilates as ejection fraction decreases. Failure of the right ventricle to compensate for the increased afterload produces hypotension and, if severe, syncope. Studies of hemodynamic profiles in patients with acute PE have demonstrated mean pulmonary artery pressures >40 mm Hg only in patients with pre-existing cardiopulmonary disease, suggesting that the normal right ventricle is incapable of generating pressures >40 mm Hg in the setting of acute pulmonary vascular bed obstruction.

Pulmonary artery catheterization may be useful to optimize therapy in the hypotensive patient, but the catheters may be difficult to pass due to high pulmonary artery resistance and low-flow state. A right atrial pressure (RAP) of approximately 15 to 20 mm Hg is probably optimal. Overdistention of the right ventricle (more likely when mean RAP is >20 mm Hg) may be problematic for several reasons. First, the right ventricle may be made ischemic due to decreased coronary perfusion related to the high RV pressure since perfusion pressure of the right ventricle is approximated by aortic diastolic pressure minus mean RV pressure. With high right-sided pressures, LV compliance may also be decreased as the interventricular septum shifts into the left ventricle.

Based on the above, volume therapy is typically ineffective and may be deleterious, with resultant overdistension of the right ventricle. RV ischemia may be a primary cause or a major contributing factor to hypotension. Therapy should be targeted toward reducing RV afterload (RV work) by reducing pulmonary clot burden, avoiding volume-induced RV overdistension (RAP >20 mm Hg), and maintaining adequate aortic diastolic pressure (upstream filling pressure for the left and right ventricles).

RV contractility may be improved by the use of inotropic drugs. Dopamine at doses beginning at 5 μg/kg/min is the recommended inotrope in the presence of hypotension. Dobutamine may be preferred in the presence of hypoperfusion but absence of hypotension.

Vasopressors may also be beneficial by increasing aortic diastolic pressure when it is critically low. Combination inotrope/vasoconstrictor therapy such as dopamine or norepinephrine is recommended in the hypotensive patient. Vasoconstriction of systemic vascular bed with selective vasodilation of pulmonary vascular bed would be ideal. Inhaled nitric oxide has anecdotally been demonstrated to improve hemodynamics in PE by this mechanism. Benefit could only occur through vasodilation of PE-released humorally mediated vasoconstriction because clot burden-induced increase in pulmonary vascular resistance is not reversible except through dissolution of clot.

Surgical thrombectomy may be considered in situations of severe hemodynamic instability with a contraindication to thrombolytic therapy and close proximity to the operating room. Bypass capability is necessary, and the clinical scenario should indicate a certain or almost certain clinical diagnosis of massive PE. It should also be considered when hemodynamic instability persists despite thrombolytic therapy. Interventional radiology use of mechanical fragmentation may be an alternative to surgery in patients with severe hemodynamic instability and contraindication to thrombolytic therapy.

Prevention of PE

The most powerful statement that can be made for prophylaxis is that, of the patients who die of pulmonary emboli, most patients survive <30 min after the event, which is not long for most forms of treatment to be effective. Without prophylaxis, the frequency of fatal PE is approximately 7% for emergency hip surgery, 2% after elective hip surgery, and 1% after elective surgery. Length of surgery, age, and type of surgery (hip, pelvis, knee, prostate) are important considerations for risk of emboli. Autopsy findings demonstrate that PE causes 5% of deaths in patients receiving mechanical ventilation. The frequency of PE after myocardial infarction in the absence of prophylaxis may be ≤5%. The great majority of patients in the ICU should receive heparin prophylaxis for thromboembolic disease. The dose for general surgical patients or in medical patients is typically 5,000 U bid or tid of unfractionated heparin subcutaneously or LMWH once daily. Hemorrhagic side effects of low-dose heparin are rare (<2%) in patients without hemorrhagic diathesis. High-risk patients or those who have contraindications for heparin should receive intermittent pneumatic venous compression (IPVC), additively or as a replacement, respectively. Low-dose LMWH is the heparin of choice in knee surgery patients, hip surgery patients, and CNS trauma patients. It also offers the advantage of one injection vs three in all patients.

Recent reports of epidural hematoma after LMWH use in patients who have had epidural puncture should alert the physician to this potential complication with any anticoagulation in place, independent of type. IPVC is a nonpharmacologic prophylaxis alternative for knee surgery. IPVC is contraindicated in the face of arterial compromise of extremity. IPVC can be added to heparin prophylaxis in patients with additive risk factors. In high-risk patients such as those undergoing elective hip surgery, the use of either LMWH, adjusted-dose unfractionated heparin targeting heparin to prolong mid-dosing prothrombin time measurement by 4 to 5 s, or low-dose warfarin is recommended. Low-dose warfarin can be instituted at 1 mg/d beginning 21 days before elective surgery and continuing through the postoperative hospitalization. For hip fracture surgery, LMWH or full-dose warfarin (international normalized ratio, 2.0 to 3.0) is recommended.

Clinically significant DVT develops in many trauma cases. Risk factors include advanced age, prolonged immobilization, severe head trauma, paralysis, pelvic and lower-extremity fractures, direct venous trauma, shock, and multiple transfusions. Low-dose heparin or IPVC may not be effective in the highest-risk patient. In trauma patients at high risk for bleeding and those at high risk for pulmonary emboli, prophylactic IVC filter placement has been recommended by some investigators, especially if leg injury prevents application of pneumatic compression devices. Similar rationale has been offered when PE is diagnosed in advanced malignancy. Neither of these uses has been validated.

One study demonstrated that only 52% of hospitalized patients who had documented PE had received prophylactic therapy. Obviously, better prophylactic alternatives are needed.

Summary

PE is a treatable condition with a nonspecific clinical presentation that makes diagnosis difficult. CT scanning has become the primary diagnostic test. Predictive capability of negative CT findings in higher-risk patients is enhanced by additional studies (nonelevated d-dimer, negative leg ultrasound, and low-probability perfusion scan). Occasionally, pulmonary angiography is necessary. Thrombolytic therapy is indicated in patients with hemodynamic instability and no contraindications.

Annotated Bibliography

ACCP Consensus Committee on Pulmonary Embolism. Opinions regarding the diagnosis and management of venous thromboembolic disease. Chest 1998; 113:499–504
Question-and-answer format for controversial areas of VTE management.

Arcelus JI, Monreal M, Caprini JA, et al. Clinical presentation and time-course of postoperative venous thromboembolism: Results from the RIETE Registry. Thromb Haemost 2008; 99:546–551
Getting a grasp on incidence and timing of post-operative pulmonary embolism.

Baile EM, King GG, Müller NL, et al. Spiral computed tomography is comparable to angiography for the diagnosis of pulmonary embolism. Am J Respir Crit Care Med 2000; 161:1010–1015
Pig model using colored methacrylate beads and postmortem methacrylate casting showing no difference in diagnosis of subsegmental clot between angiography and spiral CT.

Bernardi E, Camporese G, Buller HR, et al. Serial 2-Point ultrasonography plus D-dimer vs whole-leg-color-coded Doppler ultrasonography for diagnosing suspected symptomatic deep vein thrombosis. A randomized controlled trial. JAMA 2008; 300:1653–1659
Mixing and matching ultrasound and D-dimer. Where is the value?

Böttiger B, Eike M. Thrombolytic therapy during cardiopulmonary resuscitation and the role of coagulation activation after cardiac arrest. Curr Opin Crit Care 2001; 7:176–183

Brender E. Use of emboli-blocking filters increases, but rigorous data are lacking. JAMA 2006; 295:989–990
Retrievable IVC filters are experiencing increased utility despite limited trials that would allow higher level of evidence for their utility. This is a nice concise review of where we stand with retrievable filters.

Dalen JE, Banas JS, Brooks HL, et al. Resolution rate of acute pulmonary embolism in man. N Engl J Med 1969; 280:1194–1199
No resolution of PE by angiogram before day 14.

Dong B, Jirong Y, Wag Q, et al. Thrombolytic therapy for pulmonary embolism. Cochrane Database Syst Rev 2006; (2):CD004437
This is a Cochrane metaanalysis of thrombolytic therapy for PE that, although heavy with methods, still offers significant clinical information.

Elliott CG, Goldhaber SZ, Visani L, et al. Chest radiographs in acute pulmonary embolism. Chest 2000; 118:33–38
Review of chest radiographs in 2,454 patients with diagnosis of PE. Cardiomegaly (27%) was most common abnormal finding, as well as the most common finding; 24% were normal.

Fedullo PF, Tapson VF. The evaluation of suspected pulmonary embolism. N Engl J Med 2003; 349:1247–1256
General review on diagnosis with algorithms.

Gibson NS, Sohne M, Gerdes VEA, et al. The importance of clinical probability assessment in interpreting a normal d-Dimer in patients with suspected pulmonary embolism. Chest 2008; 134:789–793
Pre-test clinical probability important for D-dimer interpretation as well.

Giordano A, Angiolillo DJ. Current role of lung scintigraphy in pulmonary embolism. Q J Nucl Med 2001; 45:294–301
A view on utility of perfusion lung scanning from the nuclear medicine side.

Goldhaber SZ. Pulmonary embolism. N Engl J Med 1998; 339:93–104
Medical intelligence review article of PE management.

Goldhaber SZ. Unsolved issues in the treatment of pulmonary embolism. Thromb Res 2001; 103:V245–V255
Highlights areas of ongoing uncertainty.

Goodacre S, Sutton AJ, Sampson FC. Meta-analysis: the value of clinical assessment in the diagnosis of deep venous thrombosis. Ann Intern Med 2005; 143: 129–139
This article evaluates the potential utility of individual single clinical variables vs pooled estimates of risk for DVT; it supports use of pooled estimates, such as the Wells score and limited value of individual variables.

Goodman LR. Venous thromboembolic disease: CT evaluation. Q J Nucl Med 2001; 45:302–310
Points to improving ability to use CT results in decision making.

Goodman LR, Lipchik RJ, Kuzo RS et al. Subsequent pulmonary embolism: risk after a negative helical CT pulmonary angiogram: prospective comparison with scintigraphy. Radiology 2000; 215:535–542

Grifoni S, Olivotto I, Cecchini P, et al. Short-term clinical outcome of patients with acute pulmonary embolism, normal blood pressure, and echocardiographic right ventricular dysfunction. JAMA 2000; 101: 2817–2822
Demonstrated significant morbidity and mortality developing in patients with PE, acute RV dysfunction, and initial hemodynamic stability.

Hamel E, Pacouret G, Vincentelli D, et al. Thrombolysis or heparin therapy in massive pulmonary embolism with right ventricular dilation: results from a 128-patient monocenter registry. Chest 2001; 120:6–8
Two retrospective cohort massive PE groups were matched with the exception of thrombolytic therapy. Although lung scan improved more rapidly in the thrombolytic group, there were no differences in recurrent PE with increased bleeding deaths in the thrombolytic group.

Hermsen JL, Ibele AR, Faucher LD, et al. Retrievable inferior vena cava filters in high-risk trauma and surgical patients: factors influencing successful removal. World J Surg 2008; 32:1444–1449
Useful information on safety data as well as thought on timing of removal.

Janata K, Holzer M, Kürkciyan I, et al. Major bleeding complications in cardiopulmonary resuscitation: the place of thrombolytic therapy in cardiac arrest due to massive pulmonary embolism. Resuscitation 2003; 57:49–55

Jerges-Sanchez C, Ramirez-Rivera A, Garcia M, et al. Streptokinase and heparin versus heparin alone in massive pulmonary embolism: a randomized control trial. J Thromb Thrombolysis 1995; 2:227–229
Paper occasionally used to justify utility of thrombolytic therapy in massive PE and value of streptokinase in particular; however, there were only four patients in each group. Furthermore, all four patients in the thrombolytic therapy group had PE diagnosed in the emergency department of the hospital performing the study, while all four patients in the heparin-only group were transferred to that institution from other hospitals with recurrent PE receiving heparin.

Johnson MS. Current strategies for the diagnosis of pulmonary embolus. J Vasc Interv Radiol 2002; 13: 13–23
General review of diagnostic modalities available for diagnoses and their severity and specificity.

Kearon C, Kahn SR, Agnelli G, et al. Antithrombotic therapy for venous thromboembolic disease. Chest 2008; 133(suppl):454S–545S

Konstantinides S. Acute pulmonary embolism. N Engl J Med 2008; 359:2804-2813
A very good case based study highlighting key concepts of management.

Konstantinides S, Geibel A, Heuset G, et al. Heparin plus alteplace compared with heparin alone in patients with submassive pulmonary embolism N Engl J Med 2002; 347:1143–1150
Primary thrombolytic therapy decreased subsequent death and use of vasopressors/mechanical ventilation/secondary thrombolysis as a combined end point but no difference in mortality.

Kürkciyan I, Meron G, Sterz F, et al. Pulmonary embolism as cause of cardiac arrest. Arch Intern Med 2000; 160:1529–1535
These three articles address the issue of the use of thrombolytic therapy in the situation of cardiac arrest. PE is one of the primary diagnoses in the differential diagnosis of unexpected cardiac arrest in the hospital. Thrombolytic therapy

not only might offer potential utility if the arrest was due to PE but also with acute myocardial infarction. These three articles assess the empiric use of thrombolytic therapy in patients who do not quickly respond to resuscitation;10% salvage rate when rTPA is administered to patients with either confirmed PE or those highly likely to have PE.

Landefeld CS. Noninvasive diagnosis of deep vein thrombosis. JAMA 2008; 300:1696-1697

Concise update on value and limitations of ultrasound diagnosis of DVT.

Lorut C, Ghossains M, Horellou MH, et al. A non-invasive diagnostic strategy including spiral computed tomography in patients with suspected pulmonary embolism. Am J Respir Crit Care Med 2000; 162:1413–1418

A protocol was used for evaluation and decision as to presence or absence of PE using CT, Q scan, and d-dimer. Ultrasound was used in middle-ground situation as a final decision maker. Only 1.7% of untreated patients had PE over next 3 months.

McConnell MV, Solomon SD, Fayan ME, et al. Regional right ventricular dysfunction detected by echocardiography in acute pulmonary embolism. Am J Cardiol 1996; 78:469–473

The finding of abnormal wall motion in RV mid-free wall and normal motion in apex was very predictive of PE among patients with acute symptoms and evidence of pulmonary artery hypertension.

Meneveau N, Séronde MF, Blonde MC, et al. Management of unsuccessful thrombolysis in acute massive pulmonary embolism. Chest 2006; 129:1043–1050

This article offers a perspective on surgical embolectomy following failed thrombolysis.

Miniati M, Pistolesi M, Maseri C, et al. Value of perfusion lung scan in the diagnosis of pulmonary embolism: results of the Prospective Investigative Study of Adult Pulmonary Embolism Diagnosis (PISA-PED). Am J Respir Crit Care Med 1996; 154:1387–1393

Studied the use of perfusion scanning/chest radiograph analysis without ventilation scanning in 890 consecutive patients with suspected PE. Abnormal scan findings were considered PE positive if scans demonstrated one or more wedge-shaped perfusion defects, and PE if they did not. Sensitivity was 92% (most patients with angiographically proven PE had PE-positive scans) and specificity was 87% (most patients without angiographically proven PE had PE-negative scans). The addition of pretest clinical probability further heightened predictive capability.

Molina JE, Hunter DW, Yedlicka JW, et al. Thrombolytic therapy for post-operative pulmonary embolism.

Am J Surg 1992; 163:375–380

Thirteen patients within 2 weeks of surgery (mean, 9.6 days) used modified urokinase regimen to demonstrate complete lysis of PE with no bleeding complications.

Musset D, Parent F, Meyer G, et al. Diagnostic strategy for patients with suspected pulmonary embolism: a prospective multicentre outcome study: Lancet 2002; 360:1914–1920

Nijeuter M, Hovens MM, Davidson BL, et al. Resolution of thromboemboli in patients with acute pulmonary embolism. Chest 2006; 129:192–197

For the first time in 30 years, another look at thromboemboli resolution; this could be of great utility in patients referred from another institution, already having received therapy, and with the diagnosis of PE in doubt.

Pandey AS, Rakowski H, Mickleborough LL, et al. Right heart pulmonary embolism in transit: a review of therapeutic considerations. Can J Cardiol 1997; 13:397–402

This article presents the challenges of reacting to the presence of right-heart clot on ultrasound as it is pertinent to decision making in patients with PE. This finding is particularly problematic in the unstable patient and the patient with contraindication to thrombolytic therapy.

Perrier A, Howarth N, Didier D, et al. Performance of helical computed tomography in unselected outpatients with suspected pulmonary embolism. Ann Intern Med 2001; 135:88–97

Quinlan DJ, McQuillan A, Eikelboom JW. Low-molecular-weight heparin compared with intravenous unfractionated heparin for treatment of pulmonary embolism. Ann Intern Med 2004; 140:175–183

Quinn DA, Fogel RB, Smith CD, et al. D-dimers in the diagnosis of pulmonary embolism: Am J Respir Crit Care Med 1999; 159:1445–1449

Nonelevated d-dimers make PE very unlikely, while elevated d-dimers were not useful.

Rathbun SW, Raskob GE, Whitwett TL. Sensitivity and specificity of helical computed tomography in the diagnosis of pulmonary embolism: a systematic review. Ann Intern Med 2000; 132:227–232

A review of the 15 prospective English-language studies of use of helical (spiral) CT in the diagnosis of PE found that only two studies had consecutive patients, 8 studies had independently interpreted angiogram and CT, and only 1 study included a broad spectrum of patients; the review concluded that there are not currently enough data to support withholding of heparin after negative spiral CT findings without additional testing. Large prospective trials are needed.

Rathburn SW, Whitsett TL, Veseley SK, et al. Clinical utility of d-dimer in patients with suspected pulmonary embolism and nondiagnostic lung scans or negative CT findings. Chest 2004; 125:851–855

This study, done at an academic health center, supports the limited use of plasma d-dimer for decision making in patients with clinically suspected PE and nondiagnostic lung scans or negative helical CT studies.

Ryu JH, Swensen SJ, Olson EJ, et al. Diagnosis of pulmonary embolism with use of computed tomographic angiography. Mayo Clin 2001; 76:59–65

General review of role of CT scanning in PE.

Segal JB, Strieff MB, Hoffman LV, et al. Management of venous thromboembolism: a systematic review for a practice guideline. Ann Intern Med 2007; 146: 211–222

This is a systematic review done as a practice guideline that addresses numerous important, but infrequently addressed questions with PE, such as outpatient therapy, utility of LMWH, catheter-directed thrombolysis, and recurrence of PE after IVC filter placement.

Severi P, LoPinto G, Doggio R, et al. Urokinase thrombolytic therapy of pulmonary embolism in neurosurgical patients. Surg Neurol 1994; 42:469–470

Nine neurosurgery patients (mean, 19 days following surgery) received urokinase; all survived; no intracranial hemorrhage; one subgaleal hemorrhage.

Stein PD, Afzal A, Henry JW, et al. Fever in pulmonary embolism. Chest 2000; 117:39–42

Demonstrated no source of fever (temperature > 100.0°F) other than PE in 14% of patients with angiographically documented PE. Fever correlated with DVT but not with infarction. Only 2 of 268 patients had temperatures > 103.0°F.

Stein PD, Athanasoulis C, Alavi A, et al. Complications and validity of pulmonary angiography in acute pulmonary embolism. Circulation 1992; 85:462–468

Interobserver radiologist agreement on angiographic diagnosis of PE: lobar, 98%; segmental, 90%; subsegmental, 66%.

Stein PD, Fowler SE, Goodman LR, et al. Multidetector computed tomography for acute pulmonary embolism. N Engl J Med 2006; 354:2317–2327

This is the report of the PIOPED II study, which looked at the positive and negative predictive power of spiral CT in predicting presence or absence of PE. The "gold standard" was diagnosis by high-probability or normal ventilation/perfusion scan, positive leg ultrasound, or positive to negative digital subtraction angiography. This report points to the value of spiral CT with the exception of discordance between clinical suspicion and test results.

Stein PD, Huang H, Afzal A, et al. Incidence of acute pulmonary embolism in a general hospital. Chest 1999; 116:909–913

Women > 50 years old, but not women < 50 years old, have greater incidence of PE than men.

Tajima H, Murata S, Kumazaki T, et al. Hybrid treatment of acute massive pulmonary thromboembolism: mechanical fragmentation with a modified rotating pigtail catheter, local fibrinolytic therapy, and clot aspiration followed by systemic fibrinolytic therapy. AJR Am J Roentgenol 2004; 183:589–595

Mechanical fragmentation of clot with local fibrinolysis and manual clot aspiration are interventions that may be of utility in some patients with life-threatening PE. This article offers perspective on how this technology might be utilized.

Tapson VF, Carroll BA, Davidson BL, et al. The diagnostic approach to acute venous thromboembolism: clinical practice guidelines. Am J Respir Crit Care Med 1999; 160:1043–1066

Comprehensive clinical practice guideline for the diagnosis and treatment of DVT and PE; extensive discussion of DVT diagnostic strategy; also very good review on utility and risk of pulmonary angiography.

The PIOPED Investigators. Value of the ventilation/perfusion scan in acute pulmonary embolism: results of the Prospective Investigation of Pulmonary Embolism Diagnosis (PIOPED). JAMA 1990; 263:2753–2759

The article includes a discussion of the use of Bayes theorem, as well as the role of the previous cardiopulmonary disease and previous PE in reliability of scanning.

van Strijen MJL, de Monye W, Schiereck J, et al. Single-detector helical computed tomography as the primary diagnostic test in suspected pulmonary embolism: a multicenter clinical management study of 510 patients. Ann Intern Med 2003; 138:307–314

Verstraete M, Miller GAH, Bounameaus H, et al. Intravenous and intrapulmonary recombinant tissue-type plasminogen activator in the treatment of acute massive pulmonary embolism. Circulation 1988; 77:353–360

Demonstrated no beneficial effect of thrombolytic therapy infused into pulmonary artery versus peripheral administration.

Wells PS, Owen C, Doucette S, et al. Does this patient have deep vein thrombosis? JAMA 2006; 295:199–207

D-dimer of limited value with high clinical suspicion.

Wiegand UKH, Kurowski V, Giannitsis E, et al. Effectiveness of end-tidal carbon dioxide tension for monitoring of thrombolytic therapy in acute pulmonary embolism. Crit Care Med 2000; 28:3588–3592

End-tidal CO_2 decreases as thrombolytic therapy improves hemodynamics as indicator of decreased dead space.

Wood KE. Major pulmonary embolism: review of a pathophysiologic approach to the golden hour of hemodynamically significant pulmonary embolism. Chest 2002; 121:877–905

Excellent general review devoted to massive PE.

Notes

Weaning From Ventilatory Support

Scott K. Epstein, MD, FCCP

Objectives:

- Learn readiness testing using clinical factors and weaning predictors
- Discuss use of spontaneous breathing trials to test readiness
- Review causes of weaning failure
- Understand use of modes of progressive withdrawal and application of weaning protocols
- Describe weaning patients with prolonged mechanical ventilation

Key words: extubation; mechanical ventilation; reintubation; respiratory failure; weaning

Invasive mechanical ventilation reverses some causes of acute respiratory failure while providing crucial ventilatory support as the respiratory system recovers from the initial insult. There is a tradeoff because invasive mechanical ventilation is associated with substantial complications including ventilator-associated pneumonia, sinusitis, airway injury, thromboembolism, and gastrointestinal bleeding.[1] Increasing duration of mechanical ventilation is associated with increased mortality.[2] Once significant clinical improvement occurs, the clinician should focus on rapidly removing the patient from the ventilator.

The terms *weaning, liberation,* and *discontinuation* have been used to describe the process of freeing the patient from the ventilator.[3,4] The weaning process can be further described as a continuum stretching from onset of acute respiratory failure through discharge from the hospital.[5] An early step is "readiness testing," recognizing that respiratory failure has partially or totally resolved, respiratory muscle function has improved, and the patient is ready to breathe spontaneously. A number of studies demonstrates that respiratory therapists and ICU nurses can effectively implement readiness testing. Approximately three of every four patients meeting readiness criteria tolerate spontaneous breathing (without ventilator assistance or on low levels of support) indicating

that mechanical support is no longer required.[6–8] Approximately one in four patients fail to tolerate spontaneous breathing and require a more prolonged process. For these patients, weaning consumes 40 to 60% of the total ventilator time.[9,10] Successful weaning depends on identifying and correcting treatable causes for weaning failure. Once the patient tolerates spontaneous breathing, the clinician must address whether the patient is ready for extubation (Fig 1).

A new classification of the weaning process had been suggested, although not yet prospectively validated.[5] *Simple weaning* refers to those who tolerate their first spontaneous breathing trial (SBT) and are successfully extubated, all without difficulty. Approximately 70% of patients fall into this category. *Difficult weaning* refers to failure to tolerate the initial SBT with a need for up to three SBTs or taking up to 7 days from first SBT to successful weaning. Prolonged weaning is defined by a failure of at least three SBTs or taking >7 days after the first SBT. Thirty percent experience difficult and prolonged weaning and these patients experience higher mortality than simple weaning.

A considerable evidence base is now available to assist the clinician in making weaning and extubation decisions. Readers are referred to the published results of two recent consensus conferences.[5,11]

Readiness Testing: Using Clinical Factors and Weaning Predictors

Rapid weaning must be weighed against the risks of allowing a patient to breathe spontaneously before he or she is ready. Those risks include precipitating cardiac dysfunction, psychological discouragement, and respiratory muscle fatigue or structural injury. When mechanical ventilation results from a rapidly reversible cause such as drug overdose or cardiogenic pulmonary edema, readiness testing can start within hours of intubation. In contrast, with other causes of acute respiratory

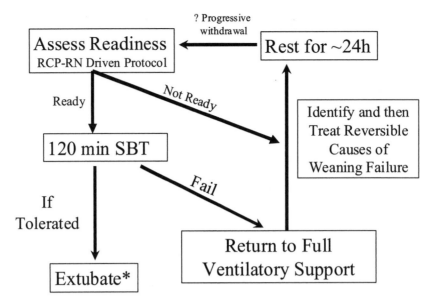

Figure 1. Overview of weaning. *Extubation is carried out if the patient has no evidence of upper airway obstruction, is without excessive airway secretions, and has an adequate cough (see text for details). RCP = respiratory care practitioner; ICU-RN = intensive care unit nurse; SBT= spontaneous breathing trial.

failure the clinician should employ full ventilatory support and respiratory muscle rest for 24 to 48 h before readiness testing. Because subjective assessment is notoriously inaccurate in determining readiness, objective criteria are used as surrogate markers of recovery (Table 1). Objective criteria should serve as guidelines rather than inflexible standards as many patients *never* satisfying objective readiness criteria are still successfully weaned.[12] Similarly, studies have noted that neither depressed neurologic status nor anemia necessarily preclude successful liberation from the ventilator.

Many objective physiologic tests (weaning parameters) have been studied as predictors of readiness for spontaneous breathing (Table 2). Numerous design problems, inflating the accuracy of weaning predictors, have been identified.[11,13,14] These problems include, for example, weaning predictors were used *a priori* to determine which patients undergo weaning, methodology of predictor measurement differs between studies and displays large coefficients of variations, insufficient blinding of physicians determining weaning tolerance, and absence of objective criteria to determine weaning tolerance.

To be clinically useful weaning predictors should accelerate liberation from mechanical ventilation while avoiding the adverse consequences of

Table 1. *Criteria Used to Determine Readiness for Trials of Spontaneous Breathing**

Required Criteria

1. Pao_2/Fio_2 ratio, $\geq 150^{\dagger}$ or $Sao_2 \geq 90\%$ on $Fio_2 \leq 40\%$ and (PEEP), ≤ 5 cm H_2O
2. Hemodynamic stability (no or low-dose vasopressor medications)

Additional Criteria (optional criteria)

1. Weaning parameters: respiratory rate ≤ 35 breaths/min, spontaneous tidal volume > 5 mL/kg, negative inspiratory force < -20 to -25 cm H_2O, f/Vt, 105 breaths/L/min
2. Hemoglobin, ≥ 8–10 mg/dL
3. Core temperature, ≤ 38–38.5°C
4. Mental status awake and alert or easily arousable

---

*Sao_2 = arterial oxygen saturation.
†A threshold of $Pao_2/Fio_2 \geq 120$ can be used for patients with chronic hypoxemia. Some patients require higher levels of PEEP to avoid atelectasis during mechanical ventilation.

failed weaning trials. Unfortunately, an evidence-based systematic review identified few predictors associated with clinically significant changes in the probability of weaning success or failure.[11,13,14] Only five predictors measured during ventilatory support had possible value in predicting weaning outcome, but predictive capacity was either relatively weak or inadequately studied.[14] The frequency/tidal volume ratio, f/Vt, measured during the initial few minutes of spontaneous unassisted breathing, was more accurate but,

Table 2. *Weaning Predictors**

Measurements of oxygenation and dead space
 Pao_2/Fio_2
 Pao_2/Pao_2
 Dead space (V_D/V_T)
Simple tests of respiratory load and muscular capacity
 Negative inspiratory force (maximal inspiratory pressure)[†]
 Respiratory system compliance and resistance
 Minute ventilation[†]
 Maximal voluntary ventilation
 Vital capacity
 Respiratory frequency[†]
 Tidal volume[†]
Tests that integrate more than one measurement
 f/V_T[†]
 CROP index (compliance, respiratory rate, oxygenation, pressure)[†]
Complex measurements (usually require special equipment)
 Airway occlusion pressure
 P0.1/MIP[†]
 Esophageal pressure measurements
 Oxygen cost of breathing, work of breathing
 Gastric intramucosal pH

*Pao_2 = partial pressure of arterial oxygen; MIP = maximal inspiratory pressure.
[†]Predictors found to be most accurate in a systematic review.[14]

Table 3. *Criteria Indicating That a Patient Is Not Tolerating a Trial of Spontaneous Breathing**

Objective criteria
 $Sao_2 < 0.90$ or $Pao_2 < 60$ mm Hg on $Fio_2 > 0.40$–0.50 or $Pao_2/Fio_2 < 150$
 Increase in $Paco_2 > 10$ mm Hg or decrease in pH > 0.10
 Respiratory rate > 35 breaths/min
 Heart rate > 140 beats/min or an increase $> 20\%$ of baseline
 Systolic BP < 90 mm Hg or > 160 mm Hg or change of $> 20\%$ from baseline
Subjective criteria
 Presence of signs of increased work of breathing, including thoracoabdominal paradox or excessive use of accessory respiratory muscles
 Presence of other signs of distress such as diaphoresis or agitation

*Sao_2 = arterial oxygen saturation.

unfortunately, associated with only a moderate change in the probability of success or failure. Performance of a weaning predictor also depends on how the test is performed. As an example, the f/V_T measured during pressure support or continuous positive airway pressure will be lower than that determined on T-piece.[15] An analysis of studies of the f/V_T found a sensitivity of 0.87 and concluded that the wide range of pretest probability of success explained much of the heterogeneity in performance of this test.[16] Yet the more important question is whether the f/V_T, or any weaning predictor, facilitates weaning decision making and improves outcome. One study randomized 304 patients who required mechanical ventilation for at least 24 h.[17] All patients underwent a five-component daily screen, including, Pao_2/fraction of inspired oxygen (Fio_2), positive end-expiratory pressure (PEEP), hemodynamic stability, mental status, adequate cough, and the f/V_T. Those passing the screen automatically underwent a 2-h SBT, and were then considered for extubation if the SBT was tolerated. Based on randomization, in one group the f/V_T was not used for weaning decision making, while in the other only patients with

$f/V_T < 105$ breaths/L/min underwent an SBT. The group randomized to use of the f/V_T experiences took longer to wean from the ventilator. This result may derive either from the limited predicted value of weaning predictors or from the inherent safety of a closely monitored SBT. Along those lines, Laghi et al[18] used phrenic nerve stimulation and found that low-frequency fatigue did not occur in patients failing a T-piece trial. The key is that patients were returned to ventilatory support as soon as signs of weaning intolerance occurred (Table 3). It is likely that fatigue, and possibly structural respiratory muscle injury, would ensue if the failed weaning trial was unduly extended.

Support for the principle outlined here comes from the recently published Awakening and Breathing Controlled (ABC) trial.[19] The authors successfully used SBT screening criteria that did not include weaning predictors. Indeed, they used very liberal oxygenation criteria (oxygen saturation measured by pulse oximetry, $\geq 88\%$ on $Fio_2 \leq 0.5$; PEEP ≤ 8 cm H_2O) finding that $> 50\%$ tolerated the resulting SBT. These findings strongly indicate that patients are ready to breathe on their own earlier than detected by conventional criteria.

Readiness Testing: The Spontaneous Breathing Trial

Direct extubation after satisfying readiness criteria alone is unwise, as 40% of such patients require reintubation.[20] Therefore a *trial of spontaneous breathing (SBT) is strongly recommended.* The SBT can be performed on low-level pressure support (PSV, ≤7 mm Hg), continuous positive airway pressure (CPAP), or unassisted through a T-piece. Advocates of T-piece maintain that it best estimates work of breathing after extubation. In contrast, it has been argued that PSV more effectively counterbalances endotracheal tube-related resistive workload, although the level required varies from 3 to 14 cm H_2O and is challenging to determine noninvasively.[21] Not surprisingly, a given PSV level may either over- or undercompensate for imposed work. CPAP can improve ventilator triggering in the setting of significant intrinsic PEEP. Automatic tube compensation (ATC) has been advocated as it adjusts PSV level based on tube characteristics. Randomized controlled trials (RCTs)[6,22,23] comparing pressure support to T-piece and CPAP to T-piece have shown the techniques to be essentially equivalent in terms of successful weaning and extubation. One study[25] found no difference comparing ATC, PSV, and T-piece,[24] while another found a trend for better SBT success for ATC (96% vs 85% with CPAP). An observational study[26] examined 31 patients who failed a 30-min T-tube trial and were immediately placed on a 30-min trial of PSV at 7 cm H_2O. Ten of these patients failed the PSV trial, but 21 could be extubated, 17 of them successfully. Practical advantages to conducting an SBT through the ventilator include there is no additional equipment is required, ventilator alarm and monitoring systems promptly identify weaning intolerance, and there is rapid reinstitution of ventilatory support, if needed.

In general, tolerance for a 120-min SBT indicates that a patient no longer requires ventilatory support. One study, examining only the initial SBT attempt, found no difference in success rate comparing patients randomized to either 30 or 120 min of T-piece breathing.[7] A smaller study compared 30 or 120 min SBT of PSV at 7 cm H_2O after a weaning strategy of progressive decrease in pressure support.[27] There was no difference in the percentage of patients passing the SBT; although it did not reach statistical significance, twice as many patients were extubated after 30 min of PSV required reintubation. The ideal duration for the SBT may depend on the duration of ventilation or

the underlying cause for respiratory failure. As an example, a study of 75 patients with COPD, ventilated for at least 15 days, found a *median* time to trial failure of 120 min.[28]

Careful assessment during an SBT is based on both objective and subjective criteria, although these have not been rigorously validated (Table 3). Some criteria are nonspecific (tachypnea, tachycardia) and may reflect processes other than physiologic weaning intolerance (*eg*, anxiety). The criteria may be insufficiently sensitive in detecting incipient respiratory failure: some patients satisfying criteria for weaning tolerance may demonstrate more sophisticated indicators of respiratory dysfunction followed by postextubation respiratory failure.[29]

Pathophysiology of Weaning Failure

Fifteen to 35% of patients fail their initial SBT and should undergo a thorough investigation trying to identify, and treat, reversible factors (Fig 2). Adequate oxygenation (*eg*, Pao_2/Fio_2 ratio >150) is a prerequisite for initiating SBTs; thus, hypoxemia is an unusual cause for weaning failure. When hypoxemia ensues during weaning, another underlying mechanism for failure should be sought.

Depressed central respiratory drive (oversedation, neurologic process) can delay weaning initiation or lead to weaning intolerance. Indeed, as a consequence of capacity-load imbalance, patients with weaning failure usually manifest elevated respiratory drive, detected by an elevated airway occlusion pressure (P0.1).[30] Excessive load may be imposed by the endotracheal tube, heat and moisture exchange devices, or the ventilator tubing and valves.[31,32] Intrinsic factors are more commonly responsible. As an example, a study of 31 patients with COPD found that the patients failing the SBT had higher loads (increased resistance, elastance, and intrinsic PEEP) at SBT onset, and these progressively increased until the trial was terminated.[33] Rapid shallow breathing was noted, resulting in more dynamic hyperinflation, intrinsic PEEP, and increased inspiratory work. Another investigation of 30 patients with acute respiratory failure used each patient as his or her own control and observed markedly elevated inspiratory loads and reduced respiratory muscle capacity

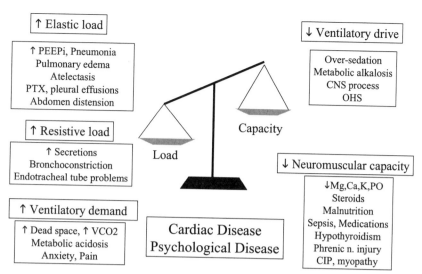

Figure 2. Potential causes of weaning failure. PEEPi = intrinsic positive end-expiratory pressure; PTX = pneumothorax; V_{CO_2} = carbon dioxide production; CNS = central nervous system; OHS = obesity hypoventilation syndrome; Mg^+ = magnesium; Ca^{++} = calcium; K^+ = potassium; PO_4^- = phosphorus; CIP = critical illness polyneuropathy.

during weaning failure compared with observations made at the time of weaning success.[34]

Reduced respiratory muscle strength is frequently seen in patients with weaning intolerance. This may occur from decreased diaphragmatic pressure generation secondary to dynamic hyperinflation, phrenic nerve injury after cardiac surgery, critical illness neuromyopathy,[35,36] respiratory muscle remodeling secondary to inactivity or muscle atrophy (especially with neuromuscular blocking agents),[37,38] the effects of endocrinopathy (*eg*, hypothyroidism, adrenal insufficiency), or malnutrition.[39,40]

Older studies[11] have suggested that respiratory muscle fatigue was an important manifestation of weaning failure. But rapid shallow breathing and thoracoabdominal paradox have been observed to appear immediately after ventilator disconnection and do not progress during failed weaning, suggesting a response to increased loading rather than fatigue.[41] This hypothesis is supported by the observation that healthy subjects breathing against an inspiratory load develop thoracoabdominal paradox in the absence of fatigue.[42] In contrast, other studies[33,34] noted that patients with weaning intolerance demonstrated a tension-time index above the 0.15 threshold at which respiratory muscle fatigue occurs in healthy subjects. Using the twitch occlusion and magnetic stimulation, Laghi et al[18] found that patients intolerant of a

well-monitored SBT failed to develop evidence for low-frequency respiratory muscle fatigue.

Cardiac disease can cause weaning intolerance via a number of mechanisms. Increased work of breathing, or the associated release in catecholamines, can cause myocardial ischemia (detected by nuclear technique or continuous ECG monitoring).[43-45] The transition from positive-pressure ventilation to spontaneous (negative pressure) breathing can increase left ventricular preload and afterload, elevating transmural pulmonary artery occlusion pressure and causing pulmonary edema.[46] Patients intolerant of SBTs often fail to appropriately increase cardiac output and stroke volume during the trial.[47,48]

Patients at risk for the latter may demonstrate an elevated brain natriuretic peptide (BNP)[49] or N-terminal pro-BNP50 prior to the weaning trial or an elevated N-terminal pro-BNP at the end of the trial. In one study,[49] a pre-SBT BNP of > 275 pg/dL correlated with a longer duration of weaning. A decrease in left ventricular ejection fraction has been observed in COPD patients undergoing T-piece trials, an effect that can be partially offset by the use of pressure support.[51] The stress of weaning is considerable as it results in increased levels of plasma insulin, cortisol, and glucose.[52] Lastly, positive fluid balance has been associated with weaning failure.[53]

Psychological factors can limit weaning but few data exist to define how often this occurs.

Delirium is present in the majority of ventilated patient and its presence is correlated with prolonged duration of intubation.[54] A confounding factor is that criteria used to indicate weaning intolerance (eg, agitation, diaphoresis, tachycardia, and tachypnea) are also manifestations of anxiety or psychological distress. Nevertheless, small uncontrolled reports found that biofeedback, relaxation techniques, hypnosis, or therapy for depression contributed to successful weaning.[55]

Modes of Progressive Withdrawal

Once the reversible factors causing weaning intolerance have been addressed, further efforts to discontinue mechanical ventilation are indicated (Table 4). One issue is how long to rest a patient after a failed weaning effort. In the most common clinical scenario, when clinical evidence of respiratory muscle fatigue is absent, multiple daily attempts may be appropriate. As an example, a large RCT found no difference in outcome for patients given multiple daily SBTs and those given a single daily trial.[56] In contrast, if evidence for fatigue is evident, then 24 h of rest

on full support should precede the next weaning effort.[57] Interestingly, comparison of data from two international surveys indicates that fewer ICUs are employing multiple daily SBTs than in the past.[2,58]

The clinician must next decide whether to perform another SBT or whether to more gradually reduce ventilatory support (progressive withdrawal). The latter approach theoretically slowly shifts work from ventilator to patient. It remains unproven whether this process reconditions (or trains) the respiratory muscles or simply allows time needed for recovery (eg, reduction in respiratory load or increased respiratory muscle strength and endurance). Two large multicenter RCTs directly compared progressive withdrawal techniques in patients who satisfied readiness criteria but failed to tolerate a 2-h SBT.[56,59] One study found T-piece to be superior and the other found PSV the most efficient. Differences in patient populations and study design may explain the contrasting results. These studies demonstrate that synchronized intermittent mandatory ventilation (SIMV) alone slows the process, a finding that is concordant with physiologic investigations

Table 4. *Examples of Reversible Causes of Weaning Failure and Their Associated Treatments*

Cause	Examples of Treatment	Comment
↑ Ventilatory demand	↓ CO_2 production by suppressing fever and avoiding overfeeding; ↓ dead space by treating hypovolemia; treat sepsis; give $NaHCO_3$ for severe metabolic acidosis	Presence suggested by VE > 15 L/min
↑ Resistive load	Administer bronchodilators or steroids; antibiotics for respiratory tract infection; airway suctioning for secretions; place larger endotracheal tube	Presence suggested by measured airway resistance of > 15–20 cm H_2O/L/s[†]
↑ Elastic load	Diuretics for increased lung water; drainage of pleural fluid and air; decompression of abdomen with NG tube, paracentesis; bronchodilators to reduce PEEPi; treat pneumonia	Presence suggest by clinical examination, chest radiograph, and respiratory system compliance < 50–70 mL/cm H_2O[†]
↓ Neuromuscular capacity	Correct electrolyte abnormalities; minimize use of NMB agents; provide adequate nutrition; treat sepsis and hypothyroidism	Presence suggested by poor maximal inspiratory pressure (MIP > -20 to -30 cm H_2O)[†]
↓ Ventilatory drive	Sedation algorithm to avoid oversedation; correct metabolic alkalosis with acetazolamide	Presence suggested by unexplained hypercapnia, respiratory frequency < 12 breaths/min

*NG = nasogastric; PEEP = inspiratory PEEP; NMB = neuromuscular blocking.
[†]An imbalance between respiratory load and neuromuscular capacity is also suggested by an elevated f/VT ratio (> 100 breaths/L/min) or increased airway occlusion pressure ($P_{0.1}$ > 4–6 cm H_2O).

Weaning From Ventilatory Support (Epstein)

demonstrating that the degree of respiratory muscle rest on SIMV is *not* proportional to the level of ventilatory support. The neuromuscular apparatus poorly adapts to changing loads because respiratory muscle contraction during lower levels of SIMV is similar during both intervening (unsupported) and mandatory (supported) breaths.[60] This effect can be overcome by adding PSV to the unsupported breaths during SIMV.[61] Indeed, one small RCT of 19 patients with COPD noted a trend toward shorter weaning duration with SIMV/PSV compared with SIMV alone.[62] One study[63] randomized patients to 2-h SBTs with T-piece or PSV and found the latter associated with decreased weaning time, duration of mechanical ventilation, and ICU length of stay. These results must be interpreted cautiously as the study was unblended, the weaning protocol not explicitly stated, and the randomization unequal.

Finally, one RCT[64] examined the use of a closed-loop, knowledge-based system compared with usual care in 144 patients. The computer-driven ventilator continuously adjusts the level of pressure support based on respiratory rate, minimal tidal volume, and maximal end-tidal carbon dioxide to keep the patient in a "zone of comfort." A trial of spontaneous breathing is automatically conducted at the point a minimal level of PSV is achieved. If the SBT is successful, the physician is prompted about extubation. Using this design, computer-driven ventilation decreased duration of weaning, total duration of ventilation, and median ICU stay without adverse event or increased reintubation. In contrast a subsequent, single-center study,[65] involving the same computerized system, did not find the closed-loop system to be superior. To date, there is no RCT that indicates that modes such as volume support, volume-assured pressure support, and adaptive support ventilation facilitate the process of weaning compared with the techniques previously discussed.

Noninvasive ventilation (NIV) effectively treats acute respiratory failure complicating COPD and also benefits select patients with acute hypoxemic failure. Six RCTs have explored the use of NIV in patients having trouble weaning from mechanical ventilation. Nava et al[66] studied 50 COPD patients with acute-on-chronic hypercapnic respiratory failure (mean $Paco_2$, approximately 90 mm Hg)

who failed an initial T-piece trial. Patients were randomized to standard PSV weaning *or* immediate extubation to NIV (PSV mode) delivered via a full-face mask and standard ICU ventilator. The NIV group had statistically significant reductions in duration of mechanical ventilation, length of ICU stay, and 60-day survival. Another investigation of 53 acute-on-chronic respiratory failure patients found NIV reduced duration of invasive mechanical ventilation, although other outcomes were unchanged.[67]

Finally, Ferrer et al[68] randomized 43 patients who had failed three SBTs, 77% of whom had chronic lung disease. This study was stopped at an interim analysis finding that NIV was associated with shorter duration of mechanical ventilation, shorter ICU stay, shorter hospital stay, fewer tracheostomies, higher ICU survival, and a lower incidence of nosocomial pneumonia and septic shock. Two additional studies, one presented in preliminary form[69] and the other a quasi-randomized study in the Chinese literature,[70] indicate that NIV is equal or superior to invasive weaning. A metaanalysis[71] of these five studies (80% of patients with COPD) found that NIV was associated with decreased mortality, ventilator-associated pneumonia, duration of invasive ventilation, and length of stay in ICU and in hospital. A subsequent RCT (only one-third of patients with COPD) found no difference in survival, duration of intubation, and length of stay when comparing invasive weaning with NIV, although the latter was associated with fewer complications.[72]

Taken together, these studies indicate that NIV is a reasonable approach in patients with COPD for whom the treatment has not allowed weaning. Important caveats include the following: SBT readiness criteria must be satisfied, extubation criteria must be satisfied (*eg*, adequate mental status, effective cough, and manageable volume of respiratory secretions), and the patient must be a good candidate for NIV (able to breath spontaneously for at least 5 to 10 min and not deemed to have difficulty in reintubation). The benefits of NIV include a reduction in the acquisition of pneumonia, lower sedation requirements, and better recognition of readiness for extubation, particularly when psychological factors or the imposed work of breathing is contributing to weaning failure.

Application of Weaning Protocols

Uncontrolled investigations and RCTs demonstrate improved outcome with weaning driven by a protocol and implemented by physicians or by respiratory care practitioners and ICU nurses. Protocols can be used to perform a daily screen to determine readiness for an SBT, to determine the pace of weaning using methods of progressive withdrawal, or to direct a search for treatable causes for weaning failure. Of these three applications, the first is more important than the second; the third strategy has yet to be fully investigated.

One study[73] randomized mechanically ventilated medical patients to an intervention strategy combined daily readiness testing with SBTs compared to standard care. Control patients were screened daily but the information was not used to make weaning decisions. Intervention patients passing the daily screen underwent a 120-min SBT and if the trial was passed, the managing clinicians received a prompt for extubation. The intervention group experienced significant reductions in weaning time, duration of mechanical ventilation, complication rate, and ICU costs; no differences were noted in ICU or hospital length of stay, hospital costs, or mortality. Subsequent RCTs in medical and surgical ICUs[74,75] found that respiratory care practitioner/ICU nurse-directed protocols are also able to shorten the duration of mechanical ventilation. Nevertheless, protocols must be tailored to the environment in which they will be employed. This entails modifying the protocol for application to a distinct patient population. Studies performed in a neurosurgical ICU,[76] a pediatric ICU,[77] and in a medical ICU at a leading academic medical center found no superiority to a protocolized approach.[78] Although a protocol may serve as the default approach to weaning, flexibility and clinical judgment are highly recommended as too rigid an approach needlessly prolongs weaning and extubation.

Most randomized trials demonstrate that protocols directed at minimizing the use of sedative infusions decrease the duration of mechanical ventilation. Strategies designed to avoid oversedation by limiting the use of continuous infusions, either through sedation assessment scoring[79] or by daily cessation of sedative infusions,[80] decrease

duration of mechanical ventilation and duration of ICU stay. In contrast, at least one study[81] found that a sedation protocol did not hasten weaning from mechanical ventilation. Girard et al[19] recently published the results of a trial that employed a "wake up and breathe" strategy (the ABC trial). Patients randomized to a daily awakening trial followed by an SBT (vs SBT alone) experienced increased time off of mechanical ventilation, decreased time in coma, decreased ICU and hospital length of stay, and improved survival at 1 year. Interestingly, the two groups progressed to the point of passing an SBT at the same rate. Therefore, the improved outcome of combining a daily awakening trial and SBT resulted from patients being awake and ready for extubation once they passed the SBT.

Additional factors are important as studies show reduced duration of mechanical ventilation when nurse/patient ratios improve[82] and when a bedside weaning board and flow sheet are used to enhance communication between critical care practitioners.[83]

Extubation

When a patient has tolerated an SBT the clinician must next determine whether the endotracheal tube is still required. Approximately 10 to 15% of patients fail extubation (require reintubation) within 24 to 72 h of extubation.[84] A number of risk factors for extubation failure have been identified (Table 5). Reintubated patients suffer increased hospital mortality, prolonged ICU and hospital stays, and more frequently need long-term acute care.[6,7,85,86] On the other hand, unnecessary delays in extubation prolong ICU stay, heighten the risk for pneumonia, and increase hospital mortality.[87]

Table 5. *Risk Factors for Extubation Failure*

Medical, pediatric, or multidisciplinary ICU patient
Older age
Pneumonia as cause for mechanical ventilation
Higher severity of illness at the time of extubation
Use of continuous IV sedation
Abnormal mental status, delirium
Semirecumbent positioning
Transport out of ICU for procedures
Physician and nurse staffing in the ICU

As both extubation delay and extubation failure are linked to adverse outcomes, importance has shifted to developing strategies to more accurately predict and prevent postextubation respiratory failure. Measuring blood gases at the end of the SBT has not been shown to accurately predict extubation outcome.[88,89] In general, weaning predictors perform poorly in predicting extubation outcome.[90] Examining the f/V_T at SBT conclusion[91] or the time needed to return to baseline minute ventilation after resumption of full ventilatory support[92] shows promise. This is not unexpected as extubation failure often results from inability to protect the airway and manage respiratory secretions.[93] The upper airway can be assessed by identifying an audible air leak when the endotracheal tube balloon is deflated (cuff-leak test). Air leak can be quantified as the difference between the inspired and expired tidal volume during assist-control ventilation. False-positive test findings result from secretions adhering to the external surface of the endotracheal tube or when an undetected increase in inspired volume (machine tidal volume plus spontaneous gas inspired around the tube) contributes to an elevated exhaled tidal volume. Because these confounders are difficult to detect prior to extubation, an expert in airway management should be available immediately when extubating the patient with a positive cuff-leak test. Recently, several RCTs have demonstrated that systemic corticosteroids can reduce postextubation stridor, especially in high-risk patients.[94-96] For example, Cheng et al[94] randomized 128 high-risk patients (cuff-leak volume, <24% of tidal volume) to placebo or methylprednisolone injection (multiple or single dose) during the 24 h prior to extubation. Treatment with methylprednisolone significantly reduced the risk for postextubation stridor and need for reintubation.

The ability to protect the airway also depends on cough strength and volume of respiratory secretions (eg, suction requirement more than every 2 h), parameters that can be qualitatively and quantitatively measured. Mental status is also important, although studies looking exclusively at this parameter have come to conflicting conclusions. More recently, the integration of parameters has been found most useful. For example, Salam et al[97] found that measuring peak cough flow rates (cutoff, <60 L/min), secretions (cutoff, >2.5 mL/h), and abnormal mental status (inability to complete four simple commands) was highly predictive of extubation outcome. Failing all three criteria led to certain extubation failure, and the absence of all three was associated with only a 3% risk for reintubation.

Despite these advances, accurate prediction of extubation outcome remains challenging. The success of NIV for acute respiratory failure and its recent successful application in facilitating weaning has led to renewed interest in application to prevent extubation failure. RCTs indicate that *routine* use of nasal intermittent positive pressure ventilation after extubation[98] or application in heterogeneous populations with *overt*[99] or those with *early signs* of extubation failure[100] does not decrease need for reintubation or improve survival. In contrast, one case-control study[101] found that NIV effectively reduced reintubation in COPD patients with early evidence of postextubation hypercapnic respiratory failure. Two recently published RCTs[102,103] indicate that immediate postextubation application of NIV in patients at *highest risk* for extubation failure is effective in preventing reintubation and may reduce mortality.

Weaning Patients Supported by Prolonged Mechanical Ventilation

Approximately 10 to 20% of patients with acute respiratory failure require prolonged ventilatory support (>21 days). Once stable, these patients are often transferred to a chronic ventilator or long-term acute care unit. A recent multicenter observational study[104,105] of >1,400 patients transferred to long-term care hospitals found that 50% could be successfully weaned from mechanical ventilation. As in the acute ICU setting, standard weaning predictors perform poorly in foretelling outcome for patients supported by prolonged mechanical ventilation.[106] Weaning efforts should start as soon as possible after transfer as nearly 30% of patients supported by prolonged mechanical ventilation will tolerate their initial SBT and be liberated.[28] For the remaining patients, an imbalance between respiratory load and neuromuscular capacity often forms the basis of ventilator dependence.[107] Therefore, continued efforts to identify, and reverse, factors that either increase work of breathing or contribute to respiratory muscle weakness should be undertaken.

An RCT[28] in prolonged mechanical ventilation found no difference between PSV weaning and tracheotomy collar trials of increasing duration in 52 COPD patients. Compared with historic controls, weaning protocols in this setting are associated with shorter weaning duration than that of traditional approaches.[108]

References

1. Epstein S. Complications in ventilator supported patients. In: Tobin M, ed. Principles and practice of mechanical ventilation. New York, NY: McGraw Hill, 2006; 877–902

2. Esteban A, Anzueto A, Frutos F, et al. Characteristics and outcomes in adult patients receiving mechanical ventilation: a 28-day international study. JAMA 2002; 287:345–355

3. Hall JB, Wood LD. Liberation of the patient from mechanical ventilation. JAMA 1987; 257:1621–1628

4. Manthous CA, Schmidt GA, Hall JB. Liberation from mechanical ventilation: a decade of progress. Chest 1998; 114:886–901

5. Boles JM, Bion J, Connors A, et al. Weaning from mechanical ventilation. Eur Respir J 2007; 29:1033–1056

6. Esteban A, Alia I, Gordo F, et al. Extubation outcome after spontaneous breathing trials with T-tube or pressure support ventilation. The Spanish Lung Failure Collaborative Group. Am J Respir Crit Care Med 1997; 156(2 Pt 1):459–465

7. Esteban A, Alia I, Tobin MJ, et al. Effect of spontaneous breathing trial duration on outcome of attempts to discontinue mechanical ventilation. Spanish Lung Failure Collaborative Group. Am J Respir Crit Care Med 1999; 159:512–518

8. Vallverdu I, Calaf N, Subirana M, et al. Clinical characteristics, respiratory functional parameters, and outcome of a two-hour T-piece trial in patients weaning from mechanical ventilation. Am J Respir Crit Care Med 1998; 158:1855–1862

9. Esteban A, Alia I, Ibanez J, et al. Modes of mechanical ventilation and weaning. A national survey of Spanish hospitals. The Spanish Lung Failure Collaborative Group. Chest 1994; 106:1188–1193

10. Nevins ML, Epstein SK. Predictors of outcome for patients with COPD requiring invasive mechanical ventilation. Chest 2001; 119:1840–1849

11. MacIntyre NR, Cook DJ, Ely EW Jr, et al. Evidence-based guidelines for weaning and discontinuing ventilatory support: a collective task force facilitated by the American College of Chest Physicians; the American Association for Respiratory Care; and the American College of Critical Care Medicine. Chest 2001; 120(6 Suppl):375S–395S

12. Ely EW, Baker AM, Evans GW, et al. The prognostic significance of passing a daily screen of weaning parameters. Intensive Care Med 1999; 25:581–587

13. Epstein SK. Weaning parameters. Respir Care Clin North Am 2000; 6:253–301

14. Meade M, Guyatt G, Cook D, et al. Predicting success in weaning from mechanical ventilation. Chest 2001; 120(6 Suppl):400S–424S

15. El-Khatib MF, Zeineldine SM, Jamaleddine GW. Effect of pressure support ventilation and positive end expiratory pressure on the rapid shallow breathing index in intensive care unit patients. Intensive Care Med 2008; 34:505–510

16. Tobin MJ, Jubran A. Variable performance of weaning-predictor tests: role of Bayes' theorem and spectrum and test-referral bias. Intensive Care Med 2006; 32:2002–2012

17. Tanios MA, Nevins ML, Hendra KP, et al. A randomized, controlled trial of the role of weaning predictors in clinical decision making. Crit Care Med 2006; 34:2530–2535

18. Laghi F, Cattapan SE, Jubran A, et al. Is weaning failure caused by low-frequency fatigue of the diaphragm? Am J Respir Crit Care Med 2003; 167:120–127

19. Girard TD, Kress JP, Fuchs BD, et al. Efficacy and safety of a paired sedation and ventilator weaning protocol for mechanically ventilated patients in intensive care (Awakening and Breathing Controlled trial): a randomised controlled trial. Lancet 2008; 371:126–134

20. Zeggwagh AA, Abouqal R, Madani N, et al. Weaning from mechanical ventilation: a model for extubation. Intensive Care Med 1999; 25:1077–1083

21. Brochard L, Harf A, Lorino H, et al. Inspiratory pressure support prevents diaphragmatic fatigue during weaning from mechanical ventilation. Am Rev Respir Dis 1989; 139:513–521

22. Farias JA, Retta A, Alia I, et al. A comparison of two methods to perform a breathing trial before extubation in pediatric intensive care patients. Intensive Care Med 2001; 27:1649–1654

23. Jones DP, Byrne P, Morgan C, et al. Positive end-expiratory pressure vs T-piece. Extubation after mechanical ventilation. Chest 1991; 100:1655–1659

24. Haberthur C, Mols G, Elsasser S, et al. Extubation after breathing trials with automatic tube compensation, T-tube, or pressure support ventilation. Acta Anaesthesiol Scand 2002; 46:973–979

25. Cohen JD, Shapiro M, Grozovski E, et al. Extubation outcome following a spontaneous breathing trial with automatic tube compensation versus continuous positive airway pressure. Crit Care Med 2006; 34:682–686

26. Ezingeard E, Diconne E, Guyomarc'h S, et al. Weaning from mechanical ventilation with pressure support in patients failing a T-tube trial of spontaneous breathing. Intensive Care Med 2006; 32:165–169

27. Perren A, Domenighetti G, Mauri S, et al. Protocol-directed weaning from mechanical ventilation: clinical outcome in patients randomized for a 30-min or 120-min trial with pressure support ventilation. Intensive Care Med 2002; 28:1058–1063

28. Vitacca M, Vianello A, Colombo D, et al. Comparison of two methods for weaning patients with chronic obstructive pulmonary disease requiring mechanical ventilation for more than 15 days. Am J Respir Crit Care Med 2001; 164:225–230

29. Wysocki M, Cracco C, Teixeira A, et al. Reduced breathing variability as a predictor of unsuccessful patient separation from mechanical ventilation. Crit Care Med 2006; 34:2076–2083

30. Del Rosario N, Sassoon CS, Chetty KG, et al. Breathing pattern during acute respiratory failure and recovery. Eur Respir J 1997; 10:2560–2565

31. DeHaven CB, Kirton OC, Morgan JP, et al. Breathing measurement reduces false-negative classification of tachypneic preextubation trial failures. Crit Care Med 1996; 24:976–980

32. Girault C, Breton L, Richard JC, et al. Mechanical effects of airway humidification devices in difficult to wean patients. Crit Care Med 2003; 31:1306–1311

33. Jubran A, Tobin MJ. Pathophysiologic basis of acute respiratory distress in patients who fail a trial of weaning from mechanical ventilation. Am J Respir Crit Care Med 1997; 155:906–915

34. Vassilakopoulos T, Zakynthinos S, Roussos C. The tension-time index and the frequency/tidal volume ratio are the major pathophysiologic determinants of weaning failure and success. Am J Respir Crit Care Med 1998; 158:378–385

35. De Jonghe B, Bastuji-Garin S, Sharshar T, et al. Does ICU-acquired paresis lengthen weaning from mechanical ventilation? Intensive Care Med 2004; 30:1117–1121

36. Garnacho-Montero J, Amaya-Villar R, Garcia-Garmendia JL, et al. Effect of critical illness polyneuropathy on the withdrawal from mechanical ventilation and the length of stay in septic patients. Crit Care Med 2005; 33:349–354

37. Anzueto A, Peters JI, Tobin MJ, et al. Effects of prolonged controlled mechanical ventilation on diaphragmatic function in healthy adult baboons. Crit Care Med 1997; 25:1187–1190

38. Le Bourdelles G, Viires N, Boczkowski J, et al. Effects of mechanical ventilation on diaphragmatic contractile properties in rats. Am J Respir Crit Care Med 1994; 149:1539–1544

39. Datta D, Scalise P. Hypothyroidism and failure to wean in patients receiving prolonged mechanical ventilation at a regional weaning center. Chest 2004; 126:1307–1312

40. Huang CJ, Lin HC. Association between adrenal insufficiency and ventilator weaning. Am J Respir Crit Care Med 2006; 173:276–280

41. Tobin MJ, Guenther SM, Perez W, et al. Konno-Mead analysis of ribcage-abdominal motion during successful and unsuccessful trials of weaning from mechanical ventilation. Am Rev Respir Dis 1987; 135:1320–1328

42. Tobin MJ, Perez W, Guenther SM, et al. Does rib cage-abdominal paradox signify respiratory muscle fatigue? J Appl Physiol 1987; 63:851–860

43. Chatila W, Ani S, Guaglianone D, et al. Cardiac ischemia during weaning from mechanical ventilation. Chest 1996; 109:1577–1583

44. Frazier SK, Brom H, Widener J, et al. Prevalence of myocardial ischemia during mechanical ventilation and weaning and its effects on weaning success. Heart Lung 2006; 35:363–373

45. Hurford WE, Lynch KE, Strauss HW, et al. Myocardial perfusion as assessed by thallium-201 scintigraphy during the discontinuation of mechanical ventilation in ventilator-dependent patients. Anesthesiology 1991; 74:1007–1016

46. Lemaire F, Teboul JL, Cinotti L, et al. Acute left ventricular dysfunction during unsuccessful weaning from mechanical ventilation. Anesthesiology 1988; 69:171–179

47. Frazier SK, Stone KS, Moser D, et al. Hemodynamic changes during discontinuation of mechanical ventilation in medical intensive care unit patients. Am J Crit Care 2006; 15:580-593; quiz 594

48. Jubran A, Mathru M, Dries D, et al. Continuous recordings of mixed venous oxygen saturation during weaning from mechanical ventilation and the ramifications thereof. Am J Respir Crit Care Med 1998; 158:1763–1769

49. Mekontso-Dessap A, de Prost N, Girou E, et al. B-type natriuretic peptide and weaning from mechanical ventilation. Intensive Care Med 2006; 32:1529–1536

50. Grasso S, Leone A, De Michele M, et al. Use of N-terminal pro-brain natriuretic peptide to detect acute cardiac dysfunction during weaning failure in difficult-to-wean patients with chronic obstructive pulmonary disease. Crit Care Med 2007; 35:96–105

51. Richard C, Teboul JL, Archambaud F, et al. Left ventricular function during weaning of patients with chronic obstructive pulmonary disease. Intensive Care Med 1994; 20:181–186

52. Koksal GM, Sayilgan C, Sen O, et al. The effects of different weaning modes on the endocrine stress response. Crit Care 2004; 8:R31–34

53. Upadya A, Tilluckdharry L, Muralidharan V, et al. Fluid balance and weaning outcomes. Intensive Care Med 2005; 31:1643–1647

54. Ely EW, Gautam S, Margolin R, et al. The impact of delirium in the intensive care unit on hospital length of stay. Intensive Care Med 2001; 27:1892–1900.

55. Epstein S. Weaning from ventilatory support. In: Crapo J, Glassroth J, Karlinsky J, et al, eds. Textbook of pulmonary diseases. Philadelphia, PA: Lippincott, Williams & Wilkins, 2003; 1089–1101

56. Esteban A, Frutos F, Tobin MJ, et al. A comparison of four methods of weaning patients from mechanical ventilation. Spanish Lung Failure Collaborative Group. N Engl J Med 1995; 332:345–350

57. Laghi F, D'Alfonso N, Tobin MJ. Pattern of recovery from diaphragmatic fatigue over 24 hours. J Appl Physiol 1995; 79:539–546

58. Esteban A, Ferguson ND, Meade MO, et al. Evolution of mechanical ventilation in response to clinical research. Am J Respir Crit Care Med 2008; 177:170–177

59. Brochard L, Rauss A, Benito S, et al. Comparison of three methods of gradual withdrawal from ventilatory support during weaning from mechanical ventilation. Am J Respir Crit Care Med 1994; 150:896–903

60. Imsand C, Feihl F, Perret C, et al. Regulation of inspiratory neuromuscular output during synchronized intermittent mechanical ventilation. Anesthesiology 1994; 80:13–22

61. Leung P, Jubran A, Tobin MJ. Comparison of assisted ventilator modes on triggering, patient effort, and dyspnea. Am J Respir Crit Care Med 1997; 155:1940–1948

62. Jounieaux V, Duran A, Levi-Valensi P. Synchronized intermittent mandatory ventilation with and without pressure support ventilation in weaning patients with COPD from mechanical ventilation. Chest 1994; 105:1204–1210

63. Matic I, Majeric-Kogler V. Comparison of pressure support and T-tube weaning from mechanical ventilation: randomized prospective study. Croat Med J 2004; 45:162–166

64. Lellouche F, Mancebo J, Jolliet P, et al. A multicenter randomized trial of computer-driven protocolized weaning from mechanical ventilation. Am J Respir Crit Care Med 2006; 174:894–900

65. Rose L, Presneill JJ, Johnston L, et al. A randomised, controlled trial of conventional versus automated weaning from mechanical ventilation using SmartCare/PS. Intensive Care Med 2008; 34:1788–1795

66. Nava S, Ambrosino N, Clini E, et al. Noninvasive mechanical ventilation in the weaning of patients with respiratory failure due to chronic obstructive pulmonary disease. A randomized, controlled trial. Ann Intern Med 1998; 128:721–728

67. Girault C, Daudenthun I, Chevron V, et al. Noninvasive ventilation as a systematic extubation and weaning technique in acute-on-chronic respiratory failure: a prospective, randomized controlled study. Am J Respir Crit Care Med 1999; 160:86–92

68. Ferrer M, Esquinas A, Arancibia F, et al. Noninvasive ventilation during persistent weaning failure: a randomized controlled trial. Am J Respir Crit Care Med 2003; 168:70–76

69. Hill N, Lin D, Levy M, et al. Noninvasive positive pressure ventilation (NPPV) to facilitate extubation after acute respiratory failure: a feasibility study [abstract]. Am J Resp Crit Care Med 2000; 161:A263

70. Chen J, Qiu D, Tao D. Time for extubation and sequential noninvasive mechanical ventilation in COPD patients with exacerbated respiratory failure who received invasive ventilation [in Chinese]. Zhonghua Jie He He Hu Xi Za Zhi 2001; 24:99–100

71. Burns KE, Adhikari NK, Meade MO. A meta-analysis of noninvasive weaning to facilitate liberation from mechanical ventilation. Can J Anaesth 2006; 53:305–315

72. Trevisan CE, Vieira SR. Noninvasive mechanical ventilation may be useful in treating patients who fail weaning from invasive mechanical ventilation: a randomized clinical trial. Crit Care 2008 Apr 17 [Epub ahead of print]

73. Ely EW, Baker AM, Dunagan DP, et al. Effect on the duration of mechanical ventilation of identifying patients capable of breathing spontaneously. N Engl J Med 1996; 335:1864–1869

74. Kollef MH, Shapiro SD, Silver P, et al. A randomized, controlled trial of protocol-directed versus physician-directed weaning from mechanical ventilation. Crit Care Med 1997; 25:567–574

75. Marelich GP, Murin S, Battistella F, et al. Protocol weaning of mechanical ventilation in medical and surgical patients by respiratory care practitioners and nurses: effect on weaning time and incidence of ventilator-associated pneumonia. Chest 2000; 118:459–467

76. Namen AM, Ely EW, Tatter SB, et al. Predictors of successful extubation in neurosurgical patients. Am J Respir Crit Care Med 2001; 163(3 Pt 1):658–664

77. Randolph AG, Wypij D, Venkataraman ST, et al. Effect of mechanical ventilator weaning protocols on respiratory outcomes in infants and children: a randomized controlled trial. JAMA 2002; 288:2561–2568

78. Krishnan JA, Moore D, Robeson C, et al. A prospective, controlled trial of a protocol-based strategy to discontinue mechanical ventilation. Am J Respir Crit Care Med 2004; 169:673–678

79. Brook AD, Ahrens TS, Schaiff R, et al. Effect of a nursing-implemented sedation protocol on the duration of mechanical ventilation. Crit Care Med 1999; 27:2609–2615

80. Kress JP, Pohlman AS, O'Connor MF, et al. Daily interruption of sedative infusions in critically ill patients undergoing mechanical ventilation. N Engl J Med 2000; 342:1471–1477

81. Bucknall TK, Manias E, Presneill JJ. A randomized trial of protocol-directed sedation management for mechanical ventilation in an Australian intensive care unit. Crit Care Med 2008; 36:1444–1450

82. Thorens JB, Kaelin RM, Jolliet P, et al. Influence of the quality of nursing on the duration of weaning from mechanical ventilation in patients with chronic obstructive pulmonary disease. Crit Care Med 1995; 23:1807–1815

83. Henneman E, Dracup K, Ganz T, et al. Effect of a collaborative weaning plan on patient outcome in the critical care setting. Crit Care Med 2001; 29:297–303

84. Epstein SK. Decision to extubate. Intensive Care Med 2002; 28:535–546

85. Epstein SK, Ciubotaru RL. Independent effects of etiology of failure and time to reintubation on outcome for patients failing extubation. Am J Respir Crit Care Med 1998; 158:489–493

86. Epstein SK, Ciubotaru RL, Wong JB. Effect of failed extubation on the outcome of mechanical ventilation. Chest 1997; 112:186–192

87. Coplin WM, Pierson DJ, Cooley KD, et al. Implications of extubation delay in brain-injured patients meeting standard weaning criteria. Am J Respir Crit Care Med 2000; 161:1530–1536

88. Pawson SR, DePriest JL. Are blood gases necessary in mechanically ventilated patients who have successfully completed a spontaneous breathing trial? Respir Care 2004; 49:1316–1319

89. Salam A, Smina M, Gada P, et al. The effect of arterial blood gas values on extubation decisions. Respir Care 2003; 48:1033–1037

90. Frutos-Vivar F, Ferguson ND, Esteban A, et al. Risk factors for extubation failure in patients following a successful spontaneous breathing trial. Chest 2006; 130:1664–1671

91. Kuo PH, Wu HD, Lu BY, et al. Predictive value of rapid shallow breathing index measured at initiation and termination of a 2-hour spontaneous breathing trial for weaning outcome in ICU patients. J Formos Med Assoc 2006; 105:390–398

92. Martinez A, Seymour C, Nam M. Minute ventilation recovery time: a predictor of extubation outcome. Chest 2003; 123:1214–1221

93. Epstein SK. Etiology of extubation failure and the predictive value of the rapid shallow breathing index. Am J Respir Crit Care Med 1995; 152:545–549

94. Cheng KC, Hou CC, Huang HC, et al. Intravenous injection of methylprednisolone reduces the incidence of postextubation stridor in intensive care unit patients. Crit Care Med 2006; 34:1345–1350

95. Francois B, Bellissant E, Gissot V, et al. 12-h pretreatment with methylprednisolone versus placebo for prevention of postextubation laryngeal oedema: a randomised double-blind trial. Lancet 2007; 369:1083–1089

96. Lee CH, Peng MJ, Wu CL. Dexamethasone to prevent postextubation airway obstruction in adults: a prospective, randomized, double-blind, placebo-controlled study. Crit Care 2007; 11(4):R72

97. Salam A, Tilluckdharry L, Amoateng-Adjepong Y, et al. Neurologic status, cough, secretions and extubation outcomes. Intensive Care Med 2004 Mar 4 [Epub ahead of print]

98. Jiang JS, Kao SJ, Wang SN. Effect of early application of biphasic positive airway pressure on the outcome of extubation in ventilator weaning. Respirology 1999; 4:161–165

99. Keenan SP, Powers C, McCormack DG, et al. Noninvasive positive-pressure ventilation for postextubation respiratory distress: a randomized controlled trial. JAMA 2002; 287:3238–3244

100. Esteban A, Frutos-Vivar F, Ferguson ND, et al. Noninvasive positive-pressure ventilation for respiratory failure after extubation. N Engl J Med 2004; 350:2452–2460

101. Hilbert G, Gruson D, Portel L, et al. Noninvasive pressure support ventilation in COPD patients with postextubation hypercapnic respiratory insufficiency. Eur Respir J 1998; 11:1349–1353

102. Ferrer M, Valencia M, Nicolas JM, et al. Early noninvasive ventilation averts extubation failure in patients at risk: a randomized trial. Am J Respir Crit Care Med 2006; 173:164–170

103. Nava S, Gregoretti C, Fanfulla F, et al. Noninvasive ventilation to prevent respiratory failure after extubation in high-risk patients. Crit Care Med 2005; 33:2465–2470

104. Scheinhorn DJ, Hassenpflug MS, Votto JJ, et al. Post-ICU mechanical ventilation at 23 long-term care hospitals: a multicenter outcomes study. Chest 2007; 131:85–93

105. Scheinhorn DJ, Hassenpflug MS, Votto JJ, et al. Ventilator-dependent survivors of catastrophic illness transferred to 23 long-term care hospitals for weaning from prolonged mechanical ventilation. Chest 2007; 131:76–84

106. Nevins ML, Epstein SK. Weaning from prolonged mechanical ventilation. Clin Chest Med 2001; 22:13–33

107. Purro A, Appendini L, De Gaetano A, et al. Physiologic determinants of ventilator dependence in long-term mechanically ventilated patients. Am J Respir Crit Care Med 2000; 161(4 Pt 1):1115–1123

108. Scheinhorn DJ, Chao DC, Stearn-Hassenpflug M, et al. Outcomes in post-ICU mechanical ventilation: a therapist-implemented weaning protocol. Chest 2001; 119:236–242

Trauma and Thermal Injury

David J. Dries, MD, MSE, FCCP

Objectives:

- Identify the multisystem manifestations of trauma
- Recognize common patterns of presentation for cardiopulmonary injury
- Recognize evolving management of secondary brain injury
- Identify patients at high risk for venous thromboembolism following injury
- Recognize burn injury of various degrees and associated treatment options
- Assess and manage inhalation injury
- Review the latest available data regarding the outcome of burn injury

Key words: blunt cardiac injury; duplex ultrasonography; hemothorax; inhalation injury; low-molecular-weight heparin; pneumothorax; secondary brain injury; venous thromboembolism

Trauma

Principal decision making in the management of multiple organ injury rests with the trauma surgeon. The intensivist, however, is a critical component of the management team, particularly in the setting of blunt injury with multiple system dysfunction and less need for acute operative intervention. Certain types of injury have implications for all members of the trauma care team, both emergency department management and critical care support. All team members should therefore be able to identify and act immediately on identification of injury and complications of initial treatment. The international process for injury identification and treatment is discussed in the *Advanced Trauma Life Support Course* published by the American College of Surgeons Committee on Trauma. This chapter reviews recent developments and discusses common patterns of injury or complications of injury according to organ system.

Airway and Spine

The initial priority in the management of any injured patient is assessment and management of the airway. At the same time, care is taken to prevent movement of the cervical spine. All patients with blunt trauma are at risk for cervical spine injury. Patients with unknown cervical spine status and need of emergency airway control may be intubated safely by temporary removal of the immobilizing cervical collar, while inline stabilization is maintained during intubation. After securing the airway, the collar is reapplied and the patient remains on log-roll precautions until the complete spine status has been assessed. The choice of nasotracheal vs orotracheal intubation technique is based on provider preference and experience. Nasotracheal intubation, however, requires spontaneous respiration. In addition, no tubes should be passed through the nose of a patient who has midfacial trauma with a risk of cribriform plate fracture. When other means of airway control have failed, a surgical airway may be required.

Neurologic examination alone does not exclude a cervical spine injury. The integrity of the bony components of the cervical spine may be assessed in various ways. A variety of plain radiographs, CT scans, or MRI scans may be obtained. The following patients are excluded from examination: (1) those who cannot relate neurologic examination changes; (2) those who are unresponsive due to either primary injury or the effects of pain medication; and (3) those who receive muscle relaxants. Thus, recommendations were developed to determine the presence or absence of cervical spine instability. The following recommendations were made for patients at risk for cervical spine injury:

- Patients who are alert, awake, and without mental status changes and neck pain and who have no distracting injuries or neurologic deficits may be considered to have a stable cervical spine and need no radiologic studies.
- All other patients should have at least a lateral view of the cervical spine, including the base of the occiput to the upper border of the first

thoracic vertebra, and anteroposterior view showing the spinous processes of the second cervical through the first thoracic vertebra; and an open-mouth odontoid view indicating lateral masses of the first cervical vertebra and the entire odontoid process. Axial CT scans with sagittal reconstruction may be obtained for any questionable level of injury or any area that cannot be adequately visualized on plain radiographs.

- Flexion and extension views of the cervical spine may be appropriate in patients complaining of significant neck pain with normal plain radiograph results.
- Patients with neurologic deficits that may refer to a cervical spine injury require subspecialty consultation and MRI evaluation. MRI may also facilitate clearance of ligamentous injury.
- Patients with an altered level of consciousness secondary to traumatic brain injury or other causes may be considered to have a stable cervical spine if adequate three-view plain radiographs and thin-cut axial CT images through C1 and C2 are normal.
- Most recent work suggest that CT scans may facilitate evaluation of the cervical spine in any head-injured or intubated patient. More and more centers are adding CT scans of the cervical spine when scans of the head are obtained after injury.

Cervical spine injury following blunt trauma reportedly occurs at a frequency of 4 to 6%. In the literature of cervical spine injury, there is little supporting evidence that defines the criteria for determining who gets cervical spine radiographs and who does not. Long-term follow-up to identify all cases of cervical spine injury missed in the acute setting is frequently unavailable. The true incidence of cervical spine injury is thus not known. The three-view plain spine series (anteroposterior, lateral, and open-mouth odontoid view), supplemented by thin-cut axial CT imaging with sagittal reconstruction through suspicious areas or in adequately visualized areas, provides a false-negative rate <0.1% if the studies are technically adequate and properly interpreted.

The lessons of cervical spine evaluation have also been applied to injuries to the thoracic and lumbar regions. While plain radiographs in the majority of patients are adequate to screen in individuals with high-risk mechanisms, helical CT allows reconstruction of the thoracic and lumbar spine from various views. This information can be obtained in patients receiving chest and abdominal CT scanning protocols for other visceral injuries. A dedicated spine CT examination is no longer required. In our center, adjacent spine reconstructions are obtained in any patient receiving torso scans as a part of evaluation for injury. When the use of helical CT was compared to conventional radiographs of the thoracic and lumbar spine, improved sensitivity and specificity were obtained.

Tracheobronchial Injury

Tracheal or laryngeal disruption or fracture most commonly occurs at the junction of the larynx and the trachea. Signs and symptoms may include hoarseness, subcutaneous air, edema, or crepitus at the neck, but the patient may have minimal evidence of injury. The patient should be allowed to assume the position of comfort; this position may include sitting if spinal injury is unlikely during the patient's initial assessment. Airway management by an experienced physician may include an awake tracheostomy. Cricothyroidotomy should be avoided.

Injury to the proximal trachea may be caused by blunt or penetrating trauma. Blunt injury to the cervical trachea occurs in <1% in all patients with blunt trauma to the trunk. Injury to the larynx is the most common blunt injury. A direct blow to the trachea may cause compression or fracture of the cartilaginous ring, hematoma formation, bleeding, or airway obstruction. Injury to the trachea may also occur from the shoulder restraint harness of a seat belt. Proximal tracheal injuries may be caused by gunshot wounds or stab wounds to the neck. Hemoptysis and airway obstruction indicate the need for urgent access to the airway. Patients with subcutaneous air or dissecting air within the cervical fascia should be suspected for tracheal and/or esophageal injury.

Patients presenting with massive subcutaneous or mediastinal emphysema are suspected to have a distal tracheal or bronchus injury. Hemoptysis, hemopneumothorax, or a collapsed lung on a plain chest radiograph confirm injury in the major intrathoracic airways. When chest tubes are placed and there is constant air loss, major airway disruption must be suspected. In this situation, bronchoscopy should be done as soon as possible to exclude a tracheal or large bronchial tear or proximal bronchial obstruction by a foreign body or secretions. More than 80% of traumatic tracheobronchial tears occur within 2.5 cm of the carina; lobar or segmental bronchi are seldom injured. Injury to the distal trachea is associated with severe compression trauma to the chest, particularly when the glottis is closed.

Airway control and ventilation may be difficult in these patients. A double-lumen endotracheal tube may be required. Placement of these tubes requires skill, and secretion management may be difficult. Surgical repair must be prioritized. If an airway can be established and maintained, other life-threatening problems, such as intra-abdominal hemorrhage, may be addressed. Repair of distal tracheal or bronchial injuries typically requires a thoracotomy. Postoperative management of these patients has several components. Repeat bronchoscopy may be required for secretion control. Mechanical ventilation should be provided to minimize the pressure within the airways. Use of pressure control modes of ventilation may be optimal.

Intrabronchial bleeding, manifest as hemoptysis and air hunger, is poorly tolerated and may lead rapidly to death due to alveolar flooding. Bleeding is typically caused by injury to bronchial arteries or fistulas between pulmonary veins, pulmonary arterial branches, and the bronchus. These patients may rapidly become hypoxic before other evidence of respiratory failure is apparent. In general, these patients should be positioned to facilitate drainage of blood out of the trachea. The uninvolved lung must be free of blood, if possible. Nasotracheal suctioning or bronchoscopy may be necessary to keep the bronchial tree clear and the contralateral lung expanded. For severe bleeding, a double-lumen endotracheal tube may be inserted to confine the bleeding and protect the uninvolved lung. Where severe bleeding continues, thoracotomy should be performed with clamping of the involved bronchus at the hilum.

Recognizing the paucity of literature on tracheobronchial injuries, Richardson reviewed a single institution experienced with a single lead surgeon in the management of tracheobronchial injuries. He classified injuries into those involving the larynx and trachea and those involving the mainstem bronchus. In all, 60 patients were treated from 1976 to 2001 for blunt and penetrating injuries. Six injuries involved the larynx and trachea, while 27 tracheal wounds and 27 injuries to the mainstem bronchus were identified. Only one of six laryngotracheal wounds had a good result. One patient required tracheal resection, and another required permanent tracheostomy. Of tracheal injuries, patients surviving tracheal resection and end-to-end anastomosis had good outcomes. Two granuloma complications were caused by the use of a permanent suture. One patient treated by a primary tracheal repair had stenosis requiring resection. Of patients with injuries to the mainstem bronchus, 14 pneumonectomies were performed with eight survivors. Three of these patients had stump leaks with empyema, and three of these individuals had cor pulmonale on follow-up. Ten patients had repair of blunt mainstem bronchial injuries; in two cases, bronchial stenosis required pneumonectomy. Clearly, these patients frequently have suboptimal outcome. Where end-to-end tracheal repairs can be created and direct repair of mainstem bronchus injuries provided, improved outcome can be anticipated.

Rib and Pulmonary Parenchymal Injury

Rib fractures are frequently not detected on chest radiographs; the fracture may be documented by tenderness on physical examination. Pain control is essential for ensuring adequate spontaneous ventilation. Where multiple adjacent rib segments are fractured, a flail chest may occur. The clinical manifestation of flail chest is paradoxical movement of the involved portion of the chest wall (ie, inward movement of the segments during inhalation). Frequently, flail chest is associated with contusion of the underlying lung, pain, and hypoxemia. Less common is pneumothorax associated with an open thoracic wound. Open pneumothorax is generally associated with soft-tissue deficit requiring dressings or closure and chest tube placement to reexpand the involved lung. Another complication of rib injury is hemothorax. Massive hemothorax is suggested by physical examination and the chest radiograph. Rapid loss of 1,000 to 2,000 mL of blood or ongoing blood loss > 200 mL/h through a chest tube is an indication for thoracotomy. In general, pneumothorax is associated with rib fractures and requires chest tube placement. Suction is applied routinely at approximately 20 cm H_2O. Any patient with a pneumothorax who requires a general anesthetic should have a chest tube in place. Perhaps the most feared complication of rib fracture is tension pneumothorax. Air is under pressure in the pleural space, resulting in hemodynamic embarrassment and pulmonary dysfunction. This emergency should not be diagnosed using a chest radiograph. This clinical diagnosis is based on absent breath sounds, respiratory distress, jugular venous distention, and cardiovascular compromise. The trachea may deviate away from the side, requiring tube thoracostomy. Needle catheter placement into the pleural space at the second intercostal level in the midclavicular line may be necessary for urgent decompression of the involved hemithorax.

A common result of rib and chest wall injury is pulmonary contusion. Patients with penetrating trauma may have areas of hemorrhage surrounding a missile tract. The patient sustaining pulmonary contusion from blunt trauma may have a more globular or diffuse pattern of injury. Pulmonary contusion is usually diagnosed on the basis of the history of blunt chest trauma and findings of localized opacification on chest radiographs. The extent of pulmonary contusion is usually underestimated on plain film radiographs. CT scans evaluate and quantify pulmonary contusions. A scan demonstrating a large contusion (>20%) increases the likelihood of prolonged ventilatory support for acute respiratory failure.

CT may also be useful in confirming the diagnosis of pulmonary contusion. One third of pulmonary contusions do not manifest on plain radiographs until 12 to 24 h after injury. More frequently than previously noted, CT scans have also demonstrated traumatic pneumatocele and parenchymal lacerations to the lung. Hypoxia may be the first evidence of severe pulmonary contusion. If the contusion is large enough or is bilateral, a significant decrease in lung compliance may also occur with associated increase in shunt fraction. The overall mortality rate of patients with pulmonary contusion is 15 to 16%. When chest wall injury is associated with this problem, particularly flail chest, the mortality rate approaches 45%.

Treatment is directed primarily at maintaining ventilation and preventing pneumonia. Progressive respiratory therapy to promote deep breathing, coughing, and mobilization is critical. Pain relief is essential for chest wall injuries. To this end, epidural analgesia is superior to intrapleural medication administration or rib blocks. The patient should be euvolemic, not dehydrated. Mechanical ventilation may be required in the hypoxic patient. This therapy may also be necessary in the patient with shock, increased work of breathing, coma, or significant preexisting lung disease.

An intriguing clinical series from the University of Oregon Health and Science University describes use of absorbable prostheses for rib fracture fixation in 10 patients. These individuals underwent rib fracture fixation with absorbable plates and screws. Indications included flail chest with failure to wean (five patients), acute pain with rib instability (four patients), and a significant chest wall defect. All patients with flail chest were weaned successfully from mechanical ventilation. Patients with pain and instability reported subjective improvement or resolution of symptoms. The patient with a chest wall defect returned to full athletic activity within 6 months. Muscle-sparing incisions were used, and thoracoscopic assistance was employed in three cases. Two patients with screw fixation only had loss of rib fracture reduction, and one patient had a wound infection. Given the frequency of rib fractures and the morbidity associated with this problem, absorbable plates are an option that warrants further evaluation for rib fracture repair in selected patients. This technique may be enhanced with further refinements in minimally invasive surgical methods.

ICU Resuscitation

Patients sustaining major trauma without brain injury who survive the first 6 h after injury are at risk for multiple organ failure. A statistical model suggests that age, injury severity score, and severity of shock are independent risk factors for this complication. The University of Texas-Houston Medical School has developed a shock resuscitation protocol applied to major torso trauma patients at known risk for multiple organ

Trauma and Thermal Injury (Dries)

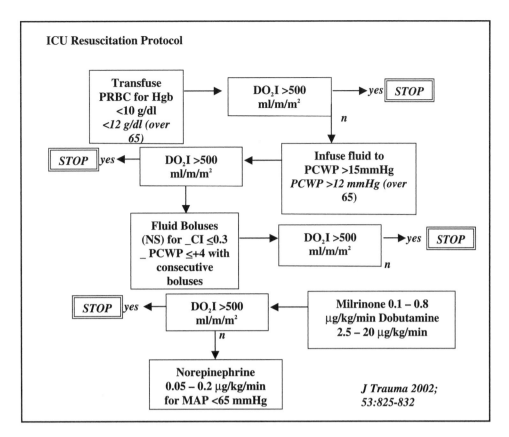

ICU Resuscitation Protocol

Transfuse PRBC for Hgb <10 g/dl <12 g/dl (over 65) → $DO_2I > 500$ ml/m/m² → yes → STOP

n

STOP ← yes ← $DO_2I > 500$ ml/m/m² ← Infuse fluid to PCWP >15mmHg *PCWP >12 mmHg (over 65)*

Fluid Boluses (NS) for _CI ≤0.3 _ PCWP ≤+4 with consecutive boluses → $DO_2I > 500$ ml/m/m² → yes → STOP

n

STOP ← yes ← $DO_2I > 500$ ml/m/m² ← Milrinone 0.1 – 0.8 µg/kg/min Dobutamine 2.5 – 20 µg/kg/min

n

Norepinephrine 0.05 – 0.2 µg/kg/min for MAP <65 mmHg

J Trauma 2002; 53:825-832

Figure 1. Shock resuscitation protocol applied to major torso trauma patients at known risk for multiple organ failure.

failure (Fig 1). This standardized process employs much of the contemporary thinking regarding protocol-driven resuscitation and comes from a group with an extensive database in this area.

Patients likely to require this resuscitation were those with injuries including two or more abdominal organs, two or more long bone fractures, a complex pelvic fracture, flail chest, and/or major vascular injury. Blood loss is a marker of need for aggressive resuscitation. Where patients are anticipated to need ≥6 U of packed RBCs during the first 12 h after hospital admission and demonstrate an arterial base deficit ≥6 mEq/L during the first 12 h after hospital admission, shock resuscitation is employed. Trauma victims ≥65 years old are also at increased risk if they have any two of the previous criteria. Notably, patients with severe brain injury (Glasgow coma scale [GCS] score ≤8 or abnormal brain CT scan results) were not resuscitated by this protocol.

The resuscitation strategy employed is a goal-directed, rule-based process emphasizing hemoglobin and volume loading to attain and maintain oxygen delivery for the first 24 h of hospital stay. A hierarchy of five therapies including RBC

transfusion, lactated Ringers infusion, creation of Starling curves for oxygen transport determination, inotrope, and vasopressor administration with data managed in a database.

Use of invasive hemodynamic monitoring and related end points of resuscitation remains controversial. In the late 1980s, unrecognized flow-dependent oxygen consumption was a suspected cause of late organ failure, and it was thought that oxygen delivery should be pushed until oxygen consumption plateaued. Shoemaker and coworkers, noting that survivors of severe injury increased oxygen delivery to supranormal levels compared with nonsurvivors, proposed that supranormal oxygen delivery be used as a resuscitation goal. In a series of publications, these workers provided data to support the concept that early management to supranormal oxygen delivery improved outcome. These publications prompted controversy that has persisted for >20 years and has led to a host of trials offering conflicting results. A more recent metaanalysis of goal-directed resuscitation suggests that the concept of achieving supranormal values for oxygen delivery does not work in patients in whom organ failure has developed. Shortly after this metaanalysis, a rebirth of early goal-directed resuscitation driven by the emergency department work of Rivers and others appeared. Optimal results in high-risk patients, it appears, come when hemodynamic optimization takes place before significant organ dysfunction occurs. As evidence of major inflammation with organ failure progresses, the attempt to achieve high oxygen delivery is not beneficial and may be harmful. Early use of invasive monitoring and aggressive resuscitation is supported by a recent retrospective assessment of the National Trauma Data Bank for outcome associated with management of the pulmonary artery catheter. After stratification for injury severity, pulmonary artery catheter use was associated with survival benefit in patients aged 61 to 90 years, with arrival base deficit worse than −11 and injury severity score of 25 to 75. The role of supranormal targets for oxygen transport remains unclear.

Moore and coworkers in Houston address this issue by comparing two cohorts of patients. The control patients were resuscitated to an oxygen delivery index of 600 mL/min/m² as compared to a more modest, but acceptable, resuscitation end point of 500 mL/min/m². Comparing a wide range of hemodynamic variables, these workers suggest that outcome with the more modest resuscitation goal was comparable in patients with critical injury and that patients could be resuscitated with a smaller resuscitation fluid volume for a lower target oxygen delivery index. Other observations from this group suggest that female patients have a comparable if not better response to resuscitation after trauma, and trauma during the later years of life is not inevitably associated with resuscitation futility. While acceptance of the invasive hemodynamic monitoring strategy and fluid resuscitation end points of Moore and coworkers is not uniform among the trauma community, this is some of the best recent data incorporating an ICU resuscitation strategy after injury. An interesting concern with such aggressive protocols is an increased recognition of abdominal compartment syndrome, both as a primary consequence of injury and as a secondary effect of resuscitation strategy. Clearly, we still need to strike a balance.

In an effort to optimize blood product administration in critically injured patients, a massive transfusion policy is being introduced in trauma centers in the United States to allow expedient and appropriate blood component replacement during acute patient management. Individuals presenting *in extremis* typically receive non–cross-matched blood in the resuscitation room while specific component replacement begins in the ICU, operating room, or angiography suite. On presentation of a patient deemed likely to need massive transfusion, a blood sample is sent to the laboratory for a type and cross-match of products. Consistent with recent data supporting increased administration of fresh frozen plasma (FFP), 6 to 8 U of FFP are provided as well as platelets for each 10 U of packed RBCs used, a departure from previous strategies, which included later administration of plasma and platelet products. An administration cycle providing 4 to 5 U of packed RBCs at a time with appropriate amounts of FFP and platelets continues with activation of this protocol until discontinued by the trauma team.

Stimulated by recent work suggesting the efficacy of recombinant activated factor VII in hemophilia, factor deficiency states, and off-label administration in surgery and trauma, trauma centers are incorporating administration of recombinant activated factor VII with massive transfusion protocols. In general, this material is employed in doses approximating 100 µg/kg after administration of 8 to 10 U of packed RBCs in <6 h. Use of recombinant activated factor VII assumes prior administration of appropriate amounts of FFP, platelets, and cryoprecipitate (for fibrinogen <100 mg/dL). Contraindications to use of recombinant activated factor VII include pH <7, GCS score <8, cardiac arrest, pregnancy, and possibly prior venous thromboembolic disorders, myocardial infarction (MI), or cerebral vascular accident (CVA) [if recent]. Recombinant activated factor VII binds to platelets, and effects are concentrated at the site of injury where bleeding and hemostatic alterations occur. Thrombin generation is enhanced, and tissue factor-dependent and -independent activation of factor X is seen. Factor IX is activated, and platelet activation and aggregation are focused at sites of injury. While available multicenter data does not support widespread use of recombinant activated factor VII in the setting of injury, contemporary practice patterns support administration of this material in a controlled fashion within institutional massive transfusion protocols (Table 1).

Trauma and Thermal Injury (Dries)

Table 1. *Use of Recombinant Factor VIIa in Surgery and Trauma*†*

Indications for use of recombinant factor VIIa
  Active bleeding following the use of two massive
    transfusion packs: 8 U packed RBCs in <6 h, and
  Appropriate use of clotting factor replacement:
    8 U FFP
    1 U pheresis platelets if platelet count <100, 2 U if
      platelet count <50
    12 U of cryoprecipitate if fibrinogen <100
  Massive transfusion pack 1 will have:
    4 U packed RBCs
    4 U FFP
  Following administration of pack 1, the following
    laboratory investigations are needed:
    Partial thromboplastin time; prothrombin time
    Complete blood examination and platelet count
    Fibrinogen
  Massive transfusion pack 2 will have:
    4 U packed RBCs
    4 U FFP
    1 U apheresis platelets
Contraindications for use of recombinant factor VIIa
  pH <7
  Preceding cardiac arrest
  Patient not salvageable
  Pregnancy
  Recent VTE, MI, or CVA, <3-mo relative CI
Dose of recombinant factor VIIa
  90 µg/kg rounded to the nearest vial size
  Can repeat once if bleeding not controlled in 3 h

*CI = contraindications.
†Transfusion Committee, Regions Hospital, 2007.

Table 2. *Use of Recombinant Factor VIIa in ICH Patients Receiving Warfarin**

Indications for use of recombinant factor VIIa
  Active life-threatening bleeding in a patient receiving
    warfarin, and
  International normalized ratio >1.4
Treatment
  Recombinant factor VIIa, 1.2 mg, single dose
  Vitamin K, 10 mg slow IV
  FFP, 15 mL/kg
  If international normalized ratio is >1.4 at >2 h after
    recombinant factor VIIa and FFP have been
    administered, repeat FFP dosing
Monitoring
  International normalized ratio before and at 1, 2, 4, 8,
    12, 18, and 24 h
Contraindications to recombinant factor VIIa
  Deep vein thrombosis, pulmonary embolism, CVA, or MI
    within 30 days prior to the event
Relative contraindications
  Pregnancy

*Transfusion Committee, Regions Hospital, 2007.

Table 3. *Indications for Damage Control*

Inability to achieve hemostasis due to coagulopathy
Inaccessible major venous injury
Time-consuming procedure in a patient with suboptimal
  response to resuscitation
Management of extra-abdominal life-threatening injury
Reassessment of intra-abdominal contents

Another important, but investigational, application of recombinant activated factor VII comes in the patient sustaining intracranial hemorrhage (ICH) while receiving warfarin therapy. In this patient group with an elevated international normalized ratio, recombinant activated factor VII may be administered in a low dose along with FFP, vitamin K, and other products as appropriate. This aggressive approach is warranted due to high morbidity in patients sustaining head injury while receiving various anticoagulant therapies. Contraindications to administration of recombinant activated factor VII include pregnancy, venous thromboembolic disorders, CVA, or MI within 30 days before onset of symptoms for ICH. There is a significant need for further data in this area (Table 2).

Damage Control

In use for over a decade, the concept of damage control has become an accepted, proven surgical method with wide applicability and success. Damage control is no longer confined to the abdomen, and its principles cross surgical disciplines, including thoracic, urologic, orthopedic, and vascular surgery. The concept is most often used in the massively injured exsanguinating patient with multiple competing surgical priorities (Tables 3–6). With growing experience and application, the technique continues to evolve. The group at the University of Pennsylvania Trauma Center first published on the contemporary experience with damage control in 1993. This experience included 24 abdominal injury patients. This group has noted an improvement in survivability when abbreviated laparotomy and abdominal packing are combined with physiologic resuscitation and more extensive visceral repair at later operations.

The patient receiving damage control treatment is *in extremis* and undergoes a truncated laparotomy, followed by physiologic optimization in the ICU and eventual restoration of GI, orthopedic,

Table 4. *Stages of Damage Control*

Abbreviated resuscitative surgery
  Hemorrhage control
  Control of fecal spillage
  Packing
  Temporary abdominal closure
  Splinting, external fixation
Critical care unit resuscitation
  Rewarming
  Control acidosis
  Treat coagulopathy
  End-organ support
Definitive reconstructive surgery
  GI continuity
  Removal of packs
  Abdominal closure
  Definitive stabilization of fractures, other injuries

Table 5. *Complications of Damage Control*

Type	Rate, %
Wound infection	5–100
Abdominal abscess	0–83
Dehiscence	9–25
Bile leak	8–33
Enterocutaneous fistula	2–25
Abdominal compartment syndrome	2–25
Multisystem organ failure	20–33
Mortality	12–67

Table 6. *Damage Control Approach to Specific Organ Injury*

Organ	Treatment
Liver	Packing, embolization
Spleen	Splenectomy, not splenorrhaphy
Duodenum	Treat associated vascular injury drain succus
Pancreas	Treat associated vascular injury drain pancreatic bed
Urology	Rapid nephrectomy if hematoma expanding; pack stable hematoma; transurethral or suprapubic bladder catheter; ureteral stents (internal/external)
Pelvic fracture	Pelvic compression (military anti-shock trousers, sheet); external fixator; embolization (5–10%)
Extremity fracture	External fixator; temporary soft-tissue coverage

or thoracic integrity at a subsequent operation. In general, the decision to proceed with a damage control approach comes from the operating surgeon prompted by the patient's presenting pathophysiology and response to resuscitation.

With the escalation of gun violence in the late 1980s and early 1990s, trauma centers accumulated significant experience in treating severely injured patients. They found that efforts to proceed with definitive repair at initial operation often led to patient demise despite control of anatomic bleeding. Many of the damage control techniques used today were developed during this period. Various descriptors have been used to describe the procedure: *temporary abdominal closure* ("bailout surgery"), *abbreviated laparotomy*, *planned reoperation*, and *staged laparotomy*. *Damage control* is a term used by the US Navy to describe the capacity of a ship to absorb damage and maintain mission integrity. It has become the preferred descriptor of this modern, three-phase surgical approach to the catastrophically injured patient. Damage control is neither a bailout procedure nor an abandonment of proper surgical technique. It is a deliberate and calculated surgical approach requiring mature surgical judgment. The decision to use damage control is now often made on presentation on the basis of patient pathophysiology (coagulopathy, hypothermia, and acidosis), subsequent response to fluid therapy, and magnitude of blood loss. Classic triggers for damage control are well described and may include pH <7.30, transfusion of ≥10 U of packed RBCs (estimated blood loss >4 L), and temperature ≤35°C. Success with damage control requires its application prior to onset of profound acidosis when rapid control of hemorrhage, simultaneous resuscitation, and reversal of hypothermia can best limit coagulopathy.

Damage control philosophy has undergone maturation with involved personnel understanding the pathophysiology and supporting the steps necessary to reverse the cascade of events leading to resuscitation failure. It has become increasingly apparent that damage control does not simply describe the initial truncated operation but the entire process from the first moment of patient contact in the field until definitive repair has been successfully completed.

The best prospective data on the impact of damage control surgery came from the Shock Trauma Center at the University of Maryland. These investigators gathered data prospectively on 56 consecutive patients admitted from May 2000 to January 2002. After stratifying patients based on physiologic parameters, readmissions, complications, and long-term outcome were recorded. Blunt and penetrating injuries were seen in equal proportions. Liver injuries were the most common solid-organ injury, followed by bowel, spleen, great-vessel, and pancreatic injuries. Initial management entailed four abdominal surgical procedures per patient. The mortality rate during the initial admission to the trauma center was 27%. Hospital length of stay was 30 days. Seventy-four readmissions and 58 subsequent surgical procedures took place in the 41 patients during the follow-up interval of this study. Seventy-six percent of damage control patients were readmitted at least one time. Infection, ventral hernia repair, and fistula management were the most common reasons for readmission. No patient who survived index hospitalization died during the follow-up interval. The initial patient group managed with damage control intervention had a 58% survival in 1993. Two reports in 2001 and 2007 document survival of 73% and 90%, respectively.

Abdominal Closure

A variety of methods to accomplish temporary abdominal closure have evolved with damage control techniques. Most operators now do not close skin or fascia after the initial operation. A variety of temporary dressings including the "vacuum pack" technique are used for temporary abdominal closure in damage control patients. In our center, the nonadherent aspect of a small bowel bag is placed on the intestine with interposition of omentum between the dressing and intestine if possible. Our temporary abdominal dressing allows rapid and effective temporary abdominal coverage and increase in abdominal capacity. Controlled egress of fluid from the abdomen is permitted by drains, which are laid within the layers of the dressing, and the sterile barrier created in the operating room is maintained. Prior to use of temporary abdominal closure techniques, which increase the abdominal domain, intra-abdominal hypertension (IAH) was a common complication in patients receiving standard closure of the abdomen after massive fluid resuscitation. During this earlier time period, abdominal compartment pressures were

not routinely measured and abdominal compartment syndrome less well recognized as a cause of refractory shock.

Contemporary approaches allow rapid detection of IAH and abdominal compartment syndrome when clinical signs (distended abdomen, elevated peak inflation pressures, decreased urine output, elevated bladder pressures) are suggestive of its presence. The use of temporary abdominal closure does not eliminate the possibility of abdominal compartment syndrome, but these techniques allow sufficient expansion of the abdominal domain that makes this problem infrequent.

Abdominal Compartment Syndrome

IAH has a variety of physiologic effects. In experimental preparations, animals die from congestive heart failure when abdominal pressure passes a critical threshold. Increased intra-abdominal pressure (IAP) significantly decreases cardiac output and left and right ventricular stroke work and increases central venous pressure, pulmonary artery wedge pressure, and systemic and pulmonary vascular resistance. Abdominal decompression reverses these changes. As both hemidiaphragms are displaced upward with increased IAP, decreased thoracic volume and compliance are seen. Decreased volume within the pleural cavities predisposes to atelectasis and deceases alveolar clearance. Pulmonary infections may also result. Ventilated patients with abdominal hypertension require increased airway pressure to deliver a fixed tidal volume. As the diaphragm protrudes into the pleural cavity, intrathoracic pressure increases with reduction of cardiac output and increased pulmonary vascular resistance. Ventilation and perfusion abnormalities result and blood gas measurements demonstrate hypoxemia, hypercarbia, and acidosis. Elevation of IAP also causes renal dysfunction. Control of IAP leads to reversal of renal impairment. IAP as low as 15 to 20 mm Hg may produce oliguria. Anuria is seen with higher IAPs. Clearly, deterioration in cardiac output plays a role in diminished renal perfusion, but even when cardiac output is maintained at normal or supranormal values by blood volume expansion, impairment of renal function persists in the setting of IAH. Renal dysfunction is also caused by

Table 7. *Causes of Abdominal Hypertension**

Peritoneal tissue edema
  Diffuse peritonitis
  Severe abdominal trauma
Fluid overload secondary to hemorrhagic or septic shock
Retroperitoneal hematoma
Reperfusion injury after bowel ischemia
Inflammatory edema secondary to acute pancreatitis
Ileus and bowel obstruction
Intra-abdominal masses
Abdominal packing for hemorrhage
Closure of the abdomen under tension
Intra-abdominal fluid accumulations

---

*Modified from Wittman DH. Compartment syndrome of the abdominal cavity. In: Irwin RS, Rippe JM, eds. Intensive care medicine. 5th ed. Philadelphia, PA: Lippincott, Williams & Wilkins, 2003; 1694–1709.

compression of the renal vein, which creates partial renal blood outflow obstruction. Compression of the abdominal aorta and renal arteries may contribute to increased renal vascular resistance. Direct pressure on the kidneys may also elevate cortical pressures (Table 7).

Other organs affected by increased IAP include the liver, where hepatic blood flow has been demonstrated to decrease with abdominal hypertension. It may be assumed that hepatic synthesis of acute phase proteins, Igs, and other factors of host defense may be impaired by reduced hepatic flow. Other GI functions may be compromised by increased IAP. Splanchnic hypoperfusion may begin with IAP as low as 15 mm Hg. Reduced perfusion of intra-abdominal arteries, veins, and lymphatics may create changes in mucosal pH, translocation, bowel motility, and production of GI hormones. Finally, intracranial hypertension is seen with chronic increase in IAP. Intracranial hypertension has been demonstrated to decrease when IAP is reduced in morbidly obese patients. Abdominal hypertension significantly increases intracranial pressures at IAPs routinely used during laparoscopy.

A recent international conference has attempted to standardize definitions of intra-abdominal hypertension and abdominal compartment syndrome. IAP should be expressed in millimeters of mercury and measured at end-expiration in the complete supine position after ensuring that abdominal muscle contractions are absent with a transducer zeroed at the level of the midaxillary line. The current reference standard for IAP measurement is the pressure measured via an indwelling urinary drainage catheter within the bladder. Using a bladder catheter, the aspiration port may be connected to a pressure transducer, and IAP read from the bedside monitor. An alternative and less expensive technique is to read the height of the urine column in urinary catheter drainage tubing (for either pressure measurement, 50 mL of sterile room temperature saline solution is instilled in the bladder, and a stabilization period of 30 to 60 s is allowed). Abdominal perfusion pressure (APP) assesses not only severity of IAH but also the adequacy of the systemic perfusion. APP = mean arterial pressure minus IAP. IAH is the pathologic evaluation of IAP. IAH is defined by sustained or repeated IAP $\geq$ 12 mm Hg or an APP $\leq$60 mm Hg. Grades of IAH have been proposed: grade I, IAP from 12 to 15 mm Hg; grade II, IAP from 16 to 20 mm Hg; grade III, IAP from 21 to 25 mm Hg; and grade IV, IAP >25 mm Hg. IAH may be divided into two types. Acute IAH develops within hours as a result of trauma, intra-abdominal hemorrhage, or over days as a result of sepsis, capillary leak, or other critical illness. Chronic IAH develops over months to years as a result of morbid obesity, intra-abdominal tumor growth, chronic ascites, or pregnancy, and is characterized by progressive abdominal wall adaptation to increase in IAP.

Abdominal compartment syndrome (ACS) is present when organ dysfunction occurs as a result of IAH. ACS is defined by sustained or repeated IAP > 20 mm Hg and/or APP <60 mm Hg in association with new-onset single or multiple organ failure. ACS is not graded but rather considered as an all-or-none phenomenon. ACS may be further divided into three types. Primary ACS develops due to conditions associated with injury or disease in the abdominal/pelvic region requiring emergent surgical or angioradiographic intervention. Secondary ACS develops due to conditions outside the abdomen, such as sepsis, capillary leak, major burns, or other conditions requiring massive fluid resuscitation. Recurrent ACS develops following initial successful surgical or medical treatment of either primary or secondary ACS or following closure of a previous decompressive laparotomy.

Operative decompression is the method of choice in the patient with severe abdominal hypertension and evidence of intra-abdominal organ

Trauma and Thermal Injury (Dries)

dysfunction. After decompression, improvements in hemodynamics, pulmonary function, tissue perfusion, and renal function have been demonstrated in a variety of clinical settings. To prevent hemodynamic decompensation during decompression, intravascular volume should be restored, oxygen delivery maximized, and hypothermia and coagulation defects corrected. The abdomen should be opened under optimal conditions in the operating room, including hemodynamic monitoring with adequate venous access and controlled ventilation. Adjunctive measures to combat expected reperfusion wash out from byproducts of anaerobic metabolism include prophylactic volume loading and use of vasoconstrictor agents to prevent sudden changes in BP. After decompression, the abdomen and the fascial gap is left open using one of a variety of temporary abdominal closure methods.

Abdominal Organ Injury

The focus on management for intra-abdominal organ injury remains nonoperative. The practitioner must be aware, however, of patients at greater risk for failure of that approach. Nonoperative management should be entertained only in hemodynamically stable patients. Identifying hemodynamically stable patients may be challenging in the setting of multiple injuries. A recent multicenter study of blunt splenic injury from the Eastern Association for the Surgery of Trauma (EAST) included > 1,400 patients (age <15 years) from 26 centers. Nonoperative management was attempted in 61% of these patients, with a resulting failure rate of 10.4%. Failure was associated with increasing age, injury severity score, GCS, grade of splenic injury, and quantity of hemoperitoneum. Interestingly, other studies of nonoperative management of splenic injury suggest that many patients in high-risk categories can be managed nonoperatively, and that there is no increased mortality with failure of this approach.

Advances in nonoperative management have indicated differences between the spleen and liver. A high percentage of liver injuries appear to be manageable nonoperatively, and a somewhat lower proportion of liver injuries fail nonoperative management in comparison with blunt injury to the spleen. It has been speculated that liver injuries are more commonly associated with low-pressure venous injuries, and a greater proportion of spleen injuries are associated with arterial or arteriolar injury. Planned nonoperative management of the liver may be attempted in as many as 85% of patients with liver injuries; a failure rate of only 7% was found. In addition, significant improvement in outcome with nonoperative management was identified compared to operative management with respect to abdominal infection rates, transfusions, and length of hospital stay. Patients requiring operation due to hemodynamic instability may be successfully treated with packing. Evolution to nonoperative management in stable patients with high-grade injury results in lower mortality. In another major report from the University of Louisville, death secondary to blunt liver injury dropped from 8 to 2%; this improvement was attributed to improved methods of managing hepatic venous injuries. Proposed improvements in the management of hepatic venous injury include nonoperative management in stable patients and willingness to employ gauze packing in unstable individuals.

As nonoperative management of abdominal solid-organ injury continues to advance, missed blunt bowel injury has received increased attention. The sensitivity of CT scanning in defining bowel injury has been assessed by a variety of investigators. Recent reports suggest that sensitivity with latest-generation CT scans is as high as 94% for bowel injury particularly if unexplained free fluid is considered a critical finding. A number of patients explored after CT scanning, however, undergo nontherapetic laparotomies for bowel hematomas or contusions.

Late-generation CT scanners, contrast-enhanced CT scans, and angiography support are changing the face of management for injury to the solid abdominal and retroperitoneal organs. As abdominal CT scans replace laparotomy as the definitive diagnostic procedure in injury, the contrast blush is a useful tool in identification of slow bleeding sites associated with lacerations to solid organs. In patients who are hemodynamically stable, these sites may then be embolized with a high degree of success in both the liver and the spleen. Aggressive application of CT scanning and angiographic intervention has increased the rate of salvage and decreased length of stay and resource consumption for patients with these solid-organ injuries. It is important to note that patients with significant solid-organ injury may present without significant free intraperitoneal blood. Therefore, up to 5% of patients with significant trauma may not be appreciated with abdominal ultrasound, which is designed to examine the abdomen for the fluid stripe indicative of free intraperitoneal blood. Many investigators now recommend that abdominal ultrasound not be used as the sole diagnostic modality in stable patients at risk for blunt solid-organ injury. Finally, it appears that the approach to blunt organ injury may vary with the type of hospital treating the patient. A recent multicenter study in Pennsylvania suggested that patients treated at level II trauma centers had a higher rate of operative treatment and lower rate of failure for nonoperative management than level I trauma centers. Mortality for patients managed nonoperatively was lower at level I trauma centers. Level I trauma centers were also more likely to repair rather than remove the spleen.

Perforation of the GI tract, whether due to blunt or penetrating injury, is being managed with direct repair rather than diverting ileostomy or colostomy in an increasing number of patients. Indications for consideration of primary repair of injury perforating the GI tract include good response to resuscitation, lack of acidosis, limited blood loss, limited fecal spillage, and a small number of associated injuries. Where additional life-threatening injuries that complicate evaluation or limit available time for primary bowel repair are present, immediate control of spillage from the gut is appropriate with diversion of the fecal stream at the primary operation or during staged repair in the patient receiving damage control management.

Traumatic Brain Injury

Traumatic brain injury accounts for 40% of all deaths from acute injuries. It is the single most important factor in determining the outcome of various forms of trauma. Two hundred thousand victims with such injuries require hospitalization each year and often are permanently disabled. Many more persons suffer mild traumatic brain injury resulting in a physician visit or temporary disability. Individuals at greatest risk for traumatic

brain injury are typically young and at the beginning of potentially productive life. Thus, loss of potential income, cost of acute care, and continued expenses of rehabilitation and medical care are enormous. These realities mandate aggressive attention to the management of brain injury. Clinical factors associated with poorer outcome with head injury include the following: (1) midline shift on CT scan; (2) systolic BP <90 mm Hg; (3) intracranial pressure (ICP) >15 mm Hg; (4) age >55 years; and GCS score <8. Notably, head injury outcomes are determined by the number of secondary insults, not the injuries to other organ systems or body regions.

Given these realities, the most important concept in the recent treatment of brain-injured patients is the distinction between primary and secondary brain injury. Primary injury is injury that occurs at the time of the traumatic incident and includes brain lacerations or other mechanical injuries to the brain at the moment of impact. After impact, the brain continues to be injured by various mechanisms including the mechanical injury from cerebral edema or intracranial hematomas, ischemia from hypotension, cerebral edema or cerebral vascular dysregulation, hypoxia from inadequate ventilation, and secondary damage from a wide array of inflammation mediators. While prevention is the only strategy to avert primary brain injury, secondary injury can be prevented or at least blunted. Thus, the management of traumatic brain injury now includes increasing emphasis on the prevention of secondary insults.

The most important feature of the initial neurologic examination, the GCS, is designed to identify rapidly the severity of patient injury. Patients with GCS scores of 13 to 15 are considered to have mild head injuries. These individuals have an excellent prognosis and may not require hospitalization. They have a 3% chance of deteriorating into coma, and serial neurologic examinations make this deterioration easy to detect. Individuals with GCS scores of 8 to 12 have moderate head injury. These patients do not have normal neurologic examinations, but the severity of their injuries usually is not appreciated until the full GCS score is obtained. This group of patients has a 20% chance of declining into coma (GCS score ≤8). Patients with severe head injury have the worst prognosis and require the most immediate care.

All of these individuals require head CT scanning; except for select subpopulations, all of them require ICP monitoring. As a group, there is a >50% chance of an increased ICP; their depressed clinical examinations often preclude detection of changing neurologic status until their condition reaches catastrophic deterioration.

Evacuation of mass lesions has been the traditional focus of brain injury management throughout this century. The goal of removing space-occupying lesions is to prevent cerebral herniation. In previous studies among patients who talk and die, undetected hematomas were the principal cause of death. These are examples of patients who survive primary brain injury with the ability to talk and interact at some level but who later succumb to preventable secondary brain injury. Cerebral herniation, representing the compression of critical neurologic centers against the retaining structures of the skull, is the common final pathway in these patients. Once herniation (regardless of the type) has occurred, patient outcome is dramatically affected. Studies over the last 50 years have demonstrated that once herniation occurs and the patient slips into coma, the mortality rate reaches 33 to 41%, compared with mortality rates of 0 to 21% in patients who present with herniation before coma. Once herniation occurs and the patient progresses to coma, hematomas must be evaluated within hours to avoid a significant risk of mortality.

After evacuation of mass lesions, emphasis is given to monitoring and control of ICP. ICP monitoring was introduced >40 years ago as a means to quantify the study of brain swelling and cerebral edema. While the study of ICP initially focused on prevention of herniation by preventing swelling, it was soon apparent that keeping ICP from rising was a desirable end. As ICP rises, cerebral perfusion decreases and the threat of brain ischemia increases. Data are now emerging, however, that even in patients with adequate cerebral perfusion pressure (CPP), high ICP is associated with poor outcome. In the past, a variety of guidelines have been proposed for the optimal ICP level for treatment. Most current data place 25 mm Hg as the highest acceptable level for ICP at which treatment must begin. Modern methods of ICP monitoring include the ventriculostomy and intraparenchymal fiberoptic or strain-gauge devices. Subarachnoid bolts and epidural monitoring are used rarely or in select patient populations. Ventriculostomy carries an increased risk of infection and a slightly increased risk of bleeding. It is, however, the "gold standard" for ICP measurement.

Experimental work beginning in the mid-1980s demonstrated that ischemia is a significant threat to the head-injured patient. Ischemia had long been recognized as a factor in the outcome of head injury, but recent work has changed the paradigm through which head injury was viewed. Up to this time, the treatment priority has been control of cerebral edema and prevention of cerebral herniation. Any technique reducing ICP was thought to be good for the head-injured patient. By giving equal attention to ischemia, the current approach to the head-injured patient has evolved.

Ischemia is common following head injury. Autopsy findings have indicated that 60% of head-injured patients had ischemia. Cerebral blood flow on the first day after injury is less than half that of healthy individuals and may approach the ischemic threshold. In normal gray matter, cerebral blood flow is 50 mL/100 g/min of tissue; in white matter, cerebral blood flow is 18 mL/100 g/min of tissue. Typical blood flow to gray matter within the first 8 h after head injury is 30 mL/100 g/min of tissue; in individuals with more severe injuries, cerebral blood flow as low as <20 mL/100 g/min of tissue has been noted.

Improved recent understanding of cerebral blood flow coincides with multiple studies demonstrating disastrous consequences of hypotension in the setting of head injury. An increased death rate in head-injured patients with hypotension was documented in the National Traumatic Coma Data Bank, in which the two most important factors related to outcome from head injuries were time spent with an ICP >20 mm Hg and time spent with a systolic pressure <90 mm Hg. These data suggest that patients with only a single episode of systolic BP <90 mm Hg have a significantly worse outcome than those individuals who never experience this degree of hypotension.

Recent head injury management therefore places maintenance of adequate CPP as a goal equivalent to prevention of high ICP. The autoregulatory mechanisms in the brain are designed to maintain cerebral blood flow constant over a range of CPP ranging from 50 to 150 mm Hg. This highly adaptive capacity allows the brain to see constant blood supply, despite changes in position and activity. In the severely injured brain, cerebral blood flow passively follows CPP. In the extreme case, with cerebral autoregulation disabled, cerebral ischemia results as patients are maintained in a hypovolemic state with low mean arterial pressure to reduce cerebral blood volume and thereby ICP. In this practice, CPP was maintained below the autoregulatory threshold. Seemingly paradoxically, the best way to reduce ICP is to increase CPP into the autoregulatory range. This practice avoids hypotension and the ischemic damage that almost certainly attended the old practice of keeping patients with severe head injury "dry" and their arterial pressure low. At present, it is unclear what an adequate CPP is. Based on available data, including stepwise regression analysis, a CPP of 70 mm Hg has been suggested as a desirable level. Most head injury research protocols maintain this level.

Cerebral edema was thought to be aggravated by overzealous fluid administration, leading to increased intracranial pressure, brain ischemia and, ultimately, a poor outcome. However, in the patient with multiple injuries without head injury, aggressive volume resuscitation is a widely accepted method to maintain end-organ perfusion and adequate oxygen delivery. Traditional management strategies of the patient with severe head injury have changed with the knowledge of adverse effects of secondary brain insults. Much like the treatment of MI for which the original zone of injury cannot be restored to normal, emphasis in the management of brain injury must be placed on avoidance of secondary insults to prevent extension of injury resulting from ischemia. An analysis of the Traumatic Coma Data Bank demonstrated that hypoxia and hypotension in the immediate period after head injury resulted in mortality rates of 28% and 50%, respectively. When the combined effect of hypoxia and hypotension during resuscitation was analyzed, the mortality rate increased to 57%. Later studies by other workers, using an algorithm guided by optimization of CPP, demonstrated a lower mortality in a cohort of patients thought to be similar to those enrolled in the Traumatic Coma Data Bank.

The second important consideration after avoidance of hypotension during resuscitation of the head-injured patient is the prevention of hypoxia. Hypoxia is one of the five top predictors of poor outcome in the National Traumatic Coma Data Bank, with 30 to 60% of severely head-injured patients presenting with hypoxia. While the optimal Pao_2 level in the head-injured patient has not been determined, available data suggest that a level of <60 mm Hg (< 8.0 kPa) is associated with poor outcome.

ICP is controlled with a variety of modalities. Our views on the use of these modalities and the management of head injury continue to evolve. Hyperventilation reduces ICP by reducing cerebral blood volume with increased cerebral vascular tone and induction of hypocapnia. Reduction in cerebral blood volume leads to intracranial blood volume loss and lower ICP. For many years, hyperventilation has been a primary means of reducing ICP. Hyperventilation can cause vasoconstriction independent of the metabolic demands of the brain. Hyperventilation may, therefore, reduce blood flow to the brain even if that reduction results in an ischemic injury. Recent studies using jugular venous oximetry have indicated that hyperventilation may produce cerebral ischemia. Other studies demonstrated that desaturation found in jugular venous blood is more common with hyperventilation than with other means employed for reduction in ICP. One prospective, randomized trial evaluated severely head-injured patients managed with hypocapnia vs normocapnia. The normocapnic group had better outcome at 3-month and 6-month follow-ups. Increasing evidence indicates that hyperventilation is an ICP treatment with high cost, the threat of ischemia. Current management therefore includes use of less toxic means of reducing ICP, if available, rather than the use of hyperventilation. For example, drainage of cerebrospinal fluid (CSF) through ventricular drains should be started early with aggressive use of sedation, muscle relaxants, and administration of mannitol before resorting to hyperventilation.

Drainage of CSF and use of mannitol may be employed to control ICP and to optimize CPP. Some medical centers are facilitating drainage of CSF by placing ventriculotomy catheters when possible, as opposed to subarachnoid monitors, which do not allow for CSF removal. Drainage of CSF may be the first choice for the treatment of increased ICP. Mannitol is an osmotic diuretic administered as a bolus that develops an osmotic gradient between the blood and the brain. Mannitol may also act by improving cerebral blood flow through reduction in hematocrit and viscosity. Mannitol, however, cannot be administered to hypotensive patients because it will magnify shock states. In large doses, mannitol may lead to acute renal failure. If administered as a constant infusion, mannitol may also open the blood-brain barrier and result in rebound cerebral edema. Mannitol drips therefore are not recommended. Serum osmolarity must be monitored in individuals who receive mannitol for control of ICP and optimization of CPP.

Recent developments in the care of the head-injured patient focus on the importance of secondary brain injury as a determinant of prognosis. In studies of long-term outcome, the key elements of secondary brain injury, hypoxia, and hypotension with secondary ischemia are recognized as occurring with increasing frequency. Optimal modalities to control secondary brain injury focus on maintenance of optimal CPP with the lowest possible ICP consistent with avoidance of cerebral ischemia. To control ICP, hyperventilation is now employed as an emergency tool rather than as a primary therapy.

Injury to Thoracic Aorta

Injury to the thoracic aorta is common among victims of high-speed motor vehicle crashes with an acute deceleration mechanism. Many victims of this injury are dead at the scene. An estimated 20% of the persons who sustain deceleration injury to the thoracic aorta live to reach the hospital due to containment of aortic rupture by connective tissue covering the aorta. Without recognition and treatment of this injury, 30% of these individuals will die within 12 h and 50% within 1 week. The mechanism of injury is a combination of differential deceleration of the mediastinal contents and force provided by the steering wheel or dashboard impacting the chest. Falls may also produce this injury. Most often, disruption occurs at the aortic isthmus, just distal to the origin of the left subclavian artery at the ligamentum arteriosum.

The initial anteroposterior chest radiograph is the single most important screening tool for injury to the thoracic aorta. Arteriography is the "gold standard" diagnostic study because of its ability to demonstrate the specific injury and reveal unsuspected vascular anomalies. Unfortunately, intimal flaps are being reported in up to 10% of studies. Most of these lesions resolve spontaneously and may be managed nonoperatively. In the emergency setting, newer spiral CT scans have become useful at rapidly diagnosing thoracic aortic injuries (particularly to the descending aorta) because of their greater speed and resolution. With a suspicious mechanism of injury, a clear chest radiograph is inadequate to rule out aortic injury. While mediastinal widening warrants aortography, 80% of the time the angiogram does not show injury to the thoracic aorta as the cause of mediastinal widening. Thus, latest-generation CT imaging is becoming an acceptable method for evaluation of the widened mediastinum with aortography in cases requiring further definition.

Patients who are unstable at the scene of a crash or during the first 4 h of hospitalization have a mortality rate >90%. Hemodynamically stable patients whose systolic BP does not exceed 120 mm Hg during the first to 6 to 8 h after injury have a survival rate >90%. Of the operative procedures for repairing injuries to the descending aorta, the most dreaded complication is paraplegia. Unfortunately, no one causative or preventative factor has been identified.

Various reports have suggested that operative management of injury to the descending aorta may be delayed in stable patients for a period that can range from hours to months. These individuals should receive an afterload-reducing agent or a drug to alter dP/dT (change in pressure over time), have their BP maintained at or <120/80 mm Hg, and have a stable mediastinal hematoma. Delayed reconstruction of chronic posttraumatic aneurysm of the descending aorta, using endovascular stented grafts, is also being reported. At this time, expeditious repair of injury to the descending aorta remains the most cost-effective approach with no additional risk of complications in adequately resuscitated patients.

Esophageal Perforation

Esophageal perforation is a true emergency and therapeutic challenge because delay affects survival. Broad-spectrum antibiotics, improved nutrition, and improved critical care have led to better results. Iatrogenic esophageal disruption (60%), spontaneous perforation (15%), and external trauma (20%) are responsible for the majority of esophageal ruptures. Esophageal perforation from penetrating or blunt trauma is frequently obscured by associated injuries and has a poor prognosis if diagnosis is delayed. Self-induced esophageal injury by acid or alkali may cause extensive necrosis and esophageal destruction.

Symptoms and signs vary with the cause and location of perforation as well as the time delay between perforation and diagnosis. Pain is the most consistent symptom, present in 70 to 90% of patients, and it is usually related to the site of disruption. Neck ache and stiffness suggest perforation after endoscopy. In the abdomen, dull epigastric pain radiating to the back may occur if the disruption is posterior and communicates with the lesser sac. Severe chest pain suggests thoracic perforation. Misdiagnosis of dissecting thoracic aneurysm, spontaneous pneumothorax, or MI is common. Acute pain in the epigastrium often suggests perforated peptic ulcer disease or acute pancreatitis. Dysphasia appears late and is generally related to thoracic perforation. Tachycardia and tachypnea are documented in 50 to 70% of patients. Hypotension and shock are present when sepsis or significant inflammatory third spacing occurs. Subcutaneous emphysema is seen frequently when perforation is cervical and less often with thoracic or abdominal injury.

Plain chest radiography suggests the diagnosis in 90% of patients with esophageal perforation. However, immediately after disruption, chest radiographic findings may be normal. Pneumomediastinum, subcutaneous emphysema, mediastinal widening, or a mediastinal air fluid level must prompt investigation to rule out esophageal perforation. Perforation of the distal third of the esophagus leads to hydropneumothorax on the left. Contrast esophagogram with water-soluble material followed by dilute barium reveals primary sites or areas of leakage and determines whether perforation is confined to the mediastinum or communicates freely with the pleural or peritoneal cavities. Unfortunately, the rate of false-negative esophagogram results may be as high as 10%. CT of the chest can often show the site of perforation and is used when presentation is atypical, when signs or symptoms are vague or misleading, or when perforation involves the lesser sac. Mediastinal fluid and air on CT of the chest are strongly suggestive of esophageal perforation. Esophagoscopy can easily miss a perforation or enlarge a hole. This test is usually not performed to identify perforation.

Three factors affect management of esophageal perforation: origin, location, and delay between rupture and treatment. For example, postemetic perforation with massive contamination is the most morbid, whereas pharyngeal perforation rarely ends in fatality because of relative ease of diagnosis, drainage, and repair. Morbidity and mortality increase as perforation extends into the thorax. Patients with perforations of the cervical esophagus have an 85% survival, whereas thoracic disruption is associated with survival rates of 65 to 75%. Abdominal esophageal perforation is associated with 90% survival.

Conservative management is associated with a 22 to 38% mortality. The difficulty with nonoperative management is determination that perforation will remain contained and not cause continued contamination with subsequent uncontrolled infection. Surgery remains the mainstay of treatment. Early surgical reinforced repair with drainage of contaminated spaces provides the best chance of survival after esophageal perforation. Before repair, all nonviable and grossly contaminated tissue in the mediastinum and around the esophagus is debrided. Decortication of trapped lung tissue may be necessary.

Sepsis, shock, pneumothorax, pneumoperitoneum, mediastinal emphysema, and respiratory failure are absolute indications for rapid surgical intervention. Preoperative preparation includes nasogastric intubation for gastric decompression, broad-spectrum antibiotics, and IV fluid resuscitation. Cervical perforation is best treated by direct suture closure and drainage of the neck. Thoracic esophageal perforation requires right thoracotomy for exposure of the upper two thirds and left thoracotomy for control of the lower third. Lesions at the esophagogastric junction are approached by left thoracotomy or upper midline laparotomy, and repairs may be buttressed by gastric fundoplication. Late perforations usually can be repaired primarily with muscle or pleural reinforcement. If repair is not possible, most operators favor esophageal resection, cervical esophagostomy, and enteral feeding tube placement with later reconstruction. Perforations encountered late may initially be treated by wide drainage of the mediastinum by opening the pleura along the length of the esophagus. Patients with complex perforations should preferably be administered a jejunostomy, enteral nutrition, or parenteral hyperalimentation because gastrostomy should be avoided for later reconstruction. Alternative procedures (esophageal exclusion, T-tube drainage, and esophageal resection) have been proposed for patients with late esophageal disruption. Exclusion of the perforated esophagus by division of the esophagus adjacent to the stomach and at the neck allows partial or total exclusion of the perforation. One of the major disadvantages of this approach is the obligation to perform a second major reconstructive procedure. T-tube drainage of the perforation creates a controlled esophagocutaneous fistula, but continued leakage may progress to mediastinal and pulmonary sepsis. If extensive mediastinitis and sepsis are present with continued contamination, resection of the esophagus with delayed reconstruction is preferable.

In summary, treatment of esophageal perforation is directed toward fluid resuscitation, control of sepsis, operative drainage of the mediastinum and pleural cavity, suture repair of the esophagus if possible, and reinforcement of the suture line with vascularized tissue particularly muscle. Delay in diagnosis makes repair more difficult because of friability and necrotic tissue at the site of the tear. Primary repair may be possible, but cervical diversion with esophageal exclusion and long-term tube feeding may be necessary. Postoperative care emphasizes control of infection and nutrition support until healing of an esophageal injury is demonstrated.

Blunt Cardiac Injury

Cardiac injuries from blunt chest trauma are usually the result of high-speed motor vehicle crashes. Falls from heights, crushing injuries from motor vehicle crashes and falling objects, blast injuries, and direct violent trauma from assault are less common causes of blunt cardiac injury. Blunt trauma to the heart ranges from minor injuries to frank cardiac rupture. Minor injury is a nonspecific condition frequently termed *cardiac contusion*, or *myocardial contusion*. Moderately severe lesions may include injury to the pericardium, valves, papillary muscles, and coronary vessels. The most severe of blunt cardiac injuries is the dramatic and often fatal condition of cardiac rupture.

The reported incidence of blunt cardiac injury depends on the modality and criteria used for diagnosis. The occurrence rate ranges from 8 to 71% in patients sustaining blunt chest trauma. The true occurrence rate remains unknown because there is no diagnostic "gold standard." The lack of such a standard leads to confusion with respect to making the diagnosis, thereby making the available literature difficult to interpret. Key issues involve identification of a patient population at risk for adverse events from blunt cardiac injury and then appropriately monitoring and treating these individuals. Conversely, patients who are not at risk for complications could be discharged from the hospital with appropriate follow-up.

EAST has recently reviewed studies that focused on the identification of blunt cardiac injury. Based on randomized, prospective data, they recommend that an admission ECG should be performed in all patients in whom blunt cardiac injury is suspected. Additional recommendations included continuous ECG monitoring for 24 to 48 h in patients in whom the initial ECG was abnormal. Similarly, if patients are hemodynamically unstable, evaluation should proceed with transthoracic echocardiography followed by transesophageal echocardiography if an optimal study cannot be obtained. Finally, patients with coexisting cardiac disease and those with an abnormal admission ECG finding may undergo surgery if they are appropriately monitored. These individuals may require placement of a pulmonary artery catheter. The presence of sternal fracture does not predict the presence of blunt cardiac injury. To date, enzyme analysis is inadequate for identifying patients with blunt cardiac injury.

Pelvic Fracture

Substantial blunt force is required to disrupt the pelvic ring. The extent of injury is related to the direction and magnitude of the force. Associated abdominal, thoracic, and head injuries are common. Forces applied to the pelvis can cause rotational displacement with opening or compression of the pelvic ring. The other type of displacement seen with pelvic fractures is vertical, with complete disruption of the pelvic ring and the posterior sacroiliac complex.

Patients with pelvic ring injuries are easily subclassified into two groups on the basis of clinical presentation: (1) those who are hemodynamically stable; and (2) those who are hemodynamically unstable. There is a dramatic difference in the mortality rates between pelvic fracture patients who are hypotensive (38%) and those who are hemodynamically stable (3%). Hemodynamic instability and biomechanical pelvic instability are separate though related issues, which tend to confuse the clinical picture. The source of bleeding may be multifactorial and not directly related to the pelvic fracture itself. However, pelvic fracture blood loss that contributes to hemodynamic instability is a significant risk factor. Early fracture diagnosis and stabilization, using external skeletal fixation, are extremely important in the acute phase of patient management. Treatment of the patient is also directed by response to initial fluid resuscitation. It is essential to examine for other sources of hemorrhage (intrathoracic, intraperitoneal, external) in patients with evidence of ongoing bleeding. Retroperitoneal bleeding in a pelvic fracture patient usually arises from a low-pressure source, the cancellous bone at the fracture site or adjacent venous injury. Significant retroperitoneal arterial bleeding occurs in only approximately 10% of patients. Clinical evidence has suggested that provisional fracture stabilization using a simple anterior external fixator or even "wrapping" in a bed sheet can control low-pressure bleeding. Continued unexplained bleeding after provisional fracture stabilization suggests an arterial source. Angiography with embolization of the involved vessel is then indicated. Therapeutic angiography may also be required after abdominal exploration if a rapidly expanding or pulsatile retroperitoneal hematoma is encountered. In general, definitive operative stabilization of pelvic fractures is delayed 3 to 5 days to allow the patient to recover from acute injury.

Deep Venous Thrombosis and Thromboembolism

That deep venous thrombosis and thromboembolism occur after trauma is incontrovertible. The optimal mode of prophylaxis has yet to be determined. Low-dose heparin (5,000 U subcutaneously bid or tid) represents one pharmacologic treatment modality used for prophylaxis against deep venous thrombosis and pulmonary embolism. A metaanalysis of 29 trials and >8,000 surgical patients demonstrated that low-dose heparin significantly decreased the frequency of deep venous thrombosis from 25.2% in patients with no prophylaxis to 8.7% in treated individuals. Similarly, pulmonary embolism was halved by low-dose heparin treatment (0.5% with treatment compared with 1.2% in control subjects). In double-blind trials, the occurrence rate of major hemorrhage was higher in patients treated with anticoagulation than in control subjects, but the difference in incidence was not significant. Minor bleeding complications, such as wound hematomas, were more frequent in low-dose heparin treatment patients (6.3%) than in control subjects (4.1%).

Unfractionated low-dose heparin has not been shown to be particularly effective in preventing venous thromboembolism (VTE) in trauma patients. Two recent prospective trials demonstrated that low-dose heparin was not better in preventing deep venous thrombosis than no prophylaxis in patients with an injury severity score of >9. Sample sizes in these studies were small, and statistical error could not be excluded. The results of low-dose heparin administration after injury with regard to pulmonary embolism were even more vague.

Defining the trauma patient at risk for VTE is subjective and variable in the literature. The following injury patterns appear to differentiate high-risk patients for VTE: closed-head injury (GCS score <8), pelvis plus long-bone fractures (multiple long-bone fractures), and spinal cord injury. Greenfield and associates have developed a risk factor assessment tool for VTE; preliminary evidence supported this risk factor assessment tool as a valid indicator of the development of VTE. In this scale, risk factors are weighted; scores of <3 represent low risk, scores of 3 to 5 represent

Table 8. *Risk Factors Associated With VTE in Trauma**

Underlying condition
  Obesity
  Malignancy
  Abnormal coagulation factors on hospital admission
  History of VTE
Iatrogenic factors
  Central femoral line >24 h
  >4 transfusions in first 24 h
  Surgical procedure >2 h
  Repair or ligation of major vascular injury
Injury-related factors
  Abbreviated injury scale >2 for chest
  Abbreviated injury scale >2 for abdomen
  Abbreviated injury scale >2 for head
  Coma (GCS score <8 for >4h
  Complex lower-extremity fracture
  Pelvic fracture
  Spinal cord injury with paraplegia or quadriplegia
Age (sequential increased risk with age)
  >40 but <60 yr
  >60 but <75 yr
  >75 yr

*From J Trauma 1997; 42:100–103.

moderate risk, and scores of >5 represent high risk (Table 8).

There is a wealth of randomized, prospective data supporting the use of low-molecular-weight heparin as VTE prophylaxis in orthopedic surgery. This literature is derived primarily from total hip replacement and knee replacement patients. We now have data suggesting that low-molecular-weight heparin is superior to unfractionated heparin for prophylaxis in moderate- to high-risk trauma patients. Most data in many different types of patients confirm improved efficacy of low-molecular-weight heparin with the same or even less bleeding risk compared with prophylaxis with unfractionated heparin. Low-molecular-weight heparin should be the standard form of VTE prophylaxis in trauma patients with complex pelvic and lower-extremity injuries as well as in those patients with spinal cord injuries. This agent is also safe for patients receiving craniotomy or nonoperative management of solid organ injury if started 24 or 72 h after injury respectively. Finally, the literature is beginning to support the use of inferior vena cava filters in high-risk trauma patients without a documented occurrence of deep venous thrombosis or pulmonary embolism and who cannot receive prophylactic therapy.

For established deep venous thrombosis or pulmonary embolism, anticoagulation is a well-established treatment. Current evidence suggests that a 3- to 6-month period provides adequate treatment for the first episode of deep venous thrombosis or pulmonary embolism in a patient without clotting abnormality. Patients in whom the risk of recurrent VTE extends >6 months may have anticoagulation extended indefinitely. In addition, patients whose injuries preclude the use of anticoagulants because bleeding would exacerbate their injury should have consideration given to placement of a vena cava filter. Recent evidence also supported initial treatment of VTE with low-molecular-weight heparin.

Evaluation for deep venous thrombosis in the setting of injury receives continued study. Early identification of this complication would allow treatment to be initiated, thus decreasing the frequency and severity of complications. Studies in the nontrauma literature support the accuracy of both Doppler and duplex ultrasonography in the detection of deep venous thrombosis in the symptomatic patient. The overall accuracy of screening ultrasonography in the asymptomatic patient is less clear. Similarly, impedance plethysmography has high sensitivity and specificity in the detection of proximal deep venous thrombosis in symptomatic patients. Its low sensitivity in detecting deep venous thrombosis in asymptomatic patients precludes use as a surveillance technique in trauma patients at high risk for deep venous thrombosis. Logistical problems and complications associated with venography make the procedure less appealing than other noninvasive diagnostic measures. Venography still has a role in confirming deep venous thrombosis in trauma patients if diagnostic studies are equivocal. At present, it appears that future investigational efforts are best directed at developing the role of duplex ultrasonography in screening for deep venous thrombosis in the setting of injury.

Antibiotic Management

Much of the data surrounding antibiotic use in patients following injury comes from studies of patients with penetrating abdominal trauma. There are a wide variety of randomized prospective data available, which support clear recommendations regarding the use of antibiotics in this patient group. While antibiotic therapy must be initiated prior to operation or in the emergency department, the intensivist should be aware of available recommendations regarding appropriate agents, duration of therapy, and the impact of shock and resuscitation.

In a clinical management update produced by the Practice Management Guidelines Workgroup of EAST, evidence regarding antibiotic use in penetrating abdominal trauma was reviewed. These writers suggest that there are sufficient randomized prospective data to recommend the use of only a single preoperative dose of prophylactic antibiotics with broad-spectrum aerobic and anaerobic coverage as a standard of care for trauma patients sustaining penetrating abdominal wounds. If no hollow viscus injury is noted subsequently, no further antibiotic administration is warranted. The second issue addressed is the duration of therapy in the presence of injury to any hollow viscus. Based on available prospective randomized data, there is sufficient evidence to recommend continuation of prophylactic antibiotics for only 24 h even in the presence of injury to any hollow viscus. Unfortunately, there are insufficient data to provide meaningful guidelines for reducing infection risks in trauma patients with hemorrhagic shock. Vasoconstriction alters the normal distribution of antibiotics, resulting in reduced tissue penetration. To alleviate this problem, administered antibiotic doses may be increased twofold to threefold and repeated after every tenth unit of blood transfusion until there is no further blood loss. As the patient is resuscitated, antibiotics with activity against obligate and facultative anaerobic bacteria should be continued for periods dependent on the degree of identified wound contamination. Notably, aminoglycosides have been demonstrated to exhibit suboptimal activity in patients with serious injury, probably due to altered pharmacokinetics of drug distribution. Finally, a metaanalysis has examined studies assessing effectiveness of a single agent vs combination therapy containing aminoglycosides for penetrating wounds. This report concludes that single β-lactam agents were as effective as combination therapy in the setting of penetrating abdominal trauma.

Controversy continues regarding appropriate antibiotic therapy for open fractures. Where lesser degrees of soft-tissue injury are present, a first-generation cephalosporin with 24 h of coverage is appropriate. The most difficult open fracture is the tibial fracture with significant soft-tissue damage. These wounds require Gram-negative as well as Gram-positive coverage. The likelihood of infection is generally associated with the degree of soft-tissue injury. Antibiotic support may be continued until closure is accomplished.

Fewer data are available regarding the use of antibiotics in patients following blunt injury. In the absence of monitoring device placement or the use of tube thoracostomy, antibiotics are not warranted. Many practitioners, however, believe Gram-positive antibiotic coverage is appropriate in the patient with tube thoracostomy or with invasive monitors of ICP. There are no randomized prospective data or multidisciplinary guidelines available to address this issue.

Thermal Injury

Thermal injury is a major public health problem for 2 to 2.5 million people who seek medical treatment in the United States each year. Thermal injury results in 100,000 to 150,000 hospitalizations and 6,000 to 12,000 fatalities. Death rates are highest in the very young and the very old. Scalds are the most common form of childhood thermal trauma, while electrical and chemical injuries affect adults in the workplace. Factors shown to relate to mortality in thermal injury include the size of cutaneous involvement, age, and the presence or absence of inhalation injury.

Nearly 70% of burn patients in the recent iteration of the National Burn Repository (2005) were men. Mean age for all cases was 33 years. Infants accounted for 10% of cases, and patients ≥ 60 years old represented 14% of individuals. Sixty-two percent of reported total burn sizes were <10% total body surface area (TBSA). Inhalation injury was present in 7% of the total reported cases but played a significant role in increasing hospital length of stay and risk of death. The two most common reported etiologies were flame burns and scalds, accounting for almost 80% of cases. There were >6,000 scald injuries in patients <2 years of age, making up 28% of all scald injuries, and 70% of all reported injuries to the population <2 years old. Forty-three percent of burn injuries occurred in the home.

Wound

Characteristics of skin affect patterns of cutaneous injury. Skin is very thin in infants and increases in thickness until 30 to 40 years of age. After this, skin progressively thins. Male subjects have thicker skin than female subjects. Average skin thickness is 1 to 2 mm. In general, the dermis is 10-times thicker than the associated epidermis. Cell types in the epidermis are predominately keratinocytes and melanocytes. The latter cells provide pigment generation against ultraviolet radiation. The predominant cell type in the underlying dermis (derived from the mesoderm) is the fibroblast, which produces collagen and elastin, ground substance of glycosaminoglycans and proteoglycans. The dermis itself consists of a superficial papillary dermis and a thicker reticular dermis.

The skin serves a number of critical functions. Unfortunately, all of these functions may be lost with thermal injury. Most importantly, the skin is a principal barrier against infection. Sebum has noted antibacterial properties. Skin also helps to maintain antigen presentation to immune cells and protects fluid, protein, and electrolyte homeostasis. Skin has various sensory functions, affects heat preservation, and is associated with vitamin production.

In thermal injury, damage to the skin results from temperature of the thermal source and the duration of exposure. At 40 to 44°C, enzymatic failure occurs within the cell with rising intracellular sodium concentration and swelling due to failure of the membrane sodium pump. At exposure to 60°C, necrosis occurs in 1 h with release of oxygen free radicals. Three cutaneous zones of injury have been described:

- The *zone of coagulation* is the site of irreversible cell death with new eschar formation from local degradation of protein.
- The *zone of stasis* is the site of local circulatory impairment with initial cell viability. If ischemia follows in this zone, cell death will occur. Impaired circulation is thought to be secondary to platelet and neutrophil aggregates, fibrin deposition, endothelial cell swelling, and loss of erythrocyte deformability. These tissues are susceptible to secondary insults such as dehydration, pressure, overresuscitation, and infection. Measures implemented to minimize further tissue loss include nondesiccating dressings, careful fluid resuscitation, and topical antimicrobials.
- The *zone of hyperemia* is characterized by minimal cellular injury but prominent vasodilation and increased blood flow. Cell recovery generally occurs in this zone.

Neutrophils are a major source of oxidants released in the burn wound and arrive during early inflammation. Neutrophils are part of the ischemia reperfusion injury, which occurs in the burn wound as suggested by increases in xanthine oxidase activity. Neutrophils are present in large numbers in the dermis within hours after a superficial burn, peaking at 24 h then beginning to resolve by 72 h. The rate of neutrophil sequestration in the deeper burn is slower but persists for a longer time. The longer time to accumulation in the deeper burn is the result of occlusion of superficial vessels in the upper dermis and damage to deeper vessels. Lymphocytes begin to accumulate in the superficial burn at 12 h as well as macrophages. Lymphocytes do not appear to accumulate in the deeper burn. Therefore, superficial burns have more inflammatory cells earlier but progressive damage usually does not occur, whereas measurable progression of dermal microvascular damage occurs in deeper burns but with fewer initial neutrophils.

Cellular Changes

Baxter described the cellular changes that provide the foundation of our present resuscitation strategies. He noted a decrease in cell membrane potential involving burned and unburned tissues. This potential change is associated with increased intracellular sodium, probably due to a decrease in sodium-adenosine triphosphate activity. Resuscitation only partly restores normal intracellular sodium and membrane potentials. Inadequate resuscitation leads to further decline in cell membrane potential and cell death. Later work on burn shock concluded that this phenomenon is due not only to intravascular hypovolemia but also extracellular sodium depletion.

Table 9. *Pathophysiologic Changes in Burn Tissue Leading to Edema**

Marked immediate and sustained increase in the rate of fluid and protein crossing from the capillary to the interstitial space
Rate of edema formation is extremely rapid in the first 1–2 h
Early disruption of the integrity of the interstitial space with disruption of collagen and hyaluronic acid scaffolding
Progressive increase interstitial space compliance as edema forms
Marked transient decrease in interstitial pressure caused by the release of osmotically active particles, causing a vacuum effect "sucking" in fluid from the plasma space
Marked and sustained increase in capillary permeability in the burn wound
Decrease in plasma proteins and oncotic pressure and increase in interstitial protein and oncotic pressure due to increased capillary permeability to protein
Inability to maintain a plasma to interstitial oncotic gradient
Likely a transient increase in capillary hydrostatic pressure in the burn capillaries
Marked and sustained decrease in the surface area of the perfused capillaries and lymphatics, especially in the deep burn
Increase in the ease of fluid accumulation in the interstitium (increase in hydraulic conductivity)

*From J Burn Care Rehabil 2005; 26:207–227.

Edema

Tissue edema after thermal injury is a well-recognized entity. Clinical edema, as seen after burns, is an expansion of the interstitial liquid volume. The interstitium is the intervening space between the vascular and cellular compartments. It binds together structural and cellular elements into a tissue such as the skin dermal matrix. Complications of edema formation are familiar to all who treat burn patients. The edema process is responsible for losses of intravascular fluid. Hypovolemia will occur after large burns if massive volume resuscitation is not provided, particularly in the initial hours after injury when edema formation is most rapid. Hypoproteinemia occurs from the loss of protein in the edema fluid. Edema itself results in tissue hypoxia and increased tissue pressure with circumferential injuries, which can result in further downstream damage. Increased interstitial pressure in burn soft tissue compartments often requires escharotomy or even fasciotomy. It is not unusual to see patients with a 20% increase in body weight after a major burn, owing to the large fluid loads employed in resuscitation. Edema formation is found in burned and unburned tissue.

Peak burn edema formation after a 10% partial-thickness burn occurs at approximately 3 h, whereas after a 40% burn, peak edema does not occur until after 12 h. Total edema is usually less after a larger burn. This is because intravascular volume depletion, which occurs after a larger burn, decreases blood volume and blood flow to burned tissue, allowing less edema. If volume

Table 10. *Mediators Involved With Burn Edema**

Marked early and sustained increase in oxidant activity leading to oxidant damage to the following: interstitial gel, fragmenting collagen, and hyaluronic acid; capillary membrane, leading to increased permeability; distant nonburn tissues
Local increase in a large number of vasoactive mediators that can damage the capillary and interstitium
Prostaglandins, leukotrienes
Cytokines, protease
Histamine, bradykinin
Neuropeptides
Complement components

*From J Burn Care Rehabil 2005; 26:207–227.

resuscitation keeps up with losses in large burns, severe edema formation occurs. Even with massive fluid infusion, hematocrits of 55 to 60% are not uncommon in the early post-burn period, indicating continued loss of plasma volume into burn soft tissues. Where fluid flux has been studied, rate of edema production was matched by rate of fluid clearance after 12 h. Increased protein permeability persists for several days after burn injury. Additional edema is not visible because clearance appears to keep up with fluid deposition (Table 9).

Virtually all components controlling fluid and protein loss from the vascular space are altered after burns. Marked increase in fluid flux into the interstitium is seen due to a combination of decrease in interstitial pressure, an increase in capillary permeability to protein, and further imbalance in hydrostatic and oncotic forces favoring fluid movement into the interstitium. Increased vascular permeability causes marked increase in

AREA	0 to 1	1 to 4	5 to 9	10 to 15	ADULT	% TOTAL
Head	19	17	13	10	7	
Neck	2	2	2	2	2	
Anterior Trunk	13	17	13	13	13	
Posterior Trunk	13	13	13	13	13	
Right Buttock	2.5	2.5	2.5	2.5	2.5	
Left Buttock	2.5	2.5	2.5	2.5	2.5	
Genitalia	1	1	1	1	1	
Right Upper Arm	4	4	4	4	4	
Left Upper Arm	4	4	4	4	4	
Right Lower Arm	3	3	3	3	3	
Left Lower Arm	3	3	3	3	3	
Right Hand	2.5	2.5	2.5	2.5	2.5	
Left Hand	2.5	2.5	2.5	2.5	2.5	
Right Thigh	5.5	5.5	8.5	8.5	9.5	
Left Thigh	5.5	5.5	8.5	8.5	9.5	
Right Leg	5	5	5.5	6	7	
Left Leg	5	5	5.5	6	7	
Right Foot	3.5	3.5	3.5	3.5	3.5	
Left Foot	3.5	3.5	3.5	3.5	3.5	

Trauma and Thermal Injury

LUND & BROWDER CHART   TOTAL

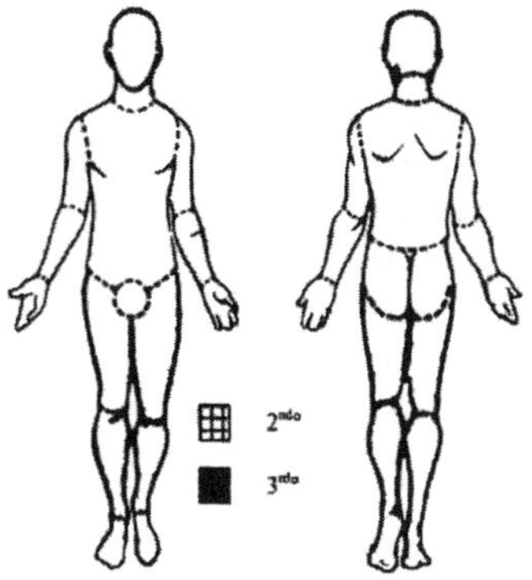

Figure 2. Rule of "nines."

protein content of edema fluid. The combination of abnormalities favoring edema further accelerates plasma protein losses. Some of these changes are transient, such as negative interstitial pressure, whereas other abnormalities such as increased permeability persist as noted above. As edema forms, the interstitium is altered such that more edema is easier to accumulate for the same intravascular and interstitial physical changes. In all probability, this reflects breakdown of the matrix molecules in the interstitium.

There is overwhelming evidence that biochemical mediators released into the burn also play a significant role in the edema process. These mediators are released from injured cells as well as from neutrophils, which rapidly accumulate in injured dermis. These agents are numerous, and it remains difficult to sort out the most important agents, cause, and effect (Table 10).

Wound Care

The degree of injury is assessed by the well-known rule of "nines" (Fig 2). Anatomic criteria can also be employed to recognize the depth of injury and coincident likelihood of healing (Table 11). Partial-thickness injuries should heal within 3 weeks and leave the stratum germinosum intact. Third-degree or full-thickness injuries involve all layers of epidermis and dermis. Some authors

Table 11. *Classification of Burn Depth**

Degree of Burn	Depth of Tissue	Penetration Characteristics
First degree	Partial thickness	Injury to the superficial epidermis, usually caused by overexposure to sunlight or brief heat flashes; classically described as sunburn.
Second degree	Superficial partial thickness	Injury is to the epidermis and upper layers of the dermis. Wounds characteristically appear red, wet, or blistered, blanchable, and extremely painful. Will heal within 3 wk from epidermal regeneration from remaining remnants found in the tracts of hair follicles.
	Deep partial thickness	Injury is through the epidermis and may affect isolated areas of the deep thermal strata from which cells arise. This wound may appear red and wet or white and dry, depending on the extent of deep dermal damage. It heals without grafting but requires >3 wk with suboptimal cosmesis. Excision and split-thickness skin grafting are recommended.
Third degree	Full thickness	Injury has destroyed both the epidermis and the dermis. The wound appears white, will not blanch, and is anesthetic. Tough, nonelastic, and tenacious coagulated protein (eschar) tissue may be present on the surface. This wound will not heal without surgical intervention.

*Reproduced with permission from the Society of Critical Care Medicine.

Table 12. *Topical Antimicrobial Agents**

Agents	Advantages	Disadvantages
Silver sulfadiazine	Painless application; broad spectrum; easy application	May produce transient leukopenia; minimal penetration of eschar; some Gram-negative species resistant
Mafenide acetate	Broad spectrum; easy application; penetrates eschar	Painful application; promotes acid-base imbalance; frequent sensitivity
Bacitracin,	Painless application	No eschar penetration
Polysporin	Nonirritating; transparent; may be used on nonburn wounds	
Silver nitrate (0.5% solution)	Painless application; broad spectrum; rare sensitivity; must be kept moist	No eschar penetration; electrolyte imbalances; discolors the wound and environment
Povidone-iodine	Broad spectrum	Painful application; systemically absorbed; requires frequent reapplication; discolors wounds
Gentamicin	Painless application; broad spectrum	Oto/nephrotoxic; encourages development of resistant organisms

*Reproduced with permission from the Society of Critical Care Medicine.

speak also of fourth-degree injuries, which involve deep structures such as tendon, muscle, and bone.

Local care begins with serial debridement of nonviable tissue and blisters. Topical antimicrobials, one of the major advances in burn wound care, are applied once or twice daily after washes with antiseptic solutions (Table 12). These topical antimicrobials are applied in occlusive dressings that also help maintain fluid balance. The burn wound affords a warm, moist, protein-laden growth medium to Gram-positive and later Gram-negative bacteria. In general, systemic antibiotics are not employed in the initial days after injury.

Biological dressings (cadaver allograft, porcine xenograft) are used for relatively clean wounds to reduce pain, bacterial colony counts, and fluid and protein loss. Rate of epithelialization is also increased, more so than with topical antimicrobials, which tend to cause relative inhibition of wound epithelialization.

- Biological dressings may be placed on newly debrided partial-thickness wounds in anticipation of healing without surgery.
- Biological dressings cover granulating excised wounds awaiting autografts.
- Biological dressings gauge readiness of a wound for autografting (via early "take").
- Biological dressings may facilitate removal of necrotic tissue from granulating wounds.

Where circumferential injury with second-degree or third-degree depth exists, the wound may need to be divided at the lateral aspects of extremities or on the torso to facilitate extremity perfusion or chest wall movement respectively. Division of wound eschar for this purpose is termed *escharotomy*. Usually, the need for escharotomy is clear within 48 h of injury. Progressive tissue edema during resuscitation creates the need for escharotomy even if initial perfusion of circumferential torso burns is adequate. Abdominal wall escharotomy or laparotomy for abdominal compartment syndrome with respiratory embarrassment is sometimes required.

Wound Excision

Excision of burned tissue that will clearly not heal (determined by clinical assessment) is generally performed within 3 to 5 days of injury. Generally, we do not excise >20% TBSA at a time. If possible, wounds are covered with sheet or meshed autograft, harvested 3/ to 10/1,000-inch thickness with a power dermatome from unburned sites. Good harvest sites are the thighs, back, and scalp. Grafts can be meshed onto the burn area in a ratio from 1:1 to 1:9 to increase coverage with the assumption that the wound will re-epithelialize within the mesh network. We generally do not use meshing >1:3 due to increased incidence of contractures and graft shear. Cadaveric allograft can be used to cover excised areas where donor skin is unavailable.

Sequential layered tangential excision of burned tissue is employed to reach viable tissue with visible punctate bleeding. While blood loss is greater with this method, cosmetic outcome is improved and the maximum amount of viable tissue is preserved. Excision to fascia is limited to large, full-thickness injuries, where the risks of blood loss and potential graft compromise from a suboptimal recipient bed may cause increased mortality.

Management of deeper thermal injury has always been complicated by loss of dermal tissue. Because the body does not naturally regenerate dermal tissue, surgeons are often left with few choices for wound coverage that will eventually result in minimal contraction and scarring. In addition, open wounds lead to fluid loss and an increase in metabolic rate that may impact overall physiologic condition of the patient.

Over the past decade, burn treatment has evolved to include early excision of necrotic tissue and immediate coverage of excised open wounds. A recent option for permanent wound coverage is a commercially available crosslinked collagen and chondronitin sulfate dermal replacement covered by a temporary silicone epidermal substitute. Within 2 to 3 weeks of application of this material, a new dermis forms and ultrathin autografts may then be placed over the neodermis. After healing, the synthetic dermis-supported skin graft appears to have histologic structure and physical properties similar to those of normal skin.

A large postapproval study of this material was performed involving >200 burn patients at 13 burn care centers. These patients had large injuries (average 36.5% TBSA). A low incidence of invasive infection or early application of the dermal substitute was noted (3.1%). Excellent mean rate of take for the dermal substitute was noted at >75%. Median take rate was 95%. Mean rate of healing for epidermal overlying autografts was 87%, with a median healing rate of 98%. This large study supports the role of dermal substitutes as a standard of care for reconstruction of deep, large thermal injuries.

Hemodynamic Response

Global hemodynamic changes include a decrease in extracellular fluid of as much as 30 to 50% in unresuscitated animal models by 18 h after burn. In one study, cardiac output decreased to 25% of control at 4 h after injury and increased to only 40% of control at 18 h after a 30% TBSA injury. The principal site of volume loss was the functional extracellular intravascular fluid.

- Subsequent studies with salt solutions confirmed a variety of approaches to minimize extracellular fluid loss and maximize hemodynamic response in the first 24 h after burn.
- During the first 24 h, the work of Baxter showed that plasma volume changes were independent of the fluid type employed. Thus, colloids should not be used in the first 24 h of burn resuscitation.

- After 24 h, infused colloids can increase plasma volume by anticipated amounts as capillary integrity is restored.
- Peripheral vascular resistance was actually very high in the initial 24 h after burn but decreased as cardiac output improved to supranormal levels coincident with the end of plasma and blood volume losses.

Burn wound edema is caused by dilation of precapillary arterioles and increased extravascular osmotic activity due to various products of thermal injury. All elements in the vascular space except RBCs can escape from this site during the initial period of increased permeability.

Burn Resuscitation Strategies

In burn injury, intracellular and interstitial volume increase at the expense of plasma and blood volume. Edema formation is affected by resuscitation fluid administration. Thus, two principles are agreed on: (1) administer the least amount of fluid necessary to maintain adequate organ perfusion (as determined by vital signs, urine output, or function studies); and (2) replace extracellular salt lost into cells and burned tissue with crystalloids and lactated Ringers solution.

Probably the most popular resuscitation approach utilizes a modified Parkland formula, giving 4 mL/kg/percentage of TBSA burn of fluid (lactated Ringers solution) with half of the 24-h volume required administered in the first 8 h. A variety of other formulas have been described (Table 13). All represent guidelines for the initiation of resuscitation. Continuation of this process requires perfusion as indicated by a urine output of 30 to 50 mL/h in the adult. Hypoproteinemia and edema formation complicate the use of isotonic crystalloids for resuscitation. Hypertonic resuscitation solutions have the theoretical advantages of improved hemodynamic response and diminished overall fluid needs as intracellular water is shifted into the extracellular space by the hyperosmolar solution. A clear role for hypertonic resuscitation has not yet been defined. Some groups add colloid to resuscitation fluids as protein formulations or dextran after the first 8 h when much of the capillary leak has subsided. Groups most likely to benefit from supplemental colloid are the elderly, patients with large burns (>50% TBSA), and/or patients who have inhalation injury. Inhalation injury increases the overall fluid requirement of the burned patient from volume and total salt requirement standpoints.

Overall, patients in good health with burns of <40% TBSA can be resuscitated with crystalloids alone. Where coexistent injury, comorbid conditions, limited cardiac reserve, and inhalation injury complicate burn trauma, a combination of crystalloid and colloids may be optimally employed. The resuscitation target is generally 30 to 50 mL/h of urine output with acceptable vital signs. In the patient with complicated trauma or thermal injury management, a pulmonary artery catheter may be needed.

Patients receiving crystalloid resuscitation will frequently require supplemental colloid during the second 24 h after burn injury. Maintenance fluids must include allowance for evaporative losses. This fluid may come from IV repletion or enteral

Table 13. *Resuscitation Formulas**

Formula	Calculation: First 24 Hours	Calculation: Thereafter
Parkland	4 L/kg/% TBSA burn lactated Ringers solution; administer 50% total volume during first 8 h after burn and the remaining 50% over the subsequent 16 h	% dextrose in water, potassium, plasma to maintain normal serum sodium and potassium levels and colloid oncotic pressure Maintain urine output 0.5 to 1.0 mL/kg/h
Brooke	2 mL/kg/% TBSA burn lactated Ringers solution; administer 50% total volume during the first 8 h after burn and the remaining 50% over the subsequent 16 h	
Shrine	5,000 mL/m² TBSA burn + 2,000 mL/m² BSA lactated Ringers solution; administer 50% total volume during the first 8 h after burn and the remaining 50% over the subsequent 16 h	3,750 mL/m² TBSA burn + 1,500 mL/m² BSA; may replace IV fluid with enteral feedings if GI function is normal

*Reproduced with permission from the Society of Critical Care Medicine.

Trauma and Thermal Injury (Dries)

feeding. Evaporative losses = (25 + percentage of TBSA burn) × body surface area (BSA) [in meters squared] × 24 h. Potassium, calcium, magnesium, and phosphorus losses should be monitored and aggressively replaced. After 24 to 48 h, a urine output of 30 to 50 mL/h is an inadequate guide to perfusion due to relative osmotic diuresis with the metabolite loss of burns and deranged antidiuretic hormone metabolism. Adults require 1,500 to 2,000 mL/24 h of urine output to excrete the osmolar products of large burns. Serum sodium concentration, weight change, intake and output records, and physical examination also guide ongoing fluid administration.

Inhalation Injury

Inhalation injury has emerged as a persisting cause of increased mortality in burn victims. Upper airway injury is frequently due to direct heat exposure, while laryngeal reflexes protect the lung from thermal injury in all cases except possibly high-pressure steam exposure. The upper airway is also an extremely efficient heat sink. Lower airway injury is predominantly due to chemical products of combustion carried to the lung on particles of soot (particle size, 5 μm). To a degree that varies unpredictably among affected patients, inhalation injury causes several physiologic derangements including:

- Loss of airway patency secondary to mucosal edema
- Bronchospasm secondary to inhaled irritants
- Intrapulmonary shunting from small airway occlusion caused by mucosal edema and sloughed endobronchial debris
- Diminished compliance secondary to alveolar flooding and collapse with mismatching of ventilation and perfusion
- Pneumonia and tracheobronchitis secondary to loss of ciliary clearance endotracheal bronchial epithelium
- Respiratory failure secondary to a combination of the above factors

Injuries evolve over time and parenchymal lung dysfunction is often minimal for 24 to 72 h.

- Aldehydes, oxides of sulfur and hydrochloric acid, combine with water in the lung to yield corrosive acids and oxygen radicals. Degradation of polyvinyl chloride, for example, yields up to 75 toxic compounds.
- Carbon monoxide exposure is also associated with inhalation injury but does not define this process because the true degree of exposure to carbon monoxide is frequently not detected. The half-life of carboxyhemoglobin in room air is 4 h, 30 min at 100% oxygen. Therefore, increased carboxyhemoglobin levels are not often found.
- Diagnosis of inhalation injury is most commonly made with bronchoscopy, which reveals airway edema, erythema, soot accumulation, and sometimes mucosal sloughing. This test picks up far more injuries than standard clinical criteria including history of closed-space burn injury, facial burns with nasal hair singeing, wheezing, and soot in the sputum. Chest radiography is frequently normal on hospital admission, and hypoxia on blood gases is not frequently seen.

Chemical injury to the lung stimulates release of substances including histamine, serotonin, and kallikreins with recruitment of leukocytes to airways and lung parenchyma. Edema of airway mucosa and sloughing can combine with formation of plugs of fibrin and purulent material to create casts, which obstruct small airways. Neutrophils and other activated inflammatory cells also release oxygen radicals and lytic enzymes, which magnify tissue change. Pulmonary edema is also seen due to increased capillary permeability, which is magnified by cutaneous burns if present. Patients with cutaneous injury alone do not increase extravascular lung water.

Three stages of clinical inhalation injury have been identified. Acute hypoxia with asphyxia typically occurs at the fire scene, sometimes in association with high carbon monoxide exposure, and is followed by acute upper airway and pulmonary edema. Pulmonary edema with acute airway swelling usually resolves by the passage of the first several days after injury. Later complications are infections with the morbidity of pneumonia complicating that of inhalation exposure to heat and chemical irritants.

Optimal initial management of inhalation injury requires directed assessment and ensurance of airway patency. Prophylactic intubation is not indicated for a diagnosis of inhalation injury alone. However, if there is concern over progressive edema, intubation should be strongly considered. Intubation is indicated if upper airway patency is threatened, gas exchange or compliance mandate mechanical ventilatory support, or mental status is inadequate for airway protection. Prophylactic use of steroids and antibiotics is not indicated in the initial management of inhalation injury. In patients requiring mechanical ventilatory support, transpulmonary inflating pressures >40 cm H_2O should be avoided except in exceptional circumstances (eg, pH <7.2 or Pao_2 <60 mm Hg), or if impaired chest wall compliance suggests that inflating pressures measured at the endotracheal tube did not reflect transpulmonary pressures. Any mode of mechanical ventilation consistent with these limits is appropriate. Survivors of inhalation injury may have permanent pulmonary dysfunction, late endobronchial bleeding from granulation tissue, and upper airway stenosis. While there is no specific therapy for inhalation injury, proper initial management can have a favorable influence on outcome. Management goals during the first 24 h are to prevent suffocation by ensuring airway patency, to ensure adequate oxygenation and ventilation, to forego the use of agents that may complicate subsequent care, and to avoid ventilator-induced lung injury.

In any situation where carbon monoxide exposure is possible, 100% oxygen should be provided to eliminate carbon monoxide. Resuscitation fluid administration should not be delayed or withheld in inhalation injury patients. These individuals may, in fact, require additional fluid. Humidification of inhaled gases may help to reduce desiccation injury. The role of early hyperbaric oxygen is minimized in the burn care community but remains popular among pulmonologists; prospective randomized clinical data are limited. Heparin nebulization is now employed in some centers over the initial days after inhalation injury due to presumed mucolytic and antiinflammatory effects. This process may stimulate expectoration of accumulated proteinaceous material.

Carbon Monoxide Poisoning

Carbon monoxide poisoning is a serious health problem resulting in approximately 40,000 visits to emergency departments annually in the United States. In thermal injury, it may be a significant source of additional morbidity. Cognitive sequelae (memory, attention span or concentration, and affect) may occur immediately after exposure and persist or can be delayed. In general, neurologic changes occur within 20 days after carbon monoxide exposure. Cognitive sequelae lasting >1 month appear to occur in 25 to 50% of patients with loss of consciousness or carboxyhemoglobin levels $>25\%$. Recommended treatment for acute carbon monoxide intoxication is 100% normobaric oxygen. This is commonly delivered through a face mask or endotracheal tube. Hyperbaric oxygen therapy is sometimes recommended for patients with acute carbon monoxide poisoning, particularly if they have lost consciousness or have high carboxyhemoglobin levels.

Carbon monoxide is an odorless, tasteless, and nonirritating gas. It is a product of incomplete combustion. Carbon monoxide poisoning is a major source of early morbidity in the burn-injured patient with many fatalities occurring at the scene of injury. Carbon monoxide levels may be $>10\%$ in a closed space fire (significant injury may occur in a short period of time with exposure to as little as 1% carbon monoxide). With affinity for hemoglobin 200 times greater than for oxygen, carbon monoxide effectively competes with oxygen for hemoglobin binding. This competition not only shifts the oxyhemoglobin dissociation curve to the left but it alters its shape. Oxygen delivery to tissues is severely compromised as the result of both reduced oxygen carrying capacity of blood and less efficient dissociation of oxygen from hemoglobin at the tissue level. Carbon monoxide competitively inhibits intracellular cytochrome oxidase enzyme systems, most notably cytochrome P-450 resulting in an inability of cellular systems to use oxygen. Inhaled hydrogen cyanide, produced during combustion of household materials, also inhibits the cytochrome oxidase system and may have a synergistic effect with carbon monoxide. Cerebral oxygen consumption and metabolism are decreased.

Carbon monoxide poisoning may be difficult to detect. As the absorbent spectrum of carboxyhemoglobin and oxyhemoglobin are very similar, pulse oximeters cannot distinguish between the two forms of hemoglobin. Oximeter readings will be normal even if lethal amounts of carboxyhemoglobin are present. The Pao_2 measured from an arterial blood gas reflects the amount of oxygen dissolved in the plasma but does not quantitate hemoglobin saturation, which is the most important determinant of oxygen carrying capacity of the blood. Carboxyhemoglobin levels may be measured directly, but this test is rarely available at the scene of injury. Because of the delay between exposure and testing, levels measured on arrival at a health-care facility will not reflect the extent of poisoning, particularly when the patient has been breathing high concentrations of oxygen.

The half-life of carboxyhemoglobin is 250 min for the victim breathing room air; this is reduced to 40 to 60 min with inhalation of 100% oxygen. If the patient is unconscious or cyanotic, intubation for administration of high oxygen concentrations is indicated. Although hyperbaric oxygen will further reduce the half-life of carboxyhemoglobin, the hyperbaric chamber is a difficult environment in which to monitor the patient, perform resuscitation, and provide early burn care. Most burn experts reserve hyperbaric oxygen for the patient with minimal to no other injuries.

In the setting of pregnancy, greater sensitivity of the fetus to harmful effects of carbon monoxide has been noted. Data from animal studies suggest a lag time in carbon monoxide uptake between the mother and the fetus. Fetal studies state that carbon monoxide levels occur up to 40 h after maternal steady-state levels are achieved. Final carboxyhemoglobin levels in the fetus may significantly exceed levels in the mother. Exaggerated leftward shift of the fetal carboxyhemoglobin dissociation curve makes tissue hypoxia more severe by causing even less oxygen to be released to fetal tissues.

Hyperbaric oxygen has been proposed as a treatment for acute carbon monoxide exposure. Reported advantages include increased dissolved oxygen content in the blood and accelerated elimination of carbon monoxide. Potential benefits of hyperbaric oxygen treatment include prevention of lipid peroxidation in the CNS and preservation of adenosine triphosphate levels in tissue exposed to carbon monoxide. Significant disadvantages of hyperbaric oxygen therapy include the risks associated with transport of patients and maintenance of critically ill individuals in the hyperbaric setting. Recent work with patients with significant carbon monoxide exposure in the

absence of significant thermal injury suggests that neurologic outcome measured at 6 weeks and 12 months after acute exposure will improve with acute hyperbaric oxygen administration. Notably, the patient sustaining significant thermal cutaneous injury is not represented in these studies. The optimal management of carbon monoxide exposure in the setting of significant thermal cutaneous injury remains unclear, and the challenges of early administration of hyperbaric oxygen in the setting of multisystem trauma remain daunting.

Electrical Injury

In 2001, the American Burn Association published a set of practice guidelines for various aspects of burn care. Guidelines for the management of electrical injury were not included. This shortcoming is now being addressed by the American Burn Association with additional guidelines for the management of electrical injuries.

The critical care practitioner should be aware that an ECG should be performed on all patients sustaining electrical injuries (high and low voltage). Children and adults sustaining low-voltage electrical injuries, having no ECG abnormalities, no loss of consciousness, and no other indications for admission can be discharged from the emergency department. In the presence of loss of consciousness or documented dysrhythmia either before or after admission to the emergency department, telemetry monitoring and hospital admission are recommended. Cardiac monitoring is also advised for patients with ECG evidence of ischemia. Creatine kinase levels are not reliable indicators of cardiac injury after electrical burns and should not be used in decisions regarding patient disposition. There are insufficient data regarding troponin levels to formulate a guideline. Beyond recommendations pertaining to ECG, the duration of monitoring and role of other testing has not been established. Additional recommendations from the American Burn Association regarding management of electrical injury are in preparation.

Outcome

Three contemporary articles detail outcome of burn patients. The most recent comes from the National Burn Repository, which published a 10-year review in 2006. In all, >125,000 acute burn admissions to US burn centers were described. Seventy percents of hospital admissions were male (mean age, 33 years). Infants accounted for 10% of cases, and patients aged ≥70 years comprised 8.5% of cases. Thirty-two percent of admissions were <20 years old. Sixty percent of patients were from 5 to 50 years old. Sixty-two percent of patients had a total burn size <10% TBSA, with 21% of patients having a burn size between 10% and 19.9% of TBSA. Only 10% of patients had a burn size >30% TBSA. Inhalation injury was reported in 6.5% of patients. In patients sustaining inhalation injury, mortality was 30% as opposed to 5% for the patient group as a whole. Thus, inhalation injury continues to have a disproportionate effect on mortality following burns.

Flame and scald burns accounted for 78% of total cases, with the largest fraction of injuries occurring in the home (43%). Work-related injuries comprised 17% of all cases. Intentional injuries accounted for 5% of cases. Survival in the study cohort has remained constant over recent years (approximately 94.5%). Deaths from burn injury increased with advanced age and burn size and in the presence of inhalation injury. The leading cause of death was multiple organ failure. Leading complications were pneumonia, wound infection, and cellulitis. During the 10-year period from 1995 to 2005, average length of stay declined from 13 days to 8 days.

A second review of >1,600 patients admitted to Massachusetts General Hospital and the Schriners' Burn Institute in Boston was published in early 1998. Logistic progression analysis was employed to develop probability estimates for mortality based on a small set of well-defined variables. Mean burn size and survival were similar to the larger report above. The following three risk factors for death were identified: age >60 years; TBSA burned >40%; and inhalation injury. The mortality formula developed from these data predicts 0.3%, 3%, 33%, or 90% mortality depending on whether 0, 1, 2, or 3 risk factors are present, respectively.

Trends in mortality according to age among adult burn patients have recently been examined over a 25-year period. In this important study, patients admitted to a regional burn center between 1973 and 1997 were classified into three

Table 14. *Case Fatality Rates* *

Patient Age, yr	Case Fatality Ratios	
	Mid 1970s	Mid 1990s
18–34	11.6	3.9
35–54	22.9	6.6
≥55	51.0	20.8

*From J Burn Care Rehabil 2003; 24:21–25.

age groups (18 to 34 years, 35 to 54 years, and ≥55 years), and mortality rates were examined over time (Table 14).

Examination of relative rates of mortality suggests a reduction in death among adult burn patients across the age spectrum over the 25-year study. Reduction in mortality is greatest for young patients at approximately 3%/yr, while the middle-aged group saw an annual change in mortality of approximately 2%/yr, and the older patients saw a decline in mortality of approximately 1%/yr.

Suggested Readings

General Trauma Management

Moore EE, Feliciano DV, Mattox KL, eds. Trauma. 5th ed. New York, NY: McGraw-Hill, 2004

Trunkey DD, Lewis FR, eds. Current therapy of trauma. 4th ed. St Louis, MO: Mosby, 1999

Chest Trauma

Cohn SM. Pulmonary contusion: review of the clinical entity. J Trauma 1997; 42:973–979

Malhotra AK, Fabian TC, Croce DS, et al. Minimal aortic injury: a lesion associated with advancing diagnostic techniques. J Trauma 2001; 51:1042–1048

Mayberry JC, Terhes JT, Ellis TJ, et al. Absorbable plates for rib fracture repair: preliminary experience. J Trauma 2003; 55:835–839

Miller PR, Croce MA, Bee TK, et al. ARDS after pulmonary contusion: accurate measurement of contusion volume identifies high risk patients. J Trauma 2001; 51:223–230

Richardson JD. Outcome of tracheobronchial injuries: a long-term perspective. J Trauma 2004; 56:30–36

Sheridan R, Peralta R, Rhea J, et al. Reformatted visceral protocol helical CT scanning allows conventional radiographs of the thoracic and lumbar spine to be eliminated in the evaluation of blunt trauma patients. J Trauma 2003; 55:665–669

ICU Resuscitation

Balogh Z, McKinley BA, Cocanour CS, et al. Supranormal trauma resuscitation causes more cases of abdominal compartment syndrome. Arch Surg 2003; 138:637–643

Friese RS, Shafi S, Gentilello LM. Pulmonary artery catheter use is associated with reduced mortality in severely injured patients: a National Trauma Data Bank analysis of 53,312 patients. Crit Care Med 2006; 34:1597–1601

Kern JW, Shoemaker WC. Meta-analysis of hemodynamic optimization in high-risk patients. Crit Care Med 2002; 30:1686–1692

McKinley BA, Kozar RA, Cocanour CS, et al. Normal vs supranormal oxygen delivery goals in shock resuscitation: the response is the same. J Trauma 2002; 53:825–832

McKinley BA, Kozar RA, Cocanour CS, et al. Standardized trauma resuscitation: female hearts respond better. Arch Surg 2002; 137:578–584

McKinley BA, Marvin RG, Cocanour CS, et al. Blunt trauma resuscitation: the old can respond. Arch Surg 2000; 135:688–695

Rivers E, Nguyen B, Havstad S, et al. Early goal-directed therapy in the treatment of severe sepsis and septic shock. N Engl J Med 2001; 345:1368–1377

Transfusion

Dutton RP, Carson JL. Indications for early RBC transfusion. J Trauma 2006; 60:S35–S40

Malone DL, Hess JR, Fingerhut A. Massive transfusion practices around the globe and a suggestion for a common massive transfusion protocol. J Trauma 2006; 60: S91–S96

Factor VII

Boffard KD, Riou B, Warren B, et al. Recombinant factor VIIa as adjunctive therapy for bleeding control in severely injured trauma patients: two parallel randomized, placebo-controlled, double-blind clinical trials. J Trauma 2005; 59:8–18

Mayer SA, Brun NC, Begtrup K, et al. Recombinant activated factor VII for acute intracerebral hemorrhage. N Engl J Med 2005; 352:777–785

Meng ZH, Wolberg AS, Monroe DM, et al. The effect of temperature and pH on the activity of factor VIIa: implications for the efficacy of high-dose factor VIIa in hypothermic and acidotic patients. J Trauma 2003; 55:886–891

Damage Control

Johnson JW, Gracias VH, Schwab CW, et al. Evolution in damage control for exsanguinating penetrating abdominal injury. J Trauma 2001; 51:261–271

Rotondo MF, Schwab CW, McGonigal MD, et al. "Damage control": an approach for improved survival in exsanguination penetrating abdominal injury. J Trauma 1993; 35:375–383

Shapiro MB, Jenkins DH, Schwab CW, et al. Damage control: collective review. J Trauma 2000; 49:969–978

Sutton E, Bochicchio GV, Bochicchio K, et al. Long-term impact of damage control surgery: a preliminary prospective study. J Trauma 2006; 61:831–836

Abdominal Compartment Syndrome

Cheatham ML, White MW, Sagraves SG, et al. Abdominal perfusion pressure: a superior parameter in the assessment of intra-abdominal hypertension. J Trauma 2000; 49:621–627

Malbrain ML, Cheatham ML, Kirkpatrick A, et al. Results from the International Conference of Experts on intra-abdominal hypertension and abdominal compartment syndrome: I. Definitions. Intensive Care Med 2006; 32:1722–1732

Schein M, Wittmann DH, Aprahamian C, et al. The abdominal compartment syndrome: the physiologic and clinical consequences of elevated intra-abdominal pressure. J Am Coll Surg 1995; 180:745–753

Abdominal Organ Injury

Bee TK, Croce MA, Miller PR, et al. Failures of splenic nonoperative management: is the glass half empty or half full? J Trauma 2001; 50:230–236

Haan J, Ilahi ON, Kramer M, et al. Protocol-driven non-operative management in patients with blunt splenic trauma and minimal associated injury decreases length of stay. J Trauma 2003; 55:317–322

Harbrecht BG, Zenati MS, Ochoa JB, et al. Management of adult blunt splenic injuries: comparison between level I and level II trauma centers. J Am Coll Surg 2004; 198:232–239

Killeen KL, Shanmuganathan K, Poletti PA, et al. Helical CT of bowel and mesenteric injuries. J Trauma 2001; 51:26–36

Malhotra AK, Fabian TC, Katsis SB, et al. Blunt bowel and mesenteric injuries: the role of screening CT. J Trauma 2000; 49:991–1000

Mohr AM, LAvery RF, Barone A, et al. Angiographic embolization for liver injuries: low mortality, high morbidity. J Trauma 2003; 55:1077–1082

Ochsner MG, Knudson MM, Pachter L, et al. Significance of minimal or no intraperitoneal fluid visible on CT scan associated with blunt liver and splenic injuries: a multicenter analysis. J Trauma 2000; 49:505–510

Omert LA, Salyer D, Dunham M, et al. Implications of the "contrast blush" finding on CT scan of the spleen in trauma. J Trauma 2001; 51:272–278

Peitzman AB, Heil B, Rivera L, et al. Blunt splenic injury in adults: multi-institutional study. J Trauma 2000; 49:177–189

Richardson JD, Franklin GA, Lukan JK, et al. Evolution in the management of hepatic trauma: a 25-year perspective. Ann Surg 2000; 232:324–330

Velmahos GC, Toutouzas K, Radin R, et al. High success with nonoperative management of blunt hepatic trauma. Arch Surg 2003; 138:475–481

Management Guidelines for Common Problems in the Initial Care of Injury

Luchette FA, Borzotta AP, Croce MA, et al. Practice management guidelines for prophylactic antibiotic use in penetrating abdominal trauma: the EAST practice management guidelines workgroup. J Trauma 2000; 48:508–518

Pasqulae M, Fabian TC. EAST Ad Hoc Committee on Practice Management Guideline Development: practice management guidelines for trauma from Eastern Association for the Surgery of Trauma. J Trauma 1998; 44:941–957

Head Injury

Brain Trauma Foundation. Management and prognosis of severe traumatic brain injury. J Neurotrauma 2000; 17:449–627

Gress DR, Diringer MN, Green DM, et al, eds. Neurologic and neurosurgical intensive care. Philadelphia, PA: Lippincott Williams & Wilkins, 2004

Letarte P. Brain and spinal cord injury. In: Roberts PR, ed. Multidisciplinary critical care board review course. Anaheim, CA: Society of Critical Care Medicine, 1998, 613–630

Marion DW, ed. Traumatic brain injury. New York, NY: Thieme, 1999

Rosner MJ, Daughton S. Cerebral perfusion pressure in the management of head injury. J Trauma 1996; 30:933–941

Sarrafzadeh AS, Peltonen EE, Kaisers U, et al. Secondary insults in severe head injury-do multiply injured patients do worse? Crit Care Med 2001; 29:1116–1123

General Burn Management

Arnoldo B, Klein M, Gibran NS. Practice guidelines for the management of electrical injuries. J Burn Care Res 2006; 27:439–447

Demling RH. The burn edema process: current concepts. J Burn Care Rehabil 2005; 26:207–227

Herndon DN, ed. Total burn care. 2nd ed. London, UK: WB Saunders, 2002

Monafo WW. Initial management of burns. N Engl J Med 1996; 335:1581–1586

Sood R, Achauer BM. Achauer and Sood's burn surgery: reconstruction and rehabilitation. Philadelphia, PA: Saunders Elsevier, 2006

Burn Outcome

Heimbach DM, Warden GD, Luterman A, et al. Multicenter postapproval clinical trial of Integra® dermal regeneration template for burn treatment. J Burn Care Rehabil 2003; 24:42–48

McGwin G, Cross JM, Ford JW, et al. Long-term trends in mortality according to age among adult burn patients. J Burn Care Rehabil 2003; 24:21–25

Miller SF, Bessey PQ, Schurr MJ, et al. National Burn Repository 2005: a ten-year review. J Burn Care Res 2006; 27:411–436

Ryan CM, Schoenfield DA, Thorpe WP, et al. Objective estimates of the probability of death from burn injuries. N Engl J Med 1998; 338:362–366

Hyperbaric Oxygen/Carbon Monoxide

Ernst A, Zibrak JD. Carbon monoxide poisoning. N Engl J Med 1998; 339:1603–1608

McCall JE, Cahill TJ. Respiratory care of the burn patient. J Burn Care Rehabil 2005; 26:200–206

Tibbles PM, Edelsberg JS. Hyperbaric oxygen therapy. N Engl J Med 1996; 334:1642–1648

Wang C, Schwaitzberg S, Berliner E, et al. Hyperbaric oxygen for treating wounds: a systematic review of the literature. Arch Surg 2003; 138:272–279

Weaver LK, Hopkins RO, Chan KJ, et al. Hyperbaric oxygen for acute carbon monoxide poisoning. N Engl J Med 2002; 347:1057–1067

Notes

Postoperative Critical Care Management and Selected Postoperative Crises

Jonathan S. Simmons, DO, MSc, FCCP

Objectives:

- Review basic postanesthesia care including awakening, delayed emergence, sedation, and postoperative hypothermia
- Understand basic aspects of postoperative extubation
- Review and understand general postoperative and post-trauma management including deep vein thrombosis prophylaxis, timing and route of nutrition, drain care, wound care, and postoperative hemorrhage
- Review the definition, pathophysiology, and treatment of malignant hyperthermia
- Discuss the mechanisms, clinical signs, and treatment of several postoperative cardiac surgery crises

Key words: acute pulmonary hypertension; awakening; cardiac tamponade; deep vein thrombosis; delayed emergence; enteral nutrition; malignant hyperthermia; parenteral nutrition; postoperative agitation; postoperative atrial fibrillation; postoperative extubation; postoperative hypothermia; right ventricular failure; surgical drains; vacuum assisted-closure devices; wound care

Overview

The general postoperative management treatment guidelines and postoperative emergencies have been historically glossed over in critical care board review courses. Any critical care provider who cares for surgical, cardiothoracic, and/or trauma patients should be acutely aware of their general management and be able to recognize and respond to postoperative emergencies. As with all aspects of patient care, communication with nursing, ancillary personnel, and other health-care providers is essential to appropriate care. Communication with the surgical team bringing the patient to the ICU should occur to ensure that the critical care provider understands what surgical procedure occurred, what events may be expected, and what potential complications may occur. General aspects of the postoperative anesthesia care and postoperative extubation will be discussed because this may

differ from the nonsurgical patient. Malignant hyperthermia (MH) will be discussed because patients with this condition require care in an ICU following the initial event; plus, the understanding of the disease and how it is treated is imperative to good outcomes. Following this, postsurgical deep vein thrombosis (DVT) prophylaxis, timing and route of nutrition, postoperative bleeding, establishing an understanding of drains, and postoperative wound care will be discussed. Finally, I will discuss several postoperative crises involving cardiac surgery patients. This discussion is not all inclusive because many aspects are discussed in other chapters within this text; instead, this discussion covers the first several postoperative days from surgical intervention. Care has been taken to avoid duplication of more common postoperative problems, such as sepsis, ARDS, and renal failure, which are covered throughout this text.

Awakening From Anesthesia

When the patient presents to the ICU following surgery, he or she is unconscious because of a variety of medications, including volatile anesthetics, benzodiazepines, narcotics, and neuromuscular blockers. Volatile anesthetics tend to dissipate quickly but can maintain their effects for 20 to 60 min postoperatively. The speed of emergence is directly proportional to alveolar ventilation, but inversely proportionate to solubility of the agent within the blood. The longer the anesthesia time, the more total tissue uptake occurs, which can affect the duration of time it takes to emerge from the anesthesia. Recovery is generally fastest with desflurane and nitrous oxide and slowest with isoflurane. If the patient has been hypoventilated during and after the surgery, this may also lead to delayed emergence from anesthesia.[1] Narcotics and benzodiazepines have variable duration of action depending on the amount administered during surgery. Recovery from IV anesthetics is mainly dependent on redistribution rather than the elimination half-life of the drug. As the total dose administered during an anesthetic application increases, cumulative effects become apparent and lead to prolonged emergence; the half-life will become more involved in the duration of emergence. Propofol and remifentanil lead to the shortest emergence time. Advanced age, renal impairment, and/or hepatic disease can all affect duration of action of IV anesthetics.[1] An adequate amount of time should be given for these to wear off before becoming unduly concerned about mental status. The anesthetic record is an excellent resource, as well as the verbal report from the anesthesia team, which is imperative to obtain on patient arrival to the ICU. Neuromuscular blockade can have prolonged duration of action in some cases and should be considered when a patient is unable to move adequately or cannot hold up the head for 10 s. In some instances, a false sense that the blockade has worn off can be seen and, following extubation, the patient has difficulty maintaining ventilation without assistance. A train-of-four twitch monitor can assist with determining whether or not paralysis has been reversed. If paralysis is persistent, neostigmine (0.5 to 2 mg) and glycopyrrolate can be used to reverse the action of the neuromuscular blockers.[2]

Delayed emergence can occur because of several reasons, the most common being residual anesthetic, sedative, and analgesic drug effects. Emergence can also be delayed by electrolyte abnormalities such as hyperglycemia and hyponatremia. A basic metabolic profile should be checked if emergence appears delayed. Use of other sedating or interacting agents such as alcohol or recreational drugs prior to anesthesia may also contribute. If the length of emergence becomes prolonged, then naloxone in 0.04-mg increments and/or flumazenil in 0.2 mg-increments can be given to rule out opioid or benzodiazepine effects, respectively.[1]

Agitation and CNS Depression

Patients may become restless before they are fully responsive or they may experience disorientation, anxiety, and pain. Generally, this is self-limited; however, hypoxemia, acidosis, hypotension, bladder distention, or other complications should be considered and evaluated.[1] Much of the time, despite this restlessness, it is possible to have patients follow commands and participate in working toward extubation. Small doses of narcotics and/or benzodiazepines may be necessary to help relax the patient enough to avoid self-harm, self-extubation, or other complications. This usually can be accomplished without causing further sedation.[2] Generally, the use of low-dose fentanyl or morphine for pain and/or 0.5 to 1 mg of midazolam intermittently can control agitation.[1] In most cases, agitation or somnolence should improve within 30 to 60 min with appropriate management and monitoring. If not, then conditions such as sepsis, shock, and encephalopathy should be considered. In these patients, decisions regarding extubation can be difficult. In general, although controversial, patients should be able to protect their airway before extubation should occur.

Postoperative Hypothermia

Patients returning from the operating room frequently have moderate-to-severe hypothermia. The causes are multifactorial and include IV fluids and blood products that are not warmed prior to infusion, cool air temperature for operating personnel comfort, vasodilation from the use of volatile anesthetics, large open wounds and raw surfaces, and, finally, evaporation. Although there may be times when hypothermia is useful, such as in postcardiac arrest or traumatic/anoxic brain injury, the majority of postoperative patients should be returned to normothermia.[3] Postoperative hypothermia has been shown to worsen coagulopathy, increase transfusion requirements, increase susceptibility to infection, increase risk of cardiac ischemia, and increase shivering and overall discomfort.[4] The goal should be rewarming during emergence and on presentation to the ICU. Forced-air rewarming devices should be used to normalize temperature (36°C) and reduce shivering, which will reduce the risk of further complications.[5]

Postoperative Extubation

In the immediate postoperative period, many patients can be extubated quickly following

Postoperative Critical Care Management and Selected Postoperative Crises (Simmons)

surgery; however, several factors may necessitate increased weaning time. In patients who undergo major surgery, extubation may need to be delayed if there are plans to return to the operating room within the next 24 h. The overall ease of intubation and any complications during the initial intubation need to be considered in the assessment. Patients should be adequately resuscitated; hemostasis should be ensured and maintained; significant metabolic acidosis resolved; and any vasoactive agents should be minimized. Patients requiring vasoactive agents because of hypotension from inadequate fluid resuscitation and/or any form of shock would most likely benefit from remaining intubated until these issues are resolved. Patients should be assessed for their ability to protect their airway. Postoperative neurosurgical patients or patients who have recently suffered a stroke should be able to understand and respond to requests to follow commands, and a gag/cough reflex should be present. The previous statement is controversial in the medical community, but studies indicate that those patients extubated with a decreased neurologic status suffer increased rates of reintubation and increased risks of morbidity.[5a] Finally, anesthetic agents should be adequately cleared and gas exchange abnormalities should be corrected to reduce risk of postextubation complications.[6]

If patients are unable to be extubated within a short time following surgery, daily reassessment should be performed. Assessments of physiologic reserve are paramount to ensure successful extubation. Patients should breathe without mechanical assistance to allow assessment of respiratory rate, vital signs stability, end-tidal carbon dioxide levels, and comfort. If trauma is involved, especially if the chest wall has been damaged, assessment of coordination of the chest wall with the respiratory pattern is important. If patients were not intubated prior to the surgery, the patient has been stable for 60 to 90 min after surgery, tachypnea is not present, and vital signs are relatively stable, then extubation can be performed. In general, these are many of the factors involved with consideration of extubation of any patient. One main difference in the postoperative patient is the assessment of when the diaphragm is ready for respiration without mechanical assistance. The diaphragm has been shown to be the last muscle

that is paralyzed during an anesthetic application and tends to be the first to recover. Pavlin et al[7] found that patients who were able to hold either their head or leg up for 5 s were able to perform all airway-protection tests necessary for postoperative extubation.

MH

MH was first reported in 1962 after Denborough described a series of anesthetic deaths within a particular family.[1] MH is a hypermetabolic crisis that is induced by certain anesthetic agents, including succinylcholine, sevoflurane, isoflurane, desflurane, and halothane. A familial relationship does seem to exist but is not a reliable indicator, and the overall incidence is relatively rare (approximately 1 in 15,000 patients).[1] Approximately 50% of those who experience an MH crisis have had a previous anesthetic agent without any complications. The frequency is more prevalent in men than women and seems to be reduced after the age of 50 years. Pediatric patients seem to be most affected.[1]

Patients who fall into groups with musculoskeletal disorders have the highest prevalence. These diseases include myotonia, osteogenesis imperfecta, King-Denborough syndrome, and Duchenne muscular dystrophy. Certain surgical procedures have also been identified as being at increased risk, including repair of cleft palate, tonsillectomy and adenoidectomy, repair of ptosis, strabismus correction, and orthopaedic procedures.[1] The mortality rate, if the condition is not recognized, is approximately 80%. If treated aggressively, the mortality rate is < 10%.

Clinical and Laboratory Findings

The earliest indication that an MH crisis is developing is an increase in end-tidal carbon dioxide levels. Once other reasons are ruled out, the MH crisis must be aggressively treated. Fever, tachycardia, tachypnea, and rigidity of the masseter muscle (known as *trismus*) will generally develop in patients. Patients will then quickly become unstable if not aggressively treated; further symptoms and findings will include hypotension, cyanosis, cardiac arrhythmias, and severe hyperpyrexia. As the crisis develops, temperature may rise as much as 1 to 2°C every 5 min.[8]

Treatment

The Association of Surgical Technologists maintains an active Web site focusing on MH, and in 2005 they developed a guideline statement to assist with treatment recommendations.[9] Treatment includes:

1. Immediate discontinuation of anesthesia and the paralytic succinylcholine. If the surgery is life threatening or cannot be immediately stopped, then continue with use of different anesthetic agent and machine.
2. Hyperventilate with 1.0 fraction of inspired oxygen at high flow rate to treat hypercapnia, metabolic acidosis, and increased oxygen consumption.
3. Dantrolene at a dose of 2.5 mg/kg IV immediately and every 5 min until symptoms subside.
4. Change ventilator tubing and soda lime canister. Newer research indicates this may not be necessary with aggressive oxygen delivery.
5. Administer sodium bicarbonate, 1 to 2 mEq/kg IV, because of significant metabolic acidosis from increased lactate.
6. Apply ice packs to the groin, axillary region, and sides of the neck.
7. In some instances, ice lavage of the stomach and rectum can be performed, but be cautious not to induce hypothermia. Cooling measures should be stopped when the core body temperature reaches 38°C.
8. Administer mannitol at 0.25 g/kg IV and/or furosemide at 1 mg/kg IV, up to four doses of each, in order to promote and maintain urinary flow to help reduce the amount of myoglobin in the kidneys. It is recommended to maintain urinary output of at least 2 mL/kg/h to help reduce the incidence of renal failure.
9. If cardiac arrhythmias develop, the use of procainamide, 200 mg IV, may be helpful.
10. Monitor potassium closely because hyperkalemia can develop rapidly from destruction of muscle cells. Treat hyperkalemia with dextrose, 50 g IV, and regular insulin, 10 U IV, as well as sodium bicarbonate, as previously mentioned.
11. Insert a Foley catheter, if not already in place, to monitor urinary output.
12. Monitor potassium, sodium chloride, calcium, phosphate, and magnesium levels every 10 min until symptoms subside.
13. Check arterial blood gases every 5 to 10 min to monitor oxygenation and acidosis.
14. Insert arterial and central lines if not already present. Dantrolene should be administered via a central line. Monitor end-tidal carbon dioxide levels through a ventilator.

Dantrolene is a skeletal muscle relaxant that must be administered IV; it was developed specifically for use in an MH crisis. In an average 70-kg patient, thirty-six 20-mg vials will be needed for stabilization. Dantrolene comes in powder form and must be reconstituted. After the patient is stabilized, dantrolene is administered at 1 mg/kg every 6 to 8 h for 24 to 72 h to prevent recurrence. Patients generally require ICU care for 2 days following an event.[1]

Several anesthetic agents are considered nontriggering in patients with a history of MH crisis. These agents include thiopental sodium, pancuronium, droperidol, benzodiazepines, and ester-type local anesthetics. Nitrous oxide and ketamine are relatively safe for use.[1]

Prevention of DVT

All postsurgical patients requiring the ICU should have consideration given for chemical anticoagulation in addition to mechanical mechanisms for DVT because they are inherently at risk for the development of this complication. Numerous guidelines exist for assistance with determining which anticoagulation is best for certain patient populations; however, in general, prevention should be anticoagulant based for any general surgery patient who is considered to be at moderate-to-high risk for DVT.[10] Major risk factors include physical immobility, the fact that the patient has had an operation, age, malignancy, obesity, and smoking history.[11] Low-dose unfractionated heparin or low-molecular-weight heparin should be used. Low-molecular-weight heparin can be administered in most cases, unless obesity is a factor. Recent evidence suggests that low-dose unfractionated heparin should be administered three times daily (instead of twice daily, as previously recommended).[10] In very high-risk patients, mechanical devices should be used in addition to anticoagulation. If the postoperative bleeding risk is considered too high to administer chemical prophylaxis, mechanical prophylaxis should be used until chemical agents can be started.

DVT prophylaxis in the neurosurgical patient is imperative but routinely is not started within an appropriate time frame. This is generally because of the hesitation of the neurosurgeons, rather than the intensivists. Because of the increased risk in this patient population, mechanical prophylaxis should be used routinely and initiated immediately. Frim et al[12] published an article suggesting that the use of heparin (5,000 U subcutaneously q12h) significantly reduced the risk of DVT in neurosurgical patients without increasing the risk of bleeding, as long as there is no active hemorrhage or bleeding problems at the time it is initiated. In general, chemical prophylaxis should be added within 24 h of surgery. In many cases, this will have to be worked out on a case-by-case basis with the neurosurgeons. One caveat is that chemical prophylaxis should not be administered while an epidural catheter is being placed or removed. Unfractionated heparin administered subcutaneously can be administered while an epidural catheter is in place, but close monitoring for signs of complications should be performed.[13]

Trauma patients are a group that is at significant risk for the development of DVT and its complications. It is also one of the most difficult groups for which to provide adequate prophylaxis to prevent DVT from occurring. Risk factors for DVT are numerous and debated; they include spinal fractures, traumatic brain injury, spinal cord injuries, prolonged mechanical ventilation, multiple operative procedures, and pelvic fractures. Although there are few studies validating specific anticoagulation practices in patients with these factors, there is ample evidence that low-dose unfractionated heparin offers no benefit at all in trauma patients.[14] Low-molecular-weight heparin, in comparison, has been shown to reduce the incidence of DVT in trauma patients, but it must be administered twice daily and patients should be monitored closely for bleeding complications.[15] Despite several studies[16] with good evidence and creation of guidelines, the low-molecular-weight heparin prophylaxis is underused in many trauma centers. Patients with active bleeding or at high risk for bleeding complications should

receive mechanical prophylaxis; however, there are no data proving efficacy in this population. Sequential compression devices are also contraindicated or difficult to place with lower- extremity fractures, fasciotomies, or external fixators. Patients who are at high risk for venous thromboembolism who cannot receive anticoagulation should be considered for inferior vena cava filter placement. Use of removable filters should be considered.[17]

Timing and Route of Nutrition in Surgical Patients

A review of nutritional guidelines and recommendations is covered by another chapter in this text. This chapter will discuss timing and route of nutrition support in postsurgical patients. Postoperative patients have increased nutritional needs because of wound healing, changes in bowel motility, swallowing, and support of surgical anastomoses. In most postoperative patients who are relatively well nourished, enteral or parenteral support may not be needed unless it is anticipated that oral nutrition cannot be started within 7 days after surgery. In the critically ill patients, in whom metabolic demands are increased, nutritional support may be needed earlier than in hospitalized patients on regular wards.[18] In patients, including many critically ill patients, in whom the duration of illness is expected to be >10 days, nutritional support should be considered early. Examples of patients include those with severe intraabdominal sepsis, pancreatitis, major trauma, or burns.

In general, enteral nutrition should be the route of choice when oral feeding is not feasible. Parenteral nutrition has not been shown to reduce morbidity or mortality,[19] and it is associated with increased risk of catheter- and non-catheter-related infections.[20] Enteral nutrition may also reduce gut mucosal atrophy and bacterial translocation; however, there is still not sufficient evidence to state that this aspect has any outcome advantage.[21] Early enteral nutrition has been shown to decrease length of stay and decrease risk of infection compared with delayed initiation.[22] Enteral nutrition, in general, is associated with lower rates of infection and should be used when possible.[23] The combination of parenteral nutrition and early enteral nutrition has also been studied, and no benefit has been found in those who are not malnourished.[24] In general, patients who are not expected to be able to tolerate oral feeding within 7 days or have baseline malnutrition should begin enteral nutrition as soon as bowel function allows. Patients who cannot assume normal nutritional requirements by oral feeding may need some enteral nutritional support.

In trauma patients, those with penetrating and blunt abdominal injuries should be fed enterally because there is a lower incidence of infection with this route, unless the enteral route is not available or is not feasible. Beginning nutrition within 24 h has no outcome advantage to starting it within 72 h. In patients with severe head injuries, early enteral nutrition should be used because it is unlikely they will be able to take oral feeding within 7 days. The use of parenteral nutrition should be used only when bowel function or injury will not allow enteral nutrition. In those with severe injuries, if enteral nutrition cannot be started within 7 days or is not anticipated to be able to start in this period, parenteral nutrition should be used. If patients fail to reach at least 50% of their goal enteral rate by day 7, parenteral nutrition should be started. In burn patients, enteral nutrition should be started immediately as studies[25] have shown that delaying initiation >18 h results in a higher rate of parenteral nutrition requirement.

The use of intragastric vs postpyloric feeding has also been evaluated by the Eastern Association for the Surgery of Trauma (EAST) group and certain recommendations have been made.[25] In patients who have not had adequate resuscitation, the use of direct small-bowel feeding may lead to intestinal necrosis. If patients with severe head injury do not tolerate intragastric feeding within 48 h, they should have postpyloric feeding initiated. If patients who have penetrating or blunt abdominal trauma undergo laparotomy, direct small-bowel access should be obtained and enteral nutrition started immediately once resuscitation is complete. In most critically injured patients, except those previously described, gastric feeding is well tolerated and easier to accomplish than small-bowel feeding.[25]

In most postoperative patients who have undergone a laparotomy, bowel function will return and enteral nutrition can be initiated. Gastroparesis can occur and will delay gastric emptying. Clinical signs of gastroparesis include abdominal distention, 500 mL/d of nasogastric tube output, or high residual volumes in the stomach after feeding of >300 mL. One method to combat this would be to initiate postpyloric feeding. However, postpyloric feeding has not been shown to decrease ICU length of stay, mortality rate, or pneumonia rate when compared with gastric feeding.[26] Prokinetic agents, such as metoclopramide and erythromycin, can be used with some positive results.[27] Gastric residual volumes should be checked frequently while enteral nutrition is being used. Continuation of feeding can occur even with residual volumes of 150 to 300 mL as long as there is no evidence of abdominal distention and/or nausea and vomiting.

Special Circumstances

In those patients with an enterocutaneous fistula, enteral nutrition can worsen fistula output. In general, these patients should have complete bowel rest and parenteral nutrition. In addition, nutritional requirements may need to be adjusted by 1.5 to 2 times the normal nonprotein calorie complement.[28] In cases of acute pancreatitis, the degree of inflammation plays a role in route of nutrition. In mild pancreatitis, enteral nutrition will not be needed unless oral feeding cannot be tolerated after 5 to 7 days.[29] In patients with severe acute pancreatitis, early enteral feeding should be used. This route has been shown to have reduced infection, need for surgery, and length of stay compared with parenteral nutrition.[30] In addition, gastric feeding can be used in many patients with acute pancreatitis. If unable to advance to the goal rate of enteral feedings based on nutritional guidelines, without significant residual volumes or complications, postpyloric feeding can be used.[31] Patients with esophageal resection or repair will generally have distal feeding tubes placed during surgery to allow for early enteral nutrition. If this does not occur and the patient is unable or is not anticipated to be able to resume oral or enteral feedings by day 7, the patient should receive early parenteral nutrition. Gastric surgery can result in delay of gastric emptying. If it is anticipated that this will occur for a prolonged period, a postpyloric feeding tube should be placed during surgery. In patients with new gastrostomy tubes, delay of feeding for 24 h is generally considered in case gastric emptying is delayed.

Surgical Drains

The monitoring and management of drains in the postoperative patient is an important task that is frequently overlooked or not given the attention that it deserves. The surgical team should be queried during the handoff communication with the critical care team regarding the location, type, and purpose of each drain that is in place. Some surgeries, specifically abdominal and pelvic surgeries, can involve numerous drains in various locations. Sometimes a pictorial representation on the patient chart can help simplify the task of monitoring drain output. Each drain has a specific purpose, and either the increase in flow, change in nature of the fluid within the drain, or a decrease in flow can be significant. The knowledge of where these drains lie can aid in diagnosing problems that may be occurring with the patient.

Many different types of drains exist that have different purposes in the postsurgical patient. There are passive and active drains. Passive drains provide a route of low resistance for the movement of material out of the body. They work via capillary action and pressure gradients. An example of a passive system is a Penrose drain. Active drains use some sort of external source to create negative pressure, thus creating a pressure gradient. This external source can be either a mechanical unit or a bulb placed on suction. Examples of active drain systems include Hemovac, Jackson-Pratt, and Blake drains. The drainage of the GI tract and abscess cavities uses an active drainage system known as *sump drainage*. These drains draw air into one lumen and then remove fluid through another to avoid drawing mesentery and bowel into the drainage system.[2] Drains are generally soft and flexible and are made of either a silicon material or polyvinyl chloride. Latex is generally avoided because of the irritating nature of the rubber and the increase in associated allergies.

Drains can be either prophylactic or therapeutic in their purpose. If the drain is placed for therapeutic reasons, it is to remove pus, debris,

and fistula drainage, or to prevent premature closure of a wound. If the drain is placed for prophylactic reasons, it is designed to prevent the accumulation of bile, pus, intestinal fluid, and blood, or to monitor for complications of a difficult operation with high risk of anastomotic breakdown.[32]

The use of drains has decreased over time as there are now multiple randomized controlled trials demonstrating that routine use of drains in many intraabdominal (including appendectomy, colorectal, and hepatic) surgeries, as well as thyroid and parathyroid surgeries, do not prevent anastomotic leaks or other complications.[33,34] There exists some evidence that drains prevent seroma formation and can also aid in diagnosing anastomotic and biliary leaks following surgery. In addition to locations of drains, critical care physicians need to determine from the surgical team whether specific drains should be used for gravity or suction, and what are the expected fluid contents and output. Routine care of the drains is generally performed by critical care nurses.

The main current indications for drain placement include closure of soft-tissue wounds to minimize dead space; drainage of the pleural space resulting from air, blood, or fluid present in the pleural cavity; drainage of large pericardial effusions; removal of cerebrospinal fluid from the ventricles or spinal canal; removal of blood from the subdural space; drainage of abscess cavities; surveillance drainage of complicated abdominal surgeries; and drainage of fistulas.[2] A few common drains will be described.

Biliary tract drains are commonly placed following exploration or repair of the common bile duct. Part of the drain is left within the common bile duct, and the longer portion is brought to the skin for drainage. This is generally performed so surgeons are able to better determine when the common bile duct has healed, which is signaled by decreased drain output. In general, a cholangiogram will be performed prior to removal of the drain in order to ensure that decreased drainage is not due to obstruction.[35] Another common drain in the critical care unit is a cholecystostomy tube. These are generally placed percutaneously with ultrasound or fluoroscopic guidance via interventional radiology to decompress the gallbladder when patients are either considered critical and unlikely to tolerate surgery, or when severe inflammation leads to an increased operative risk.

Drains left in the abdominal cavity that are not in abscess cavities or designed to control fistula output should have little output on a daily basis. Clinicians should monitor both the quality and quantity of the output. Both an increase in drainage and change in content with new bile, debris, or stool may suggest a leak or anastomotic breakdown.

In the neurosurgical ICU, intraventricular catheters are used both to drain cerebrospinal fluid and monitor intracranial pressure. The drainage of cerebrospinal fluid can also be used to decrease intracranial pressure. Although this catheter is effective and necessary, several complications can occur, including hemorrhage and infection. The risk of hemorrhage is 1 to 6% and can either be immediate or delayed, and can occur at several anatomic locations. Infection can also occur in any of the spaces where the catheter passes, including skin, osteomyelitis of the calvarium, subdural empyema, meningitis, parenchymal abscess, and/or ventriculitis.[36] Infection rates have been reported from 2 to 22%.[37,38] The literature does not directly support the use of prophylactic antibiotics in patients with these catheters, but clinical practice generally employs their use. The best care for these catheters is to maintain sterile technique, remove them as soon as feasible, and avoid flushing the catheter as this increases risk of infection.[38]

In summary, when patients present to the critical care unit with drains in place, the following questions should be answered by the surgical team[2]:

1. Where is the location of the drain?
2. How can the location be confirmed, or is it necessary?
3. What is the expected quantity and quality of the drain output?
4. Is the drain functional normally, or is there something special about the drain that needs to be communicated?
5. What criteria will decide when the drain can be removed?

If the critical care clinician is able to understand these aspects of surgical drains, overall improvement in care, avoidance of infections, and identification of complications will be attained.

Wound Care

The topic of wound care is broad and far-reaching. This discussion will concentrate on initial postoperative dressings and their care, as well as the increased use of vacuum-assisted closure devices, which are becoming more abundant in ICUs across the world. Initial management of wounds involves the placement of a sterile dressing that covers the operative incision. It is recommended to keep this dressing dry and in place for the first 48 h following surgery. During this initial 48 h, an epithelial barrier develops over the wound when it has been closed by primary intention. After this initial period, the skin can be cleansed with water, and no further dressing is necessary.

Surgical wounds that are left open to heal by secondary intention or that have necrotic tissue, wound exudates, or inflammatory cells do not form this epithelial barrier. The larger, open wounds require a moist, occlusive dressing with frequent removal of exudates and necrotic tissue to allow for appropriate epithelialization. The wet-to-dry dressing provides a moist environment, traps the wound exudates, has bacteriostatic properties, and does not adhere to the wounds.[2] Dressing changes will occur at least twice daily for clean wounds, but more frequently for wounds with a greater amount of exudative and inflammatory material. Normal saline solution is used to soak the dressing prior to application.[39]

In the last decade, vacuum-assisted wound-closure devices have become popular and are being employed in more postoperative patients every day. These devices place the wound under subatmospheric pressures that increase blood flow to the affected area, reduce edema and excess fluid, and increase wound contraction. This allows for enhancement of wound granulation. It is important to ensure that wounds are not highly contaminated or have significant amounts of necrotic tissue before the use of these devices. Many of these devices use a sponge that is placed over the wound and then covered by an occlusive dressing.[40] Some advantages of this type of therapy—such as reduced frequency of dressing changes, improved patient comfort, improved efficiency of wound closure, and improved removal of edema fluid—have been cited. There are few clinical data available to support the superiority of these devices over other, simpler dressings. There is some evidence that this negative-pressure therapy may hasten time to grafting or secondary closure, and may help improve wound contraction over abdominal wounds. The use of these devices in complicated abdominal injuries, evisceration, and abdominal compartment syndrome has increased and studies[41] show some benefit; however, there is also evidence that these may increase rates of new enterocutaneous fistula formation.[41]

The overall supportive care of the patient is also important when attempting to enhance wound care. Hyper- and hypoglycemia should be avoided by controlling blood sugars, the routine use of postoperative antibiotics should be avoided (unless a surgical site infection exists), and optimization of nutrition should be employed to further enhance wound healing. Wounds should be evaluated at least daily to monitor for progression of healing and for signs of infection. Most normal surgical wounds will have a small, dry scab and a small border of erythema that will resolve over approximately 1 week. Wounds in which develop progressive erythema and induration without purulent drainage may indicate the presence of a cellulitis in deeper structures. If the drainage is frankly purulent, this may indicate abscess or a surgical site infection. Surgical site infections will require opening the incision for irrigation and drainage and evaluation of extent of infection. In most instances, systemic antibiotics will be needed to treat the infection. It is important to ensure that the infection has not spread to the fascia and soft tissues, indicating necrotizing fasciitis, which is a surgical emergency.[42]

Postoperative Hemorrhage

A patient in whom shock develops following either trauma or surgery should be considered hemorrhagic until proven otherwise. Patients demonstrate clinical signs including tachycardia, decreased peripheral pulses, cool extremities, agitation, and hypotension. Generally, 25 to 30% of blood volume loss occurs before signs of shock are evident, but younger patients or elderly patients

receiving certain cardiovascular medications may lose a greater percentage of blood volume prior to demonstrating signs. Most adult patients can lose up to 15% of their blood volume without showing any overt symptoms. If patients lose ≥40% of their circulating blood volume, this becomes life threatening and generally will require operative (or interventional) control of the bleeding. The absolute hemoglobin and hematocrit values are not necessarily a reliable indicator of hemorrhage because this may be affected by intraoperative losses and fluid resuscitation. These values can be used with concurrent checks to follow trends that may suggest postoperative bleeding. If clinical signs of shock are present, the absolute hemoglobin and hematocrit values also may not be useful if there is acute and active bleeding.

Patients can present from the operating room with hypothermia, acidosis, and coagulopathy, which should be corrected unless an obvious source of bleeding is seen prior to returning to the operating room. In many cases, the bleeding is venous oozing that will correct once these factors are considered. Patients should be actively warmed with an external warming device (*eg*, Bair Hugger, Arizant Inc.), and fresh-frozen plasma and platelets administered to correct the coagulopathy. Consideration should be given to checking fibrinogen levels, especially if massive transfusion has occurred. This is covered in more detail in another section of this text.

In reviewing the literature on postoperative bleeding, most of the articles and reviews are related to coagulopathy and other disorders of bleeding, which is outside the scope of this chapter. The most important point for any critical care practitioner is that if clinical signs of shock develop in a postoperative or trauma patient, hemorrhage is the answer until it is proven not to be present. Assessment of the surgical wound for signs of bleeding should be performed but is not useful in most cases. In a patient who has had thoracic or cardiac surgery, monitoring of chest tube output can aid in the diagnosis of postoperative bleeding. In the trauma patient who is not postoperative, a FAST (focused assessment with sonography for trauma) examination can be performed at the bedside to look for intra-abdominal fluid. If the patient is relatively stable, a CT scan can be performed, but this takes time and, in many cases, contrast dye must be used to look for extravasation, which may put a patient who is already at risk at higher risk for acute kidney injury. In selected trauma patients, hemorrhage can be controlled by vessel coiling or embolization in the interventional radiology suite. In the postoperative patient, emergent return to the operating room is indicated if hemorrhage cannot be ruled out as the cause of shock.

Postoperative Myocardial Infarction in the Cardiac Surgery Patient

Perioperative myocardial infarction is identified in approximately 2 to 4% of patients following coronary artery bypass grafting (CABG) and is associated with increased mortality.[43] This is identified by Q waves on the ECG that were not present prior to surgery. The actual diagnosis is difficult in this patient population, and the damage can be due to either the native vessel or a problem with the coronary graft.

Biochemical markers can be used to identify myocardial injury; however, small rises in the troponin level are normal after CABG is performed. Significant increases in the troponin level can indicate myocardial infarction in this setting. Hospitals use either troponin I or troponin T level as markers. Studies have demonstrated that a troponin I value of $>20 \ \mu g/L$ is associated with increased length of stay[43a] and early graft failure.[43b] A troponin T value of $>1.58 \ \mu g/L$ at 24 h after surgery is predictive of adverse outcomes, which includes death.[44] Evaluation of creatine kinase-MB levels has not been shown to be as useful as that of troponin levels.

Patients who have undergone cardiac surgery have significant chest wall pain from the incision, which is difficult to distinguish from angina. Many patients are receiving mechanical ventilation for at least several hours following surgery, which makes assessment difficult. Urgent attention should be given to a patient in whom hypotension develops and low cardiac output with ECG changes indicative of myocardial ischemia.

As stated earlier, new Q waves may be indicative of myocardial infarction, but do not develop immediately. A patient should be monitored for ST-segment elevation and/or depression on ECG.

If this occurs throughout a majority of the leads, it is most likely normal postoperative changes. If acute changes are seen in one specific region, such as inferior, anterior, and lateral, this may be more indicative of acute ischemia.[45] If recurrent ventricular arrhythmias develop, this is strongly suggestive that ECG changes are due to ischemia.

Echocardiography will be the main diagnostic tool to verify that a myocardial infarction has occurred. All postcardiac surgery patients with suspected myocardial infarction should undergo transesophageal echocardiography to identify segmental wall motion abnormalities. As in ECG findings, some wall motion abnormalities are normal following cardiac surgery, so they should be compared with pre- and intraoperative echocardiograms to look for changes in the postoperative period.

The treatment of postcardiac surgery myocardial infarction is multifaceted. If a specific wall motion abnormality is associated with a graft, graft spasm or occlusion should be ruled out and treated. If the patient is hypertensive, a vasodilator, such as nitroglycerin or nitroprusside, should be started. If the patient is hypotensive, volume resuscitation followed by norepinephrine, should be administered. If overt cardiogenic shock develops in a patient, an intraaortic balloon pump should be placed. If the patient fails to respond to therapy, emergent coronary angiography or a return to the operating room should occur.

Cardiac Tamponade

Cardiac tamponade in the postoperative setting can be a life-threatening compression of the heart that can either occur rapidly or over time. There are multiple causes of cardiac tamponade, but traumatic tamponade is the most common following cardiac surgery. The main problem that occurs in a postoperative patient is a rapid (or rarely, slow) compression of the chambers of the heart by increasing intrapericardial pressure. The pericardium is able to stretch; however, the rate at which the filling occurs can easily overcome this ability to compensate. As the chambers become smaller and compliance is reduced, the cardiac inflow is reduced appreciably. In the postoperative period, hemorrhage into the pericardium occurs at a time when the pericardium is stiff and unable to compensate well. This can quickly lead to a life-threatening tamponade.[46]

The pressure within the pericardium initially has a slow ascent due to accumulating volume of fluid but then there is a dramatic rise in the pressure as a final increment, which produces critical cardiac compression. Conversely, when drainage occurs, the initial amount of fluid that is removed produces the most dramatic decompression. Although coronary blood flow is reduced with tamponade, it is proportional to the reduced workload and operational components of the heart, so ischemia is rare.[46]

Postoperative cardiac tamponade occurs more frequently with valve surgery than with coronary artery bypass surgery. The main cause is trauma-induced effusion and bleeding, and this occurs more frequently when postoperative anticoagulation is used.[47] Classic signs that will be described later are relatively rare findings in postoperative tamponade, so prompt echocardiographic imaging is required when tamponade is suspected. If hypotension develops in any patient >5 days following cardiac surgery, tamponade must be suspected and ruled out. Tamponade has also been known to occur ≤2 weeks following surgery and may not be recognized by physicians who are less familiar with the diagnosis in the outpatient setting.[48]

Clinical Findings

Tamponade is a form of cardiogenic shock, so the differential diagnosis is initially numerous and complex. Subjective complaints can include tachypnea and dyspnea on exertion. Patients can also have anorexia, dysphagia, and cough. However, in the postoperative period, especially in the initial hours following cardiac surgery, these symptoms may be difficult to elucidate from patients because they are still intubated and recovering from anesthetic medications.

Physical examination findings can also be relatively obscure, with tachycardia being the main finding.[46] This is also present often in the postoperative period. It is possible for people to be bradycardic when tachycardia is a preexisting condition or they have hypothyroidism. In most cases, relative or absolute hypotension will develop when significant tamponade develops. Patients may also show signs of shock, including

cool extremities and, possibly, peripheral cyanosis. Jugular venous distention is generally present but may not occur with rapid accumulation of blood. Venous waves generally lose the early diastolic y descent.

Pulsus paradoxus is a key diagnostic finding. It is defined as a fall in inspiratory systolic arterial pressure of ≤10 mm Hg during normal breathing. In the postoperative cardiac surgery patient, this may be difficult to detect. This finding is also nondiagnostic and can also be seen in pulmonary embolism, hemorrhagic shock, COPD, and severe hypotension, all of which can be factors in the postoperative setting.[49]

Diagnostic Studies

Cardiac catheterization tends to be diagnostic, but this is not feasible in most patients emergently. Catheterization will confirm equilibration of average diastolic pressures and also respiratory reciprocation, which causes pulsus paradoxus. Chest radiograph is generally nondiagnostic because at least 200 mL of fluid are required before the finding can be suggested on film.[46]

An ECG is obtained in most circumstances, but is relatively nondiagnostic for tamponade. A finding known as *electrical alternation* can be seen and can involve all of the wave or just the QRS complex. Every other QRS complex will be a smaller voltage and may also have reverse polarity.[50]

Echocardiography, specifically with the use of Doppler, is currently the main tool used to diagnose both pericardial effusion and cardiac tamponade. Echocardiography can pick up chamber collapse of the right atrium and ventricle. The classic finding is the invagination of the right ventricular free wall during early diastole, and the subsequent right atrial wall invagination during end diastole. Right ventricular collapse can also be seen and generally indicates the presence of tamponade. In approximately 25% of the patients with tamponade, the left atrium will also collapse, and this is a highly specific finding.[51]

Management of Acute Cardiac Tamponade

The primary treatment of acute tamponade is drainage of the pericardial contents. In general, this is performed using needle paracentesis;

however, in the postoperative cardiac surgery patient, tamponade is generally due to hemopericardium, and surgical drainage is warranted in most cases. The treatment of tamponade in the noncardiac surgery patient is multifaceted and can include inotropic support and adjustment of volume status; however, in the postoperative patient population, surgical drainage is the best option and discussion will be limited to this for purposes of this review. While the patient is being prepared for surgery, fluids and inotropes will be needed to ensure BP and cardiac output optimization. Positive end-expiratory pressure (PEEP) as indicated on the ventilator should be kept at a minimum to avoid decreasing venous return.[52] If a patient presents with late tamponade and the condition is emergent, needle pericardiocentesis could be attempted because the fluid may be amenable to drainage, but clot may also be present.

Right Ventricular Failure due to Acute Pressure Overload

In general, pulmonary hypertension in the perioperative period does not require treatment; however, in some perioperative and postoperative situations, volume overload can lead to acute right ventricular dysfunction. Volume overload will induce an increase in pulmonary vascular resistance, which can then lead to reduced right ventricular end-diastolic pressure and, ultimately, reduction in right ventricular perfusion pressure. This will be further complicated by hypotension. The problem will induce myocardial ischemia, right ventricular systolic dysfunction, and a decrease in cardiac output.

Clinical Findings

Patients will exhibit signs of cardiogenic shock; as in tamponade, the differential diagnosis can be large. Patients will have cool, clammy extremities, tachycardia, and hypotension. The patient most likely will have distended neck veins and a prominent murmur consistent with tricuspid regurgitation will develop. Patients may experience acute elevation in hepatic transaminases due to backflow of fluid within the liver, and right upper quadrant abdominal pain some may even develop in some patients.[53]

If central venous pressure is being followed, an acute rise will be seen and giant V waves may be present due to the acute tricuspid regurgitation. Many of these patients will have preexisting pulmonary hypertension, which may complicate diagnosis. However, if the central venous pressure is rising and hypotension is developing, right ventricular failure should be considered. Pulmonary artery catheters are used much less frequently in modern ICUs; however, if being used, a low cardiac output state will be found. Overall, there will also be a falling pulmonary arterial pressure, which can be used for following a trend, but the absolute value is nondiagnostic. The interventricular septum may become displaced, leading to a falsely elevated pulmonary artery wedge pressure.[53]

Echocardiography is the main diagnostic tool that is used. Echocardiography findings will include a grossly dilated and hypokinetic right ventricle. Severe tricuspid regurgitation is also present in many cases. The interventricular septum will be displaced to the left in late diastole, which may give the false appearance of hypovolemia.

A patent foramen ovale (PFO) is present in approximately 25% of adults. A PFO is an atrial septal defect that allows flow from right to left only. In normal circumstances, the right atrial pressure is less than that of the left atrial pressure, so no flow occurs across the PFO. When right ventricular dysfunction occurs, right atrial pressure exceeds left atrial pressure and a significant shunt occurs, which can lead to significant hypoxemia. In a patient receiving mechanical ventilation, many clinicians will automatically increase PEEP to help compensate for the hypoxia; however, this increase in PEEP may worsen right ventricular dysfunction, thereby worsening the hypoxemia through an increased shunt. A transesophageal echocardiogram may be needed to determine if a PFO is present.[53]

Treatment

General measures should include methods to reduce an increase in pulmonary vascular resistance. Patients receiving mechanical ventilation should be heavily sedated and administered appropriate analgesia. It is recommended that the fraction of inspired oxygen level be maintained

>0.50 in the early postoperative period to avoid hypoxemia because this will increase pulmonary vascular resistance. Although it has been shown that the use of mechanical ventilation can worsen right ventricular dysfunction, when hypoxemia or acidosis is present the benefits of mechanical ventilation outweigh the risks. High airway pressures and high PEEP should be avoided if possible.

The use of volume replacement may be needed when acute right ventricular failure is present; however, the overall amount of fluids should be monitored closely and increasing pressure can reduce perfusion pressure, as previously described. Right ventricular perfusion pressure must be maintained while treating right ventricular failure. This involves the use of vasopressors to maintain BP. Norepinephrine is the vasopressor of choice.[54] If systemic hypotension is controlled and right ventricular systolic dysfunction is present, an inotrope, such as milrinone or dobutamine, may be needed.

Systemic vasodilators, such as nitroglycerin or sodium nitroprusside, may be needed to reduce ventricular afterload, which can potentially reverse right ventricular failure. However, use of these agents can cause both systemic hypotension and significant hypoxemia.

Inhaled pulmonary vasodilators can be used and have several advantages, including lack of systemic hypotension and improvement of ventilator-perfusion mismatch. Inhaled nitric oxide has been used commonly to treat pulmonary hypertension following cardiac surgery. Nitric oxide will improve oxygenation, reduce pulmonary arterial pressure, and increase cardiac output in most cases.[55] Dose range for initiation of therapy is generally 20 to 40 ppm, which is reduced to the lowest effective dose if benefits are seen at all. Nitric oxide should be weaned off slowly to avoid rebound pulmonary hypertension.

Inhaled prostacyclin (epoprostenol) can also be used after cardiac surgery for treatment of pulmonary hypertension. It is significantly cheaper than nitric oxide. It has similar effects of reducing pulmonary vascular resistance, increasing cardiac output, and improving oxygenation, as in nitric oxide. The dose range is generally 5 to 50 ng/kg/min. It is administered via continuous nebulization through the inspiratory limb of the ventilator. Methods to deliver this medication

have improved significantly over the past several years. Impaired platelet function can be seen but in most cases has not led to increased bleeding. This medication does not cause rebound pulmonary hypertension.[56]

A newer analog of prostacyclin, iloprost, is also available. It has been used in postcardiac surgery with success.[53] It has a longer half-life than epoprostenol, so it can be used intermittently instead of via continuous aerosol. Dose range for iloprost is 12 to 20 µg every 4 to 6 h by nebulizer. Disadvantages to epoprostenol involve cost and the requirement to break the ventilator circuit every few hours.[57]

Postcardiac Surgery Atrial Fibrillation

Atrial fibrillation (AF) and atrial flutter are common following any type of cardiac surgery. Studies[58,59] report varying numbers, but in general, AF will develop in up to 15 to 40% of post-CABG patients, as well as 37 to 50% of valve patients, and up to 60% of those who have both a valve replacement and CABG. Heart transplantation patients are also at risk in the immediate postoperative period, with a reported rate of 11 to 24%.[60] Studies[61] differ on whether or not postoperative AF increases length of stay; however, there are numerous studies[62] suggesting a twofold increase in ICU length of stay and overall increase in hospital stay related to this common problem.

The pathophysiology behind the common occurrence of AF following cardiac surgery is complex and will not be covered in detail in this text. However, pathophysiology is thought to be generally related to age-related changes in the atrial myocardium and perioperative conditions that affect the atrium, including conduction velocities and transmembrane potentials. Inflammation may also play a role because the incidence of AF in off-pump CABG is less than that of on-pump, and off-pump CABG is associated with less inflammation. In a metaanalysis[63] of 37 randomized trials and 22 observational trials, off-pump CABG was consistently associated with reduced rates of AF. Several other factors are most likely involved, in addition to the differences in inflammation between the two types of surgery.[64] There is also some evidence that rapid focal discharges from cells within the pulmonary vein may be responsible for AF.[64a]

Clinical risk factors are varied, depending on the results of the study that was consulted; however, advancing age has been consistently shown. Other risk factors include previous episodes of AF, increased left atrial size, repeat cardiac surgery, mitral valve disease, increased bypass or cross-clamp times, absence of previous treatment with β-blockers, and obesity, among others.[60,65,66]

Prophylactic Therapy

Because of the high incidence of postoperative AF, prophylactic therapy is administered to patients with risk factors in many centers. β-Blockers are the most commonly used therapy; they reduce the overall AF incidence to 12 to 16% in CABG patients and to 15 to 20% in valve surgery patients.[67] β-Blockers should be started either before surgery or immediately following surgery for the best results. This is considered a class I recommendation based on the American College of Cardiology/American Heart Association guidelines for CABG.[68]

Amiodarone has also been shown to reduce the incidence of AF by 40 to 50%. In addition, the combination of amiodarone and β-blockers may even be more efficacious. A metaanalysis[69] in 2005 provided evidence that both AF and atrial flutter were reduced. There was a lower incidence of ventricular tachycardia and ventricular fibrillation, as well as reduced incidence of stroke. A randomized controlled trial[70] of prophylactic amiodarone use was also published in 2005. Patients were randomized to receive either 10 mg/kg po of amiodarone daily for 6 days prior to and 6 days following CABG or valve surgery or to receive placebo. Overall, there was a 48% reduction in AF and atrial flutter, which was similar across all groups, including those receiving and not receiving β-blockers. It also demonstrated fewer ventricular arrhythmias as shown in the meta-analysis. There was, however, increased risk of bradycardia and QT prolongation compared with placebo.[70] Other perioperative regimens have also been studied and have demonstrated efficacy. In 2008, a study[71] investigating cost-effectiveness of amiodarone use to prevent AF was released that demonstrated that routine use of amiodarone, administered as a bolus dose of 300 mg IV at the time of surgery, and 5 days of 600 mg po bid amiodarone, was both efficacious and cost-effective in reducing AF and its associated increased length of stay.

Sotalol is a class III antiarrhythmic that can be administered to help prevent AF in postcardiac surgery patients. If administered, it can be started either 24 to 48 h before surgery or 4 h after surgery for efficacy. The 2004 American College of Cardiology/American Heart Association guidelines on CABG give the use of Sotalol a class IIb recommendation for those who cannot tolerate β-blockers.[68]

One of the hypotheses mentioned earlier was that postcardiac surgery AF may be related to inflammation. Because of this, glucocorticoids have been studied as prophylactic therapy. A 2008 metaanalysis[73] was performed, and it was found that glucocorticoids significantly reduced the rate of postoperative AF, from about 35.5 to 24.7%. Mortality benefit data are not available, so this is currently not a first-line recommendation.[72]

Treatment

AF following cardiac surgery can occur either with hemodynamic stability or instability. Treatment is based on the same general principles of nonoperative AF. Depending on the source, the recommendations vary on what therapy is best in this patient population. In the unstable patient, cardioversion should be attempted. Some evidence exists that electrical cardioversion may not be as efficacious as in nonoperative AF.[73] Amiodarone is used frequently, and it is recommended to give either the standard 150 mg load over 10 min then IV infusion over 24 h; some sources state 5 mg/kg over 30 min (or 2 mg/min over 4 h) as an alternative. If amiodarone itself does not lead to cardioversion, electrical cardioversion can be reattempted. An amiodarone infusion at 1 mg/min should then be continued until oral medications can be tolerated. The use of atrial pacing may minimize chance of AF recurrence.[74] Some studies[58] state that even without treatment, most AF after cardiac surgery will spontaneously convert to sinus rhythm within 24 h. If all of these measures are unsuccessful, then attempted rate control with IV β-blockers and/or diltiazem may be useful.[75]

In patients who are hemodynamically stable, it is reasonable to attempt chemical cardioversion with either amiodarone or a β-blocker. If AF persists after 24 h, attempt cardioversion followed by atrial pacing. Treatment should then be continued for 4 to 6 weeks following surgery. If AF continues after 6 weeks, recommendations are for rate control and anticoagulation.[76] Anticoagulation should be prescribed in accordance with that for similar patients in whom AF develops for other reasons than cardiac surgery. This topic is covered in another chapter within this text.

References

1. Morgan GE, Mikhail MS, Murray MJ. Clinical anesthesiology. 4th ed. New York, NY: McGraw Hill, 2006

2. Hockstein MJ, Barie PS. General principles of postoperative intensive care. In: Parrillo JE, Dellinger RP, eds. Critical care medicine. Philadelphia, PA: Mosby Elsevier, 2008; 735–751

3. Sanders AB. Therapeutic hypothermia after cardiac arrest. Curr Opin Crit Care 2006; 12:213–217

4. American Society of Anesthesiologists statement regarding postoperative hypothermia. Available at: http://www.asahq.org/Washington/CPOM%20Approved%20Measures%20Oct07%20 (2).pdf. Accessed March 19, 2009

5. American Society of Anesthesiologists. Practice guidelines for postanesthetic care: a report by the American Society of Anesthesiologists Task Force on Postanesthetic Care. Anesthesiology 2002; 96:742–752

5a. Namen AM, Ely EW, Tatter SB, et al. Predictors of successful extubation in neurosurgical patients. Am J Respir Crit Care Med 2001; 163:658–664

6. MacIntyre NR, Cook DJ, Ely EW, et al. Evidence-based guidelines for weaning and discontinuing ventilator support: a collective task force facilitated by the American College of Chest Physicians, the American Association for Respiratory Care, and the American College of Critical Care Medicine. Chest 2001; 120(6 suppl):375S–395S

7. Pavlin EG, Holle RH, Schoene RB. Recovery of airway protection compared with ventilation in humans after paralysis with curare. Anesthesiology 1989; 70:381–385

8. McCarthy EJ. Malignant hyperthermia: pathophysiology, clinical presentation, and treatment. AACN Clin Issues 2004; 15:231–237

9. Guideline statement for malignant hyperthermia in the perioperative environment, October 2005. Available at: http://www.ast.org/pdf/Standards_of_Practice/Guideline_Malignant_Hyperthermia.pdf. Accessed March 17, 2009

10. Hirsch J, Guyatt G, Albers GW, et al. Antithrombotic and thrombolytic therapy, 8th edition: ACCP guidelines. Chest 2008; 133(6 suppl):110S–112S

11. Anaya DA, Nathens AB. Thrombosis and coagulation: deep vein thrombosis and pulmonary embolism prophylaxis. Surg Clin North Am 2005; 85:1163–1177

12. Frim DM, Barker FG II, Poletti CE, et al. Postoperative low-dose heparin decreases thromboembolic complications in neurosurgical patients. Neurosurgery 1992; 30:830–832

13. American Society of Regional Anesthesia and Pain Medicine. Regional anesthesia in the anticoagulated patient: defining the risks. Second annual consensus conference, April 2002. Available at: http://www.asra.com/consensus-statements/2.html. Accessed March 22, 2009

14. Rogers FB, Cipolle MD, Velmahos G, et al. Practice management guidelines for the prevention of venous thromboembolism in trauma patients: the EAST practice management guidelines work group. J Trauma 2002; 53:142–164

15. Geerts WH, Jay RM, Code KI, et al. A comparison of low-dose heparin with low-molecular weight heparin as prophylaxis against venous thromboembolism after major trauma. N Engl J Med 1996; 335:701–707

16. Devlin JW, Tyburski JG, Moed B. Implementation and evaluation of guidelines for use of enoxaparin as deep vein thrombosis prophylaxis after major trauma. Pharmacotherapy 2001; 21:740–747

17. Knudson MM, Ikossi DG, Khaw L, et al. Thromboembolism after trauma: an analysis of 1602 episodes from the American College of Surgeons National Trauma Data Bank. Ann Surg 2004; 240:490–496

18. Guidelines for the use of parenteral and enteral nutrition in adult and pediatric patients. J Parenter Enter Nutr 2002; 26(1 suppl):1SA–138SA

19. Heyland DK, MacDonald S, Keefe L, et al. Total parenteral nutrition in the critically ill patient: a metaanalysis. JAMA 1998; 280:2013–2019

20. Peter JV, Moran JL, Phillips-Hughes J. A metaanalysis of treatment outcomes of early enteral vs early parenteral nutrition in hospitalized patients. Crit Care Med 2005; 33:213–220

21. MacFie J. Enteral vs parenteral nutrition: the significance of bacterial translocation and gut-barrier function. Nutrition 2000; 16:606–611

22. Marik PE, Zaloga GP. Early enteral nutrition in acutely ill patients: a systematic review. Crit Care Med 2001; 29:2264–2270

23. Braunschweig CL, Levy P, Sheean PM, et al. Enteral compared with parenteral nutrition: a meta–analysis. Am J Clin Nutr 2001; 74:534–542

24. Dhaliwal R, Jurewitsch B, Harrietha D, et al. Combination enteral and parenteral nutrition in critically ill patients: harmful or beneficial? A systematic review of the evidence. Intensive Care Med 2004; 30:1666–1671

25. Jacobs DG, Jacobs DO, Kudsk KA, et al. Practice management guidelines for nutritional support of the trauma patient: the EAST practice management guidelines work group. Available at: http://www.east.org/Portal/Default.aspx?tabid = 57. Accessed March 15, 2009

26. Marik Pe, Zaloga GP. Gastric vs post-pyloric feedings: a systematic review. Crit Care 2003; 7:R46–R51

27. Lacy BE, Weiser K. Gastric motility, gastroparesis, and gastric stimulation. Surg Clin North Am 2005; 85:967–987

28. Gonzalez-Pinto I, Gonzalez EM. Optimising the treatment of upper GI fistulae. Gut 2001; 49(suppl 4):iv-22–iv-31

29. Meier R, Ockenga J, Pertkiewicz M, et al. ESPEN guidelines on enteral nutrition: pancreas. Clin Nutr 2006; 25:275–284

30. McClave SA, Chang WK, Dhaliwal R, et al. Nutrition support in acute pancreatitis: a systematic review of the literature. J Parenter Enter Nutr 2006; 30:143–156

31. Kumar A, Singh N, Prakash S, et al. Early enteral nutrition in severe acute pancreatitis: a prospective randomized controlled trial comparing nasojejunal and nasogastric routes. J Clin Gastroenterol 2006; 40:431–434

32. Memon Ma, Memon Mi, Donohue JH. Abdominal drains: a brief historical review. Isr Med J 2001; 94:164–166

33. Pothier DD. The use of drains following thyroid and parathyroid surgery: a metaanalysis. J Laryngol Otol 2005; 119:669–675

34. Petrowsky H, Demartines N, Rousson V, et al. Evidence-based value of prophylactic drainage in GI surgery. Ann Surg 2004; 240:1074–1080

35. Halpin V, Soper N. The management of common bile duct stones. In: Cameron J, ed. Current surgical therapy. 7th ed. St. Louis, MO: CV Mosby, 2001

36. Lang EW, Chesnut RM. Intracranial pressure: monitoring and management. Neurosurg Clin North Am 1994; 5:573–605

37. Mayhall CG, Archer NH, Lamb VA, et al. Ventriculostomy-related infections: a prospective epidemiologic study. N Engl J Med 1984; 310:553–559

38. Aucoin PJ, Kotilainen HR, Gantz NM, et al. Intracranial pressure monitors: epidemiologic study of risk factors and infections. Am J Med 1986; 80:369–376

39. Marquardt DL, Tatum RP, Lynge DC. Postoperative management of the hospitalized patient. In: Souba WW, Fink MP, Jurkovich GJ, et al, eds. ACS surgery. 6th ed. New York, NY: WebMD, 2007; 77–86

40. Moues CM, Vos MC, van den Bemd GJ, et al. Bacterial load in relation to vacuum-assisted closure wound therapy: a prospective randomized trial. Wound Repair Regen 2004; 12:11–17

41. Fischer JE. A cautionary note: the use of vacuum-assisted closure systems in the treatment of GI cutaneous fistula may be associated with higher mortality from subsequent fistula development. Am J Surg 2008; 196:1–4

42. Barie PS, Eachempati SR. Surgical site infections. Surg Clin North Am 2005; 85:1115–1135

43. Schaff HV Gersh BJ Fisher LD, et al. Detrimental effect of perioperative myocardial infarction on late survival after coronary artery bypass: report from the Coronary Artery Surgery Study-CASS. J Thorac Cardiovasc Surg 1984; 88:972–981

43a. Salamonsen RF, Schneider HG, Bailey M, et al. Cardiac troponin I concentrations, but not electrocardiographic results, predict an extended hospital stay after coronary artery bypass graft surgery. Clin Chem 2005; 51:40–46

43b. Thielmann M, Massoudy P, Marggraf G, et al. Role of troponin I, myoglobin, and creatine kinase for the detection of early graft failure following coronary artery bypass grafting. Eur J Cardiothorac Surg 2004; 26:102–109

44. Alison P, McKee A. Surgery for coronary artery disease. In: Sidebotham D, McKee A, Gillham M, et al, eds. Cardiothoracic critical care. Philadelphia, PA: Elsevier, 2007; 141–157

45. Jain U, Laflamme CJ, Aggarwal A, et al. ECG and hemodynamic changes and their association with myocardial infarction during coronary artery

bypass surgery: a multicenter study. Multicenter Study of Perioperative Ischemia (McSPI) Research Group. Anesthesiology 1997; 86:576–591

46. Spodick DH. Acute cardiac tamponade. N Engl J Med 2003; 349:684–690

47. Bommer WJ, Follette D, Pollock M, et al. Tamponade in patients undergoing cardiac surgery: a clinical-echocardiographic diagnosis. Am Heart J 1995; 130:1216–1223

48. Pepi M, Muratori M, Barbier P, et al. Pericardial effusion after cardiac surgery: incidence, site, size, and haemodynamic consequences. Br Heart J 1994; 72:327–331

49. Shabetai R. Pericardial and cardiac pressure. Circulation 1988; 77:1–5

50. Spodick DH. Truly total electric alternation of the heart. Clin Cardiol 1998; 21:427–428

51. Reydel B, Spodick DH. Frequency and significance of chamber collapse during cardiac tamponade. Am Heart J 1990; 119:1160–1163

52. Sidebotham D, Gillham M. Hemodynamic instability and resuscitation. In: Sidebotham D, McKee, A, Gillham, M, et al, eds. Cardiothoracic critical care. Philadelphia, PA: Elsevier, 2007; 295–315

53. Sidebotham D. Pulmonary hypertension. In: Sidebotham D, McKee, A, Gillham, M, et al, eds. Cardiothoracic critical care. Philadelphia, PA: Elsevier, 2007; 374–382

54. Mebazza A, Karpati P, Renaud E, et al. Acute right ventricular failure-from pathophysiology to new treatments. Intensive Care Med 2004; 30:185–196

55. Maxey TS, Smith CD, Kern JA, et al. Beneficial effects of inhaled nitric oxide in adult cardiac surgical patients. Ann Thorac Surg 2002; 73:529–532

56. Lowson SM. Inhaled alternatives to nitric oxide. Crit Care Med 2005; 33:S188–S195

57. Theodoraki K, Rellia P, Thanopoulos A, et al. Inhaled iloprost controls pulmonary hypertension after cardiopulmonary bypass. Can J Anaesth 2002; 49:963–967

58. Maisel WH, Rawn JD, Stevenson WG. Atrial fibrillation after cardiac surgery. Ann Intern Med 2001; 135:1061–1066

59. Asher CR, Miller DP, Grimm RA, et al. Analysis of risk factors for development of atrial fibrillation early after cardiac valvular surgery. Am J Cardiol 1998; 82:892-897

60. Creswell LL, Schuessler RB, Rosenbloom M, et al. Hazards of postoperative trial arrhythmias. Ann Thorac Surg 1993; 56:539–545

61. Aranki SF, Shaw DP, Adams DH, et al. Predictors of atrial fibrillation after coronary artery surgery: current trends and impact on hospital resources. Circulation 1996; 94:390–397

62. Seguin P, Signouret T, Laviolle B, et al. Incidence and risk factors of atrial fibrillation in a surgical ICUs. Crit Care Med 2004; 32:722–726

63. Wijeysundera DN, Beattie WS, Djaiani G, et al. Off-pump coronary artery surgery for reducing mortality and morbidity. J Am Coll Cardiol 2005; 46:872–882

64. Tomic V, Russwurm S, Moller E, et al. Transcriptomic and proteomic patterns of systemic inflammation in on-pump and off-pump coronary artery bypass grafting. Circulation 2005; 112:2912–2918

64a. Haissaguerre M, Jais P, Shah DC, et al. Spontaneous initiation of atrial fibrillation by ectopic beats originating in the pulmonary veins. N Engl J Med 1998; 339:659–666

65. Mathew JP, Fontes ML, Tudor IC, et al. A multicenter risk index for atrial fibrillation after cardiac surgery. JAMA 2004; 291:1720–1729

66. Deliargyris EN, Raymond RJ, Guzzo JA, et al. Preoperative factors predisposing to early postoperative atrial fibrillation after isolated coronary artery bypass grafting. Am J Cardiol 2000; 85:763–764

67. Crystal E, Connolly SJ, Sleik K, et al. Interventions for prevention of post-operative atrial fibrillation in patients undergoing heart surgery: a metaanalysis. Circulation 2002; 106:75–80

68. Eagle KA, Guyton RA, Davidoff R, et al. ACC/AHA 2004 guideline update for coronary artery bypass graft surgery: summary article. A report of the American College of Cardiology/American Heart Association Task Force on Practice Guidelines. J Am Coll Cardiol 2004; 44:1146–1154

69. Aasbo JD, Lawrence AT, Krishnan K, et al. Amiodarone prophylaxis reduces major cardiovascular morbidity and length of stay after cardiac surgery: a metaanalysis. Ann Intern Med 2005; 143:327–336

70. Mitchell LB, Exner DV, Wyse DG, et al. Prophylactic oral amiodarone for the prevention of arrhythmias that begin early after revascularization, valve replacement, or repair: PAPABEAR; a randomized controlled trial. JAMA 2005; 294:3093–3100

71. Zebis LR, Christensen TD, Kristiansen IS, et al. Amiodarone cost effectiveness in preventing atrial fibrillation after coronary artery bypass graft surgery. Ann Thorac Surg 2008; 85:28–33

72. Whitlock RP, Chan S, Devereaux PJ, et al. Clinical benefit of steroid use in patients undergoing cardiopulmonary bypass: a metaanalysis of randomized trials. Eur Heart J 2008; 29:2592–2600

73. Mayr A, Ritsch N, Knotzer H, et al. Effectiveness of direct-current cardioversion for treatment of supraventricular tachyarrhythmias, in particular atrial fibrillation, in surgical intensive care patients. Crit Care Med 2003; 31:401–405

74. Smith W, Hood, M. Arrhythmias. In: Sidebotham D, McKee, A, Gillham, M, et al, eds. Cardiothoracic critical care. Philadelphia, PA: Elsevier, 2007; 316–341

75. Martinez EA, Epstein AE, Bass EB. Pharmacological control of rhythm: American College of Chest Physicians guidelines for the prevention and management of postoperative atrial fibrillation after cardiac surgery. Chest 2005; 128:56S–60S

76. Wyse DG, Waldo AL, DiMarco JP, et al. A comparison of rate control and rhythm control in patients with atrial fibrillation. N Engl J Med 2002; 347:1825–1833

Acute Respiratory Distress Syndrome

John P. Kress, MD, FCCP

Objectives:

- Describe the epidemiology of ARDS
- Explain the pathophysiology of ARDS
- Discuss the treatment of ARDS

Key words: respiratory failure; sepsis, aspiration; mechanical ventilation; lung injury; ARDS

ARDS and the related acute lung injury (ALI) syndromes are forms of type I or acute hypoxemic respiratory failure. This form of lung dysfunction arises from diseases causing the collapse and/or filling of alveoli, with the result that a substantial fraction of mixed venous blood traverses nonventilated airspaces, effecting a right-to-left intrapulmonary shunt (Fig 1, *right, b*). In addition to the adverse consequences on gas exchange, interstitial and alveolar fluid accumulation result in an increase in lung stiffness, imposing a mechanical load with a resulting increase in the work of breathing (Fig 1, *left, a*). Uncorrected, the gas exchange and lung mechanical abnormalities may eventuate in tissue hypoxia, respiratory arrest, and death (Fig 2). When this form of respiratory failure arises from ALI with diffuse alveolar damage (DAD) and flooding, it is termed *ARDS*.

Classification and Definition

To a first approximation, the disorders causing acute hypoxemic respiratory failure may be divided into diffuse lesions, such as pulmonary edema, and focal lung lesions, such as lobar pneumonia (Table 1). Since the distribution of airspace involvement may have implications for the response to interventions such as positive end-expiratory pressure (PEEP), this nosology is of both therapeutic and didactic value.

Acute Lobar Atelectasis

Low-pressure pulmonary edema, termed *ARDS* as a clinical entity, results from injury to the lung microcirculation sustained from direct lung insults (*eg*, aspiration, inhalation, or infectious agents) or indirectly by systemic processes (*eg*, sepsis or traumatic shock with large volume blood product resuscitation). The former is termed *pulmonary ARDS*, and the latter *extrapulmonary ARDS*. Some studies have suggested different lung mechanical properties for these entities and a different response to ventilator maneuvers directed at alveolar recruitment. In addition to the distinction between pulmonary and extrapulmonary forms of ARDS/ALI, it is also useful to distinguish between the early phases of ALI and the events occurring subsequently (Fig 3).

By light microscopy, early ARDS/ALI is characterized by flooding of the lung with proteinaceous fluid and minimal evidence of cellular injury. By electron microscopy, changes of endothelial cell swelling, widening of intercellular junctions, increased numbers of pinocytotic vesicles, and disruption and denudation of the basement membrane are prominent. This early phase of DAD has been termed *exudative*; it is a period of time during which pulmonary edema and its effects are most pronounced and intrapulmonary shunt is a primary problem dictating ventilatory strategies.

Over the ensuing days, hyaline membrane formation in the alveolar spaces is prominent and inflammatory cells become more numerous. The latter phase of DAD is dominated by disordered healing. This can occur as early as 7 to 10 days after the initial injury and often exhibits extensive pulmonary fibrosis, which is not dissimilar microscopically to the case with patients with long-standing pulmonary fibrosis. This has been termed the *proliferative phase* of DAD. Pulmonary edema may not be as prominent in this latter phase of lung injury, and the clinician managing the patient is challenged by the large dead space fraction

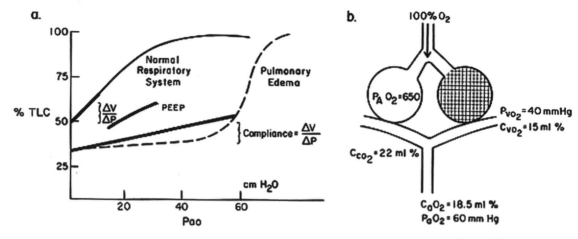

Figure 1. Gas exchange (*left, a*), and interstitial and alveolar fluid accumulation (*right, b*) in ARDS.

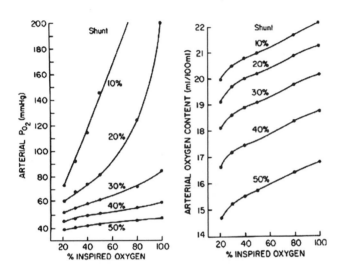

Figure 2. *Left:* the impact of shunt fraction on oxygenation. Note that when shunt is 30% and above, the response to oxygen as judged by arterial Po$_2$ is minimal. *Right:* Even though the arterial Po$_2$ changes with oxygen are minimized by large shunt fraction, the increase in arterial oxygen content are large given the steep slope of the hemoglobin-oxygen dissociation curve in this range.

and high minute ventilation requirements. These patients may also exhibit progressive pulmonary hypertension, even if the pulmonary circulation was normal at baseline, slightly improved intrapulmonary shunt that is less responsive to PEEP, further reduction in lung compliance, and a tendency toward creation of zone I conditions of the lung if hypovolemia develops in the patient.

Patients with ARDS/ALI have a large number of underlying medical and surgical etiologies, and there has been broad recognition of a need for specific definitions of these entities. The widely applied definitions offered by a joint American-European Consensus Conference published in 1994 are given in Table 2.

Table 1. *Causes of Acute Hypoxic Respiratory Failure*

Homogenous lung lesions (producing pulmonary edema)
Cardiogenic or hydrostatic edema
LV failure
Acute LV ischemia
Accelerated or malignant hypertension
Mitral regurgitation
Mitral stenosis
Ball-valve thrombus
Volume overload, particularly with coexisting renal and cardiac disease
Permeability or low-pressure edema (ARDS)
  Most common
    Sepsis and sepsis syndrome
    Acid aspiration
    Multiple transfusions for hypovolemic shock
  Less common
    Near drowning
    Pancreatitis
    Air or fat emboli
    Cardiopulmonary bypass
    Pneumonia
    Drug reaction or overdose
    Leukoagglutination
    Inhalation injury
    Infusion of biologics (*eg*, interleukin 2)
    Ischemia-reperfusion (*eg*, postthrombectomy or posttransplant)
    Edema of unclear or "mixed" etiology
    Reexpansion
    Neurogenic
    Postictal
    Tocolysis-associated
    Diffuse alveolar hemorrhage
    Microscopic angiitis
    Collagen vascular diseases
    Goodpasture syndrome
    Severe coagulopathy and bone marrow transplant
    Retinoic-acid syndrome
    Focal lung lesions
    Lobar pneumonia
    Lung contusion
    Acute lobar atelectasis

*LV = left ventricular.

Table 2. *The 1994 American-European Consensus Conference Definitions of ALI and ARDS**

Criteria	Timing	Oxygenation	CXR	PCPW
ALI	Acute onset	Pao_2/Fio_2 ratio, <300 mm Hg (regardless of PEEP level)	Bilateral infiltrates	<18 mm Hg or no clinical evidence of right atrial hypertension
ARDS	Acute onset	Pao_2/Fio_2 ratio, <200 mm Hg (regardless of PEEP level)	Bilateral infiltrates	<18 mm Hg or no clinical evidence of right atrial hypertension

*CXR = chest radiograph.

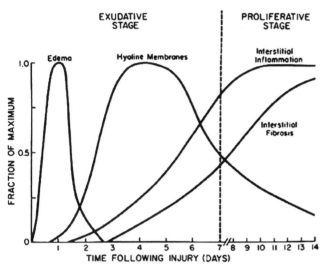

Figure 3. Depiction of the pathologic phases of ALI/ARDS.

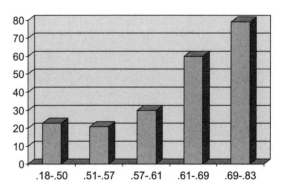

Figure 4. The observed mortality according to the quintile of dead space fraction in 179 patients with ARDS (from Nuckton et al; N Engl J Med, 2002; 346:1281).

Scoring systems have also been used to grade patients with ALI/ARDS. Despite the large derangements in lung physiology in these patients, initial measurements of gas exchange and lung mechanics have not been very useful in predicting mortality in these patients. One report, however, indicated that the dead space fraction measured during the first day of mechanical ventilation was a powerful determinant of survival; the odds ratio for mortality associated with each increase of dead space fraction of 0.05 was 1.45 (95% confidence interval, 1.15 to 1.83; p = 0.002) (Fig 4).

Treatment

This discussion will focus on ventilator and circulatory strategies for patients with ARDS/ALI, but it cannot be overemphasized that simultaneously a search for and treatment of the underlying cause of the lung failure must be conducted. Absent an identification and treatment of the underlying processes causing lung injury, supportive therapy alone will likely ultimately result in mounting complications and irreversible organ failures.

Ventilatory Management of ARDS

Lung Mechanics, Ventilator-Induced Lung Injury, and Ventilator-Associated Lung Injury

Over the past decade or more, a body of knowledge has accrued from both bench and clinical investigations that has motivated intensivists to reconsider how they ventilate patients with ARDS. Much of this work was based on early observations that mechanical ventilation using large tidal volumes (VTs) and high inflation pressures could cause lung injury in animals with normal lungs or worsen a baseline lung injury. This phenomenon was termed *ventilator-induced lung injury* (VILI). VILI is indistinguishable morphologically, physiologically, and radiologically from DAD caused by other etiologies of ALI. VILI is unique because one can identify that mechanical ventilation is the cause of lung injury, hence the term *ventilator-induced lung injury*. Ventilator-associated lung injury (VALI) is defined as lung injury that resembles ARDS and occurs in patients receiving mechanical ventilation. VALI is invariably associated with a preexisting lung pathology such as ARDS. However, while the experimental data are overwhelming in demonstrating the existence of VILI, one cannot be sure in any particular case whether and to what extent VALI is caused by a particular ventilator strategy; rather, VALI is only associated with mechanical ventilation.

Studies in animal models of VILI have demonstrated that lung injury during mechanical ventilatory support appears to be related to the distending volume to which the lung is subjected, rather than to distending pressure as measured at the mouth. For instance, in animal experiments in which the chest is banded and mechanical ventilation is conducted with high airway pressures but low Vts resulting from the restricted chest wall, lung injury is not present. Such observations have caused the term *volutrauma* to be coined for this form of microstructural injury, a refinement of the standard term *barotrauma*, which is applied to the grosser forms of extraalveolar air collections that are sought on routine radiographs obtained in patients receiving mechanical ventilation.

In addition to the detrimental effects of overdistension, numerous investigations have suggested a protective or ameliorating effect of PEEP on VILI. This protective effect has been postulated to result from the action of PEEP to avoid alveolar collapse and reopening. In the aggregate, these studies offer a view of VILI that is portrayed in Figure 5. During the respiratory cycle, alveolar

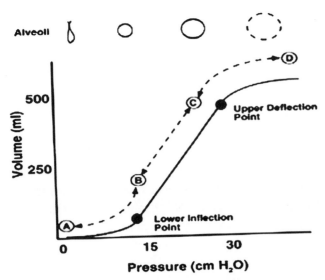

Figure 5. An idealized and simplified depiction of the PV curve of the injured lung during inflation, with the state of alveolar collapse and inflation.

opening and collapse occur if end-expiratory pressure is zero or only modestly positive, and depending on end-inspiratory lung volume, alveolar overdistension may occur.

Both in animal models of lung injury and in patients with ARDS, the respiratory system inflation pressure-volume (PV) curve exhibits a sigmoidal shape, with a lower inflection point (LIP) and an upper inflection point. Marked hysteresis is often noted when the inflation and deflation limbs are compared. The presence of the LIP is consistent with the edematous lung behaving as a two-compartment structure, one population of alveoli exhibiting near-normal compliance and another population recruitable only at higher transpulmonary pressure. As transpulmonary pressure is raised to the LIP, effecting alveolar recruitment, lung compliance improves, as reflected by the increase in the slope of the PV curve. Volume tends to increase in a nearly linear fashion as pressure is increased, until the upper inflection point is reached, with a flattening of the curve taken to represent alveolar overdistension with the attendant risks of alveolar injury.

Clinical Studies of Ventilator Strategies for ARDS

These descriptions of VILI in animals and physiologic observations in patients resulted in strategies that have been tested at the bedside and have demonstrated improved patient outcome. In the field of critical care medicine, this is one of the most substantive examples of bench-to-bedside transfer of knowledge that now provides an evidence-based approach to patient care.

Hickling and colleagues reported a favorable impact on survival of Vt reduction and permissive hypercapnea in the management of patients with ARDS, comparing their outcome to those of historical control subjects. These studies were limited by the lack of a randomized, prospective, controlled design, particularly in light of findings that the survival of patients with ARDS in the same time frame is likely improving apart from the details of mechanical ventilatory support.

The first prospective randomized trial testing a strategy of limiting Vt and utilizing PEEP to avoid alveolar recruitment-derecruitment (so-called *open lung ventilation*) was conducted by Amato and colleagues, who randomized patients with ARDS to the following two treatments: (1) assist-control ventilation with VTs of 12 mL/kg, PEEP sufficient to maintain an adequate arterial oxygen saturation on a fraction of inspired oxygen (FIO_2) of < 0.6, respiratory rates sufficient to maintain arterial carbon dioxide levels of 25 to 38 mm Hg, and no effort made to control peak inspiratory or plateau airway pressures (Pplat) [ie, the *conventional approach*]; or (2) pressure-controlled inverse-ratio ventilation, pressure-support ventilation, or volume-assured pressure-support ventilation with VTs of < 6 mL/kg, recruitment maneuver, peak pressures of < 40 cm H_2O, and PEEP titrated to maintain lung inflation above the LIP (ie, the *open-lung approach*). Patients managed with the open-lung approach demonstrated a more rapid recovery of pulmonary compliance, a decreased requirement for high FIO_2, a lower rate of barotrauma, a higher rate of liberation from the ventilator, a decreased rate of death associated with respiratory failure, and a decreased mortality rate at 28 days (although not at hospital discharge).

While these results were striking, a number of concerns regarding this study deserve consideration. The number of patients included in the study was small (only 53). Furthermore, there were multiple treatment differences between the two groups, including PEEP strategy, VT, PCO_2, minute ventilation, lung recruitment maneuvers, and mode of ventilation. Importantly, the mortality rate was extremely high in the conventional ventilation group (71%), and the early differences in mortality rate seen between the groups did not seem consistent with those of the two ventilator strategies differing by the accrual of progressive lung injury. Finally, patients with severe metabolic acidosis, which is a common feature of patients with overwhelming sepsis and ARDS, were excluded from study. Even if one accepts the results of this study, perhaps the benefit was simply due to VT reduction, not to the PEEP strategy. Even if this PEEP strategy prevented VILI, the PEEP value selected from the LIP on the inflation of edematous lungs from zero end-expiratory pressure is considerably larger than the PEEP value required to maintain alveolar recruitment during tidal ventilation while receiving PEEP. In addition, several other investigations evaluating the effect of VT manipulation on outcome did not show a similar salutary effect of low-VT ventilation.

Table 3. *ARDSnet Low-VT Protocol**

Variables	Protocol
Ventilator mode	Volume assist-control
VT	≤6 mL/kg predicted body weight
Plateau airway pressure	≤30 cm H_2O
Ventilation rate/pH goal	6–35/min, adjusted to achieve arterial pH of >7.30 if possible
Inspiratory flow	Adjust for I:E of 1.1:1.3
Oxygenation	PaO_2 ≥55 and ≤80 mm Hg or SaO_2 ≥88% and ≤95%
Combinations of FIO_2, mm Hg/PEEP, mm Hg	0.3/5, 0.4/5, 0.4/8, 0.5/8, 0.5/10, 0.6/10, 0.7/10, 0.7/12, 0.7/14, 0.8/14, 0.9/14, 0.9/16, 0.9/18, 1.0/18, 1.0/22, and 1.0/24
Weaning	Attempt by PS when FIO_2/PEEP combination is <0.4 mm Hg/ 8 mm Hg

*I:E = inspiratory/expiratory flow ratio. Predicted body weight for men: 50 + (2.3 × [height in inches − 60]) or 50 + (0.91 × [height in centimeters − 152.4]). Predicted body weight for women: 45 + (2.3 × [height in inches − 60]) or 45 + (0.91 × [height in centimeters − 152.4]).

The controversy over proper VTs for the ventilation of patients with ARDS has been largely resolved by the performance of a trial conducted by the National Institutes of Health-funded ARDSnet, a network of 10 centers in 24 hospitals comprising 75 ICUs that enrolled 861 patients. Patients were randomized to a VT strategy of either 12 or 6 mL/kg, based on ideal body weight. If Pplat, used as a surrogate of end-inspiratory lung "stretch," exceeded 30 cm H_2O pressure in the low-VT group, VT was further reduced as necessary to reduce Pplat to this target value. The experimental protocol is summarized in Table 3.

The trial was stopped sooner than the anticipated end point since the findings were striking. The strategy achieved a significant difference in VTs as intended. The mean VTs on days 1 to 3 were 6.2 and 11.8 mL/kg, respectively, in the low-VT and high-VT groups (p <0.001), and were associated with Pplat values of 25 and 33 cm H_2O, respectively (p <0.001). PEEP levels were minimally higher in the low-VT group from days 1 to 3 (averaging <1 cm H_2O, lower on day 7). The low-VT group had a modest increase in $PaCO_2$ relative to the traditional group and a very modest decrease in pH; the potential for greater degrees of respiratory acidosis between the groups was minimized by the higher respiratory rates used in the low VT group. The primary end point of the study, 28-day mortality, was significantly improved with low-VT ventilation, falling from 39.8% in the traditional group to 31.0% with low-VT ventilation (p = 0.007). In addition, the number of ventilator-free days in the first 28 days was greater in the low-VT group.

This trial is a benchmark and confirms earlier basic and clinical studies suggesting that low-VT ventilation can be protective for patients with ARDS and will improve outcome. Perhaps the best evidenced-based recommendation for the routine management of patients with ARDS undergoing mechanical ventilation is to implement the ARDSnet protocol. While questions surround other elements of ventilatory strategy (eg, the "best PEEP" level, the trade-off between F_{IO_2} and PEEP, the use of recruitment maneuvers, and patient positioning), the current evidence strongly supports the use of the ARDSnet strategy, pending additional information to guide these other components of ventilatory support.

Despite these very convincing data from a well-conducted trial and the peer review of the report of this study, some have called the results into question. A 2002 metaanalysis by Eichacker and colleagues has suggested that the ARDSnet VT trial may have "missed" the ideal VT for these patients by not testing VT in the range between 6 and 12 mL/kg, and that, while survival was better for patients with lower VT, these results point more to the detrimental effects of very high VTs and not to the superiority of lower VTs. While this argument is interesting in a theoretical sense, there are really no data to support this contention, and most experts would agree that the ARDSnet trial indeed tested the general range of VT used in managing these patients, and that the results support the low-VT approach.

Practical Points for Managing the Patient With ALI/ARDS

On presentation the patient should receive oxygen provided by high-flow or rebreather mask, although these devices rarely achieve a tracheal F_{IO_2} much >0.6 in dyspneic, tachypneic patients. The administration of supplemental oxygen is a diagnostic as well as therapeutic maneuver.

Patients whose oxygenation improves dramatically with supplemental oxygen generally have a small shunt and a larger component of ventilation-perfusion mismatch (or hypoventilation). Even when the Pa_{O_2} improves only slightly, indicating a large shunt, oxygen delivery may rise importantly, due to the steep nature of the hemoglobin saturation relationship at low Pa_{O_2} (Fig 2). The role of noninvasive positive-pressure ventilation (NIPPV) has not been established in the treatment of ARDS. Although we have used NIPPV successfully in this setting, we believe that it is generally not a good choice, and patients must be carefully selected. Since the course of ARDS is usually longer than the length of time that patients will tolerate NIPPV, and since ARDS is so often associated with hemodynamic instability, coma, and multiorgan system failure (including ileus), we believe that all but exceptional patients should be endotracheally intubated.

Intubation should be performed early and electively when it is clear that mechanical ventilation will be required, rather than waiting for frank respiratory failure. If hypoperfusion is present, as in the patient with hypotension, cardiovascular instability, or the hyperdynamic circulation of sepsis, oxygen delivery may be compromised not only by hypoxemia but by an inadequate cardiac output as well. In this circumstance, sedation and muscle relaxation should be considered as a means to diminish the oxygen requirement of the skeletal muscles. Patients with extreme hypoxemia despite ventilator management may also benefit from sedation or paralysis.

The initial ventilator settings should pursue the protocol given in Table 3. While the use of low VT is strongly supported by current evidence, the proper PEEP level is less clear. Some intensivists recommend a "least PEEP" approach, using PEEP only as necessary to achieve adequate oxygenation and avoid toxic levels of F_{IO_2} (although these thresholds are not well established). Others would recommend higher PEEP levels with a goal of achieving maximal lung recruitment and avoiding mechanical events such as collapse-reinflation that could lead to VALI. Some even advocate the use of the PV curve of the lung measured during the respiratory cycle as a guide to this PEEP titration. A trial completed by the ARDSnet comparing the PEEP strategy as implemented in the trial of low VT vs high VT against a higher PEEP level did not show a difference in survival; although, even though this study was prospective and randomized, a difference in age and severity of illness existed between the two cohorts, somewhat confounding interpretation.

Regardless of specific strategy, reducing PEEP, even for short periods of time, is often associated with alveolar derecruitment and hence rapid arterial hemoglobin desaturation. Thus, once endotracheal tube suctioning has been accomplished for diagnostic purposes, nursing and respiratory therapy staff should be instructed to keep airway disconnections to a minimum or to use an in-line suctioning system that maintains sterility and positive pressure, usually via the suctioning catheter residing in a sterile sheath and entering the endotracheal tube via a tightly sealed diaphragm. These suctioning systems are generally effective for lower levels of PEEP (ie, <15 cm H_2O) but often leak if higher levels are attempted.

Innovative Therapies for ARDS

While the general strategy described above will provide adequate ventilatory support for the majority of patients with ALI/ARDS, a fraction of patients will have severe hypoxemia or other adverse consequences of these approaches, and innovative or salvage therapies have been reported in the literature. In general, these approaches are not supported by large prospective trials (or trials have been conducted without seeing a benefit), but they may have some role in individual patient management.

Prone Position: Multiple studies have shown that a substantial fraction of patients with ARDS exhibit improved oxygenation with prone positioning. Some studies have suggested that this maneuver enhances lower lobe recruitment and thus would have the potential to not only improve gas exchange but perhaps reduced VALI and ultimate patient outcome. A large prospective trial evaluated prone positioning in patients with ALI/ARDS and did not see a benefit. In a subset analysis, there appeared to be a trend toward improved outcome in patients with more severe physiologic derangement. In addition, this study has been criticized for the relatively short periods of prone positioning that were employed. Further studies of this strategy are ongoing.

High-Frequency Ventilation: If excessive lung excursion is associated with injury to the lung, then it seems reasonable that ventilation with very small VTs at high frequencies would be associated with the least possible VILI and would be associated with improved outcome. High-frequency jet ventilation (HFV) typically employs VTs of 1 to 5 mL (or higher) and respiratory rates of 60 to 300 breaths/min. Gas exchange is poorly understood under these conditions but is thought to occur as much through augmented axial diffusion as through bulk flow. Unfortunately, multiple trials of high-frequency ventilation in adults have failed to demonstrate any benefit compared to mechanical ventilation. It is interesting to note that HFV has never been associated with improved oxygenation, reduced barotrauma, or decreased number of days of mechanical ventilation. These are all outcomes that would be reasonably expected as a logical extension of the physiology and concerns driving open lung ventilation. That they have not been observed suggests that all previous investigations of HFV were conducted using the wrong guidelines for ventilation (ie, striving to maintain normocarbia) or that some other effect not yet understood precludes benefit from this technique. Future studies of HFV should compare this technique to ventilation using the low-VT ventilation as described in the ARDSnet trial and will have to demonstrate benefit compared to these strategies to gain acceptance.

Extracorporeal Gas Exchange: The use of extracorporeal gas exchange (ie, extracorporeal membrane oxygenation) to adequately oxygenate and ventilate the blood while allowing the lung to rest remains an attractive strategy for the management of patients with ALI, but has not been supported by clinical outcome studies. There is little apparent future for this technique in adult patients with ARDS. Extracorporeal membrane oxygenation is best regarded at this time as heroic salvage therapy for patients with isolated respiratory failure in whom all other supportive measures have failed.

Inhaled Nitric Oxide: Nitric oxide (NO) is a potent endogenous vasodilator, which, when administered by inhalation, selectively vasodilates the pulmonary circulation. Inhaled NO (iNO) has several potentially salutary effects in ARDS patients. It selectively vasodilates pulmonary vessels, which subserve ventilated alveoli, diverting blood flow to these alveoli (and away from areas of shunt). The first effect, the lowering of the pulmonary vascular resistance, accompanied by a lowering of the pulmonary artery pressure, appears maximal at very low concentrations (approximately 0.1 ppm) in patients with ARDS. The beneficial effects on oxygenation take place at somewhat higher inspired concentrations of NO (1 to 10 ppm). The rapid inactivation of iNO via hemoglobin binding prevents unwanted systemic hemodynamic side effects but also mandates the continuous delivery of gas to the ventilator circuit. In numerous studies evaluating the short-term response to iNO, there has been a consistent finding of approximately 50 to 70% of patients improving oxygenation. However, two prospective trials have failed to demonstrate improved long-term outcome from iNO administration in ARDS patients receiving mechanical ventilation; thus, this remains a salvage therapy at best.

Circulatory Management of ARDS

For many years, debate has surrounded the proper circulatory management of patients with ARDS. On the one hand, animal studies and some clinical studies have suggested that edemagenesis can be reduced by reducing pulmonary microvascular pressures in patients with ALI in a fashion similar to the management of cardiogenic pulmonary edema. Of course, since these microvascular pressures are normal in these patients despite their lung flooding, the possibility of reducing cardiac preload exists, thus engendering inadequate organ perfusion in a patient population known to be at risk of multiple organ failure, and, indeed, in whom outcome appears dictated in large part by the accrual of organ failures.

In addition, the proper monitoring tools for assessing the adequacy of the circulation in these patients and whether monitoring should include invasive hemodynamic measurement was equally controversial. It seemed reasonable to state that mere monitoring with invasive measurements

that were not coupled to a strategy to achieve predefined goals would be unlikely to be helpful.

This past year, the ARDSnet completed a large multicenter trial addressing these questions. Patients were randomized to receive management with either a central venous catheter or right heart catheter, and then each group was additionally randomized to receive a liberal or conservative fluid strategy. This 2 × 2 factorial study showed no discernable benefit for the use of the right heart catheter with a protocolized management algorithm. However, the use of a conservative fluid strategy (ie, central venous pressure, <4 mm Hg; pulmonary capillary wedge pressure [PCWP], <8 mm Hg) as opposed to a liberal fluid strategy (ie, central venous pressure, 10 to 14 mm Hg; or PCWP, 14 to 18 mm Hg) was associated with improvements in oxygenation index and lung injury score, as well as with increased ventilator-free days and days not spent in the ICU. There was no difference in shock or the need for renal replacement therapy between the groups. A mortality difference between the conservative and liberal fluid strategy groups was not seen.

Management of Proliferative Phase of ARDS

A subset of patients with ARDS will progress over the first week of mechanical ventilation to disordered healing and severe lung fibrosis. This is usually characterized by increasing airway pressures or a falling VT while receiving pressure-control ventilation, a further fall in lung compliance, less response to PEEP, a "honeycomb"' appearance on chest radiograph, progressive pulmonary hypertension, and rising minute ventilation requirements (>20 L/min). Barotrauma is a prominent feature, and multiple organ failures often accrue. A number of observations regarding their supportive therapy should be made. Increased vascular permeability at this point in the course of treatment may be minimal, and strategies to reduce preload and edema are fraught with complications. Patients are prone to increases in zone I lung conditions, and attempts to reduce the PCWP may result in increased dead space and hypoperfusion. Thus, seeking the lowest PCWP providing adequate cardiac output is no longer appropriate; instead, the liberalization of fluid intake to provide a circulating volume in excess of one that is just adequate is a better strategy in this later phase of ARDS.

Interventions to directly influence the course of lung fibrosis are not well established, but high-dose corticosteroid therapy has its advocates. One prospective trial has shown an improved survival with the use of corticosteroids in patients with late ARDS, but routine use in late ARDS remains controversial. The utility of corticosteroids was studied by the ARDSnet in a randomized trial. Survival differences were not seen to be related to corticosteroid therapy.

If corticosteroids are used in this setting, aggressive measures to monitor for ventilator-associated pneumonia are warranted. This complication of mechanical ventilation has a high incidence and high mortality in patients with ARDS. In view of the abnormal chest radiograph findings and gas exchange, the multiple causes of fever and leukocytosis, and the high incidence of colonization of the airway, diagnosis is difficult and may be aided by various techniques to obtain protected specimens.

Long-term Sequelae of ARDS

There is a variability to the recovery of lung function following ALI. Patients may recover with minimal or no abnormality by routine lung function testing shortly after acute lung insult, or they may remain substantially impaired for a year or longer, if not permanently. In most studies, approximately a fourth of patients show no impairment at 1 year, a fourth of patients show moderate impairment, roughly half show only mild impairment, and a very small fraction show severe impairment. Exertional dyspnea is the most commonly reported respiratory symptom, although cough and wheezing are common as well. A reduced single-breath carbon monoxide diffusing capacity is the most common pulmonary function abnormality. Spirometry and lung volumes tend to reveal mixed restrictive-obstructive abnormalities. Determining the prognosis after ARDS may be aided by obtaining complete lung function tests at the time of hospital discharge. Those patients with substantial abnormalities should be referred for appropriate follow-up. Herridge and colleagues

also have reported that lung dysfunction may be of only minor significance in terms of regaining general function, and that weight loss, neuromuscular weakness, and neuropsychiatric dysfunction related to critical illness or supportive management may be much more significant than respiratory dysfunction *per se*.

Bibliography

Amato MRP, Barbas CSV, Medeiros DM, et al. Effect of a protective ventilation strategy on mortality in the acute respiratory distress syndrome. N Engl J Med 1998; 338:347–354

Anzueto A, Baughman RP, Guntupalli KK, et al. Aerosolized surfactant in adults with sepsis induced acute respiratory distress syndrome. N Engl J Med 1996; 334:1417–1421

Bernard GR, Artigas A, Brigham KL, et al. The American-European Consensus Conference on ARDS: definitions, mechanisms, relevant outcomes, and clinical trial coordination. Am J Respir Crit Care Med 1994; 149:818–824

Brower RG, Lanken PN, MacIntyre N, et al. Higher versus lower positive end-expiratory pressures in patients with the acute respiratory distress syndrome. N Engl J Med 2004; 351:327–336

Brower RG, Rubenfeld GD. Lung-protective ventilation strategies in acute lung injury. Crit Care Med 2003; 31(Suppl):S312–S316

Brower RG, Ware LB, Berthiaume Y, et al. Treatment of ARDS. Chest 2001; 120:1347–1367

Chastre J, Trouillet JL, Vuagnat A, et al. Nosocomial pneumonia in patients with acute respiratory distress syndrome. Am J Respir Crit Care Med 1998; 157:1165–1172

Dreyfuss D, Saumon G. Ventilator-induced lung injury: lessons from experimental studies. Am J Respir Crit Care Med 1998; 157:294–323

Eichacker PQ, Gerstenberger EP, Banks SM, et al. Meta-analysis of acute lung injury and acute respiratory distress syndrome trials testing low tidal volumes. Am J Respir Crit Care Med 2002; 166:1510–1514

Gattinoni L, Pelosi P, Suter PM, et al. Acute respiratory distress syndrome due to pulmonary and extrapulmonary disease: different syndromes? Am J Respir Crit Care Med 1998; 158:3–11

Herridge MS, Cheung AM, Tansey CM, et al. One-year outcomes in survivors of the acute respiratory distress syndrome. N Engl J Med 2003; 348: 683–693

Hickling KG. The pressure-volume curve is greatly modified by recruitment: a mathematical model of ARDS lungs. Am J Respir Crit Care Med 1998; 158: 194–199

Meduri GU, Headley AS, Golden E, et al. Effect of prolonged methylprednisolone therapy in unresolving acute respiratory distress syndrome: a randomized controlled trial. JAMA 1998; 280:159–165

Nuckton TJ, Alonso JA, Kallet RH, et al. Pulmonary dead space fraction as a risk factor for death in the acute respiratory distress syndrome. N Engl J Med 2002; 346:1281–1286

O'Connor M, Hall JB, Schmidt GA, et al. Acute hypoxemic respiratory failure. In: Hall JB, Schmidt GA, Wood LDH, eds. Principles of critical care. New York, NY: McGraw-Hill, 1998; 537–559

Rubenfeld GD. Epidemiology of acute lung injury. Crit Care Med 2003; 31(suppl):S276–S284

Slutsky AR, Tremblay LN. Multiple system organ failure: is mechanical ventilation a contributing factor? Am J Respir Crit Care Med 1998; 157:1721–1725

Steinbrook R. How best to ventilate? Trial design and patient safety in studies of the acute respiratory distress syndrome. N Engl J Med 2003; 348:1393–1401

Stewart TE. Controversies around lung protective mechanical ventilation. Am J Respir Crit Care Med 2002; 166:1421–1422

The Acute Respiratory Distress Syndrome Network. Comparison of two fluid-management strategies in acute lung injury. N Engl J Med 2006; 354:2564–2575

Ware LB, Matthay MA. The acute respiratory distress syndrome. N Engl J Med 2000; 342:1334–1347

The Acute Respiratory Distress Syndrome Network. Pulmonary-artery versus central venous catheter to guide treatment of acute lung injury. N Engl J Med 2006; 354:2213–2224

The Acute Respiratory Distress Syndrome Network. Ventilation with lower tidal volumes as compared with traditional tidal volumes for acute lung injury and ARDS. N Engl J Med 2000; 342:1301–1308

Coma, Delirium, and Prognosis

Scott K. Epstein, MD, FCCP

Objectives:

- Understand the definitions, differential diagnosis, and the diagnosis and management of coma
- Understand the definitions, differential diagnosis, and the diagnosis and management of delirium
- Understand the prognosis of patients with coma, delirium, and other syndromes of acute brain disfunction in the ICU

Key words: coma; delirium; prognosis; vegetative state

Global alteration in cognitive function develops in a high percentage of ICU patients.[1] Some patients come to the ICU with chronic brain dysfunction in the form of cognitive impairment or dementia.[2] Acute brain dysfunction develops in many other patients. A number of terms have been used to describe acute brain dysfunction including critical illness brain syndrome, critical illness-associated cognitive dysfunction, and critical illness encephalopathy. Acute brain dysfunction can occur as a consequence of direct cerebral injury (eg, traumatic brain injury, stroke, subarachnoid hemorrhage, and status epilepticus) or as a manifestation of systemic disease (eg, sepsis). No matter what the mechanism, acute brain dysfunction is associated with an increase in ICU mortality. Two forms of acute brain dysfunction are coma and delirium. Acute brain dysfunction must be distinguished from states in which consciousness is preserved such as the locked-in syndrome.

Disorders of consciousness can impact two related cerebral functions.[3] There may be an abnormality in wakefulness (eg, arousal, vigilance, and alertness), a result of dysfunction of the reticular activating system. There can also be abnormal cognitive function or awareness, manifested as disordered attention, executive function, sensation and perception, motivation, and memory. Awareness depends on the cerebral cortex and subcortical connections.[3] The relationship between wakefulness and awareness is hierarchical; that is, one cannot have awareness without wakefulness, but one can have wakefulness without awareness (eg, the vegetative state).

Definitions

Coma

Coma is defined as the total absence of wakefulness (arousal) and awareness: "unarousable unresponsiveness."[4] To distinguish coma from transient states (eg, seizure) this set of conditions must last at least 1 h. In coma, the typical sleep-wake cycle is absent, an important distinguishing characteristic from the persistent vegetative state. On physical examination the comatose patient does not open his or her eyes. The patient does not speak or move spontaneously, although reflexive movements may be present. Indeed, the patient demonstrates no purposeful movements and does not localize to noxious external stimuli.

Coma results either from injury to the brainstem (reticular activating system [RAS]) above the level of the mid pons or from bilateral cerebral hemispheric dysfunction. The RAS is a neuronal system that projects from the upper pons and midbrain to the thalamus, hypothalamus, basal forebrain, and hemispheres.

Coma can be thought of as a transitional state, rarely lasting >4 weeks.[1] If patients are to improve they will typically do so within 2 weeks, often passing through a state of delirium before attaining normal consciousness. Alternatively, patients can deteriorate to a state of brain death (see later discussion). Lastly, some patients evolve into a vegetative state, which is also transitional with some patients improving (first to a minimally conscious state and then normal consciousness) and others remaining in a persistent vegetative state.

Vegetative State

The vegetative state usually follows, within 2 to 4 weeks, severe brain injury and coma.[5] The injury typically involves the bilateral cerebral hemispheres but spares the brainstem. Prognosis is poorest when injury results from ischemia-hypoxia compared with traumatic brain injury. The vegetative state is said to be persistent when it lasts for >1 month. It is estimated that in the United States there are between 10,000 and 25,000 individuals in the vegetative state. Life expectancy for these patients is 2 to 5 years, with death resulting from pneumonia, urinary tract infection, multisystem organ failure, respiratory failure, or sudden death.

Patients in the vegetative state are awake but not aware; arousal is present but there is a total lack of cognition. There may be spontaneous eye opening to verbal stimuli. There are no discrete localized motor responses. Vegetative patients utter no comprehensible words and do not follow commands. Unlike those in the comatose state, vegetative patients have a preserved sleep-wake cycle.[1]

Other

Coma and the vegetative state must be distinguished from other conditions characterized by abnormal consciousness.[6] The minimally conscious state results from injury to the hemispheres with possible sparing of the corticospinal and corticothalamic fibers.[7] Patients with the minimally conscious state are more likely to recover than those in the vegetative state. Indeed, patients destined to recover from a vegetative state typically pass through a minimally conscious state on their way to normal consciousness. As with most syndromes of acute brain dysfunction, recovery is more likely with a traumatic compared with an anoxic mechanism of injury. Patients in the minimally conscious state demonstrate wakefulness and cyclic arousal. They may demonstrate intermittent awareness manifested as following commands, responding appropriately to yes/no questions, and uttering intelligible speech.

Akinetic mutism must be distinguished from the minimally conscious state.[8] The former is characterized by wakefulness with limited awareness. These patients demonstrate no responsiveness to commands. There may be evidence of visual pursuit, suggesting sparing of the corticospinal tracts. Physical examination reveals neither spasticity nor abnormal motor reflexes. A striking feature of this state is a lack of motivation; these patients

do not plan and do not initiate activities. There is often evidence of frontal lobe dysfunction, specifically with cingulated gyrus.

The locked-in syndrome (or pseudocoma) results from acute focal injury to the ventral pons below the level of the third nerve.[9] Injury may result from pontine infarction, hemorrhage, trauma, or central pontine myelinolysis (from too rapid correction of hyponatremia). In contrast to coma and the vegetative state, both arousal and awareness are preserved. Although it is not a disorder of consciousness, it can be confused for one. Patients demonstrate quadriplegia and anarthria. Vertical eye movements and blinking are typically preserved. If the injury involves the rostral pons and midbrain, eye movements may be lost (total locked-in syndrome). The differential diagnosis includes Guillain-Barre syndrome, botulism, neuromuscular blockade without adequate sedation, and critical illness neuromyopathy.

A number of other conditions can mimic coma and the vegetative state. These conditions generally display intact pupils, ocular movements, motor tone, and movement during sleep.

- Hypersomnia is defined as increased sleep with preserved sleep-wake cycle. Patients with this condition demonstrate a normal neurologic examination when aroused. Hypersomnia often occurs in the setting of sleep deprivation. It can also be seen in the presence of sleep disorders, narcolepsy, drug toxicity, metabolic encephalopathy, or RAS damage.
- Catatonia is manifested as a state in which the eyes are open but the patient does not speak or move spontaneously. Patients do not follow commands. The neurologic examination is normal. The EEG will display low voltage. Catatonia occurs as a complication of psychiatric illness (eg, depression, bipolar, and schizophrenia).
- The effects of general anesthesia, sedatives, or barbiturates can mimic coma.
- Seizures or the postictal state (eg, Todd paralysis) can mimic coma but the effect is short lived.

Brain Death

Brain death, or death by neurologic criteria, refers to irreversible loss of all cerebral and brainstem function.[10] There is an absence of consciousness and no response to noxious stimuli. There is an absence of cerebral metabolism. Spinal reflexes may persist, indicating some intact neuromuscular transmission. There is an absence of brainstem reflexes including cervico-ocular, vestibulo-ocular, cough, gag, corneal, and pupillary reflexes. There is no respiratory response, a condition that can be demonstrated with "apnea testing." In this test, the patient is preoxygenated with 100% oxygen or 10 cm H_2O continuous positive airway pressure with 10 L/min of oxygen delivered through a catheter in the trachea (to avoid injurious hypoxemia during the test). All ventilatory support is discontinued. Apnea is said to be present when the patient makes no respiratory efforts and the $Paco_2$ rises from 40 to 60 mm Hg.

In making a diagnosis of brain death, one must exclude (or correct) metabolic causes (*eg*, severe electrolyte abnormalities), physiologic causes (*eg*, severe hypothermia), and pharmacologic causes (*eg*, effects of sedatives, barbiturates, or narcotics). In general, confirmatory tests are not needed to make a diagnosis of brain death. One exception would be when safe apnea testing is not possible because of hypotension or hypoxemia. Available confirmatory tests include cerebral angiography (absence of cerebral blood flow), electroencephalography (isoelectric tracing), transcranial Doppler ultrasound (reverberating flow with small systolic peaks), and cerebral scintigraphy (no intracranial filling, the "hollow skull" sign).

Coma

The etiology of coma consists of bilateral (diffuse) cerebral hemispheric injury, unilateral hemispheric injury with displacement of midline structures, or injury to midline structures (pons, midbrain). Coma may occur as a result of a systemic, nonstructural process (Table 1) or direct, structural brain injury (Table 2). In the United States the most common causes of primary cerebral injury are hypoxic-ischemic encephalopathy and trauma. The most common systemic cause in the United States is drug overdose.

Prevalence of Coma

Cardiac arrest is complicated by coma in 80 to 90% of patients at some point during their

Table 1. *Nonstructural Causes of Coma*

Drugs
    Alcohol
    Amphetamines
    Anticholinergics
    Antidepressants
    Antipsychotics
    Barbiturates
    Benzodiazepines
    Drugs of abuse
    Opiates
    Salicylates
    Sedative
    Tranquilizers
Toxins
    Carbon monoxide
    Cyanide
    Ethylene glycol
    Lead
    Methanol
Metabolic
    Diabetic ketoacidosis
    Hepatic failure
    Hypercapnia
    Hypoxia
    Hypo- or hypernatremia
    Hypoglycemia
    Hypo- or hypercalcemia
    Hypo- or hyperthermia
    Hypothyroidism
    Nonketotic hyperosmolar coma
    Porphyria
    Renal failure (uremia)
    Wernicke encephalopathy
Infection
    Encephalitis
    Meningitis (bacterial, viral)
    Sepsis
Other
    Diffuse ischemia
    Fat embolism
    Hypertensive encephalopathy
    Hypotension
    Seizures, postictal

hospitalization with only 10 to 30% experiencing meaningful neurologic recovery. Five to 30% of patients remain comatose at discharge.[11,12] Heterogeneous patients who must have mechanical ventilation support because of acute respiratory failure will develop coma in 15 to 20% of cases.[13,14] As many as one in four patients who fail to wean from the ventilator, do so because of coma. Among elderly patients (age >65 years) admitted to the medical ICU, up to 33% have coma on admission and 8% will develop coma during their ICU stay.[15]

Table 2. *Structural Causes of Coma*

Brain abscess
Brain tumor
Brainstem hemorrhage
Brainstem infarction
Cerebral artery occlusion
Cerebral vasculitis
Herniation
Hydrocephalus
Intracranial hemorrhage
Multifocal leukoencephalopathy
Sagittal sinus thrombosis
Subarachnoid hemorrhage
Subdural empyema
Subdural hemorrhage
Trauma

Table 3. *Glasgow Coma Scale Score (3 to 15 points)*

Best motor response (6 points)
   6 - Obeying commands
   5 - Localizing to pain
   4 - Withdrawing to pain
   3 - Abnormal flexion (decorticate)
   2 - Extensor response (decerebrate)
   1 - None
Best verbal response (5 points)
   5 - Oriented
   4 - Confused conversation
   3 - Inappropriate words
   2 - Incomprehensible sounds
   1 - None
Eye opening (4 points)
   4 - Spontaneously
   3 - To speech
   2 - To pain
   1 - None

Sixteen percent of sepsis patients develop coma (defined as a Glasgow Coma Scale [GCS] score of ≤ 8) and this is associated with increased mortality.[16] Among patients admitted to long-term care units with chronic critical illness, 30% are in coma.[17]

Diagnosis of Coma

Diagnosis of the comatose patient can be carried out using the four-part neurologic evaluation outlined by Plum and Posner.[4] Using this approach the clinician focuses on level of consciousness, brainstem function, motor activity, and respiratory pattern.

The *level of consciousness* is best assessed using one of several scoring system. The GCS score (Table 3) was first developed by Teasdale and Jennett[18] for use in patients with traumatic brain injury. For patients without motor activity, the motor response should be assessed with a central painful (supraorbital or sternal) stimulus to avoid a misleading reflex response. The GCS has a number of limitations. It has low sensitivity to subtle changes in arousal. It does not assess brainstem function. The verbal score can be difficult or impossible to determine in patients who are intubated, sedated, or aphasic.

Another tool for assessing consciousness is the Glasgow Liege Score, which combines the Glasgow Scale with an assessment of five brainstem reflexes (points): fronto-orbicular (score 5), vertical oculocephalic or "doll's eyes" (score 4), pupillary light (score 3), horizontal oculocephalic (score 2), oculocardiac (heart rate slows with pressure applied to eye; score 1), and none (score 0).[19]

Table 4. *FOUR Score (0 to 16 points)*

Eye response (0–4 points)
   4 - Eyelids open or opened, tracking, or blinking to
      command
   3 - Eyelids open but not tracking
   2 - Eyelids closed but open to loud voice
   1 - Eyelids closed but open to pain
   0 - Eyelids remain closed with pain
Motor response (0–4 points)
   4 - Thumbs-up, fist, or peace sign
   3 - Localizing to pain
   2 - Flexion response to pain
   1 - Extension response to pain
   0 - No response to pain or generalized myoclonus status
Brainstem reflexes (0–4 points)
   4 - Pupil and corneal reflexes present
   3 - One pupil wide and fixed
   2 - Pupil or corneal reflexes absent
   1 - Pupil and corneal reflexes absent
   0 - Absent pupil, corneal, and cough reflex
Respiration (0–4 points)
   4 - Not intubated, regular breathing pattern
   3 - Not intubated, Cheyne-Stokes breathing pattern
   2 - Not intubated, irregular breathing
   1 - Breathes above ventilator rate

If the oculocephalic reflexes are absent or testing is not possible (*eg*, immobilized cervical spine), oculovestibular testing should be used. A third approach to assessing consciousness is the FOUR score (Full Outline of UnResponsiveness score), which combines assessment of eye response, motor response, brainstem, and respiration[20] (Table 4).

As previously indicated, brainstem function is best evaluated by assessing a number of

Table 5. *Brainstem Reflexes*

Reflex	Technique	Normal Response
Pupils	Response to light	Direct and consensual constriction
Oculocephalic (doll's eyes)	Turn head from side to side	Eyes move conjugately in opposite direction
Oculovestibular (cold water calorics)	Irrigate external auditory canal with cold water	Sustained deviation of eyes toward irrigated ear
Corneal	Stimulate cornea	Eyelid closure
Cough	Stimulate cough	Cough
Gag	Stimulate soft palate	Symmetric elevation

brainstem reflexes (Table 5). In performing oculovestibular evaluations, it is important that the head is at 30 degrees and the tympanic membranes are not obstructed (*eg*, cerumen) and not perforated. With an intact brainstem, there will be tonic deviation of eyes toward the irrigated ear.

The pupils are under control of the sympathetic (dilation) and parasympathetic (constriction) nervous systems. Pupillary responses are also helpful in localizing the sight of brain injury and in defining etiology. For example, intact responses suggest a toxic-metabolic cause while abnormal responses point toward injury to the reticular activating system. Small, reactive pupils suggest disease of the hypothalamus. A Horner pupil indicates injury to the unilateral diencephalon (thalamus, hypothalamus). Dorsal midbrain disease is manifest as slightly large, unreactive pupils, while central midbrain dysfunction is associated with fixed, irregular, midposition pupils. Pontine injury produces characteristic pinpoint pupils. A unilateral, fixed, and dilated pupil results from third nerve dysfunction and may be a sign of herniation. Pupillary responses can also provide insight into possible toxic-metabolic states. Opiates produce small reactive pupils that can become pinpoint pupils with severe intoxication. Large barbiturate doses can lead to unreactive pupils. Anticholinergics result in large, unreactive pupils. Anoxia can also result in fixed dilated pupils, although this can reverse if cerebral oxygen supply is rapidly reestablished.

Motor response may be assessed as part of the determination of the GCS, the Glasgow Liege score, and the FOUR score. The presence of purposeful motor movements is an important finding as it indicates that the cortex is processing and integrating information. Such movements may include reaching for the endotracheal tube or assuming "comfort" positions. Other abnormal movements may be involuntary (*eg*, seizure, myoclonus, and tremor). Reflex movements indicate a loss of descending hemispheric modulation. Abnormal motor responses provide a clue to the underlying cause of coma. For example, "metabolic coma" is often associated with tremor, asterixis, and myoclonus. Muscle tone is often decreased in metabolic coma. In contrast, conditions associated with increased motor tone (rigidity) are often not metabolic. For example, extension posturing (decerebrate rigidity) is characterized by extension of the lower extremities and adduction, extension, and pronation of the upper extremities. Decerebrate posturing is seen with injury to the caudal diencephalons, midbrain, or pons. This should be contrasted from abnormal flexion (decorticate rigidity), which is seen with injury to the hemispheres or thalamus. Decorticate posturing is manifested as extension of the lower extremities and adduction and flexion of the upper extremities. In general, patients with a decorticate response to pain have a better prognosis than those demonstrating a decerebrate response to pain.

The fourth element of the Plum and Posner[4] assessment to coma is the respiratory response with four major patterns observed: Cheyne-Stokes, hyperventilation, ataxic, and apneustic breathing. Cheyne-Stokes respiration is characterized by periodic breathing with hyperpnea alternating with apnea. Its presence can indicate bilateral hemispheric or diencephalon injury. It must be remembered that Cheyne-Stokes respiration may also be seen in heart failure and in some normal elderly patients during sleep. Hyperventilation is seen with injury to the pons or midbrain tegmentum. Apneustic breathing, a result of mid or caudal pons injury, is characterized by prolonged pauses at end-inspiration. Ataxic breathing, resulting from injury to the medulla, consists of a very irregular pattern with varying rate and tidal volume.

Herniation Syndromes

Brain herniation is a life-threatening event that can lead to irreversible brain damage or death.

Measures to emergently reduce intracranial pressure (ICP) are indicated. It must be remembered that brain tissue is highly inelastic. Therefore, in response to a mass lesion (tumor, blood, or edema) that increases ICP, brain tissue will shift to a different cranial compartment. When this shift results in compression of the reticular activating system coma will result. Three major herniation syndromes may occur. Central herniation occurs when brain tissue is forced toward the foramen magnum. This compresses the midbrain, leading to miosis and decerebrate posturing. The sixth cranial nerve is stretched, producing lateral gaze palsy. Finally, the medulla is compressed, leading to cardiovascular (hypertension and bradycardia) and respiratory (ataxic breathing) changes. Uncal herniation occurs when the medial temporal lobe is pushed across the tentorial edge affecting the lateral midbrain ("blown pupil" from compression of the third nerve and parasympathetics). The contralateral cerebral peduncle can be compressed, resulting in hemiparesis. Finally, the medulla can be compressed. Cerebellar herniation causes compression of the pons or medulla, resulting in ataxic breathing, bradycardia, and hypertension.

Management of Coma

Acute coma represents a medical emergency with resuscitation, diagnosis, and therapy all taking place rapidly and simultaneously.[3] Resuscitation takes the form of ensuring adequate airway, breathing, and circulation (ABCs) and, unless neck injury can be ruled out, cervical stabilization must be performed. Indeed, as a general rule all comatose patients should be assumed to have cervical spine injury unless ruled out by a reliable observer or diagnostic testing. In general, patients with GCS $\leq$ 8 should be intubated to protect the airway from aspiration and upper airway obstruction. If the patient is in a hard collar, nasal intubation (unless otherwise contraindicated) is preferred. If there is evidence of increased ICP, lidocaine or thiopental should be given for the intubation. Oxygen saturation must be maintained at >90%. Hypotension must be corrected with a general target of a mean arterial pressure of >70 mm Hg.

Laboratory evaluation must include a full metabolic panel (electrolytes, glucose, thyroid, and hepatic function tests), complete blood count, toxic screen, and arterial blood gas. The general strategy should be to treat common and rapidly reversible processes including hypoglycemia, hypoxemia, and hypothermia. Thiamine should be given prior to glucose to decrease the risk of Wernicke encephalopathy. Appropriate antidotes (eg, naloxone, flumazenil) should be given for suspected (or proven) intoxication and consideration should be given to administering charcoal and performing gastric lavage (once the airway is protected). Antibiotics should be administered for suspected meningitis. Anticonvulsants should be given if seizures are present or suspected. Consideration should be given to hyperventilation and mannitol if there is clinical evidence of increased ICP. Additional supportive or preventive strategies should be considered (eg, deep venous thrombosis and gastrointestinal prophylaxis, vigilance for infection, early nutrition).

Neurologic examination must rapidly assess for signs of existing or impending herniation. Focal findings on neurologic examination suggest stroke, CNS infection, tumor, intracranial hemorrhage, or increased ICP. Unfortunately the absence of focal findings on neurologic exam does not rule out these entities. In acute coma, immediate CNS imaging is indicated. CT scanning can demonstrate the presence of intracranial bleeding, hydrocephalus, brain edema, herniation, malignancy, or abscess. A negative finding on head CT suggests an alternative diagnosis including hypoxic-ischemic insult or toxic-metabolic coma. In the hyperacute phase of stroke, the CT can be unremarkable. When coma occurs during the course of ICU care, the head CT is unlikely to be abnormal unless the patient demonstrates a new neurologic deficit or has a seizure.[21] MRI may have a role when the cause of coma is unexplained and the CT is normal or equivocal.[22] MRI of the brain can demonstrate acute ischemic stroke, cavernous venous sinus thrombosis, tumor, brain edema, inflammation, abscess, and changes consistent with diffuse axonal injury. In sepsis and cardiac surgery, MRI can detect lesions not suspected from clinical examination or seen on CT. Lumbar puncture should be performed whenever meningitis is suspected. EEG should be carried out if seizure is suspected. Indeed, nonconvulsive status epilepticus may be present in up to 20% of ICU patients with an unexplained alteration in consciousness and in 8% with coma.[23,24]

Prognosis of Coma

Coma is of great prognostic significance in the setting of brain injury. Coma is an independent predictor of increased mortality when present in the setting of ischemic stroke, intracranial hemorrhage, traumatic brain injury, sepsis, and cardiac arrest. The etiology of coma is an important determinant of prognosis. For example, coma adversely affects outcome in sepsis more than it does in trauma. At 1 year, patients with coma resulting from trauma are more likely to be alive and less likely to be in a persistent vegetative state compared with those with coma from hypoxic-ischemic causes.[5]

In general, clinical examination provides a more accurate predictor of outcome in coma when compared with other modalities such as imaging, EEG, and biomarkers. Predictors tend to be less accurate in traumatic brain injury compared with other causes of coma. Factors associated with a poor prognosis (death or persistent vegetative state) include the duration of anoxia (>8 to 10 min), duration of cardiopulmonary resuscitation (>30 min), the length of time in coma, absent motor response (day 3), and signs of brainstem damage (absent pupillary response at day 1 or 3, absent corneal reflexes at day 1). The GCS score can be used to predict outcome, including both survival and neurologic function. For example, a day 3 GCS score <5 is associated with poor prognosis in head trauma, nontraumatic coma, ischemic stroke, subarachnoid hemorrhage, intracranial hemorrhage, meningitis, and in the general ICU population. That said, the GCS does not appear to be as accurate as the individual motor and brainstem reflexes listed here. The GCS is subject to limitations: it is difficult to measure in intubated and sedated patients, it is insensitive to subtle alterations in wakefulness, and brainstem findings are not detected.

When coma occurs in cardiac arrest, 90% of patients who will awaken do so within the first 3 days. A metaanalysis examined 11 studies comprising nearly 2,000 patients with cardiac arrest.[25] Five clinical signs were found to be predictive of death or poor neurologic outcome: at 24 h,

absent corneas, absent pupillary response, absent withdrawal response to pain, and absent motor response, and at 72 h, absent motor response. The analysis showed that immediately after the arrest there are no clinical findings that accurately predict outcome. Furthermore, no clinical findings were strongly predictive of a *good* neurologic outcome. Two systematic reviews [26,27] found that two day 3 clinical criteria were highly specific for a poor outcome: absent or extensor motor response or absent pupillary or corneal reflexes. These reviews did note that metabolic derangements and medications may impair the accuracy of prediction. An analysis of 596 nontraumatic coma patients in the SUPPORT trial showed that at 2 months 69% were dead, 19% were severely disabled, and just 7% survived without severe disability. The investigators identified five day 3 factors associated with poor prognosis: age ≥70 years, abnormal brainstem response (pupils, corneas), absent verbal response, absent withdrawal to pain, and creatinine ≥1.5 mg/dL.[28] When none of these factors were present, mortality at 2 months was 20% but rose to >90% when three or more factors were present.

Myoclonus affects the face, limbs, or axial skeleton and it may be incessant, myoclonus status epilepticus. Myoclonus has been associated with poor prognosis.[29] On rare occasions patients may recover if the cause is respiratory failure. Treatment with valproate or clonazepam can decrease myoclonus. Nevertheless, there is no evidence that treating myoclonus improves outcome.

Of the ancillary tests available, median nerve somatosensory evoked potentials (SSEPs; averaged electric cortical responses to somatosensory stimulation) are the most accurate. Bilateral absence of cortical responses at 24 to 72 h indicates an extremely poor prognosis. For example, among adults with hypoxic-ischemic encephalopathy there is a <1% chance of awakening (eg, 99% die or have persistent vegetative state) if there is an absent response.[30] SSEPs appear less accurate in trauma and in adolescents and children. Unfortunately the presence of SSEPs does not guarantee a good prognosis; 50% with present SSEPs die without regaining consciousness.

EEGs have been used to assess prognosis.[3] In postanoxic coma, isoelectric or burst-suppression patterns are associated with poor outcome. An alpha pattern is associated with mortality of 61 to 90% in hypoxic-ischemic coma and traumatic brain injury but only 27% in metabolic coma. There are limitations to the use of EEG in this setting, including alterations resulting from sedative drugs, sensitivity to electrical environmental noise, and an inability to assess the brainstem. The real value of an EEG is to rule out seizures.

Neuroimaging has been used to assess prognosis. In traumatic brain injury, CT diagnosis of brainstem lesions, encroachment of the basal cisterns, and diffuse axonal injury have been associated with poor prognosis. CT findings in intracranial hemorrhage and subarachnoid hemorrhage may also have prognostic value. MRI has proved predictive of outcome in several settings including coma in ischemic stroke. Finding lesions in the corpus callosum and dorsolateral brainstem is associated with poor prognosis in patients with persistent vegetative state after traumatic brain injury. That said, MRI is a less accurate predictor of outcome than clinical findings and SSEPs.

Several biomarkers, measured in the blood or in the cerebrospinal fluid, have been examined for prognostic significance.[12] For example, elevated levels of neuron-specific enolase, glial protein S100, and creatine phosphokinase isoenzyme BB isoform are associated with poor prognosis. Although these are sensitive markers for detecting brain injury, a metaanalysis concluded they are less predictive of outcome than clinical findings and SSEPs.[31] A subsequent prospective study[32] found that an elevated neuron-specific enolase performed comparably to bilaterally absent SSEPs in predicting poor outcome.

Delirium

Delirium is an acute condition characterized by impaired attention, disorganized thinking, a changing level of consciousness, and a fluctuating course. This condition is sometimes referred to as ICU psychosis, ICU syndrome, acute confusional state, septic encephalopathy, and acute brain failure. In may go unrecognized in up to 84% of ICU patients. Delirium occurs in 30% of patients on general medical wards and 10 to 60% of surgical patients (especially hip and cardiac surgery). It is present in 50 to 90% of ICU patients. Two

psychomotor types have been recognized, hyperactive and hypoactive.[33,34] Hyperactive delirium is characterized by a patient who is restless, agitated, combative, with emotional lability and pulling at catheters. Hypoactive delirium in characterized by a patient who demonstrates, lethargy, flat affect, apathy, and decreased responsiveness. Hypoactive and mixed hypo- and hyperactive delirium are much more common than isolated hyperactive delirium In surgical and trauma patients, the overwhelming majority of cases are hypoactive, with a minority having mixed or pure hyperactive delirium. In medical ICU patients, hypoactive delirium is most common in patients > 65 years and a mixed pattern is more common in those < 65.

Delirium results from many of the same systemic and metabolic processes and medications that can lead to coma. It can also result from focal brain injury including cerebrovascular accidents affecting the frontal lobe, right parietal lobe, and the basal ganglia. A common underlying mechanism is an imbalance in neurotransmitters than modulate behavior, mood, and cognition.[35] These include activation of glutamate and dopamine, excess cortisol and cytokines, both activation and deficiency of γ-aminobutyric acid, serotonin, and cholinergic activity.

A number of risk factors for delirium have been identified (Table 6). These include host factors, acute illness, and iatrogenic or environmental factors. Sepsis has repeatedly been identified as a major risk factor with delirium, developing in 21 to 73% of patients. Delirium in sepsis is associated with increased mortality compared to sepsis without delirium. If obtained, the EEG shows diffuse slowing, while neuroimaging and lumbar puncture results are normal.

A number of delirium scoring systems have been developed. The confusion assessment method (CAM) has been adapted for use in the ICU (CAM-ICU) by substituting the minimental status examination with the attention screening examination (ASE).[36] The ASE is performed by showing the patient 5 pictures and then asking the patient to recall these (eg, nod yes/no) among 10 subsequent pictures (including the five previously shown). Visually impaired patients are asked to squeeze the tester's hand when the letter "A" is heard. Delirium is present when there is acute onset of mental status change or a fluctuating course, inattention on the ASE, and either altered

Table 6. *Risk Factors for Delirium**

Host factors
  Age
  Baseline cognitive function
  Poor Functional status
  Visual or hearing impairment
  Poor nutritional status
  Low education level
  Substance or alcohol abuse
  Chronic comorbid conditions

Acute illness
  Sepsis
  Shock
  High severity of illness (*eg*, APACHE II, SAPS)
  Respiratory failure, hypoxemia
  Fever
  Hypothermia
  Electrolyte abnormalities
  Metabolic abnormalities

Iatrogenic/environmental
  Sleep deprivation
  Catheters
  Restraints
  Mechanical ventilation
  Medications (anticholinergics, sedatives, narcotics)

*APACHE II = Acute Physiology and Chronic Health Evaluation II; SAPS = Simplified Acute Physiology Score

level of consciousness (Richmond agitation-sedation score not equal to zero) or disorganized thinking (assessed by four yes or no questions and the ability to follow simple commands). The CAM-ICU has >90% sensitivity and specificity. The ICU Delirium Screening Checklist consists of eight items, with one point given for each and four or more points indicating the presence of delirium. The checklist is more sensitive (99%) than the CAM-ICU but much less specific (64%).[37] A third scoring system, the Delirium Detection Score, is composed of eight criteria including orientation, hallucination, agitation, anxiety, seizures, tremor, paroxysmal sweating, and altered sleep-wake rhythm.[38]

Delirium adversely affects prognosis. It is associated with prolonged duration of mechanical ventilation, increased risk for reintubation, increased length of stay in the ICU and in the hospital, and higher costs of care. It is associated with a threefold increased mortality at 6 months. The risks associated with delirium are cumulative: each day with delirium is associated with a 20% increased risk for prolonged hospital stay and 10% increased risk of death. One-third of ventilated patients

with delirium have prolonged cognitive impairment.[13,39-42] It remains unproven whether delirium is a marker or the cause of poor outcome.

The management of delirium can be divided into three components: prevention, identification of precipitating factors, and pharmacologic therapy. In non-ICU settings, prevention results in a 40% reduction in the incidence of delirium. Delirium-prevention efforts are aimed at reorientation, reducing noise, normalizing sleep patterns, physical therapy and mobilization, removing catheters and restraints, and improving interaction with the environment by providing (if necessary) glasses and hearing aids. Whether these approaches work in ICU patients remains to be proven. Precipitating factors can be categorized as physiologic, metabolic, pharmacologic, and environmental (Table 6).

There has been resurgent interest in the pharmacologic treatment (and prevention) of delirium. Indications for treatment include concerns for patient safety in the setting of hyperactive delirium, persistence of delirium despite elimination of precipitants, and when precipitating factors are unknown or cannot be rapidly corrected. In a retrospective study[43] of mechanically ventilated patients, haloperidol, a drug often used for hyperactive delirium, was associated with decreased mortality, although the mechanism remains speculative. In a randomized controlled trial[44] comparing haloperidol with olanzapine, both agents were found to be safe, with comparable treatment effect when assessed using the ICU Delirium Checklist. Benzodiazepines may prevent delirium when used in alcohol or sedative withdrawal. In contrast, they may exacerbate other types of delirium. A Cochrane analysis[45] found there were no adequate randomized controlled trials to support the use of benzodiazepines to treat nonalcohol withdrawal-related delirium. A randomized controlled trial[46] comparing lorazepam with dexmedetomidine in mechanically ventilated patients found the latter to be associated with an increase in days alive without delirium or coma. A subsequent randomized trial compared midazolam with dexmetedomidine, in ventilated medical and surgical patients, titrated to achieve light sedation from enrollment until extubation or a total of 30 days. Dexmetedomidine was associated with a lower incidence of delirium (54%) compared with midazolam (77%).[47]

References

1. Stevens RD, Nyquist PA. Coma, delirium, and cognitive dysfunction in critical illness. Crit Care Clin 2006; 22:787–804

2. Lee HB, DeLoatch CJ, Cho S, et al. Detection and management of pre-existing cognitive impairment and associated behavioral symptoms in the intensive care unit. Crit Care Clin 2008; 24:723–736

3. Stevens RD, Bhardwaj A. Approach to the comatose patient. Crit Care Med 2006; 34:31–41

4. Plum F, Posner J. The diagnosis of stupor and coma. 4th ed. Philadelphia, PA: FA Davis, 1995

5. Medical aspects of the persistent vegetative state (2). The Multi-Society Task Force on PVS. N Engl J Med 1994; 330:1572–1579

6. Cartlidge N. States related to or confused with coma. J Neurol Neurosurg Psychiatry 2001; 71(suppl 1):18–19

7. Giacino JT, Ashwal S, Childs N, et al. The minimally conscious state: definition and diagnostic criteria. Neurology 2002; 58:349–353

8. Ackermann H, Ziegler W. Akinetic mutism: a review of the literature [in German]. Fortschr Neurol Psychiatr 1995; 63:59–67

9. Smith E, Delargy M. Locked-in syndrome. BMJ 2005; 330:406–409

10. Wijdicks EF. The diagnosis of brain death. N Engl J Med 2001; 344:1215–1221

11. Puttgen HA, Geocadin R. Predicting neurological outcome following cardiac arrest. J Neurol Sci 2007; 261:108–117

12. Vos PE, Lamers KJ, Hendriks JC, et al. Glial and neuronal proteins in serum predict outcome after severe traumatic brain injury. Neurology 2004; 62:1303–1310

13. Ely EW, Shintani A, Truman B, et al. Delirium as a predictor of mortality in mechanically ventilated patients in the intensive care unit. JAMA 2004; 291:1753–1762

14. Esteban A, Anzueto A, Alia I, et al. How is mechanical ventilation employed in the intensive care unit? An international utilization review. Am J Respir Crit Care Med 2000; 161:1450–1458

15. McNicoll L, Pisani MA, Zhang Y, et al. Delirium in the intensive care unit: occurrence and clinical course in older patients. J Am Geriatr Soc 2003; 51:591–598

16. Eidelman LA, Putterman D, Putterman C, et al. The spectrum of septic encephalopathy. Definitions, etiologies, and mortalities. JAMA 1996; 275:470–473

17. Nelson JE, Tandon N, Mercado AF, et al. Brain dysfunction: another burden for the chronically critically ill. Arch Intern Med 2006; 166:1993–1999

18. Teasdale G, Jennett B. Assessment of coma and impaired consciousness. A practical scale. Lancet 1974; 2:81–84

19. Born JD. The Glasgow-Liege Scale. Prognostic value and evolution of motor response and brain stem reflexes after severe head injury. Acta Neurochir (Wien) 1988; 91:1–11

20. Wijdicks EF, Bamlet WR, Maramattom BV, et al. Validation of a new coma scale: the FOUR score. Ann Neurol 2005; 58:585–593

21. Rafanan AL, Kakulavar P, Perl J II, et al. Head computed tomography in medical intensive care unit patients: clinical indications. Crit Care Med 2000; 28:1306–1309

22. Sundgren PC, Reinstrup P, Romner B, et al. Value of conventional, and diffusion- and perfusion weighted MRI in the management of patients with unclear cerebral pathology, admitted to the intensive care unit. Neuroradiology 2002; 44:674–680

23. Claassen J, Mayer SA, Kowalski RG, et al. Detection of electrographic seizures with continuous EEG monitoring in critically ill patients. Neurology 2004; 62:1743–1748

24. Towne AR, Waterhouse EJ, Boggs JG, et al. Prevalence of nonconvulsive status epilepticus in comatose patients. Neurology 2000; 54:340–345

25. Booth CM, Boone RH, Tomlinson G, et al. Is this patient dead, vegetative, or severely neurologically impaired? Assessing outcome for comatose survivors of cardiac arrest. JAMA 2004; 291:870–879

26. Wijdicks EF, Hijdra A, Young GB, et al. Practice parameter: prediction of outcome in comatose survivors after cardiopulmonary resuscitation (an evidence-based review): report of the Quality Standards Subcommittee of the American Academy of Neurology. Neurology 2006; 67:203–210

27. Zandbergen EG, de Haan RJ, Stoutenbeek CP, et al. Systematic review of early prediction of poor outcome in anoxic-ischaemic coma. Lancet 1998; 352:1808–1812

28. Hamel MB, Goldman L, Teno J, et al. Identification of comatose patients at high risk for death or severe disability. SUPPORT Investigators. Understand Prognoses and Preferences for Outcomes and Risks of Treatments. JAMA 1995; 273:1842–1848

29. Wijdicks EF, Young GB. Myoclonus status in co-matose patients after cardiac arrest. Lancet 1994; 343:1642–1643

30. Robinson LR, Micklesen PJ, Tirschwell DL, et al. Predictive value of somatosensory evoked po-tentials for awakening from coma. Crit Care Med 2003; 31:960–967

31. Zandbergen EG, de Haan RJ, Hijdra A. Systematic review of prediction of poor outcome in anoxic-ischaemic coma with biochemical markers of brain damage. Intensive Care Med 2001; 27:1661–1667

32. Zandbergen EG, Hijdra A, Koelman JH, et al. Pre-diction of poor outcome within the first 3 days of postanoxic coma. Neurology 2006; 66:62–68

33. Pandharipande P, Cotton BA, Shintani A, et al. Motoric subtypes of delirium in mechanically ventilated surgical and trauma intensive care unit patients. Intensive Care Med 2007; 33:1726–1731

34. Peterson JF, Pun BT, Dittus RS, et al. Delirium and its motoric subtypes: a study of 614 critically ill patients. J Am Geriatr Soc 2006; 54:479–484

35. Flacker JM, Lipsitz LA. Neural mechanisms of de-lirium: current hypotheses and evolving concepts. J Gerontol A Biol Sci Med Sci 1999; 54:B239–B246

36. Ely EW, Inouye SK, Bernard GR, et al. Delirium in mechanically ventilated patients: validity and reliability of the confusion assessment method for the intensive care unit (CAM-ICU). JAMA 2001; 286:2703–2710

37. Bergeron N, Dubois MJ, Dumont M, et al. Inten-sive Care Delirium Screening Checklist: evalua-tion of a new screening tool. Intensive Care Med 2001; 27:859–864

38. Otter H, Martin J, Basell K, et al. Validity and reli-ability of the DDS for severity of delirium in the ICU. Neurocrit Care 2005; 2:150–158

39. Dubois MJ, Bergeron N, Dumont M, et al. Delirium in an intensive care unit: a study of risk factors. Intensive Care Med 2001; 27:1297–1304

40. Ely EW, Gautam S, Margolin R, et al. The impact of delirium in the intensive care unit on hospital length of stay. Intensive Care Med 2001; 27:1892–1900

41. Lin SM, Liu CY, Wang CH, et al. The impact of de-lirium on the survival of mechanically ventilated patients. Crit Care Med 2004; 32:2254–2259

42. Thomason JW, Shintani A, Peterson JF, et al. Inten-sive care unit delirium is an independent predic-tor of longer hospital stay: a prospective analysis of 261 non-ventilated patients. Crit Care 2005; 9: R375–R381

43. Milbrandt EB, Kersten A, Kong L, et al. Haloperi-dol use is associated with lower hospital mortality in mechanically ventilated patients. Crit Care Med 2005; 33:226-229; discussion 263–225

44. Skrobik YK, Bergeron N, Dumont M, et al. Olanzapine vs haloperidol: treating delirium in a critical care setting. Intensive Care Med 2004; 30:444–449

45. Lonergan E, Luxenberg J, Areosa Sastre A, et al. Benzodiazepines for delirium. Cochrane Database Syst Rev 2009; (1):CD006379

46. Pandharipande PP, Pun BT, Herr DL, et al. Effect of sedation with dexmedetomidine vs lorazepam on acute brain dysfunction in mechanically ventilated patients: the MENDS randomized controlled trial. JAMA 2007; 298:2644–2653

47. Riker RR, Shehabi Y, Bokesch PM, et al. Dexme-detomidine vs midazolam for sedation of criti-cally ill patients: a randomized trial. JAMA 2009; 301:489–499

Notes

Abdominal Problems in the ICU

Acute Abdomen/Pancreatitis/Biliary Infection and Injury

David J. Dries, MD, MSE, FCCP

Objectives:

- Discuss the presentation, causes, diagnosis, and treatment of acute abdomen in the critically ill patient
- Discuss the presentation, diagnosis, and treatment of acute pancreatitis in the ICU setting
- Discuss the presentation, diagnosis, and treatment of biliary tract diseases, specifically acute cholecystitis and cholangitis, in the ICU patient

Key words: abdominal pain; bowel obstruction; cholangitis; ileus; pancreatitis

The Acute Abdomen

The development of acute abdomen can result in a patient entering the ICU. Alternatively, acute abdominal pain can develop in a patient who is in the ICU for another reason. Both of these situations can present a diagnostic dilemma. In particular, patients who are already critically ill may not be able to manifest typical physical findings of peritonitis. This chapter will focus on the presentation, diagnosis, and management of patients with acute abdominal problems coincident with or resulting in ICU care.

Pain

In 1986, Zoltie and Cust described a group of inpatients with acute abdominal pain treated with a semisynthetic opiate or placebo to determine whether analgesia could alleviate discomfort without reducing diagnostic accuracy. Before the publication of this article, clinicians followed the surgical dictum in the classic monograph of Sir Zachary Cope on acute abdominal pain: avoid early analgesic administration in patients presenting with severe, acute undifferentiated abdominal pain because it would impair diagnostic accuracy. Despite moderation of this position over the subsequent 10 to 20 years, the surgical and emergency medicine literature reflect widespread reluctance to administer analgesia for patients presenting with undiagnosed acute abdominal pain.

As this issue has moved largely to the emergency medicine literature, multiple studies have demonstrated that diagnostic accuracy and outcome are not affected by administration of analgesia. Nonetheless, contemporary publications indicate the continued reluctance of many surgeons to accept analgesia administration during evaluation of acute abdominal pain.

Despite methodologic limitations, all published clinical studies indicate that early administration of analgesia does not appear to impair clinical diagnostic accuracy in patients with acute undifferentiated abdominal pain. Studies have appeared in the emergency medicine, surgical, and pediatric literature. More recent editions of Cope's monograph on abdominal pain changes initial recommendations concerning withholding analgesia in these patients: Silen, the current author of Cope's monograph, condemns withholding analgesia for patients who are in pain and suffering. Recent work in the surgical literature supports early provision of analgesia to patients with undifferentiated abdominal pain.

The available literature has focused primarily on evaluation of acute undifferentiated abdominal pain in the uncompromised adult capable of participating in a clinical trial. The role of analgesia in infants, children <5 years old, and vulnerable adults, in whom a comparable pattern of more sophisticated interaction is not possible, continues to be controversial.

Presentation

Patients with acute abdominal pain present with sudden or gradual onset of discomfort. Sudden abdominal pain may develop as a consequence of rupture of a hollow viscus, acute bleeding into the abdomen as with aortic or visceral artery aneurysm, or progressive expansion of a structure in the abdomen. Gradual or nonspecific abdominal pain may begin with an inflammatory process such as appendicitis or diverticulitis. Associated symptoms of fever, tachycardia, tachypnea, nausea, and vomiting may be associated with any of these processes. However, the critical care patient may not manifest these changes. I have frequently received surgical consultation for patients with abdominal pain culminating in respiratory failure and admission to the pulmonary service. Thus, acute abdominal conditions may frequently be reflected by remote organ dysfunction.

Peritonitis is caused by irritation of the lining of the abdominal cavity. The peritoneum has visceral and parietal surfaces. Pain is said to be better localized when a portion of the parietal rather than visceral peritoneum is involved in the intra-abdominal process. Thus, the classic presentation of appendicitis is periumbilical abdominal pain (visceral localization of the mid-gut), which progresses to right lower quadrant discomfort (parietal innervation, which is more localized). Generalized peritonitis is caused by irritation of the entire abdominal lining. Localized peritonitis reflects focal irritation of the peritoneum. Generalized peritonitis is more likely to result in a surgical emergency.

Patients with generalized peritonitis may lie quietly on the bed, as motion leads to peritoneal irritation and pain. A second type of patient is writhing in discomfort with nonspecific visceral but not parietal peritoneal irritation. These patients are classically described as having pain out of proportion to examination. Patients with an acute abdomen may have rapid shallow breathing, as diaphragmatic excursion is associated with pain. Thus, respiratory dysfunction may be a prominent presenting symptom if the location and the severity of the inciting process are not apparent. Physical findings of peritonitis include hypoactive or absent bowel sounds, rebound tenderness, and percussion tenderness.

Diagnostic Approach to the Patient With Acute Abdominal Pain

If the physical findings of an acute abdomen (diffuse peritonitis) are elicited, little other diagnostic testing is necessary. Routine laboratory tests are sent with an upright chest radiograph to enhance preoperative preparation and as a rapid screen to determine if there is free air in the abdomen. In some cases, additional plain radiographs including supine and upright abdominal films as well as lateral decubitus views are also obtained as part of a routine abdominal pain workup.

A CT scan is often obtained prior to or with a surgical consult. However, with the clinical diagnosis of generalized peritonitis, operative therapy is generally required and is delayed for additional imaging only with the consent of the surgeon. Patients with significant comorbidities may be candidates for further imaging, as the morbidity associated with negative laparotomy is significant. If the patient is otherwise stable, a CT scan may be obtained to corroborate a clinical diagnosis. A nondiagnostic CT scan in a patient with generalized peritonitis, however, should not deter operation.

Before operation in a patient with generalized peritonitis, a Foley catheter is placed and abnormalities of electrolytes, blood counts, and coagulation factors are corrected. Critical care admission may be required in those patients with comorbid conditions that require monitoring or additional treatment and those individuals whose volume status is inadequate to immediately tolerate the vasodilating effects of anesthetics and blood loss associated with anticipated surgery. Aggressive volume resuscitation is frequently required, and the arterial blood gas with base deficit can be useful in determining adequacy of resuscitation. However, in patients who are bleeding into the abdomen (the patient with a visceral artery laceration), adequate resuscitation cannot be attempted prior to achieving control of bleeding; in fact, these patients are better treated without aggressive fluid administration prior to surgery. General principles of surgical intervention are to control perforation of the GI tract and the leakage of succus, manage bleeding, drain purulence, resect bowel, and divert the fecal stream if necessary to permit treatment of an area of enteric leakage.

GI Conditions Resulting in Acute Abdominal Pain

Postoperative Ileus (Stomach, Small Bowel, Colon)

Ileus has been defined as the functional inhibition of propulsive bowel activity irrespective of pathogenic mechanisms. Postoperative ileus resolves spontaneously within 2 to 3 days, while paralytic postoperative ileus is defined as that form of ileus lasting > 3 days after surgery. In postoperative ileus, inhibition of small-bowel motility is transient and the stomach recovers within 24 to 48 h, whereas colonic function takes 48 to 72 h to return. Determination of the end of postoperative ileus is controversial. Bowel sounds are sometimes used as an end point, but they require frequent auscultation, and their presence does not indicate propulsive activity. Bowel sounds may be the result of small-bowel activity and not colonic function. Flatus also is not an ideal end point, as careful reporting is required, and there is some question as to the correlation between flatus and bowel movements. Bowel movements are a reliable end point, but may be too nonspecific or representative of distal bowel evacuation as opposed to global function.

A variety of factors contribute to postoperative ileus. In the stomach and small intestine, normal basal electrical activity is impaired after surgical procedures. The colonic electrical activity is also affected and is the last to return to normal (approximately 72 h after surgery). Sympathetic nervous system input, which is increased during the postoperative period, is an inhibitory factor for bowel activity. Neurotransmitters including nitric oxide, calcitonin gene-related peptide, and corticotropin-releasing factor may play a role. Finally, manipulation of the bowel and inflammation contribute to delayed return of postoperative bowel function.

Management of postoperative ileus begins with the choice of anesthetic. Anesthetic agents exert their strongest effects on regions of the bowel depending on neural integration. The large intestine is devoid of intercellular gap junctions, which makes the colon most susceptible to inhibitory actions of anesthetics. In theory, epidural anesthetics, which utilize local anesthesia, can block afferent and efferent inhibitory reflexes, increase splanchnic blood flow, and have antiinflammatory effects. Epidural anesthetics have the added benefit of blocking the afferent stimuli that trigger the endocrine metabolic response to surgery and thus inhibit catabolic hormones released during this process. Thoracic epidurals with local anesthetics significantly reduce ileus, as opposed

to systemic opioid therapy in patients undergoing abdominal surgical procedures. Other traditional therapies such as early postoperative feeding and the nasogastric tube are not supported by a consistent body of literature. In fact, inappropriate use of nasogastric tubes may contribute to postoperative complications such as fever, pneumonia, and atelectasis.

A number of additional drug strategies have been evaluated to improve outcomes with postoperative ileus. The most widely used are nonsteroidal antiinflammatory drugs, which can reduce the amount of opioid administered by 20 to 30%. An additional benefit in bowel motility may be derived from antiinflammatory properties of these agents. In both clinical and experimental studies, nonsteroidal antiinflammatory drugs resulted in decreasing nausea and vomiting and improved GI transit. Other stimulants including laxatives, prostaglandins, sympathetic inhibitors (edrophonium chloride) neostigmine, metaclopramide, and erythromycin have also been evaluated in small numbers of studies. Finally, hormone antagonists including cisapride (seratonin antagonist), cerulatide (cholecystokinin antagonist), and octreotide have been evaluated without consensus regarding their use.

The best treatment currently available is a multimodal regimen. Included in contemporary reports are utilization of epidural analgesia, early oral nutrition and mobilization, cisapride, and laxative stimulation. Perhaps it is best to recommend an approach that decreases factors contributing to postoperative ileus. Thus, limitation of narcotic administration and increased use of nonsteroidal antiinflammatory drugs with thoracic epidural catheter placement using local anesthetics should be employed. Nasogastric decompression is used selectively, and correction of electrolyte imbalances is also important.

Stomach

Early understanding of gastric physiology led to logical and time-tested surgical procedures aimed at acid reduction and lowering of ulcer recurrence rates. A shift in treatment occurred with the recognition and knowledge of *Helicobacter pylori*. Whereas surgery once dominated therapy for ulcer diathesis, medical therapy has now superseded. Despite a shrinking role for the surgeon in the management of this problem, several comments can be made.

Classic indications for surgery—perforation, bleeding, and gastric outlet obstruction—remain important. However, recent innovations in therapy have changed the natural history of ulcer disease. Acute perforations of the duodenum are estimated to occur in 2 to 10% of patients with ulcers. At present, simple patch closure is recommended for this patient population, and the importance of *H pylori* as a pathogen and therapeutic target has been emphasized. In addition to *H pylori* as a source of gastroduodenal perforation, cocaine ingestion has recently been reported by the Emory group. Feliciano and coworkers reported 50 patients with cocaine-related perforations in their series, representing approximately 40% of patients with juxtapyloric gastroduodenal perforations in an inner-city hospital. Omental patch closure again was most often used. More extensive ulcer surgery should be reserved for patients with an ongoing history of gastroduodenal ulceration or due to compliance issues. If *H pylori* is effectively treated, a simple patch approach should be adequate.

The incidence of gastroduodenal bleeding secondary to peptic ulcer disease and hospital admission for this complication have not changed in recent decades. Despite improvements in nonsurgical modalities such as proton-pump inhibitors and therapeutic endoscopy, operation for bleeding peptic ulcer disease has remained constant; such operations are performed on 10 to 20% of all patients hospitalized for upper-GI tract hemorrhage. Bleeding is more common as age increases. Mortality rates following ulcer bleeding have remained at approximately 10%. In general, when surgery is required, this occurs within 48 h of initial presentation with bleeding. The role of serial endoscopic procedures in reducing the need for emergency surgery continues to be discussed. At issue are delays to definitive therapy with increasing complication rates, as opposed to the reduced morbidity of early acid control operations. Factors associated with failure of repeat endoscopy for control of bleeding peptic ulcer disease include hypotension prior to the second endoscopic procedure or an ulcer known to be >2 cm in size. Of interest is a reported lower incidence of *H pylori* infection in those patients with significant upper-GI tract bleeding secondary to peptic ulcer disease than in those individuals with uncomplicated ulcers or minor degrees of hemorrhage. At this time, no role for empiric treatment of *H pylori* in this bleeding cohort is believed to be present. Thus, surgical procedures for bleeding should be more aggressive due to the lower incidence of *H pylori* infection. A minimal surgical approach would therefore leave up to 50% of the population presenting with bleeding at risk for further hemorrhage.

Benign gastric outlet obstruction secondary to peptic ulcer disease represents 5 to 8% of ulcer-related complications. Approximately 2,000 patients per year in the United States are operated on for this problem. Pyloric channel stenosis leads to stasis raising the gastric pH and resulting in gastrin release with excess acid production. Both surgical and nonsurgical approaches are available. Endoscopic pneumatic dilatation has been available since 1982 and continues to be used, often as primary therapy. Long-term data, however, are limited. Unfortunately, it is also unclear whether *H pylori* infection is prominent in this patient population. Case reports suggest resolution of symptomatic and endoscopic outlet obstruction with medical treatment directed at *H pylori* infection without concurrent pyloric manipulation. Large series as yet have not confirmed this mode of therapy. Surgical options include highly selective vagotomy with some form of pyloroplasty, truncal vagotomy with gastroenterostomy, or truncal vagotomy with resection of the gastric antrum. Good results have been reported for all of these procedures.

Small-Bowel Obstruction

Obstruction of the small bowel due to adhesive bands is a common problem presenting in the ICU in the setting of deranged GI or remote organ physiology. Adhesions will not develop overnight in patients with this problem. Rather, obstruction is a manifestation of a mismatch between the character and volume of succus for passage and the capability of the bowel. Both factors, succus and bowel performance, can be affected by critical illness, which in my opinion contributes to frequent consults for bowel obstruction in the ICU.

Abdominal Problems in the ICU (Dries)

Adhesive obstruction is a frequent complication of abdominal surgery. While the likelihood of surgical intervention in adhesive small-bowel obstruction increases with the number of episodes, the majority of patients presenting for operative management have undergone only one abdominal procedure. While surgeons frequently prefer, due to technical concerns, to manage bowel obstruction nonoperatively, at least one large study suggests that the risk of recurrence is significantly lower when the last bowel obstruction episode was treated surgically rather than without operation. Perhaps the greatest concern is bowel loss due to strangulation and destruction of blood supply. A large series of operative procedures places the rate of strangulation in bowel obstruction from 20 to 30%, with bowel resection required in 20% of cases. Surgeons are frequently concerned about creating bowel injury. Accidental enterostomy requiring repair occurs in approximately 5% of operations. The requirements for creation of colostomy or enterostomy are 0.2% and 0.8%, respectively. In patients receiving operative therapy for small-bowel obstruction, the initial episode requiring surgery occurred within 1 year of the last abdominal operation in 40% of patients and from 1 to 5 years after the last abdominal operation in 25% of patients.

It is important to note that abdominal pain presentation varies in adhesive small-bowel obstruction. Forty percent of patients reported pain greater than normal in a large survey. This group of patients described pain as moderate to fairly strong. Patients with bowel obstruction frequently report a history of abdominal pain, which can extend back months prior to the crisis precipitating ICU admission.

Malignant Bowel Obstruction

There are many primary cancers known to cause malignant bowel obstruction. Knowledge of primary disease and individual patient history are important because treatment can be affected. Bowel obstruction occurs in 5 to 43% of patients with a diagnosis of advanced malignancy or metastatic intraabdominal malignancy. The most common causes are ovarian (5 to 50%) and colorectal (10 to 28%) cancers; nonabdominal cancers including lung, breast, and melanoma occasionally lead to obstruction. Long-term survival for these individuals is poor. Lower-grade tumors can have a better outlook, warranting consideration of more invasive treatment approaches.

A "gold standard" for diagnosing bowel obstruction, both benign and malignant, is emerging with the use of CT. The American College of Radiology endorses CT as highly appropriate in the evaluation of bowel obstruction. Studies have demonstrated CT to be highly sensitive in identifying small-bowel obstruction with specificity >90%. Additionally, the greatest use of CT can be in identifying the cause of obstruction including metastases. CT can distinguish among pathologic processes resulting in bowel obstruction including tumor involvement of bowel wall, mesentery, mesenteric vessels, and peritoneum. Small- or large-bowel contrast studies can be used when patterns of motility are unclear or the CT suggests multiple potential levels of obstruction.

Malignant bowel obstructions are usually partial and rarely urgent situations. The rarity of intestinal gangrene in malignant obstruction gives all parties involved some breathing room for making difficult management decisions. It is important to note that operative mortality in this setting is frequent (5 to 32%), most often related to progression of neoplasm. Morbidity is also common (42%), and reobstruction after operation can be as high as 10 to 50%. Prognostic criteria that have been identified in patients less likely to benefit from surgery include the presence of ascites, carcinomatosis, palpable intraabdominal masses, multiple sites of obstruction, and advanced disease with poor overall clinical status.

Treatment options for malignant bowel obstruction include simple lysis of adhesions or bowel resection. However, in this setting, resection might not allow restoration of bowel continuity. Operation may leave the patient with multiple stomas. Intestinal bypass is also an option. Nonsurgical management of these patients frequently includes the use of opioids, which produce an ileus pattern and may alleviate pain and/or octreotide for control of intestinal secretions. The nasogastric tube should be considered only as a proximal means of temporary decompression. Percutaneous gastrostomy can provide significant relief as a vent in proximal small-bowel obstruction.

Short-Bowel Syndrome

Short-bowel syndrome is a potential postoperative complication after intraabdominal procedures. One fourth of patients presenting at tertiary centers with short-bowel syndrome experience this complication from previous abdominal surgery. Gynecologic and colon procedures are most frequently associated with short-bowel syndrome. As a rough rule of thumb, 100 cm of small bowel is required for adequate enteral nutrition. Even if intestinal length greater than this is available, adequate tolerance of enteral feeding may come slowly and combinations of parenteral and enteral nutrition may be required for extended periods of time.

Colon Obstruction

Colonic obstruction has three major etiologies: malignancy, diverticular disease, and torsion or volvulus. In each case, surgical resection is appropriate but resuscitation prior to operative intervention is essential. CT scanning can be invaluable in determining the site and characteristics of the obstructing lesion. CT is the key study for working through the differential diagnosis of large-bowel obstruction. Newly diagnosed malignancy is generally resected with either primary anastomosis or more commonly end-proximal colostomy or ileostomy, as adequate bowel preparation may not be possible.

Endoscopic stent placement has successfully relieved obstruction in a high percentage of patients with lower colorectal lesions (64 to 100%). This approach may be considered if necessary equipment and expertise are available. Typically, endoscopy is utilized in the high-risk patient with significant comorbidities. Risks of stent placement for colorectal disease include perforation (0 to 15%), stent migration requiring replacement (0 to 40%), or reocclusion (0 to 33%). Stents can frequently lead to adequate palliation for extended periods of time. Diverticular disease causing obstruction is typically treated with resection and reconstruction or proximal colostomy and later restoration of GI continuity.

Diverticulitis

A growing body of data suggests that early management of acute diverticulitis can be nonoperative. A recent large population study with acute diverticulitis noted a relatively low risk of recurrent diverticulitis after initial nonoperative management. The overall recurrence rate was approximately 13%, and the annual recurrence rate was 2% per year. These data argue against routine elective colectomy after an initial episode of acute diverticulitis. A higher rate of recurrent diverticulitis is found in patients <50 years old. Patients with organ system dysfunction or requiring drainage procedures are often better served by resection and elective reconstruction of the GI tract.

Notably, a large recent trial found no association between higher recurrence rates for diverticulitis and percutaneous drainage procedures. This challenges conventional teaching including the standards of the American Society of Colon and Rectal Surgeons. The traditional view presumes that patients with a drainable percutaneous abscess (*ie*, complicated diverticulitis) have worse disease. The findings in a large trial conducted in the Kaiser System suggest that patients who have undergone successful percutaneous drainage during initial hospitalization do not require subsequent elective colectomy. For the intensivist, therefore, aggressive and immediate surgical intervention should not be the expectation or the norm in patients presenting with diverticulitis even if a drainage procedure is required.

Colitis

Colitis can be broken down into ischemic and infectious etiologies. Causes of ischemic colitis are many, but the ultimate result is intestinal shock or end-organ hypoperfusion. Cardiac failure, systemic shock states, drugs, and underlying mesenteric vascular disease contribute to colonic ischemia. Initial management of ischemic colitis is nonoperative. Patients are resuscitated and placed on broad-spectrum antibiotics. This strategy is continued even if pneumatosis is identified with small amounts of free air. Where patients go on to multiorgan system dysfunction, emergent colectomy is appropriate. Patients who improve may resume enteral intake, discontinue antibiotics, and should receive endoscopy ≥6 weeks after the ischemic insult.

Patients with megarectum or megacolon can frequently present with primary or secondary colon toxicity associated with other organ dysfunction. In some cases, resection of the involved colon is the optimal approach. In patients with megacolon and a nondilated functional rectum, subtotal colectomy with ileorectal anastomosis is the procedure of choice, as a segmental colon resection results in a higher incidence of postoperative dysmotility. There is a definite mortality with this procedure and 20% morbidity, and further surgical intervention is commonly secondary to bowel obstruction. Patients with dilatation involving the entire colon and rectum may require removal of the entire affected large bowel and creation of an ileal pouch. Success rates in limited studies appear to be 70 to 80%, although this procedure is complex and may require a series of procedures in patients with multiorgan dysfunction. A coloanal anastomosis may be recommended in patients with distal large intestine dilatation or dysmotility. While patients with megabowel require complex surgical management, acute surgical intervention should be reserved for patients with intractable symptoms or acute organ dysfunction. Ideally, patients should be supported through acute illness and undergo multidisciplinary evaluation including clinical, psychological, and physiologic assessments.

Approximately 3% of healthy adults and 20 to 40% of hospitalized patients have *Clostridium difficile* colonization, which in healthy persons is inactive in the spore form. Reduction of competing flora with antibiotic use promotes conversion to vegetative forms that replicate and produce toxins. The characteristic clinical expression is watery diarrhea and cramps, with the pathologic finding of pseudomembranous colitis. Recently, *C difficile* with greater virulence has been reported in multi-institutional studies. Identified risk factors include fluoroquinolone use and age >65 years. These recent reports document the presence of more virulent strains of *C difficile* causing epidemic disease associated with more frequent and more severe presentation as indicated by higher rates of toxic megacolon, leukemoid reaction, shock, requirement of colectomy, and death.

In most cases, management of infectious colitis begins with identification of the offending organism and appropriate infection control procedures. Implicated antimicrobials must be stopped and administration of oral metronidazole or vancomycin initiated. *C difficile* is the most prominent organism associated with toxic colitis, but toxic colitis can also be seen in the absence of this organism. Again, fluid resuscitation and antibiotic management are initial steps in care of these patients, but colectomy must be considered for the patient with progressive organ dysfunction or hemodynamic instability.

Appendix

More than 250,000 appendectomies are performed in the United States each year, making appendectomy the most common abdominal operation performed on an emergency basis. While the diagnosis of appendicitis in young men with abdominal pain is usually straightforward, diagnostic considerations are far broader for premenopausal women and patients at the extremes of age. The latter group, which may be in the ICU, presents a diagnostic challenge because of delays in seeking medical care or difficulty in obtaining a history and performing accurate physical examination. As delayed diagnosis and treatment of appendicitis are associated with an increased rate of perforation with resulting increase in morbidity and mortality, timely intervention is crucial.

If laparotomy is performed on the basis of physical examination, the appendix is normal in approximately 20% of patients. When advanced age or female gender confounds the usual signs or symptoms of appendicitis, the error rate in managing pain in the right lower quadrant can approach 40%. To improve diagnostic accuracy, imaging is seeing increasing use. Nonetheless, physical examination and history remain the diagnostic cornerstone for evaluating the patient with right lower quadrant pain. No single aspect of clinical presentation predicts the presence of disease, but a combination of signs and symptoms support the diagnosis of appendicitis. Three signs and symptoms most predictive of acute appendicitis are right lower quadrant pain, abdominal rigidity, and migration of discomfort from the umbilical region to the right lower quadrant.

As plain radiographs and laboratory tests are marked by low sensitivity and specificity for the diagnosis of appendicitis, CT has become the cornerstone of diagnostic modalities. With improvements in CT, the entire abdomen can be scanned at high resolution in thin slices during a single period of breath holding. Such scanning virtually eliminates motion and misregistration artifacts and routinely results in high-quality, high-resolution images of the appendix and periappendiceal tissue. For patients with suspected appendicitis, spiral CT has sensitivity of 90 to 97%, with accuracy of 94 to 100%. CT also provides an opportunity to diagnose alternative disorders should the appendix be normal. The differential diagnosis of appendicitis is broad and includes colitis, diverticulitis, small-bowel obstruction, inflammatory bowel disease and ovarian cysts, cholecystitis, pancreatitis, and ureteral obstruction.

Treatment of appendicitis routinely involves right lower quadrant investigation through a transabdominal or laparoscopic approach. The patient with perforated appendicitis can be managed with antibiotics followed by interval appendectomy, although follow-up data suggest that antibiotic treatment may reduce the need for later removal of the appendix. In patients who are critically ill, with consultation by the surgeon, appendicitis can be managed with antibiotics when the operative risk is prohibitive. Late management of such patients is unclear, as clinical series following such individuals are small and infrequent.

Acute Pancreatitis

Acute pancreatitis frequently has rapid-onset manifest by upper abdominal pain, vomiting, fever, tachycardia, leukocytosis, and elevated serum levels of pancreatic enzymes. Common causes in the United States are gallstones and alcohol use. The two common severity-of-illness classifications for acute pancreatitis are the time-honored Ranson score and the more commonly used ICU scale, APACHE (acute physiology and chronic health evaluation) II. Severe acute pancreatitis is diagnosed if three or more of the Ranson criteria are present, if the APACHE II score is ≥8, or if shock, renal insufficiency, or pulmonary failure are present.

Pancreatitis may also be classified histologically as interstitial edematous or necrotizing disease according to inflammatory changes in pancreatic parenchyma. An international symposium in 1992 defined pancreatic necrosis as the presence of one or more diffuse or focal areas of nonviable pancreatic parenchyma. Pancreatic necrosis is typically associated with peripancreatic fat necrosis. Pancreatic necrosis represents a severe form of acute pancreatitis and is present in approximately 20 to 30% of the 185,000 new cases of acute pancreatitis reported each year in the United States.

Diagnosis

Initial evaluation reveals signs of peritonitis that are sometimes generalized. Laboratory testing is often consistent with volume contraction related to sequestration of fluid into the retroperitoneum, and vomiting. Correlating data include elevated hematocrit and bicarbonate levels, hypokalemia, and acidosis. Amylase and lipase levels are frequently sent to evaluate pancreatitis. Amylase elevation is less specific than lipase, as the former can be released by salivary glands. Bowel obstruction and other forms of small-bowel pathology are also associated with mild elevation in amylase (Table 1).

With suspicion of the diagnosis of acute pancreatitis, the cause of this problem is sought. As most cases correspond to alcohol use or gallstones, history and diagnostic testing initially are focused on these entities. Right upper quadrant

Table 1. *Etiologies of Acute Necrotizing Pancreatitis**

Most common
  Choledocholithiasis
  Ethanol abuse
  Idiopathic
Less common
  Endoscopic retrograde cholangiopancreatography
  Hyperlipidemia (types I, IV, and V)
  Drugs
  Pancreas divisum
  Abdominal trauma
Least common
  Hereditary (familial)

*Reproduced with permission from N Engl J Med 1999; 340:1412–1417.

ultrasound is the initial test for gallstones. Identification of gallstones in a patient with acute pancreatitis should lead to the presumptive diagnosis of biliary or gallstone pancreatitis. Occasionally, ultrasound will demonstrate choledocholithiasis, a stone in the common bile duct. Cholangitis is also possible in this setting. Where gallstones are absent and a history of alcohol use cannot be obtained, other etiologies of acute pancreatitis must be considered including hyperlipidemia, drugs (steroids and anticonvulsants), trauma, pancreas divisum, and other mechanical insults such as endoscopic retrograde cholangiopancreatography (ERCP).

In the presence of diagnostic uncertainty at the time of presentation, a CT scan of the abdomen with IV contrast (in the absence of contraindications) should be performed after fluid resuscitation to confirm the diagnosis. CT also allows alternative diagnoses to be ruled out. The admission CT scan may serve as a baseline for future studies. Some authors recommend delaying the initial CT to identify local complications for 48 to 72 h if possible as necrosis may not be visualized earlier.

While CT is the preferred imaging modality for the pancreas in the setting of acute pancreatitis, magnetic resonance cholangiopancreatography (MRCP) is gaining favor as a means to detect common bile duct stones with resolution of gallstone pancreatitis. Surgical authors are now suggesting that if MRCP is negative, ERCP is not required in patients with gallstone pancreatitis and cholecystectomy may be performed. In the majority of patients with mild gallstone pancreatitis, the common bile duct stones pass spontaneously into the duodenum. Thus, the morbidity of nontherapeutic ERCP may be avoided with MRCP. Only 20% of patients with resolving gallstone pancreatitis are found to have stones in the extrahepatic biliary tree.

Management

Patients with acute pancreatitis require aggressive resuscitation and are at risk for early development of organ dysfunction as a result of inadequate resuscitation as well as systemic and local complications of pancreatitis. Clinical monitoring should focus on intravascular volume

assessment including urine output and acid base status along with pulmonary function. It is important to note that aggressive fluid resuscitation may result in accumulation of ascites, pleural effusions, and hypoxemia. In severe cases, abdominal compartment syndrome may complicate resuscitation of severe pancreatitis.

Early antibiotic administration has received attention in recent years as a therapy in acute pancreatitis. Despite initial studies favoring administration of broad-spectrum antibiotics and selective gut decontamination, recent consensus reports debate the value of routine antibiotic prophylaxis or administration of antifungal agents in patients with acute pancreatitis and/or pancreatic necrosis in light of contradictory evidence. When patients are strongly suspected of having pancreatic infection, imipenem, meropenem, fluoroquinolones, and metronidazole may be considered. In general, infection of necrotic pancreas involves bacteria from the GI tract. Because of this observation, gut decontamination has been advocated by some authors. Current data do not support routine use of this practice (Table 2).

Nasogastric tube suctioning is warranted in patients with acute pancreatitis who are intubated or vomiting. Acid-suppression therapy with proton-pump inhibitors is reasonable, as stress-related ulcers are a risk and proton-pump inhibitors decrease GI tract fluid production.

Table 2. *Recognition of Clinically Severe Acute Pancreatitis**

Ranson score ≥ 3, criteria of severity
  At hospital admission
    Age > 55 yr
    WBCl count $> 16,000/mm^3$
    Blood glucose level > 200 mg/dL (11.1 mmol/L)
    Serum lactate dehydrogenase level > 350 IU/L
    Serum aspartate transaminase > 250 IU/L
  During initial 48 h
    Absolute decrease in hematocrit $> 10\%$
    Increase in blood urea nitrogen > 5 mg/dL (1.8 mmol/L)
    Serum calcium < 8 mg/dL (2 mmol/L)
    Arterial Pao_2 < 60 mm Hg
    Base deficit > 4 mmol/L
    Fluid sequestration > 6 L
APACHE II score ≥ 8
Organ failure
Substantial pancreatic necrosis (at least 30% glandular
  necrosis according to contrast-enhanced CT)

*Reproduced and modified with permission from N Engl J Med 1999; 340:1412–1417.

Enteral nutrition is used in preference to parenteral nutrition in patients with acute pancreatitis. This therapy should be initiated when initial resuscitation is completed. Placement of the feeding tube into the jejunum should be accomplished if possible. Parenteral nutrition is associated with an increased risk of infection and is used only if attempts at enteral nutrition have failed despite trials of 5 to 7 days.

Surgical Therapy

Sonographic or CT-guided fine-needle aspiration with Gram stain and culture should be obtained of pancreatic or peripancreatic tissue to discriminate between sterile and infected tissue in patients with radiologic evidence of pancreatic necrosis and clinical features consistent with infection. In general, debridement or drainage of patients with sterile pancreatic necrosis are not recommended. Pancreatic debridement or drainage are recommended in patients in whom infected pancreatic necrosis is documented and/or the presence of abscess is confirmed by radiologic evidence of gas in pancreatic or peripancreatic tissue or by results of fine-needle aspiration. The "gold standard" for pancreatic debridement is open operative debridement. Minimally invasive techniques including laparoscopy or percutaneous intervention are options in selected patients. Operative necrosectomy and/or drainage should be delayed 2 to 3 weeks to allow demarcation of necrotic pancreas. The clinical course of pancreatitis is the primary determinant of the timing of operative intervention.

Conventional surgical drainage involves removal of necrotic pancreas with placement of standard surgical drains and reoperation as required by the presence of fever, leukocytosis, or lack of improvement based on imaging studies. Open or semiopen management of the abdomen involves removal of necrotic pancreas and either scheduled repeated laparotomies or open abdominal packing allowing for frequent changes of dressing material. Closed management involves removal of necrotic pancreas with extensive intraoperative lavage of the pancreatic bed with closure of the abdomen over large-bore drains for continuous high-volume postoperative lavage of the lesser sac. Effective debridement of necrotic pancreas is important since inadequately removed necrotic tissue remains infected with mortality rates as high as 40%.

In general, frequent operations are required to remove necrotic pancreas and peripancreatic material. If the abdomen is left open, the need for repeated laparotomy is eliminated and packing may be changed in the ICU. Repeated debridement and manipulation of abdominal viscera with contemporary operative techniques results in a high rate of postoperative local complications including pancreatic fistula, small- and large-bowel injury, and bleeding from the pancreatic bed. Pancreatic or GI tract fistulas occur in up to 40% of patients after surgical removal of necrotic pancreas and often require additional surgery for closure.

ERCP

When obstructive jaundice or other evidence of acute obstruction of the biliary or pancreatic duct are present and acute pancreatitis is due to suspected or confirmed gallstones, urgent ERCP should be performed within 72 h of the onset of symptoms. This intervention showed improved outcome in patients with severe acute pancreatitis. While benefit has been attributed to relief of pancreatic ductal obstruction by impacted gallstones at the ampulla of Vater, other recent work suggests that improved outcome after endoscopic retrograde cholangiopancreatography and sphincterotomy in gallstone pancreatitis results from reduced biliary sepsis. Another theoretical concern is introduction of infection by incidental pancreatography during ERCP transforming sterile to infected acute necrotizing pancreatitis. Therefore, ERCP is used judiciously in patients with severe acute gallstone pancreatitis and should be reserved for those individuals in whom biliary obstruction is identified. MRCP, as noted above, is valuable in identifying the need for ERCP.

Complications

A variety of systemic and local complications of severe acute pancreatitis may occur. Systemic complications include ARDS, acute renal failure, shock, coagulopathy, hyperglycemia, and hypercalcemia. Local complications include GI hemorrhage, infected pancreatic necrosis, and adjacent bowel necrosis. Later local complications include pancreatic abscess and pancreatic pseudocysts. Infected necrosis develops in 30 to 70% of patients with acute necrotizing pancreatitis and accounts for >80% of deaths from acute pancreatitis. The risk of infected necrosis increases with the volume of pancreatic glandular necrosis.

The overall mortality rate in severe pancreatitis is approximately 30%. Deaths occur in two phases. Early deaths occurring within 1 to 2 weeks are due to multisystem organ failure associated with release of inflammatory mediators and cytokines. Late deaths result from local or systemic infection. If acute necrotizing pancreatitis remains sterile, overall mortality is approximately 10%. The mortality rate triples if there is infected necrosis.

Late Complications

Long-term endocrine and exocrine consequences of severe acute pancreatitis depend on a variety of factors, including severity of necrosis, etiology, whether the patient continues to use alcohol, and the degree of surgical pancreatic debridement. Persistent functional insufficiency has been noted in the majority of patients up to 2 years after severe acute pancreatitis. Use of pancreatic enzymes is restricted to patients with symptoms of steatorrhea and weight loss due to fat malabsorption. While glucose intolerance is frequent, overt diabetes is relatively uncommon. Obstructive pancreatic ductal abnormalities may account for persistent symptoms of abdominal pain or recurrent pancreatitis.

Management of pain is an important problem in patients progressing to chronic pancreatitis. Pancreatic duct obstruction is considered an important etiologic factor; thus, ductal decompression is advocated for patients with pain and pancreatic duct dilatation. Endoscopic and surgical treatment are options. Surgical drainage is accomplished by longitudinal pancreaticojejunostomy and has a complication rate of 6 to 30% and a mortality rate of 0 to 2 %. Success in achieving long-term pain relief is 60 to 85%. Endoscopic drainage includes sphincterotomy, dilatation of strictures, and removal of stones, and has a success rate of 30 to 100%.

A recent randomized prospective trial compared endoscopic and surgical drainage of the pancreatic duct in chronic pancreatitis. Thirty-nine patients were randomized, with 19 patients receiving endoscopic treatment while 20 patients underwent operative pancreaticojejunostomy. With 2 years of follow-up, patients undergoing surgery had lower pain scores and better physical health summary scores. At the end of follow-up, complete or partial pain relief was achieved in 32% of patients assigned to endoscopic drainage, as compared with 75% of patients assigned to surgical drainage. Complications, length of hospital stay, and changes in pancreatic function were similar with endoscopy or surgery. Patients receiving endoscopy required more procedures than did patients in the surgical arm of this trial.

Key Points in Management of Severe Pancreatitis, Modified From Crit Care Med 2004; 32:2524–2536

- In the presence of diagnostic uncertainty at the time of presentation, CT scan of the abdomen (with IV contrast if possible) should be performed after fluid resuscitation to confirm the diagnosis and rule out alternative diagnoses.
- When CT is employed to identify local complications of pancreatitis, this study may be delayed for 48 to 72 h if possible, as necrosis might not be visualized earlier.
- Routine antibiotic prophylaxis for bacterial and fungal pathogens is not warranted (a controversial topic!).
- Routine use of selective decontamination of the digestive tract is not warranted.
- Enteral nutrition is preferred to parenteral nutrition.
- The jejunal route should be used as possible.
- If used (after a 5- to 7-day trial of enteral nutrition fails), parenteral nutrition should be enriched with glutamine.
- Routine use of immune-enhancing enteral feeds is not recommended at this time.
- CT-guided fine-needle aspiration with Gram stains and culture of pancreatic or peripancreatic tissue is used to discriminate between sterile and infected necrosis. Debridement or drainage of patients with sterile necrosis are not recommended.

- Debridement or drainage in patients with infected pancreatic necrosis or abscess are best accomplished by open operative procedures.
- Open operative debridement of the pancreas should be delayed 2 to 3 weeks if possible to allow demarcation of necrotic pancreas.
- Gallstone pancreatitis should be suspected in all patients with acute pancreatitis, and sonography and biochemical test should be performed.
- In the setting of obstructive jaundice or other findings consistent with gallstones, ERCP should be performed within 72 h of the onset of symptoms.
- In the absence of obstructive jaundice but with acute pancreatitis due to suspected or confirmed gallstones, ERCP should be considered within 72 h of onset of symptoms.
- Aggressive, early resuscitation is important to address the inflammatory response in acute pancreatitis.
- When infection has been documented in the setting of acute pancreatitis, management according to current sepsis guidelines should be initiated.
- Immune-modulating therapies are not recommended in management of acute pancreatitis.
- Routine use of markers such as C-reactive protein or procalcitonin should not be used to guide decision making or predict clinical course of pancreatitis.

Biliary Tract Problems

Acute Cholecystitis

Acute cholecystitis is caused by obstruction of the cystic duct by an impacted gallstone or by local edema and inflammation. Obstruction results in gallbladder distension, subserosal edema, mucosal sloughing, venous and lymphatic congestion, and localized ischemia. The role of bacteria is debated, although positive culture results from bile or gallbladder wall tissue are found in most patients. If bacteria infiltrate the gallbladder wall, gangrenous or emphysematous cholecystitis may follow. Other complications include perforation, bile peritonitis, abscess, sepsis, gallstone ileus, or enteric fistula with the gallbladder. Sixty-five

percent of patients with acute cholecystitis will also have evidence of chronic cholecystitis characterized by gallbladder wall fibrosis and chronic inflammation. While acute cholecystitis is commonly a disease of women aged 30 to 60 years, the female to male ratio decreases from 3:1 after the age of 50 years to 1.5:1.

The classic presentation is right upper quadrant tenderness with fever and leukocytosis. Clinical diagnosis is verified by gallbladder wall thickening with stones. Ultrasound is most commonly used to assess patency of the biliary tree; identify stones or sludge in the gallbladder; determine whether the gallbladder wall is thickened, inflamed, gangrenous, scarred, or calcified; and evaluate surrounding structures. Pericholecystic fluid or impacted stones with a distended, thickened gallbladder are consistent with the diagnosis. The hydroxy iminodiacetic acid (HIDA) scan (cholescintigraphy) can contribute to diagnostic accuracy in cases in which ultrasound is indeterminate or additional information is required regarding the patency of the cystic duct. In a positive HIDA scan finding, obstruction of the cystic duct is evident when the radionuclide does not outline the gallbladder and flow normally into the common bile duct. HIDA scanning has high sensitivity and specificity and diagnostic accuracy of approximately 98% in patients with signs and symptoms of acute calculus cholecystitis. This test is less helpful (false-positive rates of 40%) if the patient has fasted for >5 days. CT with oral and IV contrast evaluates late complications of undiagnosed or misdiagnosed acute cholecystitis such as perforation, abscess, or enteric fistula.

In general, initial management is surgical resection of the gallbladder. Cholecystectomy is associated with a low complication rate and mortality rate < 0.2%, and a bile duct injury rate of 0.4%. Open or laparoscopic procedures may be used to remove the gallbladder. Antibiotic coverage should include aerobic Gram-negative and anaerobic organisms. Patients presenting with elevated liver function test results or dilated bile ducts (>7.0 mm on ultrasound) should be evaluated for the presence of common bile duct stones. ERCP is the traditional approach employed. In some cases, MRCP may be considered. Endoscopic sphincterotomy and stone extraction before cholecystectomy is the preferred approach, with operative intervention as a fallback position for patients with failed ERCP or retained common bile duct stones.

ICU patients with acute cholecystitis have historical mortality rates >40%. Patients with acute cholecystitis in the ICU often present with atypical or nonspecific findings of abdominal sepsis including fever, leukocytosis, distension, and acidosis. Standard diagnostic strategies including ultrasound, HIDA scanning, and CT are more difficult in this population and may be less accurate due to comorbidities or sepsis. Early operative intervention should be attempted if patients are stable enough to tolerate laparoscopic or open cholecystectomy. Percutaneous drainage is effective and less risky in the critical care population. Percutaneous approaches will be inadequate if emphysematous cholecystitis occurs.

Percutaneous transhepatic cholecystostomy is performed under CT or ultrasound guidance and has a reported success rate of 95 to 100%. Complications include bleeding, catheter dislodgement, bile peritonitis, bowel perforation, and respiratory distress. Use of percutaneous cholecystostomy in the critical care context facilitates delayed laparoscopic or open removal of the gallbladder in >50% of patients. Some surgeons never attempt removal of the gallbladder in high-risk patients after cholecystostomy if the cystic duct is patent. Another prospective, randomized trial suggested that percutaneous cholecystostomy did not decrease mortality in comparison to conservative management.

Acalculous Cholecystitis

Acalculous cholecystitis is identified in 4 to 8% of acute cholecystectomy cases. It is more common in male than female patients and has been associated with recent surgery, major trauma, burns, multiple transfusions, childbirth, sepsis, shock, total parenteral nutrition, narcotic administration, and rheumatologic disorders. Patients are typically critically ill and require advanced monitoring. Where cholecystitis occurs in the perioperative period, two thirds of the cases are acalculous. Fifteen percent of cholecystitis following major trauma is acalculous. Pathogenesis includes gallbladder ischemia, biliary stasis or sludge, and local or systemic infection.

Diagnosis is often delayed, as symptoms are difficult to appreciate in noncommunicative patients in the ICU setting. Patients with recent major surgery, multisystem trauma, or complicated clinical conditions will not show characteristic clinical findings. Signs and symptoms are generally similar to those of calculus cholecystitis with right upper quadrant tenderness, fever, abdominal distension, diminished bowel sounds, leukocytosis, and elevated hepatic enzymes. The reported accuracy of HIDA scanning in these patients is variable, with sensitivity as low as 70% and specificity of 90%. Ultrasound may show nonspecific signs of gallbladder wall thickening, sludge, or distention. Sensitivity and specificity of ultrasound are reduced in acalculous cholecystitis. These patients have a high risk of gallbladder wall gangrene and perforation as well as higher morbidity and mortality because of delayed diagnosis and comorbid conditions. Cholecystostomy or cholecystectomy are preferred interventions. If the patient has progressed to gallbladder wall gangrene, percutaneous drainage may be inadequate therapy.

Acute Cholangitis

Acute cholangitis is caused by proliferation of microorganisms in the bile ducts. Management of the patient with acute cholangitis requires restoration of bile flow from the liver and gallbladder into the GI tract. Constant unimpeded flow of bile into the GI tract and the presence of Igs in the biliary mucosa keep bile ducts almost sterile in the normal state. Cholangitis will not develop with a properly functioning sphincterotomy or biliary enteric anastomosis. Cholangitis occurs when bile stasis promotes the growth of sufficient microorganisms to damage tissue, produce systemic inflammation, and ultimately seed the circulation. Biliary stones most commonly cause cholangitis, which can have iatrogenic causes with inadvertent biliary tract injury. The classic diagnostic trial of Charcot (abdominal pain, fever, and jaundice) describes the most common presenting symptoms of acute cholangitis. The Reynold pentad includes these findings with the addition of hypotension and mental status changes.

Imaging of patients with suspected acute cholangitis begins with ultrasound to assess biliary tree dilatation, state of the gallbladder (presence or absence of stones), and occasionally identify foreign bodies in the bile ducts. Radionuclide studies are less useful in the management of patients with acute cholangitis. CT scanning is more sensitive than ultrasound in evaluation of nonbiliary causes of obstruction in cholangitis such as periportal malignancy. It is also high sensitive for early biliary dilatation. MRCP is becoming more common in the diagnosis of biliary pathology but may be less effective in the critically ill patient due to logistic challenges associated with obtaining this test. Percutaneous transhepatic cholangiography has a long track record of success but greater associated morbidity than ERCP, which is the present "gold standard" for the diagnosis of intraluminal biliary pathology.

Patients frequently require fluid resuscitation and antibiotic support. Typical pathogens include *Escherichia coli*, Klebsiella species, Enterobacter, and enterococcus. After stabilization, the type and timing of interventions are determined. The choice of interventions includes open operation, percutaneous transhepatic drainage, or ERCP. In general, surgical procedures are not preferred due to greater associated morbidity. ERCP successfully removes >90% of common duct stones. If stones cannot be safely removed at the initial procedure, a stent will allow relief of biliary obstruction, and remaining stones can be removed by subsequent ERCP, lithotripsy, or surgical common bile duct exploration. Bile duct strictures causing cholangitis can be treated with balloon dilatation utilizing ERCP or percutaneous methods. Percutaneous approaches are excellent for rapid decompression of intrahepatic bile ducts but offer fewer options for definitive, intermediate, and long-term treatment of cholangitis. For example, larger stones can only be removed after serial dilatation of the tube tract, and multiple procedures may be required to address strictures and malignancies.

ERCP combines the relative benefits of minimally invasive diagnosis and treatment with a variety of therapeutic options. Emergent stents can be placed in unstable or coagulopathic patients, and sphincterotomy allows later stone removal if initial basket procedures are unsuccessful. While all of these interventions depend on the skill of the endoscopist, in experienced hands in-hospital mortality with cholangitis is now well <10%.

Biliary Tract Injury

Following open and laparoscopic cholecystectomy, rapid recovery is commonplace, with patients returning to normal activity within 7 to 10 days after laparoscopic procedures. Patients in the early postoperative period with persisting abdominal complaints such as pain, anorexia, nausea, vomiting, and jaundice or evidence of infection require careful evaluation to rule out complications of cholecystectomy. After obtaining history and a physical examination, laboratory testing includes liver function tests, amylase, lipase, and CBC count. Iatrogenic biliary tract injuries result in significant morbidity and require further intervention. Approximately 75% of these complications go unnoticed intraoperatively. Injuries include bile duct leaks, strictures, division, or ligation.

Postoperative bile leaks occur in up to 1% of patients undergoing laparoscopy and cholecystectomy. Patients complaining of upper abdominal pain in the postoperative period must be evaluated for a bile leak. A variety of imaging methods may be utilized, beginning with ultrasound and CT scanning. Either of these modalities will identify a fluid collection adjacent to the liver. MRCP and ERCP provide greater anatomic detail but are more costly. Nuclear medicine studies of the hepatobiliary tree and percutaneous transhepatic cholangiography may also be employed. Studies demonstrating intraabdominal fluid near the liver and bile duct dilatation (ultrasound or CT) should raise suspicion of bile leakage or obstruction. ERCP then can delineate bile duct anatomy, diagnose leaks, and identify retained common bile duct stones. ERCP not only helps diagnose the site of biliary leak after bile duct injury, as a therapeutic modality it allows interventional procedures such as sphincterotomy, nasobiliary drainage, or stent placement. For example, after laparoscopy and cholecystectomy, the cystic duct stump can be the site of bile leakage. In this case, endoscopic, sphincterotomy, and stent placement to occlude the cystic duct remnant are usually adequate therapy. MRCP is less invasive but effectively demonstrates biliary tree anatomy and the presence of retained stones in the cystic, hepatic, or common bile ducts. Hepatobilary isotope imaging reveals hepatocellular function and flow of bile into the duodenum. Extrabiliary collections of radioisotope suggest duct injury with bile leakage.

Intraabdominal fluid collections in the early postoperative period may be secondary to bile, blood, or enteric contents secondary to unrecognized bowel injury. These may be drained percutaneously under ultrasound or CT guidance. Morbidity and mortality rates in patients with undrained bile collections are high. Prompt drainage is crucial to prevent sepsis and multiorgan failure. After drains have evacuated a bile collection, ERCP or percutaneous transhepatic cholangiography should be performed to define the site of a bile leak and the anatomy of the biliary tree. When major ductal injury has occurred, an operative treatment plan can be devised with this information. Once bile collections are drained, the major potential for immediate serious illness is generally eliminated. Then injury can be fully investigated with operative treatment executed in a controlled manner.

Special Problems

Anastomotic Leaks

Anastomotic disruption is perhaps the most dreaded complication after intestinal surgery. Some leaks present in dramatic fashion early in the postoperative period, leaving little doubt about the diagnosis. Many others present in a far more subtle fashion, often relatively late in the postoperative period and can be difficult to distinguish from other postoperative infectious complications.

Patients with early anastomotic disruption classically have agonizing abdominal pain, tachycardia, fever, and a rigid abdomen often accompanied by hemodynamic instability. Urgent return to the operating room for peritoneal washout and fecal diversion is generally required. The mortality rate for anastomotic leak in the literature typically is in the 10 to 15% range. Anastomotic leakage has been associated with increased local

recurrence and diminished survival after colorectal cancer surgery.

A growing number of patients ultimately found to have an anastomotic leak have a more insidious presentation, often with low-grade fever, prolonged ileus, or failure to thrive. In these patients, making the diagnosis may be more difficult because the clinical course is often similar to other postoperative infectious complications. Even with radiologic imaging, the diagnosis may be elusive or uncertain. This group of patients may escape detection in standard retrospective analyses, thus underestimating the true incidence of anastomotic leakage after intestinal anastomosis. Patients with late intestinal anastomotic leaks are often discharged from hospital without the correct diagnosis because nonspecific symptoms (poor appetite, failure to thrive) are insufficient to justify continued hospitalization. In a recent series, 42% of patients ultimately demonstrated to have anastomotic leakage had been sent home from hospital.

Distinguishing an anastomotic leak from a postoperative abscess, particularly retrospectively, is difficult. In fact, the definition of anastomotic leaks after GI surgery varies widely in the literature. A leak may be defined by the need for reoperation, clinical findings, or radiologic criteria making comparison between studies difficult. The typical cutoff for perioperative data at 30 days will fail to capture many leaks. Nonetheless, a low mortality rate (5.7%) is seen in contemporary series.

CT scanning is the key diagnostic study in patients in whom an anastomotic failure is suspected. Contrast enemas fail to identify anastomotic leakage 60% of the time. Occasionally, however, CT scan findings are negative and contrast placed in a prograde or retrograde fashion is helpful.

In general, a leak rate from 1 to 3% is reported. Higher leak rates are associated with procedures requiring pelvic anastomoses or anastomoses to the anal canal.

As patients may be admitted to nonsurgical services after discharge from hospital, awareness of anastomotic leakage becomes important. Drainage of fluid, which may precipitate peritonitis and shock, is the initial intervention of choice. Frequently, this objective can only be accomplished in the operating room. In other settings, with localized anastomotic failure, drains guided by imaging may be sufficient.

Corrosive Ingestion

In the United States, approximately 35,000 patients require treatment in a health-care facility each year after exposure to corrosives. Alkalis and acids are most likely to cause major injury and death. In past decades, liquid sodium hydroxide preparations such as drain cleaners accounted for the majority of corrosive ingestions. Successful lobbying by the medical profession resulted in the concentration of sodium hydroxide in this product being reduced from 30 to 5%.

Animal studies indicate that soon after ingested corrosives enter the stomach, there is reflex pyloric spasm, which limits passage of the damaging agent to the duodenum. Regurgitation then occurs propelling gastric contents into the esophagus against a closed cricopharyngeus muscle. This phenomenon lasts 3 to 5 min, after which there is esophagogastric atonia and the pylorus relaxes allowing gastric contents to enter the duodenum. Major corrosive injury may be followed by rapid collapse, but most patients reach the hospital. If injury is not rapidly fatal, significant destruction of esophageal and gastric mucosa is noted within 24 h. In less severe injuries, the submucosa is heavily infiltrated with inflammatory cells. Occasionally, there may be thrombosis of submucosal arteries and veins leading to gangrene of the mucosa. Within 2 weeks after injury, granulation tissue replaces necrotic material, and by the third week fibroblasts proliferate and stricturing commences. The amount of paraesophageal fibrosis developing is related to the severity of the initial injury. In longstanding corrosive esophageal strictures, squamous cell carcinoma of the esophagus may occur, and squamous cell carcinoma has also been reported in the strictured stomach. Ninety-five percent of severe strictures are situated in the distal esophagus, with frequent sparing of the lower esophageal sphincter.

The most common clinical symptoms are oropharyngeal pain, chest pain, and dysphagia. Other symptoms include vomiting, salvation, drooling, and stridor. Half of the patients with two or more of these features had major esophageal injury.

Retrosternal and epigastric pain are suggestive of full-thickness injury to the esophagus or stomach, particularly with radiation to the back. The mouth and pharynx should be inspected for evidence of burning in the form of black slough or gray opaque membranes. Absence of visible oral injury does not rule out esophageal or gastric involvement. In severe injuries, there may be abdominal tenderness and rigidity suggesting full-thickness involvement of the stomach or duodenum, or there may be respiratory distress, pleural pain, or surgical emphysema in the neck, all suggesting esophageal perforation with mediastinitis.

Immediate management is directed at securing the airway, relieving pain, and attending to fluid replacement. Laryngeal edema may cause stridor and prevent endotracheal intubation. Tracheostomy is occasionally necessary. Oral intake is prohibited. Attempts to neutralize acids or alkalis are unwise because exothermic reactions may be produced causing additional thermal damage.

Chest and abdominal films allow identification of mediastinal emphysema or free intraperitoneal air. These findings confirm full-thickness injury and the need for immediate operation. The superiority of endoscopy in detecting mucosal lesions is such that endoscopic examination has replaced contrast studies in most centers. Unfortunately, there are scant data to indicate the optimum timing of endoscopy after corrosive injury. Experimental studies suggest that mucosal injury is generally apparent by the time a patient arrives at the hospital. Thus, endoscopy can be carried out as resuscitation is completed. Fears that endoscopy may precipitate perforation are unfounded. Rather, endoscopic data are vital in planning subsequent management.

Oral antibiotics should be administered to all patients with severe corrosive injury. Corticosteroid administration has no proven benefit in recent trials, and disadvantages of steroids in masking sepsis suggest that they be avoided. Gastric acid suppression is sometimes used, although no data supports this treatment. There are no removal stents available for endoscopic insertion, and there is no uniform agreement about the role of stenting in acute injury. Oral intake is prohibited until the patient is able to swallow saliva with ease. Nutritional support is generally administered parenterally.

Early identification of patients with full-thickness injury of the esophagus, stomach, or duodenum is vital because this allows immediate resection of affected organs. Although the operative procedures may be extensive, lives are saved by prompt intervention that may limit further extension of evolving injury. Full-thickness injury to the stomach or duodenum is invariably accompanied by severe esophageal injury and is frequently an indication for resection of the esophagus and stomach. Resection should also be considered if there is extensive injury involving the full-thickness of the esophageal mucosa circumferentially even without muscle necrosis because such patients usually require later removal or bypass of the damaged area. Short segments of full-thickness mucosal loss may be managed conservatively with subsequent dilation if necessary.

The single most important factor contributing to mortality in corrosive injury is to delay in the diagnosis and treatment of transmural esophagogastric necrosis. An aggressive surgical approach is advised if this is suspected. In patients with significant injury who survive the initial crisis, the most important physical consequence is development of circumferential contracture in burned areas. These late consequences may be grouped in pharyngolaryngeal stenoses and more distal digestive tract strictures.

Although the upper digestive tract may often be relatively spared in corrosive injury, severe damage to the pharynx and larynx occurs in approximately 2% of patients and is especially likely when crystals of caustic soda are ingested. Urgent tracheotomy may be required; in the recovery phase, circumferential stenosis may be severe. Complications include fixation of the tongue, destruction of the epiglottis, and obliteration of the pharynx and trismus that may hinder examination. Most authors advise waiting at least 4 months after corrosive injury to allow initial inflammation to subside before pharyngeal reconstruction is attempted. Laryngeal injury may occur from transmural spread of corrosive material from the esophagus or by aspiration. As glottic refluxes usually protect the pharyngeal inlet, laryngectomy is rarely needed.

Esophageal stricture becomes evident as dysphagia 3 to 4 weeks after injury, when radiologic evaluation with oral contrast may be helpful. Nutritional support must be continued until esophageal patency has been restored. If surgical feeding access is desired, jejunostomy is preferable to gastrostomy, which may compromise the use of the stomach if needed for later reconstruction. If esophageal reconstruction is likely to be necessary, incidental procedures such as jejunostomy or gastrostomy are best avoided if possible because they may increase the difficulties of subsequent operations. Nasogastric feeding may be possible through a tube passed into the stomach over a guide wire passed through the stricture.

Dilation as treatment for esophageal strictures is satisfactory in less severe lesions. However, patients with more severe injury eventually require resection. In relatively young patients with less severe stricture, surgery may be more appropriate than dilation. Outcome data after dilation therapy for corrosive stricture are few, and those studies that are available contain small numbers of patients. Patients experiencing dilation of corrosive strictures have a high rate of perforation with standard bougie and balloon techniques. Lower perforation rates have recently been reported with later-generation dilators if used with fluoroscopic control. Dilation-related perforation may be fatal, and some patients treated with dilation have a poorer quality of life with dysphagia between dilations and are at risk for aspiration and its consequences.

Selected Reading

Pain

Silen W. Cope's early diagnosis of the acute abdomen. 21st ed. Oxford, UK: Oxford University Press, 2005

Tait IS, Ionescu MV, Cuschieri A. Do patients with acute abdominal pain wait unduly long for analgesia? J R Coll Surg Edinb 1999; 44:181–184

Thomas SH, Silen W, Cheema F, et al. Effects of morphine analgesia on diagnostic accuracy in emergency department patients with abdominal pain: a prospective randomized trial. J Am Coll Surg 2003; 196:18–31

Zoltie N, Cust MP. Analgesia in the acute abdomen. Ann R Coll Surg Engl 1986; 68:209–210

Ileus

Luckey A, Livingston E, Tache Y. Mechanisms and treatment of postoperative ileus. Arch Surg 2003; 138:206–214

Stomach

Behrman SW. Management of complicated peptic ulcer disease. Arch Surg 2005; 140:201–208

Callicutt CS, Behrman SW. Incidence of *Helicobacter pylori* in operatively managed acute nonvariceal upper gastrointestinal bleeding. J Gastrointest Surg 2001; 5:614–619

Feliciano DV, Ojukwu JC, Rozycki GS, et al. The epidemic of cocaine-related juxtapyloric perforations: with a comment on the importance of testing for *Helicobacter pylori*. Ann Surg 1999; 229:801–806

Lau JY, Leung WK, Wu JC, et al. Omeprazole before endoscopy in patients with gastrointestinal bleeding. N Engl J Med 2007; 356:1631–1640

Lau JY, Sung JJ, Lam YH, et al. Endoscopic retreatment compared with surgery in patients with recurrent bleeding after initial endoscopic control of bleeding ulcers. N Engl J Med 1999; 340:751–756

Ohmann C, Imhof M, Roher HD. Trends in peptic ulcer bleeding and surgical treatment. World J Surg 2000; 24:284–293

Rockall TA, Logan RF, Devlin HB, et al. Incidence of and mortality from acute upper gastrointestinal haemorrhage in the United Kingdom: Steering Committee and members of the National Audit of Acute Upper Gastrointestinal Haemorrhage. BMJ 1995; 311:222–226

Tokunaga Y, Hata K, Ryo J, et al. Density of *Helicobacter pylori* infection in patients with peptic ulcer perforation. J Am Coll Surg 1998; 186:659–663

Small Bowel

Bickell NA, Federman AD, Aufses AH Jr. Influence of time on risk of bowel resection in complete small bowel obstruction. J Am Coll Surg 2005; 201:847–854

Fevang BT, Fevang J, Lie SA, et al. Long-term prognosis after operation for adhesive small bowel obstruction. Ann Surg 2004; 240:193–201

Krouse RS, McCahill LE, Easson AM, et al. When the sun can set on an unoperated bowel obstruction: management of malignant bowel obstruction. J Am Coll Surg 2002; 195:117–128

Sosa J, Gardner B. Management of patients diagnosed as acute intestinal obstruction secondary to adhesions. Am Surg 1993; 59:125–128

Thompson JS, DiBaise JK, Iyer KR, et al. Postoperative short bowel syndrome. J Am Coll Surg 2005; 201:85–89

Colon/Appendix

Bahadursingh AM, Virgo KS, Kaminski DL, et al. Spectrum of disease and outcome of complicated diverticular disease. Am J Surg 2003; 186:696–701

Bartlett JG, Perl TM. The new *Clostridium difficile*: what does it mean? N Engl J Med 2005; 353:2503–2505

Broderick-Villa G, Burchette RJ, Collins JC, et al. Hospitalization for acute diverticulitis does not mandate routine elective colectomy. Arch Surg 2005; 140:576–583

Christopher FL, Lane MJ, Ward JA, et al. Unenhanced helical CT scanning of the abdomen and pelvis changes disposition of patients presenting to the emergency department with possible acute appendicitis. J Emerg Med 2002; 23:1–7

Gladman MA, Scott SM, Lunniss PJ, et al. Systemic review of surgical options for idiopathic megarectum and megacolon. Ann Surg 2005; 241:562–574

Loo VG, Poirier L, Miller MA, et al. A predominantly clonal multi-institutional outbreak of *Clostridium difficile*-associated diarrhea with high morbidity and mortality. N Engl J Med 2005; 353:2442–2449

Mittal VK, Goliath J, Sabir M, et al. Advantages of focused helical computed tomographic scanning with rectal contrast only vs triple contrast in the diagnosis of clinically uncertain acute appendicitis: a prospective randomized study. Arch Surg 2004; 139:495–500

Preventza OA, Lazarides K, Sawyer MD. Ischemic colitis in young adults: a single-institution experience. J Gastrointest Surg 2001; 5:388–392

Reilly PM, Wilkins KB, Fuh KC, et al. The mesenteric hemodynamic response to circulatory shock: an overview. Shock 2001; 15:329–343

Wong WD, Wexner SD, Lowry A, et al. Practice parameters for the treatment of sigmoid diverticulitis: supporting documentation; the Standards Task Force. The American Society of Colon and Rectal Surgeons. Dis Colon Rectum 2000; 43:290–297

Pancreas

Acosta JM, Katkhouda N, Debian KA, et al. Early ductal decompression versus conservative management for gallstone pancreatitis with ampullary obstruction: a prospective randomized clinical trial. Ann Surg 2006; 243:33–40

Acosta JM, Pellegrini CA, Skinner DB. Etiology and pathogenesis of acute biliary pancreatitis. Surgery 1980; 88:118–125

Baron TH, Morgan DE. Acute necrotizing pancreatitis. N Engl J Med 1999; 340:1412–1417

Buchler MW, Gloor B, Muller CA, et al. Acute necrotizing pancreatitis: treatment strategy according to the status of infection. Ann Surg 2000; 232:619–626

Cahen DL, Gouma DJ, Nio Y, et al. Endoscopic versus surgical drainage of the pancreatic duct in chronic pancreatitis. N Engl J Med 2007; 356:676–684

Dellinger EP, Tellado JM, Soto NE, et al. Early antibiotic treatment for severe acute necrotizing pancreatitis: a randomized double-blind, placebo-controlled study. Ann Surg 2007; 245:674–683

Eachempati SR, Hydo LJ, Barie PS. Severity scoring for prognostication in patients with severe acute pancreatitis: comparative analysis of the Ranson score and the APACHE III score. Arch Surg 2002; 137: 730–736

Fan ST, Lai EC, Mok FP, et al. Early treatment of acute biliary pancreatitis by endoscopic papillotomy. N Engl J Med 1993; 328:228–232

Folsch UR, Nitsche R, Ludtke R, et al. Early ERCP and papillotomy compared with conservative treatment for acute biliary pancreatitis: the German Study Group on Acute Biliary Pancreatitis. N Engl J Med 1997; 336:237–242

Guzman EA, Rudnicki M. Intricacies of host response in acute pancreatitis. J Am Coll Surg 2006; 202:509–519

Hallal AH, Amortegui JD, Jeroukhimov IM, et al. Magnetic resonance cholangiopancreatography accurately detects common bile duct stones in resolving gallstone pancreatitis. J Am Coll Surg 2005; 200:869–875

Heinrich S, Schäfer M, Rousson V, et al. Evidence-based treatment of acute pancreatitis: a look at established paradigms. Ann Surg 2006; 243:154–168

Nathens AB, Curtis JR, Beale RJ, et al. Management of the critically ill patient with severe acute pancreatitis. Crit Care Med 2004; 32:2524–2536

Ranson JH. Etiological and prognostic factors in human acute pancreatitis: a review. Am J Gastroenterol 1982; 77:633–638

Rau B, Pralle U, Mayer JM, et al. Role of ultrasonographically guided fine-needle aspiration cytology in the diagnosis of infected pancreatic necrosis. Br J Surg 1998; 85:179–184

Biliary Tree

Berber E, Engle KL, String A, et al. Selective use of tube cholecystostomy with interval laparoscopic cholecystectomy in acute cholecystitis. Arch Surg 2000; 135:341–346

Buell JF, Cronin DC, Funaki B, et al. Devastating and fatal complications associated with combined vascular and bile duct injuries during cholecystectomy. Arch Surg 2002; 137:703–710

Chang L, Moonka R, Stelzner M. Percutaneous cholecystostomy for acute cholecystitis in veteran patients. Am J Surg 2000; 180:198–202

Gupta N, Solomon H, Fairchild R, et al. Management and outcome of patients with combined bile duct and hepatic artery injuries. Arch Surg 1998; 133:176–181

Lai EC, Mok FP, Tan ES, et al. Endoscopic biliary drainage for severe acute cholangitis. N Engl J Med 1992; 326:1582–1586

Lillemoe KD, Martin SA, Cameron JL, et al. Major bile duct injuries during laparoscopic cholecystectomy: follow-up after combined surgical and radiologic management. Ann Surg 1997; 225:459–471

Lo CM, Liu CL, Fan ST, et al. Prospective randomized study of early versus delayed laparoscopic cholecystectomy for acute cholecystitis. Ann Surg 1998; 227:461–467

Murr MM, Gigot JF, Nagorney DM, et al. Long-term results of biliary reconstruction after laparoscopic bile duct injuries. Arch Surg 1999; 134:604–610

Spira RM, Nissan A, Zamir O, et al. Percutaneous transhepatic cholecystostomy and delayed laparoscopic cholecystectomy in critically ill patients with acute calculus cholecystitis. Am J Surg 2002; 183: 62–66

The Southern Surgeons Club. A prospective analysis of 1518 laparoscopic cholecystectomies. N Engl J Med 1991; 324:1073–1078

Special Problems

Hugh TB, Kelly MD. Corrosive ingestion and the surgeon. J Am Coll Surg 1999; 189:508–522

Hyman N, Manchester TL, Osler T, et al. Anastomotic leaks after intestinal anastomosis: it's later than you think. Ann Surg 2007; 245:254–258

Notes

Hypothermia, Hyperthermia, and Rhabdomyolysis

Janice L. Zimmerman, MD, FCCP

Objectives:

- Understand the physiologic responses associated with hypothermia
- Outline supportive measures and rewarming techniques for the management of hypothermia
- Describe predisposing factors for heat stroke, its clinical manifestations, and cooling methods
- Discuss the clinical presentations and management of malignant hyperthermia and neuroleptic malignant syndrome
- Describe the etiologies, clinical presentation, and treatment of rhabdomyolysis

Key words: heat stroke; hyperthermia; hypothermia; malignant hyperthermia; neuroleptic malignant syndrome; rhabdomyolysis

Temperature Regulation

The balance between heat production and heat loss normally maintains the core body temperature at a mean of $36.6 \pm 0.38°C$ ($97.9 \pm 0.7°F$). Heat is produced from the dissolution of high-energy bonds during metabolism. At rest, the trunk viscera supply 56% of the heat; during exercise, muscle activity may account for 90% of generated heat. Heat production may increase twofold to fourfold with shivering and more than sixfold with exercise. Most heat loss (50 to 70%) normally occurs through radiation. The conduction of heat through direct contact with cooler objects or loss of heat due to convection accounts for a smaller percentage of heat loss. The evaporation of sweat from the skin is the major mechanism of heat loss in a warm environment.

The anterior hypothalamus is responsible for the perception of temperature and the initiation of physiologic responses. Information is received from temperature-sensitive receptors in the skin, viscera, and great vessels, as well as receptors located in the hypothalamus. When a temperature increase is sensed, hypothalamic modulation results in increased sweating (a cholinergically mediated response), cutaneous vasodilation, and

decreased muscle tone. Conversely, a decrease in temperature results in decreased sweating, cutaneous vasoconstriction, and increased muscle tone and shivering. These homeostatic mechanisms deteriorate with age.

Hypothermia

Definition and Etiologies

Hypothermia is defined as the unintentional lowering of core body temperature (tympanic, esophageal, or rectal) to $< 35°C$ ($< 95°F$). Multiple factors may lead to increased heat loss, decreased heat production, or impaired thermoregulation (Table 1). Hypothermia may be characterized as primary (accidental), due to exposure to cold temperatures, or secondary, resulting from a disease process such as myxedema or sepsis. Exposure is often found in hypothermic patients, along with underlying chronic disease processes or impairment from ethanol, drugs, or mental illness. Immersion hypothermia is often distinguished from nonimmersion hypothermia because it occurs more rapidly and is more often accompanied by asphyxia. Hypothermia is frequently noted in trauma patients and is associated with increased mortality rates.

To facilitate management and anticipate physiologic changes, hypothermia can be classified by the degree of temperature reduction. Mild hypothermia refers to core temperatures of 32 to 35°C (90 to 95°F); moderate hypothermia, 28 to 32°C (82 to 90°F); and severe hypothermia, $< 28°C$ ($< 82°F$). The classification for trauma victims is more conservative with temperatures of $< 32°C$ (90°F) considered to be severe hypothermia related to the poor prognosis associated with hypothermia.

Pathophysiology

General Metabolic Changes: Hypothermia produces multisystemic involvement that varies with

Table 1. *Factors Predisposing to Hypothermia*

Increased heat loss
  Environmental exposure
  Skin disorders
    Burns
    Dermatitis
    Psoriasis
  Vasodilation
    Alcohol
    Drugs (phenothiazines)
  Iatrogenic
    Heat stroke treatment
    Environmental cold (operating suite)
Decreased heat production
  Endocrine disorders
    Hypopituitarism
    Hypothyroidism
    Hypoadrenalism
  Insufficient fuel
    Hypoglycemia
    Anorexia nervosa
    Malnutrition
    Extreme exertion
  Neuromuscular inefficiency
    Extremes of age
    Inactivity
    Impaired shivering
Impaired thermoregulation
  Peripheral dysfunction
    Neuropathies
    Spinal cord transection
    Diabetes
  Central dysfunction
    CNS hemorrhage/trauma
    Cerebrovascular accident
    Drugs
      Sedatives
      Alcohols
      Cyclic antidepressants
      Narcotics
    Neoplasm
    Parkinson's disease
    Anorexia nervosa
Miscellaneous states
  Sepsis
  Pancreatitis
  Carcinomatosis
  Uremia
  Sarcoidosis

core temperature (Table 2). The initial response to cold is cutaneous vasoconstriction, which results in the shunting of blood from colder extremities to the body core. Vasodilation secondary to ethanol can prevent this normal compensatory response. Vasoconstriction fails at temperatures <24°C (<75°F), and the rate of heat loss increases because of relative vasodilation. Heat production is increased twofold to fivefold by the onset of shivering with core temperatures of 30 to 35°C (86 to 95°F). Shivering continues until glycogen stores are depleted, which usually occurs when the body temperature reaches 30°C (86°F).

Cardiovascular System: An initial tachycardia is followed by progressive bradycardia. The pulse rate decreases by 50% when the core temperature reaches 28°C (82°F). Bradycardia is secondary to alterations in conductivity and automaticity that are generally refractory to standard treatment (*eg,* atropine). Cardiac function and BP also decline proportionately as the core temperature decreases. Systemic vascular resistance predictably increases.

Hypothermia produces a variety of myocardial conduction abnormalities. Atrial fibrillation is common and usually converts to sinus rhythm spontaneously during rewarming. At temperatures of <29°C (<84°F), ventricular fibrillation (VF) can occur spontaneously or be induced by movement or invasive procedures (*eg,* central line or nasogastric tube). Asystole occurs at temperatures <20°C (<68°F). VF and other arrhythmias are extremely refractory to defibrillation and drug treatment until the core temperature increases to approximately 30°C (approximately 86°F).

Although many ECG abnormalities have been described, the most characteristic of hypothermia is the J wave (also called the Osborne wave) at the junction of the QRS complex and ST segment (Fig 1). The J wave can occur in patients with core temperatures of <32°C (<90°F), and it is almost always present at temperatures of <25°C (<77°F). It has been observed that the size of the J wave may be inversely correlated with temperature. The presence of this wave is not pathognomonic for hypothermia, nor does it have prognostic value. It is important to distinguish J waves from ST-segment elevation, indicating myocardial infarction. Prolongation of the PR, QRS complex, and QT intervals may be noted.

Other Organ Systems: As temperature decreases, tidal volume and respiratory rate will decrease. The cough reflex may be blunted, and cold-induced bronchorrhea may contribute to atelectasis. Hypoxemia may develop early depending on the circumstances (*eg,* water immersion or aspiration). Although renal blood flow and the glomerular filtration rate decrease during hypothermia, there is an initial cold-induced diuresis due to

Table 2. *Manifestations of Hypothermia**

Core Temperature, °C	Musculoskeletal	Neurologic	Other
Mild hypothermia			
38			
36	Shivering begins	Slurred speech	
34	Maximal shivering	Increased confusion	
33	Decreased shivering	Stupor	Decreasing BP; respiratory alkalosis, cold diuresis
Moderate hypothermia			
32	Shivering nearly absent; onset of muscle rigidity	Pupils dilated	Arrhythmias; J waves on ECG
30		DTRs absent	Severe hypoventilation
28	Extreme muscle rigidity	No voluntary movement	Shock; inaudible heart sounds
Severe hypothermia			
26			
24	Patient appears dead		Severe risk of VF; minimal cardiac activity
22			
20		Isoelectric EEG	Asystole
18		Isoelectric EEG	Asystole

*DTR = deep tendon reflex.

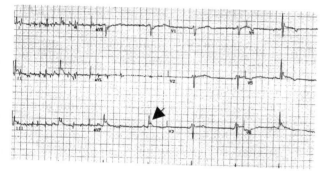

Figure 1. ECG of hypothermic patient showing J wave (arrow).

the relative central hypervolemia resulting from peripheral vasoconstriction. Additional contributory factors include the inhibition of antidiuretic hormone release and renal tubular concentrating defects. Ethanol exacerbates the diuresis. With warming, volume depletion may become evident.

With mild hypothermia, patients may exhibit confusion, lethargy, or combativeness. Below a core temperature of 32°C (90°F), the patient is usually unconscious with diminished brainstem function. Pupils dilate below a core temperature of 30°C (86°F). Intestinal motility decreases at temperatures of <34°C (<93°F), resulting in the common finding of ileus. Hepatic dysfunction affects the generation of glucose as well as drug metabolism.

Laboratory Findings: The physiologic changes described are reflected by clinical laboratory tests. An increased hematocrit is usually found, with normal or low platelet and WBC counts. The increase in hematocrit is due to hemoconcentration and splenic contraction. However, the restoration of intravascular volume and warming often result in a mild anemia. Platelet and WBC counts may drop as temperatures decrease because of sequestration. Platelet dysfunction occurs with hypothermia and may compromise hemostasis. Although disseminated intravascular coagulation (DIC) may develop, initial coagulation study results (ie, prothrombin time and partial thromboplastin time) are often normal as these laboratory measurements are performed on warmed blood. Electrolyte levels are variable, and no consistent changes are predictable. Increased values of BUN and creatinine result from hypovolemia. Hyperglycemia is common as a result of catecholamine-induced glycogenolysis, decreased insulin release, and inhibition of insulin transport. Hypoglycemia may be evident in malnourished and alcoholic patients. Hyperamylasemia is common and may be related to a preexisting pancreatitis or pancreatitis induced by hypothermia. The acid-base status is difficult to predict in hypothermia, but factors such as respiratory acidosis, lactate generation from shivering, decreased acid excretion, and decreased tissue perfusion contribute to acidemia. There is general agreement that arterial blood gas values do not need to be corrected for temperature. However, the Pao_2 should be corrected to evaluate oxygen delivery and the alveolar-arterial Po_2 gradient.

Diagnosis

The clinical manifestations of hypothermia vary with the etiology, acuteness of onset, severity, and duration. It is imperative to recognize the early signs of mild hypothermia, especially in the elderly. These patients may present with confusion, lethargy, impaired judgment, and the unusual manifestation of "paradoxical undressing." More severe hypothermia results in the following manifestations that are easily recognizable: muscle rigidity, decreased reflexes, decreased respiratory rate, bradycardia, hypotension, and even the appearance of death. The clinical suspicion of hypothermia should be confirmed with an accurate core temperature measurement. Any low temperature (35°C or 95°F) should be checked with a thermometer capable of registering lower temperatures. A rectal probe is most practical even though it may lag behind core changes. The probe should be inserted to an adequate depth (approximately 15 cm), avoiding cold fecal material. An esophageal probe is an alternative, but readings may be falsely elevated in the intubated patient who receives heated oxygen. Thermistors in bladder catheters provide readings that are similar to those of intravascular devices. The reliability of tympanic temperature devices has not been established in patients with hypothermia.

Management

Hospital Management: The severity of hypothermia, clinical findings, and comorbid conditions of the patient determine the aggressiveness of the resuscitation techniques. The following measures should be instituted as indicated:

1. *Airway management.* Intubation is often necessary for airway protection and/or the delivery of supplemental oxygen. The orotracheal route is preferred because of the risk of traumatic bleeding with the nasal route. However, muscle rigidity may preclude orotracheal intubation. Blind nasotracheal intubation in a patient with spontaneous respiration may be facilitated by topical vasoconstrictors and a smaller endotracheal tube. Endotracheal tube cuff pressures should be monitored after rewarming because volume and pressure will increase.

2. *Supplemental oxygen.* Pulse oximetry cannot be relied on to guide therapy in conditions of hypothermia and hypoperfusion.

3. *Cardiopulmonary resuscitation.* Cardiopulmonary resuscitation should be initiated if the patient is pulseless (assess for 30 to 45 s) or has a nonperfusing rhythm such as asystole or VF. Chest wall compression is often difficult and compressors may need to rotate more frequently than every 2 min.

4. *ECG monitoring. In patients with bradycardia,* avoid pharmacologic manipulation and pacing. *In patients with VF,* initial defibrillation should be attempted once even if the temperature is < 30 to 32°C (< 86 to 90°F). If the attempt is unsuccessful, institute rewarming. Defibrillation can be attempted after every 1 to 2°C (2 to 3.6°F) increase in temperature or when the core temperature reaches 30 to 32°C (86 to 90°F). Avoid the IV administration of drugs until the temperature increases to approximately 30°C (approximately 86°F) and then use the lowest effective dose. Dosing intervals should be increased in hypothermic patients. The efficacy of amiodarone has not been established in patients with hypothermia, but it is a reasonable initial antiarrhythmic drug. Magnesium sulfate has also been used successfully. Lidocaine has limited efficacy, and procainamide may increase the incidence of VF. *In patients with asystole,* follow advanced cardiac life support guidelines and administer pharmacologic agents when the temperature approaches 30°C (86°F).

5. *Core temperature monitoring.* Utilize a bladder, esophageal, or rectal thermometer device for temperature monitoring.

6. *Rewarming* (see the "Rewarming Methods" section).

7. *IV fluids.* All patients require fluids for hypovolemia. Warm normal saline solution containing glucose is a reasonable choice.

Hypothermia, Hyperthermia, and Rhabdomyolysis (Zimmerman)

Increased fluid requirements are often necessary during rewarming to prevent or treat hypotension that may occur with vasodilation. Lactated Ringer solution should be avoided because of the potential impaired hepatic metabolism of lactate.

8. *Vasopressor drugs.* Hemodynamic instability should first be managed with volume replacement. Vasopressor drugs have a minimal effect on constricted vessels and increase the risk of dysrhythmias.

9. *Nasogastric or orogastric tube.* Insert to relieve gastric distention.

10. *Urinary catheter.* Insert to monitor urine output and/or monitor bladder temperature.

11. *Venous access.* Peripheral venous catheters are preferred. The use of central venous lines (*eg,* subclavian or internal jugular) is not routinely recommended because they may precipitate dysrhythmias.

12. *Laboratory studies.* Studies should include CBC count, prothrombin time, partial thromboplastin time, electrolyte levels, creatine kinase level, and arterial blood gas levels. Thyroid function evaluation, toxicology screening, and blood cultures are obtained as warranted.

13. *Search for associated conditions* requiring urgent intervention, such as hypoglycemia, sepsis, adrenal insufficiency, and hypothyroidism.

Rewarming Methods: Choices and Controversies— Although warming is the primary treatment for hypothermia, controversy exists as to the optimal method, duration, and rate of rewarming. Rapid rewarming has not been proven to improve survival. No controlled studies comparing rewarming methods exist, and rigid treatment protocols cannot be recommended. The following three types of rewarming techniques exist: passive external rewarming (PER), active external rewarming (AER), and active core rewarming (ACR).

PER is the least invasive and slowest method. It involves placing the patient in a warm environment, providing an insulating cover, and allowing the body to regain heat. This technique should be applied as the sole method only in patients with mild hypothermia, and as an adjunct in patients with moderate and severe hypothermia. The patient must be able to generate heat for PER to be effective. Rewarming rates with PER in patients with mild hypothermia range from 0.5 to 2.0°C/h (1 to 3.6°F/h).

AER involves the external application of heat, such as warming blankets, heating pads, radiant heat lamps, or immersion in warm water. Currently, forced-air warming devices or resistive polymer blankets are the most effective and practical means of applying AER, particularly in the perioperative period. A potential disadvantage of this method is the theoretical concern of "after-drop." When a heat source is applied, peripheral vasodilation occurs and colder peripheral blood is transported to the relatively warmer core, thereby reducing the core temperature. After-drop has been hypothesized to increase the incidence of VF. In response to this concern, it has been suggested that heat be applied only to the thorax, leaving the extremities vasoconstricted. The advantages of AER are its ease of institution, ready availability, low cost, and noninvasiveness. Earlier studies showing high mortality when AER was used are not supported by more recent experience. AER is often combined with ACR techniques in patients with moderate or severe hypothermia.

ACR is the most rapid and most invasive method, and involves the application of heat to the body core. ACR is indicated in patients with a core temperature of <28°C (<82°F) or with an arrested cardiac rhythm. Techniques for ACR include heated humidified oxygen, heated IV fluids, thoracic lavage, peritoneal lavage, gastric/rectal lavage, hemodialysis, continuous arteriovenous/venovenous rewarming, and cardiopulmonary bypass.

One of the simplest methods to institute is warm, humidified, inhaled oxygen (42 to 45°C or 107.6 to 113°F), which prevents further respiratory heat loss and may result in a modest heat gain. A rewarming rate of 1 to 2.5°C/h (2 to 4.5°F/h) can be expected. This technique should be used routinely on most patients with moderate-to-severe hypothermia. Heated IV fluids (40 to 42°C or 104 to 107.6°F) are also easy to administer. If blood transfusion is indicated, it should be warmed. Although gastric, bladder, and rectal lavage with warm fluids are simple procedures, there is little information regarding the efficacy of these methods. Gastric lavage may predispose the patient to aspiration, and it cannot be performed during chest compressions. These methods should be used only as an adjunct until more effective rewarming methods can be initiated.

For patients with severe hypothermia, the following more invasive methods of ACR are preferred: peritoneal lavage, thoracic lavage, hemodialysis, continuous arteriovenous/venovenous rewarming, and cardiopulmonary bypass. These procedures require specialized equipment and intensive care. However, they are very efficient at rewarming and, in the case of cardiopulmonary bypass, may provide for hemodynamic stabilization of the patient. Peritoneal lavage can be instituted through a peritoneal dialysis catheter, using dialysate heated to 40 to 45°C (104 to 113°F). Closed thoracic lavage involves the placement of anterior and posterior chest tubes, the infusion of heated saline solution (40 to 42°C or 104 to 107.6°F) through the anterior tube, and gravity drainage from the posterior tube. Hemodialysis, using a two-way-flow catheter, may be best suited for hemodynamically stable patients. Continuous arteriovenous/venovenous rewarming uses a modified fluid warmer with 40°C (104°F) water infused through the inner chamber. Cardiopulmonary bypass (femoral-femoral or atrial-aortic) is the most invasive and labor-intensive technique for rewarming. It has the advantage of providing complete hemodynamic support and rapid rewarming rates (1 to 2°C every 3 to 5 min).

The choice of rewarming methods may combine techniques, such as AER with ACR, using heated oxygen and IV fluids. The availability of resources may be a decisive factor in choosing the method of rewarming. In all cases, the complications of rewarming, such as DIC, pulmonary edema, compartment syndromes, rhabdomyolysis, and acute tubular necrosis, must be anticipated.

Future Therapies

IV fluids heated to 65°C (149°F) have been used in animal studies and have demonstrated rewarming rates of 2.9 to 3.7°C/h with minimal intimal injury. Diathermy (ie, ultrasound or low-frequency microwave radiation) involves the conversion of energy waves into heat. It can deliver large amounts of heat to deep tissues. Further investigation is needed to determine the optimum clinical use.

Outcome From Hypothermia

There are currently no strong predictors of death or permanent neurologic dysfunction in patients with severe hypothermia. Therefore, there are no definitive indicators to suggest which patients can or cannot be resuscitated successfully. Core temperature before rewarming and time to rewarming do not predict outcome. Severe hyperkalemia (>10 mEq/L) may be a marker of death. In general, resuscitative efforts should continue until the core temperature is 32°C (90°F). However, the decision to terminate resuscitation must be individualized based on the circumstances. Patients found indoors are more severely affected and have higher mortality.

Hyperthermia

Heat Stroke

Definition: Heat stroke is a life-threatening medical emergency that occurs when homeostatic thermoregulatory mechanisms fail. This failure usually results in the elevation of body temperature to >41°C (>105.8°F), producing multisystem tissue damage and organ dysfunction. The following two syndromes of heat stroke occur: classic heat stroke (nonexertional) and exertional heat stroke. Classic heat stroke typically affects infants and elderly individuals with underlying chronic illness. The occurrence of classic heat stroke is usually predictable when heat waves occur. The syndrome develops over several days and results in significant dehydration and anhidrosis. Exertional heat stroke typically occurs in young individuals such as athletes and military recruits exercising in hot weather. These individuals usually have no chronic illness, and this syndrome occurs sporadically and often unpredictably. Dehydration is less severe, and approximately 50% of individuals will have profuse sweating.

Predisposing Factors: Heat stroke results from increased heat production and/or decreased heat loss (Table 3). Environmental factors of high heat and humidity contribute to heat production as well

Table 3. *Predisposing Factors for Heat Stroke*

Increased heat production
    Exercise
    Fever
    Thyrotoxicosis
    Hypothalamic dysfunction
    Drugs (sympathomimetic agents)
    Environmental heat stress
Decreased heat loss
    Environmental heat stress
    Cardiac disease
    Peripheral vascular disease
    Dehydration
    Obesity
    Skin disease
    Anticholinergic drugs
    Ethanol
    β-Blockers

as to the limitation of heat loss. Sympathomimetic drugs, such as cocaine and amphetamines, increase muscle activity and may also disrupt hypothalamic regulatory mechanisms. Numerous drugs interfere with the ability to dissipate heat. Drugs with anticholinergic effects, such as cyclic antidepressants, antihistamines, and antipsychotics, inhibit sweating and disrupt hypothalamic function. Ethanol may contribute to heat stroke by several mechanisms, as follows: vasodilation resulting in heat gain, impaired perception of the environment, and diuresis. β-Adrenergic blockers may impair cardiovascular compensation and decrease cutaneous blood flow. Factors that increase the risk of death include being confined to bed because of medical problems, living on the top floor of a building, lack of insulation, and living alone.

Diagnosis: The diagnosis of heat stroke requires a history of exposure to a heat load (either internal or external), severe CNS dysfunction, and elevated temperature (usually $>40°C$ or $>104°F$). The absolute temperature may not be critical because cooling measures are often instituted before the patient is admitted to a health-care facility. Sweating may or may not be present.

Clinical Manifestations: Symptoms of heat stroke vary with the rapidity of onset, severity of exposure (temperature and duration), and comorbid conditions. Profound CNS dysfunction is a defining characteristic of heat stroke. Dysfunction may range from bizarre behavior, delirium,

and confusion to decerebrate rigidity, cerebellar dysfunction, seizures, and coma. These changes are potentially reversible, although permanent deficits can occur. Lumbar puncture results may show increased protein, xanthochromia, and lymphocytic pleocytosis.

Tachycardia, an almost universal cardiovascular finding in patients with heat stroke, occurs in response to peripheral vasodilation and the need for increased cardiac output. The peripheral vascular resistance is usually low unless severe hypovolemia is present. Compensatory vasoconstriction occurs in the splanchnic and renal vascular beds. If the patient is unable to increase cardiac output, hypotension develops. A variety of ECG changes have been described in patients with heat stroke, including conduction defects, increased QT interval, and nonspecific ST-T changes.

Tachypnea may result in a significant respiratory alkalosis. However, patients with exertional heat stroke usually have lactic acidosis. Hypoglycemia may be present in patients with exertional heat stroke as a result of increased glucose use and impaired hepatic gluconeogenesis. Rhabdomyolysis and renal failure occur more commonly with exertional heat stroke and may be caused by myoglobinuria, thermal parenchymal damage, or decreased renal blood flow due to hypotension. Hematologic effects include hypocoagulability, which may progress to DIC. Hepatic injury results in cholestasis and the elevation of transaminase levels.

An inflammatory response may cause or contribute to the clinical manifestations of heat stroke. Increased concentrations of endotoxin, tumor necrosis factor, soluble tumor necrosis factor receptor, and interleukin-1 have been demonstrated in heat stroke victims. Interleukin-6 and nitric oxide metabolite concentrations correlate with the severity of illness. Endothelial cell activation/injury is suggested by findings of increased concentrations of circulating intercellular adhesion molecule-1, endothelin, and von Willebrand factor antigen.

Electrolyte concentrations are variable in patients with heat stroke. Hyperkalemia can result from rhabdomyolysis, but hypokalemia occurs more commonly. Hypocalcemia can occur, particularly with rhabdomyolysis, but usually does not require therapy.

Differential Diagnosis: The history and physical findings usually indicate the diagnosis of heat stroke. In the absence of an adequate history, other processes to be considered include CNS infection, hypothalamic lesions, thyroid storm, and other hyperthermic syndromes such as neuroleptic malignant syndrome (NMS).

Treatment: Along with resuscitative measures, immediate cooling should be instituted for any patient with a temperature of $>41°C$ ($>105.8°F$). The following two methods of cooling have been used: conductive cooling and evaporative cooling. Because definitive human studies are lacking, the optimal cooling method remains controversial.

Direct cooling by enhancing conduction of heat from the body is accomplished by immersing the patient in cold water. Skin massage to prevent cutaneous vasoconstriction in the limbs has been recommended. Shivering can result in an undesirable increase in heat production. This method requires considerable staff time and makes it difficult to treat seizures and perform other resuscitative measures. Variants of this method include ice water soaks; the application of ice packs to the axillae, groin, and neck; and ice applied to the entire body.

Evaporative cooling is a widely used practical cooling method. The patient is placed nude on a stretcher and sprayed with warm (not cold) water. Air flow is created with the use of fans to enhance evaporative cooling. This method allows personnel to institute other resuscitative measures while cooling occurs. Other cooling methods, such as peritoneal lavage, iced gastric lavage, or cardiopulmonary bypass, have not been effectively tested in humans. There are a few reports of surface and endovascular cooling devices used for induced hypothermia after cardiac arrest being used in heat stroke victims but their use cannot be recommended at this time because of cost and invasiveness. The use of antipyretic agents is not indicated, and dantrolene is ineffective.

In addition to cooling, most patients will require intubation for airway protection. Supplemental oxygen therapy should be instituted for all patients. The type and quantity of IV fluids should be individualized based on the assessment of electrolyte levels and volume status. Overaggressive hydration may result in cardiac decompensation during cooling, especially in the elderly. Hypotension usually responds to cooling as peripheral vasodilation decreases. Therapy with vasopressor agents that results in vasoconstriction can decrease heat exchange and is not recommended for the initial management of hypotension. A thermistor probe should be used for the monitoring of core temperature during cooling efforts. Cooling should be stopped at 38.0 to 38.8°C (100.4 to 102°F) to prevent hypothermic overshoot.

Outcome: With appropriate management, the survival rate of patients with heat stroke approaches 90%. However, morbidity is related to the duration of hyperthermia and to underlying conditions. Advanced age, hypotension, coagulopathy, hyperkalemia, acute renal failure, and prolonged coma are associated with a poor prognosis. Elevated lactate levels are associated with a poor prognosis in patients with classic heat stroke but not those with exertional heat stroke. In retrospective studies, rapid cooling (in <1 h) was associated with a decreased mortality.

Malignant Hyperthermia

Definition: Malignant hyperthermia (MH) is a drug-induced or stress-induced hypermetabolic syndrome that is characterized by hyperthermia, muscle contractures, and cardiovascular instability. It results from a genetic defect of calcium transport in skeletal muscle. The primary defects are postulated to be the impaired reuptake of calcium into the sarcoplasmic reticulum, the increased release of calcium from the sarcoplasmic reticulum, and a defect in the calcium-mediated coupling contraction mechanism. Sustained muscle contraction results in increased oxygen consumption and heat production. It is genetically transmitted as an autosomal-dominant trait and occurs in 1 in 50 to 1 in 150,000 adults who receive anesthesia.

Triggers: Halothane and succinylcholine have been involved in the majority of reported cases of MH. Additional potentiating drugs include muscle relaxants, inhalational anesthetic agents, and drugs such as ethanol, caffeine, sympathomimetics, parasympathomimetics, cardiac glycosides, and quinidine analogs. Less commonly, MH can be precipitated by infection, physical or emotional stress, anoxia, or high ambient temperature.

Clinical Manifestations: Manifestations of MH usually occur within 30 min of anesthesia in 90% of cases. However, onset of the syndrome may occur postoperatively. Muscle rigidity begins in the muscles of the extremities or the chest. In patients receiving succinylcholine, the stiffness most commonly begins in the jaw. The development of masseter spasm after the administration of a paralyzing agent should be considered an early sign of possible MH. Tachycardia is another early, although nonspecific, sign. The monitoring of arterial blood gas or end-tidal CO_2 levels may detect an early increase in CO_2. Hypertension and mottling of the skin also occur. The increase in temperature usually occurs later, but it is followed rapidly by acidosis, ventricular arrhythmias, and hypotension. Laboratory abnormalities include increased sodium, calcium, magnesium, potassium, phosphate, creatine kinase, and lactate dehydrogenase levels. Lactate levels are increased, and arterial blood gas levels indicate hypoxemia and an increase in $Paco_2$.

Treatment: Once the diagnosis of MH is entertained, therapy with the inciting drug should be discontinued immediately. The most effective and safest therapy is dantrolene, which prevents the release of calcium into the cell by the sarcoplasmic reticulum. Uncoupling of the excitation-contraction mechanism in skeletal muscle decreases thermogenesis. Dantrolene should be administered by rapid IV push, beginning at a dose of 2.5 mg/kg and repeated every 5 min until the symptoms subside or the maximum dose of 10 mg/kg has been reached. Decreasing muscle rigidity should be evident within minutes. Subsequent doses of 1 mg/kg every 4 to 6 h should be continued for 36 to 48 h. If dantrolene is ineffective or slowly effective, evaporative cooling methods can also be used. Calcium channel blockers are of no benefit in patients with MH and should not be used to treat arrhythmias.

The Malignant Hyperthermia Association of the United States provides a hotline for assistance in managing MH (1-800-MH-HYPER, 1-800-644-9737, or 1-315-464-7079 if outside of the United States.) The organization also maintains a Web site with useful information online (www.mhaus.org).

NMS

Definition: NMS is an idiosyncratic reaction, usually to neuroleptic drugs, that is characterized by hyperthermia, muscle rigidity, alterations in mental status, autonomic dysfunction, and rhabdomyolysis. It may occur in up to 1% of all patients receiving therapy with neuroleptic agents; it affects the young more than the old, and affected individuals are more likely to be male than female. The pathogenesis is unknown, but it is thought to be related to CNS dopamine antagonism and altered hypothalamic temperature set point.

Triggers: Although the majority of cases have been associated with haloperidol, the following agents have been associated with NMS: butyrophenones (*eg,* haloperidol), phenothiazines (*eg,* chlorpromazine and fluphenazine), thioxanthenes (*eg,* thiothixene), dopamine-depleting agents (*eg,* tetrabenazine), dibenzoxazepines (*eg,* loxapine), and withdrawal of levodopa/carbidopa or amantadine. The newer atypical antipsychotic drugs such as clozapine, risperidone, olanzapine, ziprasidone, aripiprazole, and quetiapine have also been reported to induce NMS. Rechallenge with an inciting drug may not result in the recurrence of NMS. Various diagnostic criteria have been proposed (Table 4), but NMS remains a clinical diagnosis based on exposure to neuroleptic agents

Table 4. *Diagnostic Criteria for NMS**

Major criteria
  Fever
  Muscle rigidity
  Increase in creatinine kinase level

Minor criteria
  Tachycardia
  Abnormal BP
  Tachypnea
  Altered consciousness
  Diaphoresis
  Leukocytes

*Diagnosis of NMS is suggested by the presence of all three major criteria or by the presence of two major and four minor criteria.

or other dopamine antagonists in association with characteristic manifestations.

Clinical Manifestations: NMS usually occurs 1 to 3 days after initiating therapy with a neuroleptic agent or changing the dose, and the syndrome may last for a period of 1 to 3 weeks. Hyperthermia is universally present, and the average maximal temperature is 39.9°C (103.8°F). However, NMS has been reported to occur without temperature elevation. Autonomic dysfunction includes tachycardia, diaphoresis, BP instability, and arrhythmias. Autonomic dysfunction may precede changes in muscle tone. A general increase in muscle tone or tremors occurs in >90% of patients. Early manifestations of changes in muscle tone include dysphagia, dysarthria, or dystonia. Altered mental status occurs in 75% of patients and can range from agitation to coma. Rhabdomyolysis occurs frequently with elevations of creatine kinase levels and may lead to serious electrolyte abnormalities. WBC counts are often increased (10,000 to 40,000 cells/μL) and may demonstrate a left shift. DIC has also been reported. Volume depletion or renal injury from rhabdomyolysis can result in elevated BUN and creatinine levels.

Treatment: Dantrolene is the most effective agent for reducing muscle rigidity and decreasing temperature. It is administered in the same doses as those described for MH. In addition, dopamine agonists have been reported to have beneficial effects in patients with NMS. These drugs include bromocriptine (2.5 to 10 mg tid), amantadine (100 mg bid), and levodopa/carbidopa. Supportive therapies must also be instituted as indicated. Complications may include respiratory failure, cardiovascular collapse, renal failure, arrhythmias, or thromboembolism. The Neuroleptic Malignant Syndrome Information Service (www.nmsis.org) maintains a hotline for medical professionals (1-888-667-8367) if assistance is needed.

Rhabdomyolysis

Definition

Rhabdomyolysis is a clinical and laboratory syndrome resulting from skeletal muscle injury with the release of cell contents into the plasma. Rhabdomyolysis occurs when demands for oxygen and metabolic substrate exceed availability. This syndrome may result from primary muscle injury or secondary injury due to infection, vascular occlusion, electrolyte disorders, or toxins. Table 5 provides an overview of the causes of rhabdomyolysis. Statin use is currently one of the most frequent causes of mild rhabdomyolysis but severe cases also occur. Rhabdomyolysis can develop postoperatively following bariatric surgery due to elevated deep tissue pressures.

Manifestations

Clinical manifestations of rhabdomyolysis consist of myalgias, muscle swelling and tenderness, discoloration of the urine, and features of the underlying disease. However, overt symptoms or physical findings may not be present. The results of a laboratory evaluation reflect muscle cell lysis with elevation of the levels of muscle enzymes (*ie,* creatine kinase, lactate dehydrogenase, aldolase, and aspartate aminotransferase), hyperkalemia, hyperphosphatemia, and hypocalcemia. Coagulation abnormalities consistent with DIC may occur. Renal failure may result secondary to the release of myoglobin and other toxic muscle components.

Table 5. *Causes of Rhabdomyolysis*

Traumatic	Infections	Toxins/Drugs	Metabolic Disorders
Crush syndrome	Coxsackievirus	Alcohol	Enzyme deficiencies
Muscle compression	Gas gangrene	Amphetamines	Hyperosmolar states
Hyperthermic syndromes	Hepatitis	Carbon monoxide	Hypokalemia
Burns	Influenza B virus	Cocaine	Hypomagnesemia
Electrical injury	Legionella	Phencyclidine	Hypophosphatemia
Exertion	Salmonella	Snake/spider venom	Inflammatory muscle disease
Seizures	Shigella	Statins	Thyroid disease
Vascular occlusion	Tetanus	Steroids	Vasculitis

A urine dipstick that is positive for blood and an absence of RBCs on microscopic examination suggests the presence of myoglobinuria.

Treatment

The treatment of rhabdomyolysis is aimed at treating the underlying disease and preventing complications. The maintenance of intravascular volume and renal perfusion is the most important aspect of preventing renal failure. Volume resuscitation should target a urine output of 2 to 3 mL/kg/h. Although increased urine output is beneficial, other interventions to prevent renal failure are more controversial. Alkalinization of the urine may be helpful, but clinical relevance has not been established. The greatest benefit of administering sodium bicarbonate may be the restoration of intravascular volume rather than a change in pH. Treatment with bicarbonate should be individualized, based on the patient's ability to tolerate the sodium and fluid load. Therapy with loop diuretics and osmotic diuretics has been advocated as being protective of the kidneys, but convincing clinical data are lacking. Loop diuretics theoretically can worsen renal tubular acidosis, which is thought to potentiate myoglobin-induced nephropathy. Diuresis should not be attempted without adequate volume replacement.

Electrolyte abnormalities should be anticipated and treated expeditiously. The most life-threatening abnormality is hyperkalemia. Hypocalcemia does not usually require treatment, and the empiric administration of calcium may exacerbate muscle injury.

The patient with rhabdomyolysis must be closely observed for the development of a compartment syndrome. The monitoring of intracompartmental pressures may be required. Fasciotomy is often recommended for intracompartmental pressures of >30 to 35 mm Hg.

Suggested Readings

Hypothermia

Braun R, Krishel S. Environmental emergencies. Emerg Med Clin North Am 1997; 15:451–476

Danzl DF, Pozos RS. Accidental hypothermia. N Engl J Med 1994; 331:1756–1760

Delaney KA, Howland MA, Vassallo S, et al. Assessment of acid-base disturbances in hypothermia and their physiologic consequences. Ann Emerg Med 1989; 18:72–82

Gentilello LM. Advances in the management of hypothermia. Surg Clin North Am 1995; 75:243–256

Gentilello LM, Cobean RA, Offner PJ, et al. Continuous arteriovenous rewarming: rapid reversal of hypothermia in critically ill patients. J Trauma 1992; 32:316–327

Giesbrecht GG, Bristow GK. Recent advances in hypothermia research. Ann N Y Acad Sci 1997; 813:663–675

Hanania NA, Zimmerman JL. Accidental hypothermia. Crit Care Clin 1999; 15:35–49

Hanania NA, Zimmerman JL. Hypothermia. In: Hall JB, Schmidt GA, Wood LDH, eds. Principles of critical care. 3rd ed. New York, NY: McGraw-Hill, 2005; 1679–1686

Jurkovich GJ. Environmental cold-induced injury. Surg Clin North Am 2007;87:247–267

Kimberger O, Held C, Mayer N, et al. Resistive polymer versus forced-air warming: comparable heat transfer and core rewarming rates in volunteers. Anesth Analg 2008;107:1621–1626

Kornberger E, Schwarz B, Linder KH, et al. Forced air surface rewarming in patients with severe accidental hypothermia. Resuscitation 1999; 41:105–111

Laniewicz M, Lyn-Kew K, Silbergleit R. Rapid endovascular rewarming for profound hypothermia. Ann Emerg Med 2008; 51:160–163

Plaisier BR. Thoracic lavage in accidental hypothermia with cardiac arrest: a report of a case and review of the literature. Resuscitation 2005; 66:99–104

Schaller MD, Fischer AP, Perret CH. Hyperkalemia, a prognostic factor during acute severe hypothermia. JAMA 1990; 264:1842–1845

Vassal T, Benoit-Gonin B, Carrat F, et al. Severe accidental hypothermia treated in an ICU: prognosis and outcome. Chest 2001; 120:1998–2003

Wang HE, Callaway CE, Peitzman AB, et al. Admission hypothermia and outcome after major trauma. Crit Care Med 2005; 33:1296–1301

Hyperthermia

Balzan MV. The neuroleptic malignant syndrome: a logical approach to the patient with temperature and rigidity. Postgrad Med J 1998; 74:72–76

Bouchama A, De Vol EB. Acid-base alterations in heatstroke. Intensive Care Med 2001; 27:680–685

Bouchama A, Dehbi M, Chaves-Carballo E. Cooling and hemodynamic management in heatstroke: practical recommendations. Crit Care 2007; 11:R54

Bouchama A, Knochel JP. Heat stroke. N Engl J Med 2002; 346:1978–1988

Carbone JR. The neuroleptic malignant and serotonin syndromes. Emerg Med Clin North Am 2000; 18:317–325

Caroff SN, Rosenberg H, Mann SC, et al. Neuroleptic malignant syndrome in the perioperative setting. Am J Anesthesiol 2001; 28:387–393

Gaffin SL, Gardner JW, Flinn SD. Cooling methods for heatstroke victims [letter]. Ann Intern Med 2000; 132:678

Hadad E, Rav-Acha M, Heled Y, et al. Heat stroke: a review of cooling methods. Sports Med 2004; 34:501–511

Hopkins PM. Malignant hyperthermia: advances in clinical management and diagnosis. Br J Anaesth 2000; 85:118–112

Howe AS, Boden BP. Heat-related illness in athletes. Am J Sports Med 2007; 35:1384–1396

Hubbard RW, Gaffin SL, Squire DL. Heat-related illness. In: Auerbach PS, ed. Wilderness medicine: management of wilderness and environmental emergencies. 4th ed. St. Louis, MO: Mosby, 2001; 195

Krause T, Gerbershagen MU, Fiege M, et al. Dantrolene: a review of its pharmacology, therapeutic use and new developments. Anaesthesia 2004; 59:364–373

Misset B, De Jonghe B, Bastuji-Garin S, et al. Mortality of patients with heatstroke admitted to intensive care units during the 2003 heat wave in France: a national multiple-center risk-factor study. Crit Care Med 2006; 34:1087–1092

Tomarken JL. Malignant hyperthermia. Ann Emerg Med 1987; 16:1253–1265

Varghese GM, John G, Thomas K, et al. Predictors of multi-organ dysfunction in heatstroke. Emerg Med J 2005; 22:185–187

Viejo LF, Morales V, Puñal P, et al. Risk factors in neuroleptic malignant syndrome: a case-control study. Acta Psychiatr Scand 2003; 107:45–49

Weiner JS, Khogali M. A physiological body-cooling unit for treatment of heat stroke. Lancet 1980; 1:507–509

Yarbrough B, Vicario S. Heat illness. In: Marx JA, Hockberger RS, Walls RM, eds. Emergency medicine: concepts and clinical practice. 5th ed. St Louis, MO: Mosby, 2002; 1997–2009

Zimmerman JL, Hanania NA. Hyperthermia. In: Hall JB, Schmidt GA, Wood LDH, eds. Principles of critical care. 3rd ed. New York, NY: McGraw-Hill, 2005; 1687–1692

Rhabdomyolysis

Allison RC, Bedsole L. The other medical causes of rhabdomyolysis. Am J Med Sci 2003; 326:79–88

Holt SG, Moore KP. Pathogenesis and treatment of renal dysfunction in rhabdomyolysis. Intensive Care Med 2001; 27:803–811

Thompson PD, Clarkson P, Karas RH. Statin-associated myopathy. JAMA 2003; 289:1681–1690

Ventilatory Crises

Gregory A. Schmidt, MD, FCCP

Objectives:

- Describe a systematic approach to the patient receiving mechanical ventilation in acute, life-threatening crisis
- Delineate the differential diagnosis and diagnostic plan for the agitated patient receiving mechanical ventilation
- Examine the underlying causes for high- and low-pressure alarms and acute deteriorations of gas exchange

Key words: auto-positive end-expiratory pressure; barotrauma; endotracheal tube; hypercapnia; hypoxemia; mechanical ventilation; patient-ventilator synchrony; pneumothorax ventilator alarm

An Approach to the Ventilated Patient in Crisis

The ICU course of mechanical ventilation is characterized typically by an apparently comfortable patient, quiet ventilator alarms, and adequate gas exchange. This peaceful picture may be punctuated, however, by abrupt crises of distress, alarming, or severe hypoxemia or hypercapnia. By their very nature, such crises demand a rapidly paced response. At the same time, the stakes are high: the treatment (eg, needle thoracostomy or a sedative bolus) may be lifesaving (if accurate) or life ending (if wrong). This chapter describes the most common crises during mechanical ventilation; provides a framework for rapid, bedside evaluation; and emphasizes the use of ventilator flow and pressure waveforms and bedside ultrasonography to guide therapy. This chapter is divided into the following categories: (1) the distressed patient; (2) high- and low-pressure alarms; (3) critically impaired gas exchange; and (4) high levels of auto-positive end-expiratory pressure (autoPEEP) a particular scenario that may provoke distress, alarming, or gas exchange failure.

The Distressed Patient

One of the first principles of dealing with the acutely distressed patient receiving mechanical ventilation is that either the ventilator or the patient may be the source of the distress. It is often helpful to bag ventilate the patient briefly in order to separate man from machine, potentially clarifying what is provoking the crisis. Possible machine-induced bases for the crisis include mechanical failure of the ventilator; disconnections of tubing (from source to ventilator or from ventilator to patient); endotracheal (or tracheostomy) tube malfunction, obstruction, or dislodgement; and ventilator settings that fail to match patient demands (most notably of inspiratory flow rate). Patient-related sources of distress include barotrauma; pain; myocardial ischemia; hypoxemia or hypercapnia; delirium; and anxiety.

The differential diagnosis is aided by a focused, 60-s examination, during which the patient should be bag ventilated by hand, with attention to endotracheal tube (position, patency, cuff integrity); evidence of pneumothorax (tracheal deviation; absence of breath sounds); oximetry; and vital signs. Generally, the respiratory therapist should attempt to provide ventilation sufficiently to suppress vigorous respiratory effort because this facilitates measurement of respiratory mechanical properties. Also, if bag ventilation calms the patient, the cause of distress is likely to be related to ventilator settings or function, rather than something intrinsic to the patient (such as pneumothorax or a distended urinary bladder). If the patient becomes calm, a return to machine ventilation may allow a careful measurement of respiratory mechanical properties, as detailed later, to provide further diagnostic information. If oximetry reveals new hypoxemia, both lung and circulatory function need further assessment, as discussed later.

Often, this brief, initial survey identifies the source of distress or narrows the list of possibilities sufficiently to suggest one of a few, discrete confirmatory tests. Other patients should have immediate blood gas analysis, bedside pleural ultrasound, chest radiography, and, in appropriate circumstances, ECG or other examinations.

Typically, the question of sedative administration arises from the onset of the crisis. An agitated patient presents an immediate threat to self and staff, and a sedative (occasionally to include a paralytic drug) may be just the right treatment, especially when pain or delirium is the fundamental problem. However, if agitation is merely signaling some underlying problem, a sedative may (at best) mask it or (at worst) unravel the patient's last efforts to compensate. Thus, sedative treatment must always be paired with an understanding of the cause of the crisis or with a continuing plan to solve it.

Barotrauma as the Basis for Crisis

Pneumothorax complicates approximately 3% of courses of mechanical ventilation, and most of these occur near the onset of ventilation,[1] especially in the first 24 h. Nevertheless, the risk persists even in patients receiving mechanical ventilation for weeks and, because this complication is both lethal and treatable, it should be considered in the evaluation of any distressed patient. Signs may include hemodynamic deterioration, tracheal shift, reduced chest wall movement and increased size on the affected side, a change in breath sounds, increased airway pressures (or, during pressure-preset modes of ventilation, reduced tidal volume [Vt]), and falling oxygen saturations. The sensitivity and specificity of all of these signs are unknown, so they cannot be relied on except in dire circumstances. Rather, confirmatory tests (ultrasonography or radiography) should be performed to confirm or refute the clinical impression.

Suboptimal Ventilator Settings and Patient-Ventilator Dyssynchrony

Ventilator settings may be guided by protocol (eg, to protect the lungs from overdistention) or may be tailored to achieve particular gas exchange goals. The settings achieved may or may not meet the patient's demand for flow rate, flow pattern, Vt, or minute ventilation ($\dot{V}E$). Alternatively, the settings may be adjusted primarily to attain comfort, at the cost of deleterious alveolar overdistention or autoPEEP. Most often, both comfort and safe ventilatory settings can coexist, but this often

requires sedation. Patients are at risk for distress, occasionally of crisis proportions, when sedation is interrupted or reduced, or when resolving illness allows a greater level of alertness. Evidence that ventilator settings are not meeting patient demand can be inferred readily by examining the flow and pressure waveforms. Specific examples follow.

Lung-Protective Ventilation in Acute Lung Injury/ARDS

Most patients with acute lung injury (ALI)/ARDS should receive ventilation with Vt levels of 6 mL/kg predicted body weight. At this Vt, a high respiratory rate is necessary to meet the demand for $\dot{V}E$. In the ARMA trial[2] (the Acute Respiratory Distress Syndrome Network trial of low Vt ventilation), the mean respiratory rate in the low-Vt group was 30 breaths/min, and some patients will need rates well in excess of this number. A common error in the patient with ALI is to set a low rate, such as 18 breaths/min, which may suffice in the initial hours when the patient is deeply sedated but will be insufficient on awakening. In that situation, sedative discontinuation may unmask the discrepancy between what is set and what is needed, provoking distress and agitation. This crisis can often be averted by attention to the airway pressure waveform by recognizing triggered breaths (especially double triggering), concavity of the inspiratory pressure rise, or breath-to-breath variability in pressure, as illustrated in Figure 1.

AutoPEEP and the Effort To Trigger

The presence of autoPEEP presents an inspiratory threshold load, making it difficult for the patient to trigger the ventilator. When the end-expiratory pressure greatly exceeds PEEP (as in severe airflow obstruction), the patient must exert sufficient effort to lower alveolar pressure from the autoPEEP level to the PEEP level (and further to trigger the ventilator). The work of triggering may be so high that the patient becomes distressed. This is apt to occur when ventilator rates are reduced, transitioning the patient from full ventilation (no need to trigger) to only partial support (must trigger) or, similarly, when sedatives

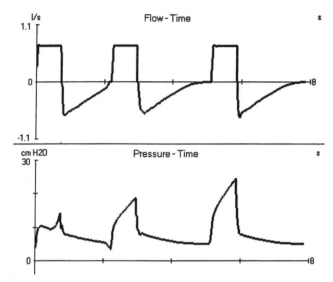

Figure 1. Airway pressure waveform with triggered breaths, concavity of the inspiratory pressure rise, and breath-to-breath variability in pressure.

are withdrawn. Recognizing this scenario entails knowing when it is likely to occur—in the patient with status asthmaticus or severe COPD exacerbation. Ventilator waveforms provide clues: end-expiratory flow, delayed triggering, and failed trigger efforts (Fig 2) all may signal the presence of autoPEEP. In passive patients, the end-expiratory port occlusion technique allows quantitation of its magnitude. One solution to the triggering difficulty of autoPEEP is to raise the PEEP level, which has the effect of reducing the inspiratory threshold load. It is worth emphasizing that changing the level of the pressure trigger, or shifting from pressure triggering to flow triggering, has no meaningful impact on the work of breathing.

Patient-Ventilator Dyssynchrony

Both examples given here involve patient-ventilator dyssynchrony, but a mismatch between the patient's desires and what the intensivist has ordered can arise in any patient receiving mechanical ventilation. Such a mismatch is often subclinical, rising to the level of crisis only when sedatives are withheld or the patient's ventilatory demand rises, such as during bathing or use of the bedpan. In both this setting and that previously described for ALI, sedating the patient again can "solve" the crisis, but a superior approach may be to adjust the ventilator instead. Patients at risk for clinically important dyssynchrony can often be identified by regular examination of ventilator waveforms, with attention to the signs exhibited in Figure 1.

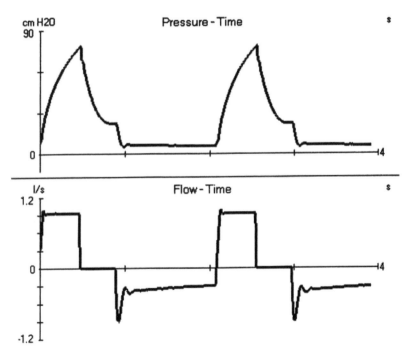

Figure 2. The end-expiratory flow is approximately 0.3 L/s (should be zero).

High Ventilator Pressure Alarm

During volume-preset modes of ventilation, the high-pressure alarm is one of the most useful clues to a new problem. At any point during inspiration, the pressure at the airway opening is the sum of pressures to (1) overcome the end-expiratory alveolar pressure (PEEP or autoPEEP); (2) drive flow across the inspiratory resistance; (3) distend the lungs and chest wall; and (4) counter any effect of expiratory muscles. Surely the most common cause of a high-pressure alarm is coughing or expiratory muscle activity during inspiration, a form of patient-ventilator dyssynchrony typically called *bucking*. Other reasons for the airway pressure to rise include biting, kinking, or occlusion of the endotracheal tube; bronchospasm; pulmonary edema; atelectasis; pneumothorax; and abdominal distention (Table 1). The basis for an elevated airway opening pressure may not be clear initially. A systematic approach to gaining useful physiologic information follows: (1) get the patient into a relatively passive state; (2) measure the peak airway pressure; (3) stop flow briefly at end-inspiration, measuring the plateau airway pressure; and (4) seek and quantitate autoPEEP.

Get the Patient Into a Passive State

Effort can greatly affect the airway pressure waveform (Fig 1), confounding the interpretation of respiratory mechanics, making it necessary that the patient become relatively passive. Many patients will already be passive as a result of illness, sedatives, paralytics, or high level of ventilator support. For those who are not, simple ventilator maneuvers (raising modestly the rate or V_T) may suffice. In others, additional sedatives would be necessary to accommodate them to the ventilator settings, and the intensivist must balance the gain from additional information against the adverse effects of sedation.

Measure the Peak and Plateau Airway Pressures

The peak airway pressure is found at end-inspiration and, in the passive patient, represents the sum of flow-related pressure, the pressure to distend lungs and chest wall, and pressure to overcome PEEP (or autoPEEP). A 0.3-s end-inspiratory pause stops flow, removing the flow-related component, so the airway pressure falls by an amount related to the flow resistance and the inspiratory flow rate. When the endotracheal tube is ≥ 7.5 and the flow is set at 60 L/min, the resistive pressure (peak pressure minus plateau pressure) is approximately 5 cm H_2O. The plateau pressure represents the sum of only the pressure to distend lungs and chest wall and the pressure to overcome PEEP.

Measure PEEP or AutoPEEP

When there is no autoPEEP, the end-expiratory pressure equals PEEP. Thus, the pressure to distend lungs and chest wall is the plateau airway pressure minus PEEP. The V_T divided by the pressure to distend lungs and chest wall is the static compliance of the respiratory system and has values normally between 70 and 100 mL/cm H_2O. The presence of autoPEEP is usually signaled by the presence of end-expiratory flow. Its magnitude can be found by stopping flow at end-expiration

Table 1. *Differential Diagnosis of Elevated Airway Opening Pressure*

Classification	Cause
Expiratory effort	Coughing, bucking
	Respiratory distress
Elevated resistive pressure	Endotracheal tube secretions, concretions
	Biting the endotracheal tube
	Bronchospasm
	Fixed airway obstruction
	Malignant or inflammatory airway masses
	Excessive inspiratory flow rate
Elevated plateau pressure due to lungs	Pulmonary edema
	Pulmonary fibrosis
	Atelectasis
	Acute lung injury/ARDS
	Severe pneumonia
	Lung cancer
Elevated plateau pressure due to chest wall	Abdominal compartment syndrome
	Massive obesity
	Pneumothorax
	Large pleural effusions
Elevated autoPEEP	Status asthmaticus
	Severe COPD
	Other obstruction or very high minute ventilation

and reading the pressure at the airway opening. Calculations of compliance must take autoPEEP into account.

By examining the airway pressure waveform and using a brief end-inspiratory pause, it becomes possible to narrow the differential diagnosis for high peak airway pressure into resistive causes, compliance-related causes, or (rarely) high autoPEEP. Moreover, by remeasuring these mechanical parameters following interventions, it becomes possible to determine the impact of the intervention.

Low Ventilator Pressure Alarm

Low-pressure alarms are uncommon and generally are due to leaks in the system (most often a disconnection between the wye connector and the endotracheal tube). A patient will rarely make so much effort as to suck the airway pressure below an alarming threshold. Leaks are readily evident with a brief bedside examination with attention to the endotracheal or tracheostomy tube, ventilator tubing, and (if present) chest tube.

Worsened Oxygenation

There are many potential explanations for acutely deteriorating oxygenation. These can be classified into three main groups: (1) a ventilator or interface problem; (2) worsened gas exchange in the lung; and (3) circulatory disruption. Many patients with severe lung derangement depend critically on the fraction of inspired oxygen (FIO_2), PEEP level, or some other inhaled gas (eg, nitric oxide or prostacyclin). Empty tanks, disconnected lines, dislodged endotracheal tubes, changes in PEEP, and various forms of ventilator malfunction may provoke acute hypoxemia.

Several forms of new or worsened lung gas exchange may present abruptly, including pulmonary edema, atelectasis, pneumothorax, pulmonary embolism, or rapid advancement of ARDS, alveolar hemorrhage, or pneumonia. At times, lung gas exchange deteriorates because of distress or increased work of breathing, without requiring any fundamental change in lung function. These conditions are most likely to follow reductions in level of sedation or some new stimulus provoking agitation. It is often useful to get the patient into a passive state and then remeasure respiratory mechanical properties to gain insight into the crisis. Bedside ultrasound testing can also be revealing[3] and is more quickly available than a portable chest radiograph (although this, too, may be useful). With this approach, many patients can be managed comfortably without performing helical CT angiography to exclude pulmonary embolism.

Finally, in patients with diseased lungs, the arterial oxyhemoglobin saturation depends, in part, on the venous oxyhemoglobin saturation. This, in turn, is a function of oxygen delivery and systemic consumption. Thus, a crippled circulation can reveal itself as worsened oxygenation. Measuring the central venous saturation (or otherwise assessing the circulation) may be useful.

When hypoxemia is severe and the FIO_2 is > 0.6, concerns arise regarding oxygen toxicity. The threshold for oxygen toxicity in humans is unknown. Further, diseased lungs and those already exposed to moderate increased oxygen may be relatively resistant to high fractions. Nevertheless, common practice stresses an attempt to get the FIO_2 to ≤ 0.6 within 24 h. Several maneuvers can help accomplish this. First, efforts should be made to accommodate the ventilator to the patient's demand or to sedate the patient to accept the ventilator settings. A trial of PEEP or recruitment maneuvers may show the capacity to open additional alveoli. Other ventilator tactics, such as high-frequency or inverse-ratio ventilation, have been tried as salvage measures. Prone positioning is often helpful in improving oxygenation, although, as with high-frequency ventilation, no effect on mortality or other relevant clinical outcomes has been demonstrated. Using the dependence of arterial saturation on venous saturation to advantage, measures to raise cardiac output or arterial oxygen content or to reduce oxygen consumption may be useful. Inhaled gases that redistribute blood flow, such as inhaled nitric oxide or prostacyclin, can raise arterial saturation and favor a reduction in oxygen fraction. Finally, it is surprising how often simply turning the FIO_2 down leads to little deterioration in saturation (recall that large shunts are relatively refractory to oxygen, both increased and decreased). This, combined with lowering the target for arterial saturation (eg, there is little reason to think that maintaining an arterial oxygen saturation of 0.92 is superior to 0.88), often allows a prompt reduction in FIO_2.

Worsening Hypercapnia

A rising PCO_2 can be explained by referring to the determinants of the arterial PCO_2, including the carbon dioxide production rate, dead space fraction, and $\dot{V}E$. An increase in the PCO_2 implies that more carbon dioxide is being produced (eg, fever, seizure, overfeeding), the dead space fraction is up (eg, higher PEEP, hypovolemia, pulmonary embolism), or $\dot{V}E$ has fallen (lower VT or rate). Examining trends in ventilator parameters, hemodynamic values, and other vital sign and laboratory data may be useful. Sometimes simply increasing the $\dot{V}E$ is sufficient to normalize the PCO_2 while the underlying problem is addressed. However, many patients receiving mechanical ventilation and who have hypercapnia have such profound lung derangement that raising the $\dot{V}E$ may be ineffective (eg, when the consequence is to raise autoPEEP, boosting the dead space fraction, and preventing any fall in PCO_2) or harmful (as when the acutely injured lung is overstretched or the dynamically inflated lung is further hyperinflated).

At the same time, it is worth emphasizing that hypercapnia is generally well tolerated in the adequately sedated patient.[4] Multiple studies[4] examining permissive hypercapnia have shown that the physiologic effects are modest and generally transient.In particular, BP and cardiac output are not depressed by hypercapnia. The tolerability of elevated PCO_2 is less certain when there is active myocardial ischemia, severe pulmonary hypertension, raised intracranial pressure, or pregnancy. Evaluation of the patient with worsening hypercapnia should focus on the endotracheal tube; ventilator settings; central drive to breathe; evidence of new or worsened systemic inflammation; radiographic changes; magnitude of autoPEEP; the intravascular volume state; and the end-tidal carbon dioxide trend.

High Levels of AutoPEEP

Persistent end-expiratory flow signals the presence of autoPEEP. In passive patients, the magnitude of autoPEEP can be quantitated with an end-expiratory port occlusion. The maneuver closes the inspiratory and expiratory limbs of the ventilator at the time that the subsequent breath is due, allowing equilibration of pressure between lung and ventilator, a pressure that can be displayed graphically.

High levels of autoPEEP are potentially harmful because they risk hypoperfusion[5] and pneumothorax. Further, a major component of the work of breathing in the severely obstructed patient is the inspiratory threshold load presented by autoPEEP. This load can be counterbalanced by externally applied PEEP, explaining the dramatic benefit of continuous positive airway pressure in patients with severe airflow obstruction. It is also appropriate to use PEEP in the intubated and ventilated patient with status asthmaticus (or COPD) for the same reason. As long as the PEEP is set at approximately $< 85\%$ of the autoPEEP, there is little to fear from further hyperinflation. Because most patients receiving mechanical ventilation tend to trigger the ventilator, PEEP should always be used. This is especially true when sedation (or paralysis) is reduced.

When autoPEEP is high, the two most important approaches to reducing it are to ease the airflow obstruction and to limit the $\dot{V}E$. For an average-sized adult, an initial $\dot{V}E$ of approximately 8 L/min (achieved by a VT between 5 and 7 mL/kg and a respiratory rate of 14 breaths/min), combined with an inspiratory flow rate of 60 L/min, is a good starting point. After making these settings (and assuming the patient is adequately sedated), the degree of lung hyperinflation should be measured. Reasonable targets are autoPEEP < 15 cm H_2O and plateau pressure < 30 cm H_2O. Occasional patients can be severely hyperinflated with low measured autoPEEP because of completely trapped, noncommunicating areas of obstructed gas.[6] Once the $\dot{V}E$ is set at a reasonable level, such as 8 L/min, further reductions in rate have only a very small impact on autoPEEP.[7]

Heliox may also be administered during mechanical ventilation and is effective in reducing autoPEEP, but many practical problems arise. The flowmeters on the ventilator that measure VT depend on gas density and will underestimate VT during heliox administration unless recalibrated. Thus, the benefit of diminished airway resistance may be confounded by adjustments of $\dot{V}_E$ upward if this phenomenon is not appreciated. Before a heliox ventilator is used, it should be validated in a lung model by the respiratory therapists and physicians who will use it clinically. A useful device is a simple spirometer on the expiratory port of the ventilator to confirm V_T during adjustments of heliox.

As long as inspiratory flow is not unusually low (or decelerating), there is little to be gained by increasing it further. To illustrate this point, consider the consequences of the following ventilator settings: V_T, 500 mL; respiratory rate, 15 breaths/ min; and peak inspiratory flow rate, 60 L/min. These settings result in an inspiratory time of 0.5 s and an expiratory time of 3.5 s. Raising the inspiratory flow rate dramatically (and unrealistically) to 120 L/min shortens inspiratory time to 0.25 s, but increases expiratory time only from 3.5 to 3.75 s, a trivial gain. On the other hand, simply lowering the respiratory rate from 15 to 14 breaths/min (without changing the flow rate or V_T) increases expiratory time to 3.8 s. When the goal is to reduce hyperinflation, it is generally more effective to reduce $\dot{V}_E$ than to change any other ventilator setting.

Hypotension Following Intubation

Postintubation hypotension in patients with severe airflow obstruction is extremely common. Causative factors are pulmonary hyperinflation, hypovolemia, and sedation. The degree of pulmonary hyperinflation is directly proportional to $\dot{V}_E$. Dangerous levels of pulmonary hyperinflation can develop if patients are "bagged" excessively in a misguided attempt to stabilize or resuscitate. With severe airflow obstruction, delivery of even a normal $\dot{V}_E$ may impair the circulation. Clinically, inspired breaths become difficult to deliver (as there is essentially no room for additional air), breath sounds are diminished, and neck veins are distended. Systemic BP and pulse pressure fall, and the pulse rate increases. In the same patients, hypovolemia related to previous dehydration, sedation, and muscle relaxation all act to decrease mean systemic vascular pressure, further decreasing venous return to the heart. This pathophysiology can be demonstrated by ceasing ventilation

temporarily: mean intrathoracic pressure falls and, within 30 to 60 s, BP rises, and heart rate falls. The treatment is augmentation of intravascular volume combined with strategies to minimize lung hyperinflation (see previous discussion). Note that the clinical features of pulmonary hyperinflation mimic tension pneumothorax; and indeed, if cessation of ventilation does not remedy the hypotension, pneumothorax should be excluded or treated empirically (bilateral chest tubes). Just as important, chest tubes should not be inserted in unstable patients until there has been a trial of hypoventilation.

References

1. Anzueto A, Frutos-Vivar F, Esteban A, et al. Incidence, risk factors and outcome of barotrauma in mechanically ventilated patients. Intensive Care Med 2004; Feb 28 [Epub ahead of print]

2. The Acute Respiratory Distress Syndrome Network. Ventilation with lower tidal volumes as compared with traditional tidal volumes for acute lung injury and the acute respiratory distress syndrome. N Engl J Med 2000; 342:1301–1308

3. Lichtenstein DA, Meziere GA. Diagnosis of acute respiratory failure: the BLUE protocol. Chest 2008; Apr 10 [Epub ahead of print]

4. Thorens JB, Jolliet P, Ritz M, et al. Effects of rapid permissive hypercapnia on hemodynamics, gas exchange, and oxygen transport and consumption during mechanical ventilation for the acute respiratory distress syndrome. Intensive Care Med 1996; 22:182–191

5. Tuxen DV, Lane S. The effects of ventilatory pattern on hyperinflation, airway pressures, and circulation in mechanical ventilation of patients with severe air-flow obstruction. Am Rev Respir Dis 1987; 136:872–879

6. Leatherman JW, Ravenscraft SA. Low measured auto-positive end-expiratory pressure during mechanical ventilation of patients with severe asthma: hidden auto-positive end-expiratory pressure. Crit Care Med 1996; 24:541–546

7. Leatherman JW, McArthur C, Shapiro RS. Effect of prolongation of expiratory time on dynamic hyperinflation in mechanically ventilated patients with severe asthma. Crit Care Med 2004; 32:1542–1545

Notes

Poisonings and Overdoses

Janice L. Zimmerman, MD, FCCP

Objectives:

- Describe physical examination and laboratory findings suggestive of intoxications
- Outline measures for the resuscitation and stabilization of the overdose patient
- Discuss the use of interventions to decrease absorption of poisons and enhance elimination
- Review indicated interventions and antidotes for poisons and substances of abuse likely to be encountered in the ICU
- Describe management of ethanol and narcotic withdrawal syndromes

Key words: antidotes; overdose; poisoning; substance abuse; toxicology

---

Intentional and accidental poisonings and substance abuse can result in the need for critical care. In many cases, only supportive care is necessary until the effects of the toxin diminish. However, some poisonings require specific antidotes or interventions to decrease morbidity and mortality. General management principles of poisonings and substance abuse that are pertinent to intensive care management are presented, as well as interventions for specific overdoses and withdrawal syndromes that the intensivist is likely to encounter. Little evidence-based information is available; current recommendations are based on animal data, volunteer studies, case reports, pharmacologic data, and/or consensus opinion.

Clinical Presentation

Patients with possible overdose may be asymptomatic or present with life-threatening toxicities. The absence of symptoms on the initial examination does not preclude potential deterioration and the development of more severe symptoms. Life-threatening toxicities that often require intensive management include coma, seizures, respiratory depression, hypoxemia, arrhythmias, hypotension, hypertension, and metabolic acidosis.

Diagnosis

The diagnosis of the exact substance involved in an overdose or poisoning does not take precedence over the resuscitation and stabilization of the patient (see the "Management" section). However, the initial evaluation of the patient may identify characteristic signs and symptoms that will enable the physician to make a specific diagnosis quickly and/or assist in directing optimal therapy.

History

Accurate information regarding the substance ingested, the quantity taken, and the time of ingestion should be collected, if possible. Establishing the time of ingestion is important to assess the significance of presenting symptoms. It is also helpful to identify the form of the drug involved (*ie*, regular or sustained-release) and the chronicity of use. Drugs that may be accessible to the patient should be determined.

Physical Examination

Vital signs and the neurologic examination findings are particularly helpful in the initial evaluation of a patient. Tables 1 and 2 list drugs that are associated with changes in vital signs and with neurologic alterations. BP may not be helpful in determining the toxin because of other systemic influences. Tachypnea is also fairly nonspecific and may be a compensatory response to metabolic acidosis or hypoxemia. Although the initial neurologic examination may be pertinent, it is also important to follow changes in neurologic function over time. The evaluation should include an assessment of level of consciousness, pupillary reactivity, ocular movements, and motor responses. Hypoactive bowel sounds may be associated with narcotic or anticholinergic agents, and hyperactive bowel sounds may result from poisoning with organophosphates.

Table 1. *Clues to Diagnosis in Poisoning: Vital Signs*

Vital Sign	Increased	Decreased
BP	Amphetamines/cocaine Anticholinergics Caffeine Ephedrine Sympathomimetics	Antihypertensives Cyanide Cyclic antidepressants Ethanol Narcotics Organophosphates/carbamates Sedative/hypnotics Barbiturates
Heart rate	Amphetamines/cocaine Anticholinergics Carbon monoxide Cyanide Cyclic antidepressants Ethanol Sympathomimetics Theophylline	β-Blockers Calcium channel blockers Cholinergics Digitalis glycosides GHB Sedative/hypnotics Organophosphates/carbamates
Respiratory rate	Amphetamines Anticholinergics Carbon monoxide Hydrocarbons Organophosphates/carbamates Salicylates Theophylline	Alcohols Barbiturates GHB Narcotics Sedative/hypnotics
Temperature	Amphetamines/cocaine Anticholinergics β-Blockers Cyclic antidepressants Salicylates Sympathomimetics Theophylline	Barbiturates Carbon monoxide Ethanol Hypoglycemic agents Narcotics Sedative/hypnotics

Table 2. *Clues to Diagnosis in Poisoning: Neurologic Findings*

Neurolgic Findings	Substances Ingested
Pupils pinpoint (miotic)	Barbiturates (late) Cholinergics Narcotics (except meperidine) Organophosphates Phenothiazine Phencyclidine
Pupils dilated (mydriatic)	Alcohol Anticholinergics Antihistamines Barbiturates Ethanol Meperidine Phenytoin Sympathomimetics
Nystagmus	Alcohols Carbamazepine Carbon monoxide Phencyclidine Phenytoin Sedative/hypnotics
Seizures	Amphetamines Anticholinergics Carbon monoxide Cocaine Cyanide Cyclic antidepressants GHB Isoniazid Lithium Organophosphates Phencyclidine Phenothiazines Salicylates Strychnine Theophylline

Toxidromes

Findings on physical examination may enable the physician to categorize the poisoning into a classic "toxidrome," or clinical syndrome of poisoning. This classification may allow the physician to direct the diagnostic evaluation and define appropriate therapy (Table 3).

Laboratory Examination

The effective use of laboratory data supplements the history and physical examination findings. An arterial blood gas measurement will detect hypoxemia, hypercarbia, and significant acid-base disorders. In combination with electrolytes, a significant anion-gap metabolic acidosis may be diagnosed. The detection of an osmolal gap (*ie*, >10 mosm) through comparison of the measured osmolality with calculated osmolality

$$(2 \times \text{Sodium} + \text{Glucose} / 18) + (\text{BUN} / 2.8)$$

may indicate the presence of methanol, ethanol, ethylene glycol, acetone, or isopropyl alcohol. An ECG should be obtained in unstable patients and when cardiotoxic drug ingestion is suspected.

Qualitative toxicology screens are performed on urine samples. These tests report only the presence or absence of a substance or class of drugs and

Table 3. *Toxidromes*

Poisoning Syndrome	Symptoms
Cholinergic (SLUDGE syndrome)	Salivation, bronchorrhea, lacrimation, urination, defecation, GI upset, and emesis; also, bradycardia, fasciculations, confusion, and miosis
Anticholinergic	Dry skin, hyperthermia, mydriasis, tachycardia, delirium, thirst, and urinary retention
Sympathomimetic	Hypertension, tachycardia, seizures, CNS excitation, mydriasis, and diaphoresis
Narcotic	Miosis, respiratory depression, depressed level of consciousness, hypotension, and hyporeflexia
Sedative/hypnotic	Depressed level of consciousness, respiratory depression, hypotension, and hyporeflexia

are limited by the testing available at an institution. Qualitative toxicology screens are helpful in evaluating coma of unknown cause, distinguishing between toxicosis and psychosis, and (rarely) choosing a specific antidote. Qualitative test results seldom change the initial management of poisoned patients. Quantitative analyses provide serum levels of a substance and may direct specific therapies in selected cases. Quantitative levels that may be useful to obtain include those for acetaminophen, carbamazepine, carboxyhemoglobin, ethanol, metha-nol, ethylene glycol, theophylline, phenytoin, lithium, salicylates, barbiturates, digoxin, valproic acid, and cyclic antidepressants. Cyclic antidepressant levels confirm antidepressant ingestion, but the levels correlate poorly with toxicity.

Management

Resuscitation and Stabilization

The initial priorities in management of poisoned patients are airway, breathing, and circulation. Intubation may be necessary to support oxygenation and ventilation or to protect the airway. Hypotension from toxins is more commonly due to venous pooling than to myocardial depression and should be treated initially with isotonic fluids, rather than vasopressor agents. Oxygen should be routinely administered to the poisoning victim, pending an assessment of oxygenation by arterial blood gas measurement or pulse oximetry.

In the patient with a depressed level of consciousness, the following additional interventions should be considered:

- 50% glucose (25 to 50 g);
- Thiamine (100 mg IV);

- Naloxone (0.4 to 2 mg IV), especially with classic findings of miosis and respiratory depression; and
- Flumazenil therapy is not routinely recommended. Consider its administration in patients who have a clinical course compatible with a sedative overdose; however, it is contraindicated in patients with known overdoses of cyclic antidepressants and in long-term users of benzodiazepine because of the risk of seizures.

Nonspecific Therapy

After stabilization, nonspecific interventions may be considered to decrease absorption of the toxin from the GI tract or to enhance elimination. GI decontamination can be attempted with gastric-emptying procedures (*ie*, induced emesis and gastric lavage), adsorption of drugs (*ie*, activated charcoal therapy), and increasing transit through the GI tract (*ie*, administration of cathartic agents or whole-bowel irrigation).

Induced Emesis: Induced emesis with ipecac is not recommended in adults or children. Ipecac is effective in inducing vomiting but is not necessarily effective in recovering toxins. Contraindications to the use of ipecac include hydrocarbon or corrosive ingestion, absent gag reflex, depressed mental status, a risk for CNS depression or seizures, and pregnancy. Potential complications include aspiration pneumonitis, Mallory-Weiss tear, and protracted emesis that delays the use of activated charcoal.

Gastric Lavage: Gastric lavage is performed in the adult with a 36F to 40F tube inserted orally. Lavage is performed with aliquots of 100 to 200 mL of normal saline solution or water. There are no definite indications for use of gastric lavage because of the lack of confirmed benefit. Current recommendations suggest that gastric lavage should not be used routinely and should be considered only in cases of life-threatening ingestion when lavage can be instituted within 1 h of ingestion. The airway must be protected in patients with a depressed level of consciousness. Lavage is contraindicated in acid or alkali ingestions because of possible esophageal perforation and in the presence of a severe bleeding diathesis. Complications of lavage include aspiration pneumonitis, esophageal perforation, and cardiovascular instability.

Activated Charcoal: Activated charcoal is probably the best intervention for orally ingested poisons. The greatest benefit occurs if charcoal is administered within the first hour after ingestion. The current recommendations for decreasing GI absorption of toxins emphasize the use of activated charcoal despite the lack of proven benefit. The appropriate dose of charcoal (1 g/kg) may be administered by an orogastric or nasogastric tube if patient cooperation is limited. Substances not adsorbed by activated charcoal include iron, lithium, cyanide, strong acids or bases, alcohols, and hydrocarbons. The only contraindication to the use of charcoal is known or suspected GI perforation.

Cathartics: Cathartic agents have been routinely administered with charcoal, based on the assumption that they decrease GI transit time, help to limit drug absorption, and serve as an adjunct to charcoal therapy. However, there is no evidence of efficacy. Sorbitol is the most commonly used cathartic. Care must be taken with very young and elderly patients because electrolyte abnormalities can ensue due to diarrhea.

Whole-Bowel Irrigation: Whole-bowel irrigation involves large volumes of polyethylene glycol electrolyte solution administered over time (1 to 2 L/h in adults) to mechanically cleanse the bowel. This method has been suggested for the treatment of ingested substances that are not adsorbed by activated charcoal (*eg*, iron and lithium), ingestions of sustained-release or enteric-coated products, and ingestions of illicit drug packets. This method may not be practical for many patients; further study is required to determine whether there is any benefit in cases of toxic ingestion.

Contraindications to this intervention include ileus, GI obstruction or perforation, hemodynamic instability, and intractable vomiting. CNS or respiratory depression and the inability to cooperate are relative contraindications.

Enhanced Elimination: Measures to increase the elimination of toxic substances attempt to use the normal detoxification mechanisms performed by the liver and kidney. Multiple doses of charcoal for the elimination of drugs with an enterohepatic circulation may have the greatest potential utility. This technique may be helpful in poisonings with barbiturates, carbamazepine, quinine, dapsone, and theophylline. Although multiple doses of charcoal have been used in the treatment of poisonings with cyclic antidepressants, digoxin, and phenytoin, proof of effectiveness is lacking. The dosing regimen has not been standardized, but currently < 12.5 g/h or an equivalent amount at other intervals is not recommended. Smaller doses administered more frequently may decrease the occurrence of vomiting. Repeat doses of charcoal should not contain a cathartic. Adequate gastric emptying must be assured before the administration of a subsequent dose.

Forced diuresis to accelerate the renal excretion of drugs has little clinical effect and may predispose the patient to volume overload. Alkaline diuresis is effective in promoting the elimination of barbiturates, primidone, and salicylates. Sodium bicarbonate (88 to 132 mEq) can be added to 1 L of dextrose 5% in a water solution; the rate of administration should be determined by the patient's ability to handle the fluid load and the maintenance of urine pH at >7. Hypokalemia is likely and requires correction to achieve urinary alkalinization. Acidification of urine has been proposed for the treatment of ingestions involving phencyclidine, strychnine, amphetamines, and quinine. However, the metabolic consequences of acidification weigh against any clinical usefulness of this measure. Dialysis is an invasive method of eliminating toxins and may be considered for life-threatening ingestions involving water-soluble substances of low molecular weight. Substances in drug overdoses for which dialysis may be beneficial include alcohols, amphetamines, phenobarbital, lithium, salicylates, theophylline, and thiocyanate. Hemoperfusion is useful in eliminating the same compounds that are dialyzable and involves the passing of blood through a filtering device that contains charcoal or a synthetic resin as an absorbent. Charcoal hemoperfusion may be helpful in the elimination of carbamazepine, phenobarbital, phenytoin, theophylline, and valproate. Hemodialysis and hemoperfusion are efficient methods of removing poisons but are costly, require trained personnel, and may be associated with complications. The use of continuous arteriovenous or venovenous hemoperfusion in the treatment of poisonings has been reported on a limited basis.

Specific Therapy

Although the management of many toxic ingestions involves only the nonspecific therapy previously outlined, ingestions of some toxins have specific interventions or antidotes. Table 4 lists toxins and their respective antidotes. Specific poisonings are discussed in detail in the following section. Attention should be directed to managing those poisonings that most frequently result in death, as follows: analgesics, sedatives and hypnotics, narcotics, antidepressants, stimulants and street drugs, cardiovascular drugs, and alcohols.

Specific Drug Poisonings

Acetaminophen

Knowledge of the appropriate management of acetaminophen ingestions is important to prevent significant toxicity and mortality. Acetaminophen levels should be obtained in all multiple-drug overdoses ≥ 4 h after ingestion. For single acute ingestions, the Rumack-Matthew nomogram determines the need for N-acetylcysteine (NAC) therapy if the level plots above the "possible hepatic toxicity" line. The oral regimen for NAC therapy includes a loading dose of 140 mg/kg followed by 17 oral maintenance doses of 70 mg/kg administered 4 h apart. A nasogastric tube may be placed for its administration, and antiemetic therapy is often needed to control vomiting. If the patient vomits the loading dose or any maintenance dose within 1 h of administration, the dose should be repeated. IV NAC is administered as a loading dose of 150 mg/kg over 15 min followed by 50 mg/kg

Table 4. *Antidotes and Interventions for Specific Toxins*

Toxin	Antidote or Intervention
Acetaminophen	NAC
Amphetamines	Benzodiazepines
Arsenic/mercury/ gold/lead	Dimercaprol
Benzodiazepines	Flumazenil
β-Blocker	Glucagon, calcium (?), and pacing
Calcium channel blocker	Calcium, glucagon, and pacing
Carbon monoxide	100% oxygen and hyperbaric oxygen
Coumarin derivatives	Vitamin K1
Cyanide	Nitrites, thiosulfate, and hydroxocobalamin
Cyclic antidepressants	Blood alkalinization, alpha agonists
Digoxin	Digoxin-specific Fab fragments
Ethylene glycol	Ethanol, fomepizole
Heparin	Protamine
Oral hypoglycemic agents/insulin	Glucose 50%, somatostatin
Iron	Deferoxamine
Isoniazid	Pyridoxine
Lithium	Hemodialysis
Methanol	Ethanol, fomepizole
Narcotics	Naloxone
Nitrites	Methylene blue
Organophosphates/ carbamates	Atropine and pralidoxime
Salicylates	Urinary alkalinization, hemodialysis
Theophylline	Multiple-dose charcoal, hemoperfusion

infused over 4 h and then 100 mg/kg infused over 16 h. Anaphylactoid reactions may occur in 14 to 18% of patients with IV NAC administration. NAC serves as a substitute for glutathione, which normally metabolizes toxic metabolites of acetaminophen. Activated charcoal adsorbs acetaminophen and many coingestants. Charcoal interferes only slightly with the effectiveness of oral NAC, and the dose of NAC does not require adjustment. NAC is most effective when administered in the first 8 h following ingestion but is recommended up to 24 h after a significant toxic ingestion. It is also reasonable to administer NAC >24 h after ingestion if toxic levels of acetaminophen are present. The late administration of NAC may also be beneficial in patients with fulminant hepatic failure due to acetaminophen toxicity.

There are no firm guidelines for the administration of NAC in chronic ingestions or multiple ingestions over time. A marker of toxicity that may be useful is the evaluation of aspartate aminotransferase and alanine aminotransferase. If enzyme levels are elevated at the time of presentation (ie, >50 IU/L) or the acetaminophen level is >10 µg/mL (66 µmol/L), a course of NAC should be strongly considered. Treatment is continued until the transaminases are stable or decreasing and the acetaminophen level is <10 µg/mL. The local poison control center should be contacted for other NAC regimens, such as shorter courses of therapy. Recommendations for the management of extended-release forms of acetaminophen include the determination of acetaminophen levels 4 and 8 h after ingestion, and the initiation of NAC therapy if either level is potentially toxic.

Alcohols

Ethylene glycol and methanol ingestions can result in significant morbidity and mortality. Clinical manifestations, metabolic derangements, and management are similar for the ingestion of both alcohols.

Cardiopulmonary and neurologic symptoms may include pulmonary edema, hypotension, ataxia, seizures, and coma. Abdominal pain, nausea, and vomiting are frequent. Visual disturbances (eg, blurred vision, photophobia, blindness, and optic disk hyperemia) suggest methanol toxicity, and the finding of urinary calcium oxalate crystals may indicate ethylene glycol ingestion. Significant symptoms may be delayed for up to 24 h after methanol ingestion. Both ingestions are classically characterized by an anion-gap metabolic acidosis and an osmolal gap. An anion-gap metabolic acidosis may not be present initially if sufficient time has not elapsed for metabolizing to toxic acids or if high levels of ethanol prevent the metabolism of other alcohols. An osmolal gap may not be present in late presentations if the alcohol has already been metabolized to acid. Many institutions are unable to provide blood levels of methanol or ethylene glycol in a timely manner, and treatment is initiated based on the clinical history and acid-base status.

Treatment of ethylene glycol and methanol ingestion includes the following:

- Maintenance of a secure airway;
- Gastric lavage may be considered within 1 h of ingestion;
- Activated charcoal, if other substances have potentially been ingested (activated charcoal does not adsorb alcohols);
- 50% glucose if indicated;
- Thiamine, folate, and multivitamin supplement;
- Folinic acid (leucovorin, 50 mg) can be administered every 4 to 6 h for 24 h in cases of methanol ingestion to provide the cofactor for formic acid elimination;
- Hydration to maintain urine output;
- Ethanol orally or IV to maintain blood levels at 100 to 150 mg/dL (ethanol is preferentially metabolized by alcohol dehydrogenase). A loading dose is followed by a maintenance infusion;
- Fomepizole (4-methylpyrazole), an inhibitor of alcohol dehydrogenase that does not cause CNS depression, may substitute for ethanol;
- Hemodialysis for visual impairment, renal failure, pulmonary edema, significant or refractory acidosis, a methanol or ethylene glycol level of >25 mg/dL; and
- Bicarbonate administration for the treatment of acidosis is advocated by some clinicians.

Isopropyl alcohol is more potent than ethanol and results in similar manifestations at lower doses. The intoxication of hospitalized patients by the ingestion of hand sanitizers that contain isopropyl alcohol in concentrations of >60% has been reported. Isopropyl alcohol ingestions are characterized by an osmolal gap and ketonemia/ketonuria but no metabolic acidosis. Treatment is supportive and may require intubation and mechanical ventilation for the treatment of respiratory depression. Hemodialysis is reserved for evidence of hypoperfusion and failure to respond to supportive therapy.

Amphetamines/Methamphetamines

Amphetamines, methamphetamines, and related agents cause the release of catecholamines, which results in a sympathomimetic toxidrome that is characterized by tachycardia, hyperthermia, agitation, hypertension, and mydriasis.

Hallucinations (visual and tactile) and acute psychosis are frequently observed. Acute adverse consequences include myocardial ischemia and arrhythmias, seizures, intracranial hemorrhage, stroke, rhabdomyolysis, renal failure, necrotizing vasculitis, and death. The long-term use of these drugs can result in dilated cardiomyopathy.

Methamphetamine hydrochloride in a crystalline form called "ice," "crank," or "crystal" is popular in this class of drugs. It can be orally ingested, smoked, insufflated nasally, or injected IV. An amphetamine-like drug, 3-4-methylenedioxymethamphetamine, is a designer drug that is associated with "rave" parties. It is commonly known as "ecstasy," "XTC," "E," and "MDMA," and acts as a stimulant and hallucinogen. It increases the release of serotonin and inhibits serotonin reuptake in the brain. Bruxism and jaw clenching are clues to the use of ecstasy. Complications are usually a result of drug effects and nonstop physical activity. Hyponatremia and liver injury progressing to fulminant failure have also been reported.

The management of amphetamine intoxication is primarily supportive. Gastric lavage has little role as absorption after oral ingestion is usually complete at the time of presentation. The patient should be carefully assessed for complications, including measuring core temperature, obtaining an ECG, and evaluating laboratory data for evidence of renal dysfunction and rhabdomyolysis. IV hydration for possible rhabdomyolysis is warranted in individuals with known exertional activities pending the measurement of creatine phosphokinase levels. Benzodiazepines, often in high doses, are useful for the control of agitation.

Benzodiazepines

Benzodiazepine overdoses rarely result in death unless other sedating drugs (*eg*, alcohol or narcotics) are also ingested. Overdose results in a typical sedative-hypnotic toxidrome that is characterized by a depressed level of consciousness, respiratory depression, hyporeflexia, and, potentially, hypotension and bradycardia. Alprazolam is one of the most common benzodiazepines found in overdose cases and may result in greater toxicity. Flunitrazepam is a potent benzodiazepine that is banned in the United States and is associated with rape. It may not be detected by most urine drug screens.

Benzodiazepine ingestions should be managed according to the clinical presentation of the patient. Activated charcoal is the primary method of GI decontamination for recent ingestion. Supportive care with intubation and mechanical ventilation may be needed for patients with significant toxicity. Hypotension should be treated initially with volume infusion. A benzodiazepine-receptor antagonist, flumazenil, is available as a diagnostic tool and for adjunctive treatment. Flumazenil should not be considered a substitute for intubation in patients with significant respiratory depression. Its use is contraindicated in patients with suspected cyclic antidepressant overdoses and in patients who are physically dependent on benzodiazepines, because of the risk of seizures. The initial dose of flumazenil is 0.2 mg over an interval of 30 s, followed by doses of 0.3 and 0.5 mg every minute up to a maximum cumulative dose of 3 mg. A flumazenil dose > 1 mg is usually not required. Resedation is likely due to the short half-life of flumazenil (0.7 to 1.3 h) compared with benzodiazepines.

β-Blockers

β-Adrenergic blockers produce toxicity primarily through bradycardia and hypotension, although a depressed level of consciousness may occur with lipid-soluble agents (*eg*, propranolol, timolol, metoprolol, and acebutolol). Hypotension often results from negative inotropic effects rather than bradycardia. Glucagon is considered to be the initial drug of choice because it produces chronotropic and inotropic effects and does not act via β-receptors. An initial dose of 2 to 5 mg of glucagon is given IV, and an infusion of 2 to 10 mg/h can be initiated, adjusted for desired clinical effects, and then tapered over 12 h as indicated. The goal of treatment is an improvement in BP and perfusion rather than an increase in heart rate. Transcutaneous pacing and transvenous pacing may be considered in patients who are refractory to treatment with glucagon. Additional drugs that have had variable efficacy in β-blocker overdoses include atropine, epinephrine, isoproterenol, and dopamine. Treatment with phosphodiesterase inhibitors such as milrinone, intraaortic balloon pump, or cardiopulmonary bypass may be considered if there is no response to the usual interventions. In some cases, therapy with calcium and insulin euglycemia (see later discussion for dosing) has been reported to be beneficial.

Calcium Channel Blockers

A diagnosis of calcium channel blocker overdose should be considered in the hypotensive, bradycardic patient, particularly if there is a history of use of antihypertensive agents. In the presence of hemodynamic instability, 10 mL of 10% calcium chloride should be administered IV. Calcium is effective in reversing negative inotropic effects and conduction abnormalities in approximately 50% of cases of overdose. Higher doses of calcium and continuous infusions may be required for beneficial effects, and ionized calcium levels should be monitored in these patients. As in β-blocker overdoses, glucagon therapy may have beneficial effects. Transcutaneous and transvenous pacing are additional options in refractory cases. Successful treatment has also been reported with amrinone and insulin euglycemia (insulin, 0.1 to 10 U/kg/h; and glucose, 10 to 75 g/h).

Carbon Monoxide

Carbon monoxide is a colorless, odorless gas that has 240 times greater affinity for hemoglobin as oxygen. Carboxyhemoglobin reduces the oxygen-carrying capacity and shifts the oxyhemoglobin dissociation curve to the left. Carbon monoxide also exerts direct cellular toxic effects. The clinical manifestations of carbon monoxide poisoning are nonspecific. The most common findings are headache, dizziness, and nausea; more severe exposure can result in chest pain, disorientation, seizures, coma, dyspnea, weakness, arrhythmias, and hypotension. Although the diagnosis of carbon monoxide poisoning is confirmed by an increased venous or arterial carboxyhemoglobin level, decisions for aggressive therapy with 100% oxygen should be based primarily on a clinical history that is suggestive of exposure. High-flow oxygen therapy or intubation with the administration of 100% oxygen should be initiated as soon as possible while confirmatory tests are performed. An ECG, chest radiograph, and arterial blood gas measurement

should be obtained to assess the severity of toxicity. The finding of metabolic acidosis implies significant exposure with inadequate oxygen availability at the tissue level. The use of hyperbaric oxygen in the setting of carbon monoxide poisoning is debated but may be considered for any patient with a depressed level of consciousness, loss of consciousness, neurologic findings other than headache, cardiac ischemia or arrhythmia, carboxyhemoglobin level of >25 to 40%, or persistent symptoms after normobaric oxygen treatment for 4 to 6 h. Hyperbaric oxygen may decrease the incidence of postexposure cognitive deficits.

Cocaine

Significant morbidity and mortality are associated with cocaine use by all routes, including nasal insufflation, IV administration, smoking, and oral ingestion. Toxicities include intracranial hemorrhage (subarachnoid and intraparenchymal), cerebrovascular accidents, seizures, noncardiogenic pulmonary edema, arrhythmias, hypertension, myocardial ischemia, barotrauma, bronchospasm, bowel ischemia, hyperthermia, and rhabdomyolysis. These potential morbidities should be considered in any critically ill cocaine abuser, and treatment should be initiated as indicated. Chest pain that is thought to be ischemic usually responds to nitroglycerin and/or benzodiazepines. Aspirin should be administered. Phentolamine and calcium channel blockers are considered to be second-line agents for the treatment of chest pain but are rarely needed. It may be appropriate to avoid the administration of β-blockers in patients manifesting acute sympathomimetic findings, but the benefits of these agents should be considered in patients with ongoing myocardial ischemia. Thrombolysis for myocardial infarction should be considered only when other interventions have failed and immediate angiography and angioplasty are not available. In patients with severe hypertension, labetalol may be considered because it has both α-adrenergic and β-adrenergic blocking properties. In most cases, IV fluid hydration should be instituted until rhabdomyolysis can be excluded. The risk of rhabdomyolysis is enhanced by high environmental temperatures and increased physical activity. The agitation and combativeness frequently associated with cocaine use can usually be controlled with benzodiazepines. If frank psychosis is present, the administration of neuroleptics such as haloperidol is indicated, although there is a potential concern with lowering the seizure threshold.

Cyanide

Cyanide exposure is rare, but may occur in occupational settings involving metal extraction, electroplating, chemical synthesis, and firefighting. Cyanide inhibits cytochrome oxidase, which halts oxidative phosphorylation. Metabolic acidosis and decreased oxygen consumption result. Symptoms include nausea and vomiting, agitation, and tachycardia. Serious poisonings can result in seizures, coma, apnea, hypotension, and arrhythmias. Additional compli-cations include rhabdomyolysis, hepatic necrosis, and ARDS. Diagnosis may be difficult in the absence of an exposure history. A cyanide antidote kit is used for management, including the following:

- Amyl nitrite pearls are an immediate source of nitrite to induce methemoglobinemia. Methemoglobin has a higher affinity for cyanide than cytochrome oxidase;
- 10% sodium nitrite IV to induce methemoglobinemia; and
- 25% sodium thiosulfate IV enhances conversion of cyanide to thiocyanate, which is excreted by the kidneys.

Hydroxocobalamin has also been used for cyanide poisoning and relies on the formation of nontoxic cyanocobalamin (vitamin B_{12}). Mixed evidence exists for the use of therapy with hyperbaric oxygen in patients with cyanide poisoning.

Cyclic Antidepressants

Deaths due to overdose with cyclic antidepressants are declining because of the increasing use of newer, safer antidepressants. Toxicities include arrhythmias, seizures, depressed level of consciousness, and hypotension. Life-threatening events usually occur within the first 6 h of hospitalization; most often, they occur within 2 h of presentation. Serum levels may confirm ingestion but do not correlate with toxicity. Altered mental status is the best predictor of a significant ingestion and the risk of complications. Cyclic antidepressants slow sodium influx into myocardial cells, resulting in intraventricular conduction delays, wide complex arrhythmias, and negative inotropy. The ECG findings may be normal in patients with significant ingestions or may demonstrate a QRS complex of >0.10 s or amplitude of the terminal R wave in lead aVR of ≥3 mm. Management should include the following measures:

- Maintain a secure airway;
- Stabilize vital signs;
- Monitor ECG;
- Consider gastric lavage if ingestion occurred within 1 h of presentation;
- Administer activated charcoal;
- Alkalinize blood and sodium loading with sodium bicarbonate to a pH of 7.45 to 7.55 for prolonged QRS complex or wide complex arrhythmias. If effective, maintain an infusion for 4 to 6 h and then taper;
- Administer mgSO$_4$ for treatment of torsades de pointes;
- Administer benzodiazepines for treatment of seizures; and
- Administer norepinephrine or phenylephrine, rather than dopamine, for the treatment of refractory hypotension.

Sodium bicarbonate uncouples the cyclic antidepressant from the myocardial sodium channels, and alkalinization therapy with bicarbonate may be superior to hyperventilation. In an animal study, hypertonic saline solution was most effective in the treatment of a wide QRS complex. The administration of hypertonic saline solution has also been reported to be effective in the treatment of patients with refractory cardiotoxicity. Bicarbonate may also be beneficial for hypotension associated with myocardial depression that is unresponsive to other interventions. Physostigmine is not indicated in patients with cyclic antidepressant overdoses.

γ-Hydroxybutyrate

γ-Hydroxybutyrate (GHB) is a naturally occurring metabolite of γ-aminobutyric acid, which was banned in 1991 because of reported toxicities. The clinical effects of GHB ingestion may include hypothermia, loss of consciousness, coma, respiratory depression (including arrest), seizurelike activity, bradycardia, hypotension, and death. The concomitant use of alcohol results in synergistic CNS and respiratory effects. More recently, γ-butyrolactone, 1,4-butanediol, and γ-hydroxyvalerate, which are precursors of GHB, have been abused with resultant manifestations similar to those of GHB. Treatment with activated charcoal offers little benefit because of the rapid absorption of these substances. Although patients usually recover spontaneously in 2 to 96 h, supportive therapy with airway protection and mechanical ventilation may be necessary. The use of physostigmine to reverse CNS effects is not recommended. A GHB withdrawal syndrome of agitation and delirium has been reported in high-dose, frequent abusers.

Isoniazid

Isoniazid toxicity produces seizures (often intractable), an anion-gap metabolic acidosis, coma, and hepatic toxicity. The treatment of choice is intensive supportive care and the use of pyridoxine (vitamin B_6, 5 g IV, or a dose equivalent to the amount of isoniazid ingested). Treatment with hemoperfusion or hemodialysis may be considered, particularly in patients with renal insufficiency.

Lithium

Although arrhythmias have been reported, neurologic abnormalities are the major manifestation of acute and chronic lithium toxicity. CNS manifestations include lethargy, dysarthria, delirium, seizures, and coma. Symptoms of GI distress, polyuria, and polydipsia may be present. A decreased anion gap is suggestive of a severely elevated lithium level. Patients with a history of chronic ingestion of lithium are more prone to toxic effects. The serum lithium level should be assessed at presentation and 2 h later to assess for increasing concentration. Serum lithium levels of >2.5 to 4 mmol/L may be considered to be life-threatening, depending on the clinical findings. Treatment with whole-bowel irrigation may be considered in patients with serious

toxicity because lithium is not adsorbed by charcoal. Volume resuscitation should be aimed at restoring adequate urine output, but forced diuresis is not effective in enhancing lithium excretion. Therapy with diuretics can worsen toxicity and should be avoided. Hemodialysis is indicated in life-threatening cases of toxicity, which may include renal dysfunction, severe neurologic dysfunction, volume overload or levels of ≥4 mmol/L in patients with short-term ingestion or ≥2.5 mmol/L in patients with long-term ingestion. The lithium level, duration of exposure, and severity of clinical symptoms should be balanced against the risks of hemodialysis. Redistribution between intracellular and extracellular compartments may result in a rebound increase in lithium level 6 to 8 h after dialysis. Improvement in neurologic status lags behind the decrease in serum lithium level. Continuous arteriovenous hemodiafiltration and venovenous hemodiafiltration have also been used to remove lithium and may be associated with less rebound. Treatment with sodium polystyrene sulfonate has been suggested to decrease lithium absorption, but evidence of clinical benefit is lacking, and complications of hypokalemia, hypernatremia, and fluid overload may result.

Narcotics

The classic clinical findings in patients with narcotic overdoses are depressed level of consciousness, respiratory depression, and miosis. However, manifestations may vary depending on the specific narcotic used and the presence of other drugs or alcohol. Miosis is not seen in patients with meperidine, propoxyphene, and tramadol toxicity. Additional clinical findings may include hypotension, pulmonary edema, bronchospasm (with heroin overdoses), ileus, nausea, vomiting, and pruritus. Methadone abuse has been associated with sudden death. Seizures may be a manifestation of toxicity with meperidine and propoxyphene. The diagnosis of a narcotic overdose is made by characteristic clinical findings, exposure history, qualitative toxicology assay, and response to naloxone.

Naloxone should be used to reverse the morbidity of respiratory depression and depressed level of consciousness that are associated with narcotic overdose. An initial dose of 0.4 to 2 mg should be administered IV, with the lower dose for patients known to be addicted and likely to develop acute withdrawal symptoms. Doses of >2 mg may be required to reverse the effects of propoxyphene, codeine, pentazocine, methadone, oxycodone, hydrocodone, and fentanyl. Naloxone can be administered at doses up to 10 mg, and occasionally up to 20 mg. Naloxone can also be administered by the IM, sublingual, and endotracheal routes if IV access is not established. Continuous infusion may be necessary because all narcotics have a longer half-life than naloxone. The initial hourly infusion dose should be one-half to two-thirds of the amount (in milligrams) that was needed to initially reverse the respiratory depression. Noncardiogenic pulmonary edema may also occur with overdoses of narcotics, and it can be managed with supportive care that may require intubation and mechanical ventilation.

Organophosphates/Carbamates/Nerve Gas

Organophosphate and carbamate poisoning producing a cholinergic syndrome is uncommon in the United States but is prevalent in developing countries. Some nerve gases (eg, sarin) that may be used in terrorist attacks produce similar toxicity. Cholinergic poisoning exerts potential deleterious effects on the following three systems: (1) the muscarinic (parasympathetic) system, inducing bronchorrhea, bradycardia, and salivation, lacrimation, urination, defecation, GI upset, and emesis (ie, the SLUDGE syndrome; Table 3); (2) the nicotinic autonomic system, resulting in muscle weakness; and (3) the CNS, including confusion, slurred speech, and central respiratory depression. Pulmonary toxicity from bronchorrhea, bronchospasm, and respiratory depression is the primary concern. Both IV atropine and pralidoxime (30 mg/kg bolus followed by an infusion of >8 mg/kg/h, which is recommended by the World Health Organization) are indicated. If there are no CNS symptoms, therapy with glycopyrrolate may be substituted for atropine. Atropine does not reverse nicotinic manifestations; therefore, patients with significant respiratory muscle weakness require the use of pralidoxime. Large amounts of atropine may be required, and the initial dose is usually 2 to 4 mg, repeated every 2 to 5 min as needed. A continuous infusion of atropine can be used. The end point of atropinization is the clearing of secretions from the tracheobronchial tree. An intermediate syndrome of respiratory paralysis, bulbar weakness, proximal limb weakness, and decreased reflexes may develop 24 to 96 h after resolution of the cholinergic crisis.

Salicylates

Salicylates are found in many over-the-counter preparations. Patients with a history of chronic ingestion of salicylates, rather than acute ingestion, are more likely to require intensive care. Symptoms of salicylate poisoning include tinnitus, nausea and vomiting, and depressed level of consciousness. In addition, fever, an anion-gap metabolic acidosis, coagulopathy, prolonged prothrombin time, transient hepatotoxicity, and noncardiogenic pulmonary edema may be present. The clinical presentation of salicylate toxicity may be mistaken for sepsis. A salicylate level should be measured initially and may need to be repeated to assess for continued absorption (especially with enteric-coated products). The Done nomogram that is used to estimate the severity of an acute salicylate overdose may not reliably correlate with observed toxicity. Acidemia predisposes the patient to more severe toxicity because more of the drug crosses the blood-brain barrier. Gastric lavage may be considered for significant ingestions, and activated charcoal should be administered. Alkalinization of the urine (ie, pH ≥7.5) is indicated to enhance salicylate excretion if serum levels are >35 mg/dL. Supplemental potassium is often needed. Hemodialysis may be indicated with levels of >100 mg/dL, refractory seizures, persistent alteration in mental status, or refractory acidosis.

Selective Serotonin Reuptake Inhibitors

Poisoning with selective serotonin reuptake inhibitors (SSRIs) is usually less severe than poisoning with cyclic antidepressants. Acute overdoses may result in nausea, vomiting, dizziness, and, less commonly, CNS depression and arrhythmias. There have been reports of cardiac toxicity responding to the administration of sodium bicarbonate. Therapeutic doses, overdoses of SSRIs alone, or overdoses of SSRIs in combination with other agents can cause serotonin syndrome, which may be life-threatening. This syndrome may be precipitated by the ingestion of SSRIs, monoamine oxidase inhibitors, serotonin precursors (eg, L-tryptophan), lithium, meperidine, and non-SSRIs (eg, imipramine, meperidine, or trazodone). Clinical manifestations include altered mental status (ie, agitation and coma), autonomic dysfunction (ie, BP fluctuation, hyperthermia, tachycardia, diaphoresis, and diarrhea), and neuromuscular abnormalities (ie, tremor, rigidity, myoclonus, and seizures). The management of an overdose should include activated charcoal, but the benefit of gastric lavage has not been determined. Intensive supportive care may be necessary, including cooling, sedatives, anticonvulsants, and mechanical ventilation. Cyproheptadine (a serotonin antagonist) in varying dose regimens (12 to 32 mg over 24 h) has been most commonly recommended as a treatment option. There is currently no role for the use of bromocriptine or dantrolene. Most cases of serotonin syndrome resolve in 24 to 72 h.

Valproic Acid

Acute and chronic valproic acid (VPA) intoxication is an increasing problem because of greater utilization of this agent. CNS depression is the most common manifestation in an acute overdose. Higher drug levels are associated with an increased incidence of coma and respiratory depression requiring intubation. Cerebral edema has been reported 48 to 72 h after ingestion and may be related to hyperammonemia, which can occur in the absence of hepatotoxicity. Massive VPA ingestions can result in refractory hypotension. Pancreatitis has been associated with both chronic ingestion and acute overdose. Metabolic abnormalities include hypernatremia, anion-gap metabolic acidosis, hypocalcemia, and acute renal failure. Serial VPA levels should be obtained because of delayed peak serum levels in patients with overdoses. Ammonia levels should also be measured in patients with an altered level of consciousness. Activated charcoal should be administered if the patient presents early after ingestion. Treatment with whole-bowel irrigation has been proposed, but further studies are needed to determine whether there is any indication for use in patients who have ingested VPA. Although a potential enterohepatic recirculation of the drug suggests that multiple doses of activated charcoal may be beneficial, routine use is not currently recommended. Hemoperfusion, combined hemodialysis-hemoperfusion, or high-flux hemodialysis may be considered in patients with persistent hemodynamic instability or metabolic acidosis. No antidote exists for VPA toxicity. L-Carnitine has been proposed for supplementation in patients with VPA toxicity and hyperammonemia.

Herbal Medicine/Dietary Supplements

Herbal medicines are the most common form of alternative therapy in the United States, and can be marketed without testing for safety or efficacy. Poisoning may result from product misuse, from contamination of the product, or through interaction with other medications. Cardiac toxicity may result from the use of aconitine and cardiac glycosides. Aconitine or related compounds are common ingredients in Asian herbal medications. Symptoms include paresthesias, hypersalivation, dizziness, nausea, vomiting, diarrhea, and muscle weakness. Sinus bradycardia and ventricular arrhythmias can occur. No antidote is available, but atropine may be considered for the treatment of bradycardia or hypersalivation. Cardiac glycosides or digoxin-like factors can be found in many herbal preparations, particularly teas and laxatives. Manifestations of toxicity are similar to those of digoxin toxicity, with visual disturbances, nausea, vomiting, and arrhythmias. Digoxin levels should be measured but may not correlate with clinical findings because numerous cardiac glycosides will not cross-react in the digoxin immunoassay. With significant toxicity, digoxin-specific antibodies should be administered. CNS stimulation is characteristic of preparations containing ephedrine and pseudoephedrine, which are often found in products marketed as "herbal ecstasy." A typical sympathomimetic syndrome can result with tachycardia, hypertension, mydriasis, and agitation. Seizures, stroke, myocardial infarction, arrhythmias, liver failure, and death have also been reported. Ephedra-free products have also been associated with cardiovascular toxicity. Supportive care is indicated as in the case of the management of other sympathomimetic syndromes. Ginkgo biloba has been reported to result in episodes of spontaneous bleeding, including subdural hematomas, which may be due to antiplatelet-activating factor effects. Treatment for bleeding includes supportive care and the administration of blood products as needed. Garlic ingestion may also result in bleeding as a result of the inhibition of platelet aggregation, and ginseng has been associated with hypoglycemia. Kava-containing dietary supplements are possibly associated with hepatic failure requiring transplantation. Contaminants such as mercury, arsenic, lead, or antihistamines that found in some products may cause toxicities.

Withdrawal Syndromes

Ethanol

Four stages of alcohol withdrawal have been described (Table 5), but symptoms are a continuum of neuropsychiatric and hemodynamic manifestations. Patients may manifest one or more of these syndromes on presentation or develop additional manifestations and progress from less severe to more severe stages while hospitalized. The presence of an intact or altered sensorium is a key distinction. Sensorium is clear with tremulousness but altered with delirium tremens (delusions, hallucinations, confusion). Delirium tremens is also associated with more severe autonomic abnormalities such as tachycardia, hypertension, hyperthermia, and diaphoresis.

The choice of treatment depends on assessment of the severity of withdrawal. Minor withdrawal symptoms can usually be treated with IV or oral benzodiazepines. Benzodiazepines act as an alcohol substitute to dampen the excitatory neuronal activity and prevent seizures and delirium tremens. The choice of benzodiazepine should take into account hepatic dysfunction, duration of action, and available routes of administration. All benzodiazepines are effective when appropriate doses are used. Scheduled dosing and symptom-triggered regimens have been used effectively. Hallucinosis also responds well to benzodiazepines. Patients with alcohol withdrawal should receive supportive measures with thiamine IV or orally to prevent Wernicke encephalopathy. Magnesium sulfate may be needed to correct hypomagnesemia.

Patients with untreated mild alcohol withdrawal symptoms may progress to seizures. Most alcohol withdrawal seizures are brief and self-limited in duration. Alcohol withdrawal seizures are usually generalized tonic-clonic but focal seizures may also occur. Multiple seizures (two to six episodes) can occur and usually occur within a 12-h period. Other causes of seizures such as hypoglycemia, metabolic abnormalities, trauma, infection, and other drug intoxication must be considered. Alcohol withdrawal seizures can be terminated with IV lorazepam or midazolam. If the seizure terminates without intervention, a benzodiazepine should be administered as soon as possible to prevent subsequent seizures. Lorazepam (2 mg) significantly reduces the risk of recurrent seizure, whereas phenytoin has no effect. Status epilepticus is infrequent and should be treated with benzodiazepines or propofol. Phenytoin is not as effective.

Patients with delirium tremens should be cared for in an ICU setting. Some patients with severe withdrawal symptoms may need intubation during treatment. High-dose IV benzodiazepines administered at frequent intervals or as a continuous infusion are needed to control hyperadrenergic symptoms. Dosing should be individualized to achieve light somnolence. High doses of lorazepam or diazepam over long periods of time can result in propylene glycol toxicity. Daily dose reductions of 25% can be initiated after the second or third day of treatment. Propofol may be an option for patients who are refractory to benzodiazepines. Cardiac monitoring is necessary to detect and treat arrhythmias. β-Blockers may be needed to treat hypertension or tachycardia but they should not be administered to treat delirium.

Table 5. *Stages of Alcohol Withdrawal*

Symptoms	Time Frame*
Tremulousness	Onset within hours, peak in 10–30 h
Seizures	Onset 6–48 h, peak 13–24 h
Hallucinations	Onset 8–48 h, may last 1–6 days
Delirium tremens	Onset 60–96 h, 48–72 h

*Time after last drink.

Narcotics

The clinical manifestations of narcotic withdrawal vary according to the drug that is abused and the temporal relationship to the last narcotic dose. Onset of symptoms can begin within 6 to 12 h of the last dose with short-acting narcotics such as heroin and within 36 to 48 h with long-acting narcotics. Early symptoms include yawning, lacrimation, rhinorrhea, and sweating. Manifestations progress to restlessness, irritability, flushing, tachycardia, fever, tremor, nausea, vomiting, abdominal pain, and diarrhea. Narcotic withdrawal alone is rarely life-threatening and usually does not require intensive care. If it is necessary to control withdrawal symptoms, most narcotics in sufficient dosage will alleviate symptoms. Clonidine (0.1 to 0.3 mg) has also been used to treat the autonomic effects of narcotic withdrawal. Side effects of clonidine are hypotension, drowsiness, dry mouth, and bradycardia.

Bibliography

Alapat PM, Zimmerman JL. Toxicology in the critical care unit. Chest 2008; 133:1006–1013

American Academy of Clinical Toxicology, European Association of Poisons Centres and Clinical Toxicologists. Position paper: gastric lavage. J Toxicol Clin Toxicol 2004; 42:933–943

American Academy of Clinical Toxicology, European Association of Poison Centres and Clinical Toxicologists. Position paper statement: single-dose activated charcoal. J Toxicol Clin Toxicol 2005; 43:61–87

American Academy of Clinical Toxicology, European Association of Poison Centres and Clinical Toxicologists. Position paper: whole bowel irrigation. J Toxicol Clin Toxicol 2004; 42:843–854

American Academy of Clinical Toxicology, European Association of Poison Centres and Clinical Toxicologists. Position statement and practice guidelines on the use of multi-dose activated charcoal in the treatment of acute poisoning. J Toxicol Clin Toxicol 1999; 37:731–751

Bailey B. Glucagon in β-blocker and calcium channel blocker overdoses: a systematic review. J Toxicol Clin Toxicol 2003; 41:595–602

Barceloux DG, Bond GR, Krenzelok EP, et al. American Academy of Clinical Toxicology practice guidelines on the treatment of methanol poisoning. J Toxicol Clin Toxicol 2002; 40:415–446

Bouchard NC, Howland MA, Greller HA, et al. Ischemic stroke associated with use of an ephedra-free dietary supplement containing synephrine. Mayo Clin Proc 2005; 80:541–545

Boyer EW, Shannon M. The serotonin syndrome. N Engl J Med 2005; 352:1112–1120

Brok J, Buckley N, Gluud C. Interventions for paracetamol (acetaminophen) overdose. Cochrane Database Syst Rev 2002;(3):CD003328

Buckley NA, Eddleston M, Szinicz L. Oximes for organophosphate pesticide poisoning. Cochrane Database Syst Rev 2005 Jan 25;(1):CD005085

Dattilo PB, Hallpern SM, Fearon K, et al. β-Blockers are associated with reduced risk of myocardial infarction after cocaine use. Ann Emerg Med 2008; 51:117–125

de la Torre R, Farré M, Roset PN, et al. Human pharmacology of MDMA, pharmacokinetics, metabolism, and disposition. Ther Drug Monit 2004; 26:137–144

De Smet PA. Herbal remedies. N Engl J Med 2002; 347:2046–2056

Domachevsky L, Adir Y, Grupper M, et al. Hyperbaric oxygen in the treatment of carbon monoxide poisoning. J Toxicol Clin Toxicol 2005; 43:181–188

Dyer JE, Roth B, Hyma BA. γ-Hydroxybutyrate withdrawal syndrome. Ann Emerg Med 2001; 37:147–153

Eddleston M, Szinicz L, Eyer P, et al. Oximes in acute organophosphorus pesticide poisoning: a systematic review of clinical trials. Q J Med 2002; 95:275–283

Glauser J. Tricyclic antidepressant poisoning. Cleve Clin J Med 2000; 67:704–719

Glauser J, Queen JR. An overview of non-cardiac cocaine toxicity. J Emerg Med 2007; 32:181–186

Goldstein RA, DesLauriers C, Burda AM. Cocaine: history, social implications, and toxicity: a review. Dis Mon 2008; 55:6–38

Heard KJ. Acetylcysteine for acetaminophen poisoning. N Engl J Med 2008; 359:285–292

Isbister GK, Bowe SJ, Dawson A, et al. Relative toxicity of selective serotonin reuptake inhibitors (SSRIs) in overdose. J Toxicol Clin Toxicol 2004; 42:277–285

Isbister GK, Buckley NA, Whyte IM. Serotonin toxicity: a practical approach to diagnosis and treatment. Med J Aust 2007; 187:361–365

Juurlink DN, Buckley NA, Stanbrook MB, et al. Hyperbaric oxygen for carbon monoxide poisoning. Cochrane Database Syst Rev 2005 Jan 25;(1): CD002041

Kalant H. The pharmacology and toxicology of "ecstasy" (MDMA) and related drugs. Can Med Assoc J 2001; 165:917–928

Lange RA, Hillis LD. Cardiovascular complications of cocaine use. N Engl J Med 2001; 345:351–358

Larson AM. Acetaminophen hepatotoxicity. Clin Liver Dis 2007; 11:525–548

Leiken JB, Thomas RG, Walter FG, et al. A review of nerve agent exposure for the critical care physician. Crit Care Med 2002; 30:2346–2354

Lineberry TW, Bostwick JM. Methamphetamine abuse: a perfect storm of complications. Mayo Clin Proc 2006; 81:77–84

McCord J, Jneid H, Hollander JE, et al. Management of cocaine-associated chest pain and myocardial infarction. A scientific statement from the American Heart Association Acute Cardiac Care Committee of the Council of Cardiology. Circulation 2008; 117: 1897–1907

McKinney PE, Rasmussen R. Reversal of severe tricyclic antidepressant-induced cardiotoxicity with intravenous hypertonic saline solution. Ann Emerg Med 2003; 42:20–24

Megarbane B, Borron SW, Baud SJ. Current recommendations for treatment of severe toxic alcohol poisonings. Intensive Care Med 2005; 31:189–195

Mokhesi B, Leiken JB, Murray P, et al. Adult toxicology in critical care: part I. General approach to the intoxicated patient. Chest 2003; 123:577–592

Mokhesi B, Leiken JB, Murray P, et al. Adult toxicology in critical care: part II. Specific poisonings. Chest 2003; 123:897–922

O'Malley GF. Emergency department management of the salicylate-poisoned patient. Emerg Med Clin North Am 2007; 25:333–346

Proudfoot AT, Krenzelok EP, Vale JA. Position paper on urine alkalinization. J Toxicol Clin Toxicol 2004; 42:1–26

Richardson WH, Slone CM, Michels JE. Herbal drugs of abuse: an emerging problem. Emerg Med Clin North Am 2007; 25:435–457

Rowden AK, Fasano CJ. Emergency management of oral hypoglycemic drug toxicity. Emerg Med Clin North Am 2007; 25:347–356

Saper RB, Kales SN, Paquin J, et al. Heavy metal content of ayurvedic herbal medicine products. JAMA 2004; 292:2868–2873

Seger DL. Flumazenil-treatment or toxin. J Toxicol Clin Toxicol 2004; 42:209–216

Snead OC, Gibson KM. γ-Hydroxybutyric acid. N Engl J Med 2005; 352:2721–2732

Sztajnkrycer MD. Valproic acid toxicity: overview and management. J Toxicol Clin Toxicol 2002; 40:789–801

Weaver LK, Hopkins RD, Chan KJ, et al. Hyperbaric oxygen for acute carbon monoxide poisoning. N Engl J Med 2002; 347:1057–1067

Wolf SJ, Lavonas EF, Sloan EP, et al. Clinical policy: critical issues in the management of adult patients presenting to the emergency department with acute carbon monoxide poisoning. Ann Emerg Med 2008; 51:138–152

Zimmerman JL. Poisonings and overdoses in the ICU: general and specific management issues. Crit Care Med 2003; 31:2794–2801

Zimmerman JL, Rudis M. Poisonings. In: Parrillo JE, Dellinger RP, eds. Critical are medicine: principles of diagnosis and management in the adult. 3rd edition. St. Louis, MO: Mosby, 2008; 1453–1474

Web Site

www.torsades.org. This Web site provides lists of medications that may cause torsades grouped by likelihood of causing the arrhythmia.

Notes

Anemia and RBC Transfusion in the ICU

Karl W. Thomas, MD, FCCP

Objectives:

- Discuss the pathophysiology, causes, and categorization of anemia in ICU patients
- Describe the indications and appropriate clinical use of commonly available RBC products
- Discuss the infectious and noninfectious complications of blood product transfusions including transfusion reactions, viral transmission, and transfusion-associated lung injury
- Discuss the role of erythropoietin and blood substitutes in the management of ICU patients

Key words: anemia; erythropoietin; hemolysis; hemorrhage; schistocyte; TRALI

Anemia, thrombocytopenia, and coagulopathies are commonly encountered in ICU patients. These disorders rarely occur in isolation and are closely associated with ICU outcomes. Rapid and efficient classification and recognition of these disorders is essential to the provision of timely and appropriate care. When present, these disorders require a clinical approach based on systematic examination of RBCs, platelets, and coagulation factor parameters. This chapter will focus specifically on the clinical evaluation and management of anemia and RBC transfusion. This chapter will review the pathophysiology, epidemiology, and management of ICU patients with anemia. This chapter will conclude with a discussion of blood substitutes and erythropoietin in ICU patients.

Epidemiology of Anemia and RBC Transfusion in ICU Patients

Observational studies have demonstrated that one-third of patients admitted to the ICU will have a baseline hemoglobin level $< 10 \, g/dL$.[2] Furthermore, two-thirds will have a baseline hemoglobin level $< 12 \, g/dL$.[1] By day 3 after admission to an ICU, below-normal hemoglobin levels will develop in $> 90\%$ of patients The average hemoglobin concentration in ICU patients will then show a measurable decline every day until discharge from the ICU. Patients in whom anemia develops or who have anemia prior to ICU admission are highly likely to have persistent anemia throughout their entire ICU stay despite treatment with transfusion.[2,3]

One-third to one-half of all patients admitted to an ICU will receive one or more RBC transfusions. The occurrence and degree of ICU anemia has a direct relationship with patient outcomes. Anemia and transfusion in critically ill patients consistently correlates with increased ICU mortality, increased ICU length of stay, prolonged mechanical ventilation, severe organ dysfunction, and higher costs.[1,3] Although transfusion is clearly associated with immediate complications, the association with worse overall outcomes is based on consistent and reproduced observational data. Direct causality between RBC transfusion and increased mortality has not been demonstrated in randomized, placebo-controlled trials.

Hemodynamic Pathophysiology and Clinical Manifestations of Anemia

The pathophysiologic effects of anemia are related to reduced oxygen-carrying capacity of the blood and the cardiovascular response to maintain the delivery of oxygen to the tissues and organs. Global delivery of oxygen (Do_2), is determined by the volume of blood delivered and the content of oxygen in that blood. This relationship can be written with cardiac output (CO) and arterial blood oxygen content (Cao_2) as follows:

$$Do_2 = Cao_2 \times CO$$

The content of oxygen in blood is determined by the formula:

$$Cao_2 = (1.39 \times Hb \times Sao_2) + (0.003 \times Pao_2)$$

where Sao_2 = hemoglobin oxygen saturation and Pao_2 = partial pressure of arterial oxygen.

The systemic oxygen consumption ($\dot{V}o_2$) is the difference between the amount of oxygen that is delivered in arterial blood minus the amount that is returned to the heart in venous blood. $\dot{V}o_2$ can therefore be represented by the following simplified formulas:

$$\dot{V}o_2 = CO\ (Cao_2 - Cvo_2)$$

$$Vo_2 = Hr \times SV \times 1.39 \times Hb \times (Sao_2 - Svo_2)$$

where Hr = heart rate, SV = stroke volume, and Svo_2 = mixed venous hemoglobin oxygen saturation.

This formula can be used to illustrate and understand the expected hemodynamic responses to anemia. This relationship predicts that the acute compensatory mechanisms for anemia are increased heart rate and increased extraction of oxygen from arterial blood (leading to lower mixed venous oxygen saturation). Chronic compensation occurs by fluid retention to increase preload and SV as well as stimulation of erythropoietin production to increase hemoglobin. Hemorrhagic shock can be viewed as a hemodynamic state with inadequate delivery of oxygen to the tissues arising from decreased hemoglobin concentration as well as loss of venous return, leading to decreased SV.

Under normal circumstances, the delivery of oxygen in arterial blood is significantly greater than tissue metabolic requirements. In the circumstance in which hemoglobin concentration, oxygen saturation, or CO is not matched to metabolic requirements, anaerobic metabolism and decreased $\dot{V}o_2$ occurs. The critical threshold for oxygen delivery is defined as the point below which oxygen delivery is inadequate and $\dot{V}o_2$ begins to decrease. Normal individuals may tolerate decreases in hemoglobin to approximately 5 g/dL.[4] However, systemic diseases, such as sepsis, that affect vasoregulation and alter cellular oxidative metabolism disrupt the normal relationship between oxygen delivery and oxygen utilization. Coexisting cardiac dysfunction also directly impairs the physiologic compensation for anemia.

The physiologic effect of anemia is clinically assessed by examination of indicators of global and organ-specific oxygen delivery. The goal of this clinical evaluation is to determine if the anemia is uncompensated and acute, or compensated and subacute/chronic. This assessment determines the need for immediate RBC transfusion and hemodynamic support (Fig 1). Serum lactate, mixed venous oxygen saturation, and oxygen extraction ratio are indicators of the adequacy of systemic oxygenation. In a cohort of patients with severe sepsis, early goal-directed therapy with RBC transfusion in anemic patients with decreased venous oxygen saturation improved survival.[5] This finding establishes some clinical utility in assessing venous oxygen saturation in acutely ill patients when considering transfusion. Organ-specific clinical indicators of anemia include confusion, headaches, fatigue, tachycardia, angina, congestive heart failure, dyspnea, and claudication. Any anemic patient with these findings that are not attributable to other factors should be considered for transfusion. RBC transfusions should only be administered to preserve or augment oxygen delivery. Patients without indicators of threatened or impaired oxygen delivery do not require immediate blood transfusion. Blood should not be used for intravascular volume expansion.

Causes of Anemia in ICU Patients

The clinical evaluation of patients with anemia should focus on determining whether the anemia is primarily the result of RBC loss, RBC underproduction, or RBC destruction. ICU patients are likely to have multiple contributing factors to anemia. Table 1 lists the most common causes of anemia in ICU patients. In general, most patients have risk factors for decreased RBC production, increased RBC loss, and increased RBC destruction.

As the result of diagnostic testing, all ICU patients are subjected to high rates of phlebotomy. This results in up to 40 to 70 mL/d average blood losses.[1,6] This high rate of RBC loss is a major contributor to ICU anemia. Conditions that predispose to ICU admission and anemia are often the same as conditions that predispose to coagulopathy and extravascular blood loss. This compounds the problem and makes ICU anemia a multifactorial condition.

Anemia and RBC Transfusion in the ICU (Thomas)

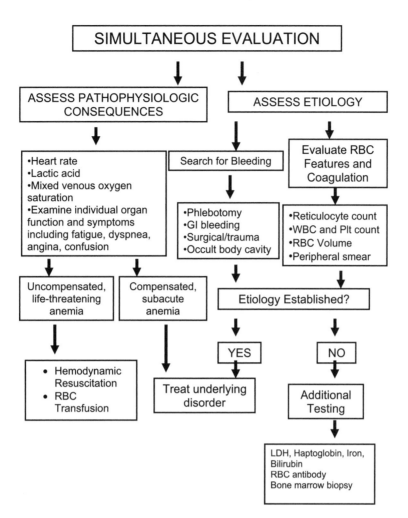

SIMULTANEOUS EVALUATION

ASSESS PATHOPHYSIOLOGIC CONSEQUENCES

ASSESS ETIOLOGY

•Heart rate
•Lactic acid
•Mixed venous oxygen saturation
•Examine individual organ function and symptoms including fatigue, dyspnea, angina, confusion

Search for Bleeding

Evaluate RBC Features and Coagulation

•Phlebotomy
•GI bleeding
•Surgical/trauma
•Occult body cavity

•Reticulocyte count
•WBC and Plt count
•RBC Volume
•Peripheral smear

Uncompensated, life-threatening anemia

Compensated, subacute anemia

Etiology Established?

YES

NO

• Hemodynamic Resuscitation
• RBC Transfusion

Treat underlying disorder

Additional Testing

LDH, Haptoglobin, Iron, Bilirubin
RBC antibody
Bone marrow biopsy

Figure 1. Clinical approach to anemia in the ICU. Plt = platelet; LDH = lactate dehydrogenase.

Table 1. *Causes of Anemia in ICU Patients*

Blood loss
    Phlebotomy
    Trauma or surgery
    GI blood loss
    Retroperitoneal, thigh, or intraabdominal hemorrhage
Decreased RBC production
    Anemia of chronic disease
    Iron deficiency
    Chronic renal disease
    Nutritional deficiencies (vitamin B_{12}, folate)
    Toxins (alcohol, drugs, chemotherapy, lead)
    Endocrinopathy (hypothyroidism, hypopituitarism)
    Myelodysplastic syndromes
RBC destruction
    Immune-mediated hemolysis
    Inherited RBC disorders (hemoglobinopathies)
    Enzyme disorders (G-6-PD deficiency)*
    Microangiopathic hemolytic anemia (disseminated intravascular coagulopathy [DIC])
    Infection (malaria)

*G-6-PD = glucose-6-phosphate dehydrogenase.

In acutely ill medical and surgical ICU patients, contributing factors for decreased RBC production include suppression of erythropoietin production, blunted erythropoietin response, nutritional deficiency, and abnormal iron metabolism. This closely resembles and is virtually indistinguishable from the pathophysiologic processes in patients with anemia of chronic disease. The characteristic laboratory features of anemia of chronic disease include low reticulocyte count, reduced serum iron, and reduced total iron-binding capacity. It is not unusual for patients with preexisting anemia of chronic disease to have acute illness develop, have additional blood loss, and require ICU care.

For most ICU patients, and particularly for those with hemodynamic instability, the clinical approach to anemia should simultaneously assess the physiologic effect of anemia and determine the primary causes of anemia. The physiologic effect should be determined by examining hemodynamic status, organ dysfunction, and markers of systemic oxygen delivery. These findings will determine the urgency of response and will determine whether or not transfusion is indicated. The etiology of anemia is determined by a systematic search for sources of blood loss and systematic laboratory analysis. The laboratory analysis of patients with anemia should include assessment of general hematopoiesis (reticulocyte, WBC, and platelet counts), and assessment of RBC features including corpuscular volume and peripheral smear. Additional testing should include assessment of coagulation function with prothrombin time and activated partial thromboplastin time. Focused testing will be performed as indicated including measurement of serum ferritin, iron, haptoglobin, lactate dehydrogenase, bilirubin, RBC antibody tests (Coombs test), and bone marrow biopsy (Fig 1).

The RBC morphology and peripheral blood smear features are a critical source of information in establishing the cause of anemia. The RBC morphology can indicate the mechanism of hemolysis or anemia (Table 2). The reticulocyte count is a critical marker of bone marrow function and

response. The majority of ICU patients will have normocytic anemia. The presence of macrocytic or microcytic anemia serves as an important indicator of a primary hematologic disease. Intravascular hemolysis is suggested by the presence of spherocytes, schistocytes, and bite cells. Spherocytes reflect destruction of the RBC membrane (eg, autoimmune hemolytic anemia). Schistocytes reflect destruction of RBC in microangiopathic hemolysis (eg, disseminated intravascular coagulation) or microangiopathic hemolysis (eg, turbulent blood flow with shear stress across an endovascular device). Finally, bite cells occur as the result of focal destruction of RBC membranes from oxidant stress or macrophage binding, as seen in methemoglobinemia and G-6-PD (glucose-6-phosphate dehydrogenase deficiency). Additional laboratory findings of hemolysis or RBC destruction include elevations in serum lactate dehydrogenase, bilirubin, and decreased haptoglobin.

RBC Transfusion

Clinical Approach

Patients being considered for RBC transfusion require an assessment of the cause of anemia

Table 2. *Morphologic Categorization of Anemia in the ICU**

	Clinical Characteristics
Macrocytic anemias (MCV > 100 fL)	
Nutritional deficiency, alcoholism (folate deficiency)	Oval macrocytes, hypersegmented neutrophils
Pernicious anemia	Cobalamin deficiency
Liver disease	Target cells, spur and burr cells
Asplenia/hyposplenism	Acanthocytes, Howell-Jolly bodies, nucleated RBCs
Microcytic anemias (MCV < 80 fL)	
Iron deficiency or reduced iron availability	Poikilocytosis, hypochromia, pencil forms
Chronic blood loss	Poikilocytosis, hypochromia
Thalassemia	Basophilic stippling, target cells, polychromasia
Chronic exposure to drugs, toxins	Basophilic stippling
Sideroblastic anemias (hereditary/idiopathic)	Dimorphic cells, reduced reticulocyte count
Normocytic and variable MCV anemias	
Anemia of chronic disease	May have microcytic features; low serum iron and TIBC
Acute extravascular blood loss	Clinical and pathophysiologic findings of hemorrhage
Hemolytic anemias	Elevated bilirubin, LDH, haptoglobin, reticulocyte count
Micro- or macroangiopathic (eg, DIC)	RBC fragmentation/schistocytes
Sickle cell anemia	Sickle cells, chronic disorder
Autoimmune hemolytic anemias	Spherocytes, direct antiglobulin test positive
Metabolic defects (eg, G-6-PD deficiency)	Bite cells
Myelodysplastic syndromes	Round macrocytes, bilobed neutrophils

*MCV = mean corpuscular volume; fL = femtoliter; TIBC = total iron-binding capacity.

and the physiologic effect of the anemia (Fig 1). The underlying etiology of anemia should be established and treated simultaneously with the consideration of blood transfusion. For virtually all ICU patients, phlebotomy for laboratory testing is a significant factor; every attempt to minimize phlebotomy should be made. The decision to administer a blood transfusion should be approached within the context of three factors: (1) the patient's known comorbidities; (2) the adequacy of hemodynamic compensation; and (3) whether or not the underlying condition leading to anemia can be treated.

The decision to give an RBC transfusion should not be made on the basis of hemoglobin concentration or hematocrit alone. For example, patients with bleeding esophageal varices and portal hypertension may require emergent transfusion before the hematocrit drops and prior to endoscopic intervention. In comparison, a patient with chronic iron deficiency anemia from peptic ulcer disease may benefit from endoscopic evaluation of the source of blood loss and iron replacement without the need for transfusion.

Review of actual transfusion patterns indicates that there is significant variation in blood transfusion practice based on medical center, individual provider, admission diagnosis, and severity of illness. Studies in North America and Europe[1,3] have demonstrated that the most common indications for transfusion include low hemoglobin level, active bleeding, and hemodynamic instability. In these studies, the mean pretransfusion hemoglobin levels were 8.4 g/dL and 8.6 g/dL. Patients who received transfusion had higher admission APACHE (acute physiology and chronic health evaluation) scores, lower admission hemoglobin levels, and longer hospital length of stay.[1,3]

Best Clinical Evidence

The most robust clinical evidence linking hemoglobin concentration, transfusion trigger, and ICU outcomes comes from the Canadian Critical Care Trials Group prospective, randomized trial of restrictive transfusion practice vs liberal transfusion practice. A mixed population of 838 medical and surgical patients with hemoglobin levels <9 g/dL were randomized in this study. Patients assigned to the restrictive group did not receive transfusion until the hemoglobin level was <7 g/dL and was maintained from 7.0 to 9.0 g/dL. The liberal transfusion group received transfusion for hemoglobin levels < 10.0 g/dL and maintained between 10.0 and 12.0 g/dL. In the overall analysis, there was no difference in 30-day mortality between the two groups. Subgroup analysis demonstrated that patients <55 years of age and those with lower APACHE scores had significantly lower mortality with restrictive transfusion. Patients with angina, acute cardiovascular disease, septic shock, and trauma had no mortality difference.[7] These results suggest that the transfusion decisions should account for the underlying comorbid conditions, the severity of illness, and presence of cardiac disease. In general, there does not appear to be a benefit of maintaining hemoglobin levels >7 to 9g/dL in the absence of significant heart disease. The restrictive transfusion strategy appears to be safe and was not associated with higher rates of adverse outcomes. Although the hemoglobin level remains an important consideration, the status of the patient should be critical factor in decisions to transfuse.

For the subset of patients with acute coronary syndromes and hemodynamically significant cardiac disease, available evidence is less definitive. A retrospective analysis of patients who entered the GUSTO IIb, PURSUIT, and PARAGON B cardiac treatment trials has provided some evidence to guide transfusion in this group.[8] This analysis of 24,000 patients demonstrated that blood transfusion for patients with acute coronary syndromes was associated with higher 30-day mortality rates for the entire patient group.[8] However, patients who received transfusion were older, had more comorbid illness, and had higher unadjusted 30-day mortality rates. This effect of higher mortality appeared most significant in patients who received transfusion but had baseline hematocrits > 25%.[8] Subgroup analysis of cardiac patients in the Canadian Clinical Trials Group restrictive vs liberal transfusion requirement demonstrated no significant benefit or harm with restrictive transfusion strategy.[7]

RBC Products

RBC transfusions may be administered in the form of packed RBCs, whole blood, leukoreduced blood, autologous stored blood, and autologous reinfused blood. Additional variations include RBC preparations selected on the basis of removal of other plasma components such as Igs or viral infections such as cytomegalovirus-seronegative blood (Table 3).

All stored RBC products must undergo component separation to remove plasma and platelets, treatment with preservatives and anticoagulants, and refrigerated storage. After collection, whole blood is subject to centrifugation to remove WBCs, platelets, and most plasma components. Each unit of RBCs is then resuspended in a storage solution that contains citrate, phosphate, dextrose, and adenine; other nutrients are added at the time of collection to give the unit a shelf life of 40 days. Although rare blood types may be frozen in solutions containing glycerol and dimethyl sulfoxide, most blood is stored at 4°C and warmed immediately prior to transfusion. Storage of packed RBCs results in mild hemolysis, release of potassium into the storage solution, decreased pH of the solution, accumulation of ammonia, and gradual depletion of RBC 2,3-diphosphoglycerate levels. These storage-related factors may become clinically relevant for patients with renal failure and in situations of massive transfusion.

Table 3. *Features and Clinical Indications for RBC Transfusion Products*

RBC Transfusion Product	Specific Features	Clinical Indication(s) and Use
Whole blood	Plasma and platelet components not removed	Rarely used and infrequently available; may be indicated for patients who have massive transfusion requirements to simultaneously replace multiple blood components
Packed RBCs	Plasma and platelet components removed	Most common in general use
Specialized RBCs	Rare donor phenotypes	Often stored frozen and shipped to hospital on demand; indicated for patients with unusual antibodies and rare blood types, and patients with IgA deficiency
Washed RBCs	RBCs are centrifuged and resuspended in saline to remove additional plasma and WBCs	Used to prevent febrile transfusion reactions and in patients with history of allergic transfusion reactions
Leukoreduced or leukofiltered blood	Blood passed through filter to remove donor leukocytes, reduces WBC contamination 99.9%	Used to prevent febrile transfusion reactions; preferred in chronically transfused patients, potential transplant recipients, some oncology patients, and CMV-seronegative patients; may reduce risk of viral disease transmission
Irradiated blood	Blood subjected to gamma or x-irradiation to eliminate donor lymphocyte proliferation	Used to prevent graft-vs-host disease (GVHD) in high-risk patients
CMV-safe blood	Packed RBCs only from donors who are CMV-negative*	CMV-negative infants, CMV-negative bone marrow. and solid organ transplant recipients, patients with immunodeficiency syndromes
Autologous stored blood	Patient donates blood for storage prior to anticipated need	Often used by patients in anticipation of operative blood loss; prepared and stored as either whole blood or packed RBCs
Autologous salvage/ rein fusion	Blood collection pumps, centrifuges, and washes used to retrieve blood from site of massive hemorrhage and rein fuse into same patient	Intraoperative blood salvage; may be acceptable to Jehovah's Witness patients; reduces need for allogenic blood products.

*CMV = cytomegalovirus.

Anemia and RBC Transfusion in the ICU (Thomas)

The Crossmatch Test and Bedside Administration of Blood

Crossmatching and pretransfusion laboratory testing must be conducted to determine three critical pieces of data: (1) the ABO/RhD blood type of the patient; (2) the presence of patient antibodies to common red cell antigens; and (3) specific crossmatch compatibility of the individual blood unit with the patient. Each of these three tests must be completed prior to transfusion and are the primary method of preventing transfusion of incompatible blood and major transfusion reactions. RhD typing is necessary to prevent exposure of RhD antigen in girls and women of childbearing age. Many steps of pretransfusion testing are performed manually and thus subject to human error. Recent development of computer-based blood-dispensing systems based on bar code verification of the patient and the individual blood unit bag may be used in place of the manual crossmatch.[9] Exceptions to pretransfusion testing exist only for patients with life-threatening hemorrhage when the delay of crossmatch testing will increase the likelihood of death of the patient. In this situation, the hierarchy of blood products is O-negative blood followed by type-specific blood that is not crossmatched followed by crossmatched blood.

Each unit of packed RBCs is delivered in 200 to 300 mL of electrolyte/nutrient/anticoagulant solution. In nonemergent conditions, RBCs may be infused over >1 to 4 h. Rapid infusion over minutes may be administered in trauma and acute resuscitation. Monitoring during blood transfusion should include continuous bedside presence of nursing staff for the first 15 min to observe for severe transfusion reactions. RBC units are typically warmed to room temperature at the time of transfusion. However, if the blood is rapidly removed from refrigeration and brought to the bedside, it may arrive below room temperature. Blood-warming devices should be considered for patients receiving >2 to 3 U/h, and attention must be given to patients receiving multiple transfusions to prevent and treat hypothermia. Optional premedication for transfusion typically includes acetaminophen as prophylaxis for febrile transfusion reactions.

Clinical Outcomes in Patients Receiving RBC Transfusion

The benefits of RBC transfusion are clearly established from a practical bedside viewpoint in patients with severe anemia, impaired oxygen delivery, and hemorrhage. However, transfusion is associated with important pathophysiologic reactions as well as negative overall ICU outcomes (Table 4). Results of an observational trial in a large US population of 4,892 patients demonstrated that 4% of all RBC transfusions were associated with complications. The most common complications in this group were fever, fluid overload, and hypotension.[3] The potential negative impact of RBC transfusions is clinically significant. Patients who receive RBC transfusions generally demonstrate worse outcomes compared with patients who do not receive transfusion. Multiple clinical observational trials show higher mortality in patients who have received blood transfusion in the ICU.[1,3,6,8] RBC transfusion may contribute to increased mortality in patients with established acute lung injury.[10] Although univariate and

Table 4. *Adverse Effects and Noninfectious Complications Associated With RBC Transfusion*

Immune and inflammatory reactions
    Acute hemolytic reaction
    Delayed hemolytic reaction
    Allergic and anaphylactic reactions
    Febrile transfusion reaction
    Posttransfusion purpura
    TRALI
    Alloimmunization to RBCs
    Relative immunosuppression/transfusion-related
     immunomodulation
    GVHD
Nonimmune adverse consequences (more commonly
    associated with massive transfusion)
    Transfusion-associated circulatory overload
    Hypothermia
    Intravascular volume overload
    Coagulopathy
    Citrate toxicity (metabolic alkalosis)
    Hypocalcemia (ionized calcium)
Patient outcomes associated with RBC transfusion (not
    directly causal)
    Increased mortality
    Longer ICU length of stay
    Higher APACHE and sequential organ failure assessment
     (SOFA) scores
    Increased rate of nosocomial infection

multivariate association analyses cannot establish a causal relationship between transfusion and mortality, at least one propensity scoring model has shown increased mortality in patients who have had blood transfusion. Additional findings in patients who require blood transfusion include higher APACHE scores, higher sequential organ failure assessment (SOFA) scores, increased length of ICU stay, and increased costs.[1,3]

Specific complications that appear to be related to immunosuppressive or immunomodulatory effects of RBC transfusion may contribute to worse clinical outcomes associated with transfusion. A prospective observational study[11] in a single medical center of 2,000 patients has demonstrated that RBC transfusion demonstrated an increase in the risk of nosocomial infection rate (14% in patients receiving transfusion vs 5.8% in those who did not receive transfusion). The adverse effects of RBC may correlate with deterioration of the donor cells with prolonged storage. An observational study[12] of patients undergoing cardiac surgery has demonstrated increased in-hospital mortality, intubation period beyond 72 h, renal failure, and sepsis in patients receiving blood stored for >14 days compared with blood stored ≤14 days.

Noninfectious Complications in ICU Patients Receiving RBC Transfusion

Acute hemolytic transfusion reactions are estimated to occur in 1 in 12,000 to 1 in 100,000 of all RBC transfusions. Fatality associated with acute hemolytic transfusion reactions occur in approximately 1 in 600,000 of RBC transfusions. In many cases, the cause of these reactions are preventable "clerical" errors in blood specimen processing, crossmatching, and blood product administration.[13,14] Hemolytic transfusion reactions occur as the result of ABO blood group, RhD, or, less commonly, other types of RBC surface antigen incompatibility. Hemolysis of donor RBCs occurs as the result of recipient antibody binding. The severity of the reaction is proportional to the volume of blood infused. Rapid clinical deterioration and organ failure results from massive cytokine release, vascular endothelial cell dysfunction, complement activation, and shock. The most severe consequences of hemolytic transfusion

reactions include renal failure, ARDS, and DIC. Clinical manifestations of acute hemolytic transfusion reaction include fever, pain at the infusion site, back pain, chest discomfort, anxiety, nausea, dyspnea, tachycardia, tachypnea, and hypotension. Hemolytic reactions may be identified in comatose or unresponsive patients by the development of hypotension, hemoglobinuria, and coagulopathy manifested by bleeding from venipuncture sites, mucosal surfaces, and surgical wounds.

Treatment of acute hemolytic transfusion reactions should include the following: (1) immediate discontinuation of the transfusion; (2) cardiopulmonary monitoring; (3) laboratory monitoring including hemoglobin, direct antiglobulin (Coombs) testing, and haptoglobin; and (3) IV fluids to maintain urine output of 100 to 150 mL/h. The role of diuretics and mannitol has not been definitively established. However, furosemide may be used if intravascular volume overload develops. There is no role for steroids or antihistamines.

Delayed hemolytic reactions occur as the result of development of alloantibodies to non-ABO RBC antigens. The alloimmunization results from prior transfusion or pregnancy of the recipient. Hemolysis may begin and continue >3 to 14 days and is related to development of an amnestic immune response. Presenting symptoms include fever, chills, jaundice, hemolytic anemia with positive Coombs test, elevated lactate dehydrogenase levels, and decreased haptoglobin. Shock, DIC, and renal insufficiency are unlikely to occur. A significant number of patients will be asymptomatic or have very subtle manifestations. There are no specific treatments for delayed hemolytic reactions; however, the occurrence should be documented for the patient. This history is important for appropriate screening and crossmatching for future transfusion requirements.

Allergic and anaphylactic reactions occur as the result of recipient antibody reaction against a noncellular protein such as Igs found in low concentration in the transfused blood. The most severe anaphylactic reactions usually result from recipient reaction against IgA found in the transfused blood when the recipient is IgA deficient. Anaphylactic reactions manifest with a range of symptoms and signs, ranging in severity from flushing, dyspnea, hypotension, bronchospasm, abdominal pain, diarrhea, and shock. Mild allergic reactions are characterized by urticaria and pruritus. Patients with anaphylaxis may require treatment with epinephrine, IV fluids, and respiratory support. Antihistamines may be used in urticarial reactions. Patients who are IgA deficient and have anaphylaxis require special attention and should receive blood products including RBCs, plasma, and Ig from IgA-deficient donors. These blood products are rare and may be difficult to obtain. Patients with urticaria reactions should be considered for washed cell transfusions if the future need arises.

Febrile nonhemolytic reactions result from donor reaction to recipient leukocytes or the presence of elevated cytokines that have accumulated in the transfused blood. These are the most common form of acute transfusion reaction and may occur in 0.5 to 5% of all transfusions. These reactions usually do not have significant consequences and require management with antipyretics. The greatest difficulty in the management of febrile nonhemolytic reactions is testing to exclude hemolytic reaction because fever is also a manifestation of that more severe complication. Patients in whom febrile reactions develop should receive WBC-filtered blood if future transfusion is necessary.

Posttransfusion purpura results from induction of platelet antibodies following transfusion. Although this complication may develop in men, it has been described more often in multiparous women, suggesting the possibility of sensitization to platelet antigens during pregnancy. The recipient may also have become sensitized to platelet antigens through prior transfusion. The reaction occurs 3 to 12 days after transfusion and is characterized by thrombocytopenia and bleeding that may be severe. The differential diagnosis for posttransfusion purpura includes DIC and heparin-induced thrombocytopenia. The diagnosis is established by the presence of platelet alloantibodies (usually to human platelet antigen-1a) in patients who have received recent transfusion.[15] Treatment includes IV Ig. Alternative proposed treatments include corticosteroids and plasmapheresis.

Transfusion-related acute lung injury (TRALI) is characterized by the development of acute lung injury following transfusion of RBCs or any other plasma-containing blood product. Given multiple confounding factors and difficulty establishing sensitive and specific clinical criteria for this reaction, the etiology has not been established. However, TRALI is likely related to infusion of antileukocyte antibodies or blood storage-related lipids. The symptoms and clinical features of TRALI are the abrupt and rapid development of dyspnea, respiratory distress, hypoxemia, and fever. Both hypertension and hypotension have been described. Chest radiography demonstrates bilateral infiltrates that have been described as *white out*. A precise definition of TRALI is the occurrence of acute respiratory distress and bilateral pulmonary infiltrates within 6 h of transfusion in patients without prior lung injury and without evidence of intravascular volume overload or cardiogenic pulmonary edema. The temporal relationship between transfusion and development of respiratory distress must be present to establish the diagnosis. The rate of TRALI is 1 in 1,000 to 1 in 2,000 transfusions and is more likely to occur in patients with sepsis and more likely to occur when blood products from female donors are given.[16,17] Treatment is supportive but respiratory failure develops in the majority of patients and they require mechanical ventilation. TRALI often resolves within several days and is associated with a lower mortality rate (estimated 5 to 10%) than other causes of acute lung injury or ARDS.[18] The main differential diagnosis for TRALI includes ARDS and hydrostatic pulmonary edema from transfusion-associated circulatory overload.

Transfusion-related GVHD results from the engraftment of immunocompetent donor lymphocytes in severely immunocompromised recipients. The donor lymphocytes proliferate and react against recipient human leukocyte antigen antigens. This reaction typically becomes evident 10 to 30 days following transfusion, and is characterized by skin rash, liver disease, GI disease, and bone marrow suppression. Specific findings include erythematous scaly rash, jaundice, elevated lung function test results, diarrhea, and cytopenias. Neonates, organ transplant patients, bone marrow transplant patients, and leukemia and lymphoma patients are at the highest risk for development of this complication. Transfusion-related GVHD is associated with high mortality rates, and treatment options are limited. Prevention of transfusion-related GVHD should include irradiation of any blood product including RBCs and platelets prior to transfusion. It is not necessary to irradiate fresh-frozen plasma or cryoprecipitate.

Infectious Complications of RBC and Blood Product Transfusion

All blood products are associated with risks of transmission of viral, bacterial, and parasitic infections. The risks are directly proportional to the origin, behaviors, and social factors of the donor. Prevention of disease transmission revolves around careful screening of donors to identify risks for infectious disease and eliminate high-risk donors from the donor pool. In general, directed donations to patients from friends and family members should not be considered to have lower risk of disease transmission than random donor products. Testing after donation testing includes a standardized series of tests to detect proteins, antibodies, and nucleic acids associated with infectious risk. The most significant limitations of disease testing are the time window for disease transmission between initial infection of the donor and development of detectable nucleic acid or antibodies in the donated product. A general principle is that pooled products (platelets and plasma components) from multiple donors are likely to have higher risk of disease transmission than single-donor products. The most important infectious etiologies and risks of transmission are listed in Table 5.[19]

Erythropoietin in ICU Patients

Recombinant erythropoietin stimulates RBC production and increases hematocrit in many subsets of patients with chronic diseases, including chronic renal failure and cancer. The effect of erythropoietin does not occur for several days following administration. This delayed effect is the primary factor that limits its role in the ICU for treatment of acute anemia and diminished oxygen delivery to the organs and tissues. Early clinical trials have demonstrated that administration of erythropoietin can significantly reduce the need for RBC transfusion, decrease the number

Table 5. *Risks of Infectious Disease Transmission With Blood Product Transfusion**

Infectious Agent	Estimated Risk Rate
HIV 1 and 2	1/2,135,000 per unit with PCR for HIV nucleic acids
Hepatitis C virus	1/1,935,000 using nucleic acid testing
Hepatitis B virus	1/205,000 using antigen/antibody testing
Hepatitis A virus	1/1,000,000
Syphilis	No cases reported since 1968
CMV	Recommended that CVM-negative patients at risk for CMV disease receive CMV-safe products or high-efficiency leukofiltration
Malaria	1/4,000,000 (depending on country of origin)

*PCR = polymerase chain reaction. Modified from Pomper GJ, Wu Y, Snyder EL. Risks of transfusion-transmitted infections: 2003. Curr Opin Hematol 2003; 10:412–418

of transfused units per patient, and increase the mean hemoglobin concentration. However, these trials[20,21] did not demonstrate an improvement in other clinical outcomes, including mortality. The most recent prospective, placebo-controlled randomized clinical trial of 40,000 U/wk of erythropoietin failed to demonstrate a decrease in the use of RBC transfusion and did not show a benefit in overall mortality except in the subgroup of patients with trauma. This trial[22] demonstrated an increase in the risk of thrombotic events in patients receiving erythropoietin.

Blood Substitutes

Considerable research has been conducted for the development of blood substitutes and oxygen-carrying solutions. There are two general categories of these replacements: cell-free hemoglobin solutions, and perfluorocarbon-based solutions. The hemoglobin solutions are derived from human or bovine sources and are partially polymerized to decrease the rate of clearance from the blood after infusion. The safety and efficacy of these cell-free hemoglobin treatments have not been clearly established in the general ICU population. There are reports[23] of efficacy of polymerized hemoglobin in surgical patients, but their efficacy has not been determined in general populations. Perfluorocarbon solutions do not have an established clinical indication in the treatment of anemia.

References

1. Vincent JL, Baron JF, Reinhart K, et al. Anemia and blood transfusion in critically ill patients. JAMA 2002; 288:1499–1507

2. Rodriguez RM, Corwin HL, Gettinger A, et al. Nutritional deficiencies and blunted erythropoietin response as causes of the anemia of critical illness. J Crit Care 2001; 16:36–41

3. Corwin HL, Gettinger A, Pearl RG, et al. The CRIT Study: anemia and blood transfusion in the critically ill: current clinical practice in the United States. Crit Care Med 2004; 32:39–52

4. Weiskopf RB, Viele MK, Feiner J, et al. Human cardiovascular and metabolic response to acute, severe isovolemic anemia. JAMA 1998; 279:217–221

5. Rivers E, Nguyen B, Havstad S, et al. Early goal-directed therapy in the treatment of severe sepsis and septic shock. N Engl J Med 2001; 345:1368–1377

6. Napolitano LM. Scope of the problem: epidemiology of anemia and use of blood transfusions in critical care. Crit Care 2004; 8(suppl 2):S1–S8

7. Hebert PC, Wells G, Blajchman MA, et al; Transfusion Requirements in Critical Care Investigators, Canadian Critical Care Trials Group. A multicenter, randomized, controlled clinical trial of transfusion requirements in critical care. N Engl J Med 1999; 340:409–417

8. Rao SV, Jollis JG, Harrington RA, et al. Relationship of blood transfusion and clinical outcomes in patients with acute coronary syndromes. JAMA 2004; 292:1555–1562

9. Chapman JF, Milkins C, Voak D. The computer crossmatch: a safe alternative to the serological crossmatch. Transfus Med 2000; 10:251–256

10. Netzer G, Shah CV, Iwashyna TJ, et al. Association of RBC transfusion with mortality in patients with acute lung injury. Chest 2007; 132:1116–1123

11. Taylor RW, O'Brien J, Trottier SJ, et al. Red blood cell transfusions and nosocomial infections in critically ill patients [quiz 9]. Crit Care Med 2006; 34:2302–2308

12. Koch CG, Li L, Sessler DI, et al. Duration of red-cell storage and complications after cardiac surgery. N Engl J Med 2008; 358:1229–1239

13. Linden JV, Paul B, Dressler KP. A report of 104 transfusion errors in New York State. Transfusion 1992; 32:601–606

14. Klein HG. Allogeneic transfusion risks in the surgical patient. Am J Surg 1995; 170:21S–26S.

15. Lubenow N, Eichler P, Albrecht D, et al. Very low platelet counts in post-transfusion purpura falsely diagnosed as heparin-induced thrombocytopenia: report of four cases and review of literature. Thromb Res 2000; 100:115–25

16. Rana R, Fernandez-Perez ER, Khan SA, et al. Transfusion-related acute lung injury and pulmonary edema in critically ill patients: a retrospective study. Transfusion 2006; 46:1478–1483

17. Gajic O, Rana R, Winters JL, et al. Transfusion-related acute lung injury in the critically ill: prospective nested case-control study. Am J Respir Crit Care Med 2007; 176:886–891

18. Moore SB. Transfusion-related acute lung injury (TRALI): clinical presentation, treatment, and prognosis. Crit Care Med 2006; 34:S114–S117

19. Pomper GJ, Wu Y, Snyder EL. Risks of transfusion-transmitted infections: 2003. Curr Opin Hematol 2003; 10:412–418

20. Corwin HL, Gettinger A, Pearl RG, et al. Efficacy of recombinant human erythropoietin in critically ill patients: a randomized controlled trial. JAMA 2002; 288:2827–2835

21. Georgopoulos D, Matamis D, Routsi C, et al. Recombinant human erythropoietin therapy in critically ill patients: a dose-response study [IS-RCTN48523317]. Crit Care 2005; 9:R508–R515

22. Corwin HL, Gettinger A, Fabian TC, et al. Efficacy and safety of epoetin alfa in critically ill patients. N Engl J Med 2007; 357:965–976

23. Levy JH, Goodnough LT, Greilich PE, et al. Polymerized bovine hemoglobin solution as a replacement for allogeneic red blood cell transfusion after cardiac surgery: results of a randomized, double-blind trial. J Thorac Cardiovasc Surg 2002; 124:35–42

Notes

Anemia and RBC Transfusion in the ICU (Thomas)

Endocrine Emergencies

James A. Kruse, MD

Objectives:

- Recognize the etiologies and clinical manifestations of endocrine crises involving the adrenal, thyroid, pancreas, and pituitary glands
- Review the confirmatory laboratory tests for these disorders in the acute care setting
- Delineate the specific initial treatment for each endocrine emergency
- Point out selected pearls and caveats related to the diagnosis and management of endocrine emergencies

Key words: adrenal failure; diabetes insipidus; diabetic ketoacidosis; hyperosmolar nonketotic dehydration syndrome; hypoglycemia; myxedema coma; pheochromocytoma; thyroid storm

Most endocrine emergencies necessitate ICU admission. Some of these endocrine crises develop in patients who are already in the ICU with a nonendocrine critical illness. Every intensivist should be able to recognize an endocrine emergency, confirm the diagnosis, ascertain the likely cause, and provide acute treatment.

A common thread running through each of the endocrine emergencies discussed herein is the concept of a precipitating factor. The precipitant may be an intercurrent medical illness, a surgical procedure, trauma, pregnancy, noncompliance with outpatient treatment, or some other factor that provokes development of the crisis. Often there is a known underlying endocrine disorder that has been under control, and the patient has been in a compensated state prior to the precipitating event. In other cases, the precipitating factor uncovers a latent endocrine disease that was not previously diagnosed.

Adrenal Failure

Critically diminished endogenous synthesis of corticosteroids constitutes adrenal failure. In primary adrenal failure, the problem lies in the adrenal glands, and the result is usually underproduction of both glucocorticoid and mineralocorticoid hormones. In secondary adrenal failure, the problem lies with the anterior pituitary or hypothalamus (*ie*, lack of sufficient adrenocorticotropic hormone [ACTH] production). There are numerous potential etiologies of adrenal failure (Table 1).

Because higher levels of cortisol are needed in times of physiologic stress, adrenal crisis is often precipitated by some type of acute illness, injury, surgery, decompensation of a chronic illness, or some other physiologically stressful event. Most of the clinical (Table 2) and laboratory (Table 3) manifestations of adrenal insufficiency are nonspecific, but finding a constellation of indicative findings in the relevant clinical context usually is enough to prompt biochemical testing to confirm or exclude the diagnosis.

Plasma cortisol concentrations <3 μg/dL signify adrenal insufficiency. In otherwise healthy subjects, levels >12 μg/dL exclude adrenal insufficiency. Critical illness physiologically necessitates higher levels, but determining the appropriate level for the degree of illness is not possible. Therefore, adrenal reserve is assessed in the ICU setting using the rapid cosyntropin stimulation test. The concept is to determine whether the adrenal glands are capable of producing extra cortisol beyond the prevailing concentration. If the glands are capable, then it can be assumed that the prevailing plasma concentration is adequate. If the glands cannot produce additional cortisol when stimulated by exogenous ACTH, there is no adrenal reserve and the prevailing cortisol level is unlikely to be adequate. In practice, the stimulation test is performed using cosyntropin, a synthetic subunit of ACTH. In the conventional version of the test, 250 μg of cosyntropin is administered by IV injection after first obtaining a plasma sample for baseline cortisol assessment. Plasma samples are then obtained at 30 min and 60 min after injection.

Although there is wide debate regarding interpretation, adequate adrenal reserve is generally signaled by a peak rise of plasma cortisol

Table 1. *Etiologies of Adrenal Insufficiency*

Primary Adrenal Failure	Secondary Adrenal Failure
Autoimmune adrenalitis	Corticosteroid withdrawal
Polyglandular autoimmune syndromes	Cranial trauma
Bilateral adrenalectomy	Panhypopituitarism
Malignancy	Craniopharyngioma
Meningococcemia	Other brain tumors
Pseudomonal infection	After pituitary surgery
Septic shock	Pituitary apoplexy
Viral infections	Other brain hemorrhage
Sarcoidosis	Postpartum pituitary infarction
Amyloidosis	Other brain infarction
Adrenal hemorrhage	Anoxic encephalopathy
Adrenal infarction	Cranial irradiation
Adrenoleukodystrophy	Lymphocytic hypophysitis
Disseminated fungal infection	Sarcoidosis
Tuberculosis	Hemochromatosis
Acquired immune deficiency	Histiocytosis
Syphilis	Tuberculosis
Trypanosomiasis	Histoplasmosis
Etomidate	Rare forms of congenital ACTH deficiency
Ketoconazole	Withdrawal of megestrol acetate

Table 2. *Manifestations of Adrenal Insufficiency*

Symptoms	Physical Findings
Malaise	Orthostatic hypotension
Fatigue	Frank hypotension
Anorexia	Tachycardia
Nausea	Abdominal tenderness
Vomiting	Weight loss
Abdominal pain	Depression
Diarrhea	Psychosis
Constipation	Confusion
Orthostatic symptoms	Hyperpigmentation
Myalgias	Vitiligo
Arthralgias	Amenorrhea
Salt craving	Auricular calcification

Table 3. *Nonspecific Laboratory Findings in Adrenal Insufficiency*

Hypoglycemia	Metabolic acidosis
Hyponatremia	Normal anion gap
Hyperkalemia	Anemia
Hypercalcemia	Neutropenia
Prerenal azotemia	Eosinophilia

level $>9\,\mu g/dL$, to an absolute concentration of $>20\,\mu g/dL$. A low baseline level and little or no response to cosyntropin signify absolute adrenal insufficiency. In the face of a high baseline cortisol level, a peak rise of $\leq9\ \mu g/dL$ after stimulation indicates relative adrenal insufficiency. Absolute adrenal insufficiency requires hormone replacement. Whether relative adrenal insufficiency is an indication for hormone treatment is less clear. In the setting of relative adrenal insufficiency associated with septic shock, information from recent clinical trials, including the Corticus trial, suggest that hormone supplementation may only be useful if there is circulatory shock that is refractory to IV volume expansion and IV vasopressor use.

Absolute adrenal insufficiency is treated with a 200-mg IV injection of hydrocortisone followed by 100 mg IV q8h. Relative adrenal insufficiency associated with refractory septic shock is treated with 50 mg of hydrocortisone IV q6h. If cosyntropin testing is to be performed, administration of hydrocortisone will invalidate the test because the cortisol assay will reflect the administered hydrocortisone. To avoid delaying hormone replacement, a one-time equivalent dose of dexamethasone may be administered initially until prompt cosyntropin testing is completed. Hydrocortisone can be started once the all blood specimens have been obtained for plasma cortisol analysis.

Adrenal crisis represents a state of critical volume contraction involving the extracellular fluid (ECF) space, such that rapid intravascular volume expansion may be lifesaving. Normal saline solution is the IV fluid of choice. Dextrose in normal saline solution should also be provided to prevent or treat hypoglycemia.

Pheochromocytoma

Pheochromocytoma is an uncommon cause of secondary hypertension that represents a chromaffin tumor, usually arising in the adrenal medulla and capable of elaborating epinephrine, norepinephrine, or dopamine, or some combination of these catecholamines. The tumor can also appear at extraadrenal sites, with the most common location being near the organs of Zuckerkandl.

The signs and symptoms of pheochromocytoma (Table 4) are due to catecholamines released from the tumor. Most commonly the manifestations are episodic and brief. Once the diagnosis

Table 4. *Manifestations of Pheochromocytoma*

Symptoms	Physical Findings
Anxiety	Hypertension
Headache	Tachycardia
Palpitations	Flushing
Chest pain	Tremors
Nausea	Diaphoresis
Vomiting	Tachydysrhythmias
Abdominal pain	Orthostatic hypertension
Visual disturbances	Orthostatic hypotension

Table 5. *Etiologies of Hypothyroidism*

Thyroidectomy with inadequate hormone replacement
Neck irradiation or ^{131}I therapy with inadequate hormone replacement
Thyroiditis (*eg*, painless, subacute, postpartum, or Hashimoto thyroiditis)
Drugs (*eg*, propylthiouracil, amiodarone, lithium, iodides, sulfonamides, ethionamide)
Thyroid infiltration (*eg*, amyloidosis, sarcoidosis, scleroderma, hemochromatosis)
Iodine related (*eg*, iodine deficiency [endemic goiter] or iodine induced)
Pituitary or hypothalamic dysfunction (<1% of cases)
Congenital (*eg*, thyroid dysplasia, thyroid agenesis, TSH unresponsiveness)

is suspected, confirmation is performed biochemically by assaying for plasma metanephrine and normetanephrine. An alternative diagnostic test is 24-h urine assay for epinephrine, norepinephrine, metanephrine, and normetanephrine. Performing these tests while the patient is in the ICU is not recommended because various acute illnesses and commonly used drugs can result in false-positive and false-negative test results. Thus, it is preferable to defer testing until the patient is sufficiently stable and discharged from the ICU. Once the diagnosis is confirmed biochemically, the tumor is localized using imaging studies such as CT, MRI, or radiolabeled *m*-iodobenzylguanidine scintigraphy.

There are two situations in which patients with pheochromocytoma may be encountered in the ICU setting. The first situation is the patient who has a hypertensive crisis due to pheochromocytoma and requires emergency management of hypertension and any resulting end-organ dysfunction. The second situation is the perioperative management of patients having surgical excision of their tumor, which is definitive treatment. There is a high risk of intraoperative and postoperative hypertensive crisis due to manipulation of the tumor. Therefore, patients must be preoperatively stabilized from the standpoint of achieving normotension, normal fluid balance, optimal treatment of comorbidities, and adequate pharmacologic α-adrenergic blockade, preferably over a period of weeks.

In an acute episode of hypertensive crisis, the conventional pharmacologic agent of choice is the short-acting α-adrenergic blocker phentolamine mesylate, administered in increments of 2 to 5 mg IV >5 min apart until the BP target is achieved. IV sodium nitroprusside has also been

used successfully. As long-term treatment, the α-blocker phenoxybenzamine is used. Supplementary treatment with a β-adrenergic blocker can be considered, but β-blockers are contraindicated unless adequate α-blockade is first achieved.

Myxedema Coma

The most severe form of hypothyroidism is that associated with profound CNS depression and is called *myxedema coma*. Although by literal interpretation, the term only refers to patients in coma ascribed to hypothyroidism, in practice any degree of obtundation ascribable to hypothyroidism should be considered myxedema coma or impending myxedema coma. There are numerous causes of hypothyroidism (Table 5), but myxedema coma can obviously occur in patients who have previously undergone radioactive iodine ablation or thyroidectomy and then stop taking their prescribed thyroid hormone replacement therapy. Among the factors that can precipitate myxedema coma in a patient with otherwise compensated hypothyroidism is the use of sedating drugs.

Any of the signs and symptoms of hypothyroidism (Table 6) may be present in myxedema coma, but significant depression of the sensorium is required. In addition to abnormal thyrotropin (thyroid-stimulating hormone [TSH]) and thyroid hormone levels, a variety of nonspecific laboratory findings may be seen (Table 7).

Critically ill patients can manifest abnormalities in thyroid function testing when there is no underlying thyroid disorder and no clinical manifestations of hyperthyroidism or hypothyroidism.

Table 6. *Manifestations of Hypothyroidism*

Symptoms	Physical Findings
Fatigue	Weakness
Cold intolerance	Hyporeflexia
Cognitive dysfunction	Apathetic affect
Somnolence	Lethargy
Constipation	Obtundation
Myalgia	Stupor or coma
Headache	Alopecia
Hearing loss	Hypothermia
	Hoarseness
	Goiter
	Bradycardia
	Distant heart sounds
	Heart block
	Periorbital edema
	Coarse dry skin
	Psychiatric disorders

Table 7. *Laboratory Findings in Hypothyroidism*

Thyroid-Related Tests	Nonspecific Laboratory Tests
↑ Thyrotropin level (may be decreased in secondary hypothyroidism)	↑ $Paco_2$ and ↓ Pao_2
↓ Free thyroxine level	↓ Serum sodium concentration
↓ Free thyroxine index	↑ Serum lipid concentration
Normal or ↓ tri-iodothyronine level	↑ Creatine phosphokinase activity

Table 8. *Etiologies of Thyrotoxicosis*

Hyperthyroidism	Non–Hyperthyroid-Related Causes
Graves disease	Excessive thyroid hormone replacement
Multinodular goiter	Transient thyrotoxicosis of thyroiditis
Toxic adenoma	Subacute thyroiditis
Iodine-induced	Thyrotoxicosis factitia
Amiodarone-induced	Struma ovarii and other teratomas
Pituitary tumor	Metastatic thyroid neoplasm
Trophoblastic disease	"Hamburger thyrotoxicosis"

This potential situation, called the *euthyroid sick syndrome*, complicates interpretation of thyroid function tests in ICU patients. The free tri-iodothyronine (T3) level is invariably depressed in critically ill patients; however, thyroxine (T4) levels may be elevated, normal, or low in the euthyroid sick syndrome. T4 levels are more likely to be elevated early in the course of a critical illness and then return to normal or fall below normal when the severity of illness worsens. The TSH level can be mildly increased or decreased in the euthyroid sick syndrome. Although not widely available, levels of reverse T3, an inactive isomer of T3, are elevated in the euthyroid sick syndrome. Treatment with thyroid hormone is not recommended for euthyroid sick syndrome.

Myxedema coma is treated with thyroid hormone replacement. This can be accomplished using a loading dose of 300 μg of thyroxine IV, followed by daily doses of 50 to 100 μg IV. Hydrocortisone, 300 mg/d IV in divided doses, is administered empirically for possible coexisting adrenal insufficiency. As an alternative to giving hydrocortisone, a single dose of dexamethasone may be administered while the rapid cosyntropin stimulation test is performed. Once the test is completed, hydrocortisone is initiated. If the stimulation test results show adequate adrenal reserve, hydrocortisone may be discontinued. Passive rewarming is used to treat hypothermia because active rewarming measures may cause hemodynamic instability by lowering systemic vascular resistance. Respiratory failure is a common complication of myxedema coma. Therefore, endotracheal intubation and mechanical ventilation are frequently required.

Thyroid Storm

Hyperthyroidism manifests clinically as a syndrome called *thyrotoxicosis*. Thyrotoxicosis can also occur without any underlying disease of the thyroid gland, for example, from oral thyroid hormone abuse or overdose, ingestion of bovine thyroid tissue, or from ectopic thyroid hormone production (Table 8).

Thyroid storm is the most extreme form of thyrotoxicosis. Any of the findings of thyrotoxicosis (Table 9) can occur, but significant cardiac manifestations, CNS manifestations, or both are required for the designation of thyroid storm. The most common cause of thyroid storm is Graves disease, an autoimmune form of hyperthyroidism. As with most other endocrine emergencies, thyroid storm is often precipitated by an acute illness, trauma, surgery, pregnancy, or some other

Endocrine Emergencies (Kruse)

Table 9. *Manifestations of Thyrotoxicosis*

Symptoms	Physical Findings
Heat intolerance	Goiter
Nervousness	Fine, friable hair
Palpitations	Skin changes
Diaphoresis	Onycholysis
Hyperphagia	Palmar erythema
Diarrhea	Pretibial myxedema
Weight loss	Tremor
Nausea or emesis	Hyperreflexia
Abdominal pain	Apathetic affect
Fatigue	Weakness
Ocular complaints	Altered mentation
Dyspnea	Delirium
Anorexia	Psychosis
Restlessness	Stupor or coma
Sexual dysfunction	Gynecomastia
	Sinus tachycardia
	Atrial fibrillation
	Atrial flutter
	Systolic hypertension
	Wide pulse pressure
	Signs of high-output heart failure
	Heart block
	Thyroid bruit
	Splenomegaly
	Thyroid stare
	Lid lag or globe lag
	Exophthalmos
	Chemosis
	Ophthalmoplegia
	Visual acuity loss

Table 10. *Laboratory Findings in Hyperthyroidism*

Thyroid-Related Tests (Exceptions Are Given in Text)	Nonspecific Laboratory Tests
↓ Thyrotropin level	Hypercalcemia and hypercalciuria
↑ Free thyroxine level	Hyperbilirubinemia
↑ Free thyroxine index	↑ Alkaline phosphatase and alanine aminotransferase
↑ Tri-iodothyronine level	Neutropenia with relative lymphocytosis

significant physiologic stress in patients with an underlying endocrinopathy, in this case hyperthyroidism. Subtotal thyroidectomy can precipitate thyroid storm if preoperative pharmacologic control of the hyperthyroidism is not achieved.

Usual laboratory findings that may be seen in thyrotoxicosis and hyperthyroidism are shown in Table 10. Most manifestations of thyrotoxicosis are attributable to high systemic levels of the thyroid hormones T3 and T4. TSH levels are low except in the rare case of central hyperthyroidism, which is due to increased TSH production by the anterior pituitary. The T3 level may be elevated; however, in severely ill patients with thyrotoxicosis, it may be low. Free T4 levels are elevated except in an uncommon form of hyperthyroidism known as *T3 thyrotoxicosis,* in which case the T4 level is normal but the T3 level is high. No cutoff levels define thyroid storm *per se,* although thyroid hormone levels tend to be higher in thyroid storm compared to thyrotoxicosis without storm.

Management can be divided into specific and nonspecific treatments. Specific treatment consists of four components. The first is pharmacologic inhibition of thyroid hormone synthesis using a thioamide drug, either propylthiouracil or methimazole. Second, some form of iodine is administered to stop the release of stored hormone from the thyroid gland. This can consist of IV sodium iodide, or oral treatment with either Lugol solution, a cholecystographic agent (*eg,* sodium ipodate or iopanoic acid), or a saturated solution of potassium iodide. Administering iodine prior to thioamide administration risks stimulating thyroid hormone synthesis. Third, a β-adrenergic blocker is administered to blunt the hyperadrenergic manifestations of thyrotoxicosis and to control tachydysrhythmias. Propranolol is the agent of choice, and it is administered IV initially. Fourth, an agent is administered to slow peripheral conversion of T4 to the biologically more active hormone T3. Several drugs have this effect, including propylthiouracil, dexamethasone, and high doses of propranolol.

Nonspecific management includes the use corticosteroids (in case of coexisting hypoadrenalism), cooling measures (if there is hyperthermia), and cardiac monitoring. Rapid cosyntropin stimulation testing may be employed in lieu of empiric hydrocortisone coverage. For antipyretic therapy, acetaminophen is used rather than acetylsalicylate. The latter displaces thyroxine from plasma-binding proteins and could exacerbate the thyrotoxicosis. However, aspirin should nevertheless be administered if there is associated acute coronary syndrome. Use of active cooling measures may be needed in some cases. High doses of β-blocker may be needed to control

Table 11. *Etiologies of Hypoglycemia*

Systemic Illness	Neoplasia	Drugs	Other Causes
Hepatic failure	β-Cell tumor	Insulin	Dumping syndrome
Renal failure	Hepatoma	Ethanol	Reactive hypoglycemia
Heart failure	Lymphoma	β-Blockers	Glycogen storage disease
Adrenal failure	Leukemia	Sulfonylureas	Hereditary fructose intolerance
Severe sepsis	Sarcoma	Disopyramide	Galactosemia
Severe inanition	Carcinoid	Quinidine	Insulin antibodies
Hypopituitarism	Adrenal tumor	Pentamidine	Insulin receptor antibodies

tachydysrhythmias. In some cases, IV diltiazem may be required adjunctively. However, the simultaneous administration of an IV β-blocker and IV diltiazem is not without risk because combined use could precipitate symptomatic heart block.

Hypoglycemia

Common causes of hypoglycemia in ICU patients are insulin administration, renal or hepatic dysfunction, adrenal insufficiency, and drug effects. Although there are many etiologies, most are either obvious or uncommon (Table 11), and therefore extensive evaluation of the cause is not required in the ICU setting unless the hypoglycemia is persistent or recurrent.

The Whipple triad defines the textbook criteria for diagnosis: (1) hypoglycemia (*ie*, a blood glucose concentration < 50 mg/dL), (2) associated manifestations of hypoglycemia, and (3) resolution of the manifestations after treatment with dextrose. Manifestations can be classified as neurologic effects of hypoglycemia and adrenergic effects triggered by hypoglycemia and mediated by counterregulatory hormones (Table 12). The adrenergic manifestations may be blunted or entirely absent in patients receiving β-adrenergic blocking drugs.

Because severe hypoglycemia can cause permanent neurologic injury, acute treatment must be instituted without delay. Laboratory confirmation can be performed using a point-of-care glucose instrument, if readily available, but IV dextrose (*eg*, 50 mL of a 50% dextrose solution) should not be delayed for more than a minute or so if the diagnosis is suspected. It should be assumed that the hypoglycemia will recur within an hour or so after administration of 25 g of dextrose, once the bolus of dextrose is metabolized. A continuous IV infusion of dextrose is therefore routinely

begun after the bolus dextrose dose. If the patient was receiving a 5% dextrose IV infusion when the hypoglycemia developed, the infusion rate should be increased, the concentration increased to 10%, or both. Finally, serial blood glucose assays should be performed on an hourly basis initially to monitor for potential recurrences and to adjust the rate of the dextrose infusion. Refractory hypoglycemia usually responds to simply administering additional dextrose, by increasing the bolus dose as well as the IV infusion concentration or rate. Glucagon, diazoxide, hydrocortisone, and octreotide are among the adjunctive agents that have been used to treat hypoglycemia refractory to IV dextrose.

Diabetic Ketoacidosis

When pancreatic endocrine function is severe enough that the gland produces essentially no insulin, hyperglycemia and ketoacidosis develop unless exogenous insulin is administered. Most of the signs and symptoms of diabetic ketoacidosis (DKA) are nonspecific (Table 13), but the diagnosis should be suspected in any acutely ill patient with known underlying insulin-dependent diabetes. DKA may also occur with new-onset (*ie*, not previously diagnosed) diabetes mellitus. The diagnosis of DKA is usually straightforward based on routine laboratory test results, which reveal hyperglycemia and a high anion gap metabolic acidosis, with evidence of ketosis (Table 14).

ECF volume depletion occurs in DKA as a result of the osmotic diuresis caused by glycosuria. This depletion can be severe, in some cases causing hypovolemic shock. IV fluid resuscitation aimed at expanding intravascular volume is therefore extremely important. Normal saline solution should be administered IV, at least until the

Table 12. *Manifestations of Hypoglycemia*

Neuroglycopenic Manifestations	Adrenergic Manifestations
Headache	Anxiety
Difficulty concentrating	Tremor
Behavioral changes	Diaphoresis
Visual disturbances	Palpitations
Confusion	Tachycardia
Stupor or coma	Nausea
Seizures	Vomiting

Table 13. *Manifestations of DKA*

Symptoms	Physical Findings
Malaise	Tachycardia
Fatigue	Orthostatic or frank hypotension
Polyuria	Abdominal tenderness
Polydipsia	Kussmaul breathing pattern
Nausea	Acetone odor on breath
Vomiting	Lethargy
Abdominal pain	Depressed sensorium

Table 14. *Laboratory Findings in DKA*

Hyperglycemia
Metabolic acidosis
Glycosuria
Ketonemia
Ketonuria
Elevated serum anion gap
Hyperkalemia (before insulin treatment)
Hypokalemia (after insulin treatment)
Hypophosphatemia
Prerenal azotemia

intravascular volume deficit is corrected, because hypotonic IV fluid does not expand intravascular volume as effectively as isotonic crystalloid solution. Regular insulin is administered as an IV bolus of 0.10 to 0.15 U/kg/h followed by a continuous IV infusion at 0.10 U/kg/h. Blood glucose is monitored hourly, and the insulin infusion is adjusted to ensure a fall in the glucose level of approximately 50 mg/dL/h. Controlling the rate of glucose correction is of particular importance in pediatric patients because cerebral edema has been observed in this population during overly rapid correction.

Although there are concomitant kaluresis and total body potassium depletion, hyperkalemia frequently occurs due to shift of potassium from the interior of cells to the interstitial and plasma compartments mediated by lack of insulin. Therapeutic administration of insulin reverses this shift and causes the potassium depletion to manifest as hypokalemia, which can be severe enough to be a threat to life. Serial serum potassium levels and administration of supplemental potassium are therefore an important part of clinical management. Hypophosphatemia can also occur in some cases, but phosphorus administration is not required unless hypophosphatemia is demonstrated. Sodium bicarbonate therapy has

conventionally been employed to lessen the severity of the metabolic acidosis; however, no evidence-based beneficial outcome effects have been demonstrated. Diagnostic evaluation of the precipitating factor responsible for the DKA episode is routinely pursued. Blood cultures are routinely considered because infection is one of the most common precipitating events.

Once the blood glucose level reaches approximately 200 mg/dL, IV fluid is changed to a dextrose-containing solution to allow continuation of the IV insulin without risking hypoglycemia. Even though the blood glucose level may be essentially normalized at this point, IV insulin must continue until the ketoacidosis resolves. This resolution is signaled by normalization of the serum anion gap. Once both hyperglycemia and ketoacidosis have resolved and the patient is receiving oral calories, IV dextrose is stopped, a subcutaneous injection of regular insulin is administered, and IV insulin is discontinued 30 min to 1 h later.

Hyperosmolar Nonketotic Dehydration Syndrome

Some patients with diabetes have severe hyperglycemia but little or no ketoacidosis. Severe hyperglycemia raises plasma osmolality and results in CNS depression, which, if sufficiently severe, can cause coma. This syndrome has various designations, including *hyperglycemic hyperosmolar nonketotic coma*, and *hyperosmolar nonketotic dehydration syndrome* (HONK). These patients are able to produce enough insulin to stave off ketoacidosis but not enough to prevent hyperglycemia. The syndrome occurs in older adults, often those with a history of type II diabetes mellitus or no prior history of diabetes at all. As a result,

Table 15. *Key Differences Between DKA and HONK**

Manifestation	DKA	HONK
Kussmaul breathing	+	0
Acetone odor on breath	+	0
Sensorium	↓–↓↓	↓↓–↓↓↓
Total body water	↓↓↓	↓↓↓↓
Blood glucose	↑↑	↑↑↑↑
Serum osmolality	↑	↑↑↑
Ketosis	+	0–trace
Metabolic acidosis	+	0–trace
Serum anion gap	↑–↑↑↑↑	0–↑
Serum sodium	↓–↓↓	↓↓↓↓–↑↑↑

*+ = present; 0 = absent; ↓ to ↓↓↓↓ = mild to severe decrease; ↑ to ↑↑↑↑ = mild to severe increase.

noncompliance is less often a precipitating factor in these patients compared to those in whom DKA develops; acute complications of chronic cardiovascular disease, including cerebral vascular accidents and acute coronary syndrome, are more common.

The signs and symptoms of HONK are similar to those encountered in DKA, with a few notable exceptions (Table 15). Similarly, there are several differences in the laboratory manifestations of HONK compared to DKA. Blood glucose concentration is >800 mg/dL in HONK and sometimes reaches extreme values (>2,000 mg/dL). Because there is commonly a degree of overlap between HONK and DKA, some patients have features of both syndromes.

ECF sodium concentration is often low in both DKA and HONK. This is due to osmotic shifting of water from the intracellular fluid (ICF) compartment to the ECF compartment mediated by ECF hyperosmolality from the hyperglycemia. This movement of water results in dilution of ECF solutes, including sodium, causing hyponatremia. Because hyperosmolality is more extreme in HONK than DKA, the hyponatremia in HONK can be extreme in some cases. Although this movement of pure water to the ECF compartment would by itself tend to expand the plasma volume, hypervolemia does not occur because of the concomitant osmotic diuresis caused by glycosuria. In some cases, marked hypotonic fluid loss predominates to a degree that surpasses the aforementioned dilutional effect on plasma sodium and results in hypernatremia, indicating a profound degree of ICF dehydration.

Hypernatremia is often used clinically as a surrogate marker for hyperosmolality to assess the degree of electrolyte-free water deficit and hence the degree of intracellular dehydration. However, the sodium concentration can be misleading in HONK because the increase in plasma osmolality is due predominately or entirely to hyperglycemia. By taking into account the degree of hyperglycemia and proportionately scaling the sodium concentration upward, the clinician can use this "corrected" sodium concentration to more accurately gauge the degree of free water deficit compared to using the measured sodium concentration alone. This is conventionally accomplished using the following equation:

$$Na\text{-}c = Na\text{-}m + 0.016 \times (Glu - 100)$$

where Na-c is the "corrected" sodium concentration, and Na-m is the measured sodium concentration, both in milliequivalents per liter, and Glu is the glucose concentration in milligrams per deciliter. Although the adjective "corrected" is often used to describe this derived value of sodium concentration, the measured sodium is not incorrect. There is no methodologic problem that results in pseudohyponatremia, as occurs in hyperlipidemia. The "corrected" value simply affords the clinician a means for assessing the degree of ICF volume depletion and hyperosmolality without measuring or deriving serum osmolality.

The initial treatment of HONK is the same as for DKA. Additional fluid replacement is often required due to the more severe fluid deficit. Normal saline solution is administered until the ECF deficit is replenished, and then half-normal saline solution is substituted. The rate of correction of the hyperglycemia may be more important in HONK than in adult patients with DKA.

Diabetes Insipidus

Water delivered to the distal nephron is reclaimed by absorption from the collecting tubule lumen. However, the luminal membrane of the collecting tubule is impermeable to water. Expression of aquaporin channels on this membrane allow water resorption, but only in the presence of the antidiuretic hormone arginine vasopressin (AVP), which is produced in the hypothalamus

Table 16. *Etiologies of DI*

Central DI	Nephrogenic DI
Congenital	Specific tubular defects
Cranial trauma	Congenital causes
Hypophysectomy	V2 receptor defect
Other brain surgery	Aquaporin gene defect
Brain neoplasms	Acquired causes
Cerebral infarction	Hypokalemia
Sheehan syndrome	Hypercalcemia
Intracranial hemorrhage	General tubular defects*
Cerebral aneurysm	Sickle-cell disease
Anoxic encephalopathy	Polycystic disease
Brain death	Medullary sponge kidney
Encephalitis	Sjögren syndrome
Meningitis	After renal infarction
Neurosarcoidosis	Sarcoidosis
Neurotuberculosis	Obstructive uropathy
Neurosyphilis	Other interstitial disease
Lymphoma	Hypergammaglobulinemia
Leukemia	Medullary gradient loss*
Hand-Scüller-Christian	Polyuria of any cause
Infundibulohypophysitis	Very low protein diet
Wegener granulomatosis	Drug-induced causes
Idiopathic	Lithium carbonate
	Demeclocycline
	Amphotericin B
	Vinblastine
	Foscarnet
	Orlistat
	Ofloxacin
	Rifampin
	Netilmicin
	Ifosfamide
	Cidofovir
	Indinavir
	Tenofovir
	Epirubicin
	Cyclophosphamide
	Methotrexate
	Streptozocin
	Cholchicine
	Methyoxyflurane
	Triamterene
	Pimocide

*See text regarding classification as DI.

Table 17. *Etiologies of Polyuria*

DI
Excessive IV fluid administration
Hyperglycemia
Diuretic administration
Primary polydipsia
Nonoliguric renal failure (recovery phase)*
After obstructive uropathy*
Renocorticomedullary gradient loss*
Generalized renotubulointerstitial disease*

*See text regarding classification.

and released at the pituitary hypophysis. Diabetes insipidus (DI) results from either lack of AVP or unresponsiveness of the distal nephron to its normal action. The former is termed *central DI*, and the latter *nephrogenic DI*. Each variety has many possible causes (Table 16).

The hallmark manifestations of DI are polyuria and polydipsia, with a propensity for dehydration, hypernatremia, and hyperosmolality to develop. Patients who can experience thirst and can obtain water will not have significant dehydration or hypernatremia. However, in patients with encephalopathy and those who are sedated or cannot obtain water, these complications can develop rapidly if adequate enteral water or hypotonic IV fluid is not supplied.

Prior to making the diagnosis of DI, other causes of polyuria must be considered and excluded (Table 17). Some DI classification systems include generalized tubulointerstitial renal disorders that result in unresponsiveness to AVP as causes of nephrogenic DI. However, other authors, including the National Kidney Foundation, restrict the rubric nephrogenic DI to tubular dysfunction that specifically involves distal nephron water reabsorption in the absence of other tubular dysfunction.

Most critically ill patients with DI tend to have hypernatremia due to the inappropriate loss of dilute urine. As long as the patient is hypernatremic, even if only slightly, the diagnosis is readily made by demonstrating inappropriately hypotonic urine. In otherwise healthy subjects, hypernatremia will be sensed by the hypothalamus, which will elaborate AVP by way of the hypophysis. The elaborated AVP will cause pure water to be reabsorbed by the distal nephron, mitigating exacerbation of the hypernatremia and producing concentrated urine with an osmolality of >800 mOsm/kg H_2O. In complete DI, urine osmolality will be dilute, *ie*, <300 mOsm/kg H_2O, in the face of mild or severe hypernatremia. Partial DI in this situation yields a urine osmolality in the range of 300 to 700 mOsm/kg H_2O.

Although the assay is generally more time consuming, AVP levels can be assessed in lieu of urine osmolality measurements. AVP measurements also allow differentiation of central from nephrogenic DI. Otherwise normal subjects who are hypernatremic will have AVP levels >2 pg/mL. Patients with complete central DI will have undetectable AVP levels. Patients with partial central DI may have AVP levels as high as 1.5 pg/mL. Nephrogenic DI will lead to high AVP values, sometimes >5 pg/mL.

Urine osmolality can be used to differentiate central from nephrogenic DI if assessed before and after providing exogenous AVP. If urine osmolality is inappropriately low in the face of hypernatremia, administration of exogenous AVP will cause the urine osmolality to increase by at least 50% if there is complete DI on a central basis. In partial central DI, the urine osmolality will increase by 10 to 50%. In nephrogenic DI, the urine osmolality will generally not increase after AVP administration. In practice, the AVP analog desmopressin is more commonly used for this purpose rather than exogenous AVP. After collecting a spot urine sample for osmolality, desmopressin is administered as a 1-μg subcutaneous dose, and a second urine collection is obtained over the next hour or so for reassessment of osmolality.

Polyuria may be >20 L/d in some cases of DI. To prevent rapid development of severe dehydration and severe hypernatremia, either the fluid deficit and ongoing fluid loss must be replaced or the polyuria stopped. The latter approach is preferred in all but the mildest cases of central DI, accomplished by administering either AVP or desmopressin. Desmopressin is the preferred agent (eg, 1 to 2 μg subcutaneously q12h) because it stimulates only V2 receptors, which are located in the collecting tubules. AVP stimulates V2 receptors in the kidney, but it also stimulates vascular V1 receptors, resulting in the potentially undesirable effect of vasoconstriction.

Even if the polyuria is completely controlled with desmopressin, IV fluid administration will likely be needed to replace any deficit that developed prior to administering desmopressin, and as maintenance. Because the urinary fluid losses in DI are hypotonic, the IV fluid is also hypotonic. The only exception is in patients who have a significant degree of concomitant intravascular volume depletion. Thus, patients who are hypotensive secondary to hypovolemia should initially receive isotonic IV fluid until intravascular volume is restored, and then hypotonic fluid can be substituted. Close monitoring of fluid intake and output, frequent measurement of serum sodium concentration, and careful adjustment of IV fluid infusion rates are key to correction and prevention of hypernatremia and dehydration.

Exogenous AVP and desmopressin are generally not useful in treating nephrogenic DI. Therefore, fluid and electrolyte monitoring and IV fluid titration assume even greater importance in managing this form of DI. Any drugs that could be causing the nephrogenic DI must be stopped. A thiazide diuretic is administered to induce mild ECF volume depletion, which causes increased water reabsorption at the proximal tubule. As a result, there is less water delivered to the distal nephron and therefore less urine is produced.

Annotated Bibliography

American Diabetes Association. Hyperglycemic crises in patients with diabetes mellitus. Diabetes Care 2001; 24:154–161
Authoritative evidence-based recommendations and treatment protocols.
Hamrahian AH, Oseni TS, Arafah BM. Measurements of serum free cortisol in critically ill patients. N Engl J Med 2004; 350:1629–1638
A study examining the use of free vs total plasma cortisol levels for assessing adrenal function: for a critical commentary, see: Dubey A, Boujoukos AJ. Free cortisol levels should not be used to determine adrenal responsiveness, Crit Care 2004; 9:E2
Kruse JA, Fink MP, Carlson RW, eds. Saunders manual of critical care. Philadelphia, PA: WB Saunders, 2003; 164–193
Contains nine succinct chapters providing practical information on the clinical management of endocrine emergencies.
Lima EQ, Aguiar FC, Barbosa DM, et al. Severe hypernatremia (221 mEq/L), rhabdomyolysis and acute renal failure after cerebral aneurysm surgery. Nephrol Dial Transplant 2004; 19:2126–2129
Describes a case of postoperative hypernatremia due to disruption of hypothalamic function.
Mohammad Z, Afessa B, Finkielman JD. The incidence of relative adrenal insufficiency in patients with septic shock after the administration of etomidate. Crit Care 2006; 10:R105
An investigation showing that etomidate administration can result in adrenal insufficiency.

Pacak K, Linehan WM, Eisenhofer G, et al. Recent advances in genetics, diagnosis, localization, and treatment of pheochromocytoma. Ann Intern Med 2001; 34:315–329

A review offering algorithmic approaches to biochemical testing and imaging selection, as well as management recommendations.

Plouin P-F, Gemenez-Roqueplo A-P. Pheochromocytoma and secreting paragangliomas. Orphanet J Rare Dis 2006; 1:49

A review of the disease, including etiologies, diagnostic methods, and preoperative and postoperative management.

Roberge RJ, Martin TG, Delbridge TR. Intentional massive insulin overdose: recognition and management. Ann Emerg Med 1993; 22:228–234

This review covers diagnostic and treatment considerations for managing hypoglycemia due to insulin overdose. The presentation includes a case report followed by a question and answer discussion.

Rodriquez I, Fluiters E, Pérez-Méndez LF, et al. Factors associated with mortality of patients with myxedema coma: prospective study in 11 cases treated in a single institution. J Endocrinol 2004; 180:347–350

A case series finding a 36% mortality rate for this illness. Average Glasgow coma scale scores were 12 in survivors and 5 in nonsurvivors.

Sands JM, Bichet DG. Nephrogenic diabetes insipidus. Ann Intern Med 2006; 144:186–194

A review of the molecular biology, congenital causes, and acquired causes of nephrogenic DI.

Service FJ. Hypoglycemic disorders. N Engl J Med 1995; 332:1144–1152

Review of the classification, evaluation, and management of hypoglycemia, including uncommon causes.

van den Berghe G, Wouters P, Weekers F, et al. Intensive insulin therapy in the critically ill patients. N Engl J Med 2001; 345:1359–1367

A randomized controlled trial showing that targeting a blood glucose level of 80 to 110 mg/dL in surgical ICU patients reduced mortality by 34% compared to standard glucose management.

Yoon S-J, Kim D-M, Kim J-U, et al. A case of thyroid storm due to thyrotoxicosis factitia. Yonsei Med J 2003; 44:351–354

Describes the presentation and clinical management of a patient who ingested 5,000 μg of levothyroxine.

Zaloga GP, Marik PE, eds. Endocrine and metabolic dysfunction syndromes in the critically ill. Crit Care Clin 2001; 17:1–252

This entire bound issue is devoted to endocrine and metabolic disturbances pertinent to the ICU setting, including individual articles on thyroid, adrenal, pituitary, and glycemic crises.

Notes

Coagulopathies, Bleeding Disorders, and Blood Component Therapy

Karl W. Thomas, MD, FCCP

Objectives:

- Distinguish and initiate appropriate treatment for common causes of thrombocytopenia including immune thrombocytopenic purpura, thrombotic thrombocytopenic purpura, and heparin-induced thrombocytopenia
- Understand and discriminate between clinical features of disseminated intravascular coagulation and the coagulopathy of liver disease
- Discuss the clinical monitoring and management of patients with coagulopathy of massive transfusion
- Determine the appropriate clinical use for platelets, fresh-frozen plasma, and cryoprecipitate
- Briefly discuss the role of blood substitutes and adjunctive treatments such as desmopressin and activated factor VII

Key words: coagulopathy; cyroprecipitate; heparin; plasma; platelet; thrombocytopenia; warfarin

Anemia, thrombocytopenia, and coagulopathies are commonly encountered in ICU patients. These disorders rarely occur in isolation and are directly related to ICU outcomes. Rapid and efficient classification and recognition of these disorders is essential to the provision of timely and appropriate care. These disorders require a clinical approach based on systematic examination of RBC, platelets, and coagulation factor parameters. This chapter will review and apply basic laboratory testing including examination of coagulation times, fibrin levels, d-dimer levels, the peripheral blood smear, and the platelet count. Disorders including thrombocytopenia, disseminated intravascular coagulation (DIC), immune thrombocytopenic purpura (ITP), thrombotic thrombocytopenic purpura (TTP), heparin-induced thrombocytopenia (HIT), and massive transfusion will be reviewed, with a focus on key identifying features. This chapter will also review the clinical indications and use of fresh-frozen plasma (FFP) and platelet transfusion.

Incidence and Clinical Significance of Thrombocytopenia

Thrombocytopenia develops in up to 45% of ICU patients; this is defined as platelet count <150,000 cells/µL. For ICU patients, observational studies have consistently associated thrombocytopenia with increased mortality, major bleeding, and increased blood product transfusion requirements. For both medical and surgical ICU patients, platelet counts typically fall and reach a nadir by days 3 to 4 of the ICU stay. Although ICU survivors typically have return of platelet counts to baseline or above, nonsurvivors more frequently have persistent thrombocytopenia. Thus, the dynamic changes of the platelet count are related to outcome, and persistent thrombocytopenia has negative prognostic value.[1,2] In the absence of other coagulopathy, significant bleeding is unlikely for patients undergoing surgery until the platelet count is <50,000 cells/µL. Spontaneous bleeding from superficial cuts or mucosal surfaces is unlikely until the platelet count decreases below 10,000 to 20,000 cells/µL.

Etiology of Thrombocytopenia

Thrombocytopenia may result from decreased production, increased destruction, or from distribution/dilution effects (Table 1). Causes of decreased platelet production include infections (eg, parvovirus, Epstein-Barr virus, HIV), drugs, and toxins (eg, chemotherapy, alcohol), nutritional deficiencies (eg, folate, cobalamin), and bone marrow diseases including myelodysplastic or myeloproliferative syndromes.

Increased platelet destruction or shortened platelet survival may result from either immune-mediated or nonimmune-mediated processes.

Table 1. *Causes and Contributing Factors in ICU Thrombocytopenia**

Decreased platelet production
    Viral infection (Epstein-Barr virus, parvovirus, HIV)
    Drugs and toxins (alcohol, chemotherapy)
    Nutritional deficiency (folate, vitamin B_{12})
    Myelodysplastic syndromes
Increased platelet destruction
    Sepsis
    DIC
    TTP
    ITP
    HIT
    Posttransfusion purpura
    Antiphospholipid antibody syndrome
    HELLP syndrome
Abnormal distribution and dilution
    Hypersplenism
    Massive blood transfusion

*HELLP = hemolytic anemia, elevated liver function tests, low platelet count.

The most common immune-mediated disorders of thrombocytopenia include HIT, TTP, and ITP. Infection, sepsis, septic shock, and chronic liver disease with hypersplenism are the underlying disorders in about one-half of all ICU patients with thrombocytopenia.[3] The mechanism for thrombocytopenia in sepsis is likely multifactorial and includes immune-mediated platelet destruction, hemophagocytic histiocytosis, and DIC.[4] Distributional thrombocytopenia has been attributed to hypersplenism and splenic sequestration resulting from portal hypertension. Dilutional thrombocytopenia commonly occurs in patients receiving massive blood transfusion on the order of 15 to 20 U of packed RBCs per 24 h.

Specific Disorders Associated With Thrombocytopenia

HIT

HIT results from the generation of antibodies to complexes of heparin and platelet factor 4 (PF4). For patients who have never received heparin, the development of HIT typically occurs 5 to 10 days after initiation of heparin. For patients who have received heparin recently or have antiheparin-PF4 antibodies, rapid declines in platelet count may occur within hours of heparin administration. The diagnosis of HIT should be considered in any patient receiving therapeutic heparin or has been exposed to heparin (*eg*, heparin line flushes) and who has an otherwise unexplained platelet count $< 150,000/\mu L$ or a decrease of $\geq 50\%$ from baseline. HIT is associated with the development of thrombotic complications—including deep venous thrombosis, pulmonary embolism, and cutaneous or limb ischemia secondary to arterial thrombosis—in 30 to 50% of patients. The risk of both HIT and thrombosis is highest in patients undergoing orthopaedic surgery or cardiac surgery, although general medical patients are also at risk. The diagnostic approach to HIT should account for the pretest probability (*eg*, presence of significant decline in platelet count, heparin exposure, acute medical, or surgical condition) and detection of antibodies directed against heparin-PF4.[5] Treatment of HIT is directed at preventing and treating thrombotic complications. Patients with HIT should be considered hypercoagulable and should receive short-term anticoagulation with direct thrombin inhibitors (*eg*, lepirudin, argatroban) followed by longer-term oral anticoagulation with warfarin.

ITP

ITP is characterized by isolated thrombocytopenia in the setting of normal coagulation time measurements and the absence of other RBC or WBC abnormalities. ITP results from the presence of autoantibodies directed against platelet glycoproteins and may be primary (idiopathic) or secondary to other systemic disorders. Secondary causes of ITP include systemic lupus, medications, HIV, lymphoproliferative disorders, and immunodeficiency syndromes. Medications associated with ITP include trimethoprim-sulfamethoxazole, thiazide diuretics, quinidine, and diphenylhydantoin. If the cause is suspected or known, every attempt should be made to remove the inciting agent or to treat the underlying disorder. First-line acute treatment for idiopathic ITP is corticosteroids. Refractory cases may be treated with IV Ig or anti-Rho(D) Ig in patients who are Rh-positive. Platelet transfusions alone do not effectively raise the platelet count in ITP, but may be necessary in combination with corticosteroids or

Coagulopathies, Bleeding Disorders, and Blood Component Therapy (Thomas)

IV Ig if the patient experiences clinically significant bleeding.

TTP-Hemolytic Uremic Syndrome

TTP-hemolytic uremic syndrome (HUS) results from the abnormal activation and intravascular aggregation of platelets accompanied by intravascular hemolysis. TTP-HUS is characterized as a thrombotic microangiopathy and is identified by the presence of hemolytic anemia and thrombocytopenia. If untreated, the mortality rate of TTP approaches 100%. Since the widespread use of plasma exchange, the mortality rate for TTP has fallen to 10 to 35%.[6,7] Epidemiologic data from the United States have demonstrated a higher rate of disease in women compared with men, and a higher mortality rate in Blacks compared with Whites.[8]

Both TTP and HUS are thrombotic microangiopathies characterized by platelet activation, microvascular platelet thrombi, and microangiopathic hemolytic anemia. Traditional definitions of TTP and HUS are based on slightly different clinical presentations. TTP has been characterized by the clinical pentad of hemolysis, thrombocytopenia, neurologic defects, fever, and renal dysfunction. TTP may be idiopathic, congenital, or may occur secondarily in systemic infections. Neurologic defects tend to be more prominent in TTP and include a spectrum of manifestations such as headache, mental status abnormalities, focal defects, seizures, or coma. Renal defects ranging from mild renal insufficiency to acute renal failure may be found in both TTP and HUS, but are more prominent in HUS. HUS has been described more frequently in childhood and younger adults; it typically presents immediately following bacterial infection. Common infection syndromes that proceed thrombotic microangiopathy include gastroenteritis from enterotoxin-producing bacteria including *Escherichia coli* O157:H7 or *Shigella* and acute bacterial infection in patients with HIV disease.[9] TTP-HUS also occurs sporadically and has been well described in postpartum patients, patients with recent viral infection including HIV, transplant patients receiving immunosuppression, cancer patients receiving chemotherapy, and patients with collagen vascular disease.

The underlying causes of TTP are congenital or acquired defects in the von Willebrand factor cleaving protease (ADAMTS13) and massive systemic vascular endothelial injury.[10] The laboratory features of TTP-HUS include thrombocytopenia, anemia, and schistocytes on peripheral blood smear. The thrombocytopenia in TTP-HUS tends be severe, with levels usually <50,000 cells/μL. Additional features include elevations of lactate dehydrogenase and serum bilirubin, which result from hemolysis. Urinalysis may demonstrate decreased creatinine clearance, proteinuria, and hematuria. Unlike DIC and liver disease, TTP-HUS is not associated with consumption of coagulation proteins. In TTP-HUS, the prothrombin time (PT), activated partial thromboplastin time (aPTT), and fibrinogen levels remain within the normal range (Table 2). From a clinical standpoint, TTP-HUS may be distinguished from DIC by the absence of clinical syndromes of trauma, shock, and sepsis that are typically associated with DIC (see the section on "DIC").

The treatment of TTP-HUS requires emergent initiation of plasma exchange and ICU monitoring. Plasma infusion alone is less effective and is limited by the volume of plasma required to produce clinical effect.[7,11] Shock may develop in patients with TTP-HUS; they may also experience respiratory failure or neurologic deterioration. Although plasma exchange may be performed through peripheral venous access, central venous hemodialysis catheters are often used. Treatment

Table 2. *Distinguishing Features of Complex Coagulopathies*

Coagulopathies	PT/aPTT	Platelets	Fibrinogen	d-Dimer
TTP-HUS	Normal	Decreased	Normal	Normal
DIC	Prolonged	Decreased	Decreased	Elevated
Liver disease	Prolonged	Normal to decreased	Normal to decreased	Normal to mild elevation
Massive transfusion	Prolonged	Decreased	Decreased	Normal

with daily plasma exchange is indicated until the patient has rising platelet counts, resolving anemia, resolution of renal failure, and normalization of neurologic deficits. Other indicators of therapeutic response include decreases in serum lactate dehydrogenase level and resolution of the abnormal peripheral blood smear. Patients will typically require 1 to 2 weeks of plasma exchange treatments tapered from daily treatments to every other day to every third day. Refractory cases, late-responding patients, and relapsed patients may require treatment for 4 to 6 weeks. Patients who fail to respond to plasma exchange should be considered for high-dose steroid therapy, rituximab, or splenectomy.

Coagulation Protein Defects, Complex Coagulopathy Syndromes, Heparin, and Warfarin

Clinically significant coagulopathies may occur as the result of defects in platelets, serum coagulation factors, or both. Platelet disorders may be quantitative (see the previous discussion of thrombocytopenia) or qualitative. Qualitative or functional platelet disorders (thrombocytopathy) result from exposure to nonsteroidal anti-inflammatory agents, aspirin, glycoprotein IIb/IIIa inhibitors, or may occur in uremia. In general, bleeding primarily associated with thrombocytopenia is cutaneous (eg, petechiae and superficial ecchymosis) or mucosal (eg, epistaxis or gingival bleeding). In distinction, disorders of coagulation protein quantity and function are typically associated with large palpable ecchymosis and deep-tissue hematomas, hemarthrosis, and severe, often delayed, postsurgical bleeding.

Coagulopathies related to disorders of coagulation protein function share the common final defect of abnormal generation of fibrin. These disorders may be the result heparin, warfarin, isolated factor deficiencies, combined factor deficiencies, coagulation protein inhibitors, or complex combined defects involving both platelets and coagulation proteins (Table 3).

DIC

DIC is characterized by systemic activation of the clotting cascade, fibrin deposition throughout the microvasculature, fibrinolysis, and consumption of clotting factors. The pathophysiology of DIC involves a primary component of thrombosis and a secondary bleeding diathesis from depletion of clotting components and active fibrinolysis. Organ failure and hemodynamic collapse occur as the result of tissue ischemia from thrombosis or hemorrhagic complications. The mechanisms that trigger DIC act through a final common pathway of massive thrombin generation and diffuse fibrin formation. This occurs as the result of exposure of the blood to procoagulants such as tissue factor and tissue thromboplastins. Predisposing factors for DIC include massive tissue injury, extensive vascular endothelial injury, shock of any cause, amniotic or fat embolism, traumatic brain injury, malignancy, severe infection with exposure to endotoxin, and massive release of inflammatory cytokines. Systemic activation of thrombosis results in a compensatory state of fibrinolysis characterized by rapid dissolution of thrombosis, multifocal sites of bleeding, and accumulation of plasma fibrin degradation products. The rate of development of organ failure in patients with DIC is highly variable and ranges from 20 to 75%.[12] Specific complications of DIC include bleeding, renal insufficiency, hepatic dysfunction, shock, respiratory failure, and thromboembolism.[13]

Clinical and laboratory features of DIC include abnormalities in all aspects of blood and coagulation including hemostasis, RBC, platelets, coagulation factors (Table 2). Petechiae, ecchymosis, and bleeding from venipuncture sites,

Table 3. *Disorders of Fibrin Formation*

Isolated factor deficiency
  Hemophilia A (factor VIII deficiency)
  Isolated factor VII, XI, XII, X, V, or II deficiency
  von Willebrand factor deficiency
Combined factor deficiencies
  Warfarin administration
  Vitamin K deficiency
  Hepatic disease
Coagulation factor inhibitors
  Lupus anticoagulant (usually hypercoagulable)
Complex combined coagulopathies
  DIC
  Massive transfusion
  Hepatic disease

Coagulopathies, Bleeding Disorders, and Blood Component Therapy (Thomas)

surgical wounds, and uninjured mucosal surfaces may develop. Peripheral blood smear may demonstrate microangiopathic hemolysis with schistocytes. Thrombocytopenia occurs through diffuse intravascular activation and consumption of platelets. The diagnosis of DIC is established through the presence of clinical conditions that predispose the patient to DIC in combination with biochemical evidence of thrombosis, thrombolysis, and clotting factor depletion. Both the aPTT and PT are prolonged and reflect consumption of clotting factors in the common, intrinsic, and extrinsic coagulation cascade. A characteristic of DIC is the presence of fibrin degradation products and elevated d-dimer levels. Because plasma fibrinogen is an acute-phase reactant, patients with inflammation, pregnancy, or malignancy may have an elevated baseline fibrinogen level. Thus, fibrinogen alone has a poor discrimination value, and patients with DIC may have a normal or decreased fibrinogen level. Other markers of DIC include detectable plasma fibrin monomers, decreased plasma antithrombin activity, and decreased levels of individual clotting factors, particularly factor VIII.

The presence of DIC is associated with increased ICU mortality in all patient subgroups. Furthermore, combined indexes for DIC, which include d-dimer, platelet count, PT, and fibrinogen levels, correlate well with acute physiology and chronic health evaluation (APACHE)-II score and are predictive of mortality in general ICU populations.[14] The treatment of patients with DIC is focused on treatment of the underlying disorder. Hemostatic deficiencies should be treated with transfusions of RBCs, platelets, and cryoprecipitate if bleeding develops or if there is a high risk of bleeding (eg, recent trauma, surgery, or planned invasive procedure). The benefit of prophylactic transfusion of blood products for patients with DIC without active bleeding or with low risk for bleeding has not been established. High-risk patients or actively bleeding patients should receive platelets to maintain a concentration of at least 20,000 to 50,000 cells/μL and FFP and cryoprecipitate to maintain a reasonable PT and a fibrinogen concentration of >50 mg/dL. Heparin treatment is indicated for patients with DIC in whom clinically apparent thrombosis develops. However, routine use of heparin in patients with DIC without clinical evidence of large vein or arterial thrombosis remains controversial. Patients with fulminant DIC or purpura fulminans should be considered for heparin or activated protein C infusion. Evidence supporting these interventions remains limited, and these treatments have high risk of hemorrhage if profound thrombocytopenia is present. Heparin for DIC should be administered as a continuous infusion without a loading bolus dose and with target PTT two to three times baseline. Monitoring for patients with DIC should include frequent reassessment for bleeding complications and serial measurements of platelet counts and fibrinogen.

Hepatic Disease

Acute liver failure and severe chronic hepatic disease are associated with multiple simultaneous defects in hemostasis and coagulation. The liver produces clotting factors including fibrinogen and prothrombin, as well as factors V, VII, IX, X, XII, and XIII. Liver disease is unlikely to contribute to significant decreases in fibrinogen, but there may be severe decreases in the vitamin-K dependent factors (II, VII, IX, and X) as indicated by prolonged PTs. In addition to coagulation proteins, the liver produces thrombopoietin. For patients with advanced liver disease, thrombopoietin deficiency, in combination with hypersplenism and toxic effects of viral hepatitis or alcohol on the bone marrow, combine to produce thrombocytopenia. Laboratory features of coagulopathy in liver disease include thrombocytopenia, prolonged PT and aPTT, and normal or low fibrinogen levels. Primary fibrinolysis associated with mildly elevated d-dimer levels may also develop in patients with liver disease. Coagulopathy associated with liver disease is distinguished from DIC by the presence of only small-to-moderate elevations in d-dimer levels and preservation of factor VIII levels. Factor VIII is not synthesized in the liver and is consumed only in DIC (Table 2). Treatment for patients with coagulopathy of liver failure includes platelet transfusion, vitamin K supplementation, and, if bleeding is present, FFP or cryoprecipitate.

Heparin and Warfarin

Heparin therapy produces a prolonged aPTT and thrombin time. If a patient requires invasive procedures while receiving heparin, it is recommended that unfractionated heparin be discontinued 6 h prior to the procedure and low-molecular-weight heparin be discontinued 12 to 24 h prior to the procedure. For patients who require urgent intervention or who develop severe bleeding complications, protamine may be administered to neutralize the effect of unfractionated heparin.

Warfarin administration results in prolonged PT, which may persist for 2 to 5 days following its discontinuation. Patients with mild elevations (<5) in international normalized ratio (INR) and with no evidence of bleeding should have their next warfarin dose withheld and be followed up with more frequent PT monitoring. Patients with higher elevations of INR (>5.0) should be treated with 1 to 2 mg of oral vitamin K. Patients with extreme elevations in INR (>9) are at elevated risk of life-threatening hemorrhage and should be hospitalized and treated with 5 to 10 mg of oral vitamin K. Patients in whom severe, hemodynamically significant bleeding develops at any level of INR while receiving warfarin should be treated with slow infusion of 10 mg of IV vitamin K. These patients should also receive FFP or prothrombin complex concentrate.[15] Recombinant activated factor VII should be considered for these patients if hemorrhage persists despite these initial interventions, although this is not a US Food and Drug Administration-approved indication for the drug.

Massive Transfusion and Coagulopathy of Trauma

Massive transfusion has been clinically defined as replacement of >50% of a patient's blood volume within 24 h. Alternative definitions range from replacement of 100% blood volume within 12 h to administration of >10 U of packed RBCs within 24 h. The primary cause of complex coagulopathy in patients receiving massive transfusion is dilution of coagulation factors by crystalloid and packed RBC solutions as well as consumption of existing coagulation factors and platelets

by the underlying disorder. Hypothermia and acidosis may exacerbate the coagulopathy. The coagulopathy of trauma and massive transfusion is characterized by bleeding from mucosal lesions, serosal surfaces, surgical wounds, and vascular access sites.[16] Risk factors for the development of severe coagulopathy in trauma include metabolic acidosis, hypothermia, hypotension, and severe injury.[17] Patients who require massive transfusion for treatment of hemorrhagic shock or major trauma are also at high risk for DIC. Thus, the distinction between coagulopathy associated with massive transfusion and DIC may be difficult. In general, massive transfusion is not associated with elevated d-dimers or decreases in factor VIII (Table 2).

The clinical approach to monitoring and treating massive transfusion is focused on three main priorities: establishment of hemostasis and hemodynamic stability, maintenance of adequate coagulation function, and mitigation of side effects of massive transfusion. Hemodynamic stability must be established by control of the underlying bleeding source, replacement of adequate intravascular volume, and maintenance of adequate hemoglobin concentration to support tissue oxygenation. Coagulation factors and platelets may become rapidly diluted or depleted in patients receiving massive transfusion. It is estimated that transfusion of approximately 10 U of RBCs in an average adult is associated with decreases in plasma coagulation proteins to 20 to 30% of baseline levels. Recommendations for resuscitation include anticipation of coagulopathy and close monitoring of the PT, aPTT, fibrinogen levels, and platelet count. Platelet transfusion and replacement of coagulation proteins with FFP and cryoprecipitate should be guided by laboratory results obtained after transfusion of every 5 to 10 U of packed RBCs. Although protocols have been proposed for replacement of blood, plasma, and platelets in fixed ratios in major trauma victims, these protocols have not been systematically evaluated in general medical patient populations.[18]

A wide range of metabolic and electrolyte abnormalities requires the monitoring and treatment of massive transfusion patients. Citrate used as an anticoagulant in packed RBCs may result in hypocalcemia through binding of serum calcium. Massively transfused patients should have routine monitoring of serum ionized calcium at regular intervals and replacement with calcium gluconate if necessary. Additional electrolyte disorders related to citrate and packed RBCs include metabolic alkalosis from metabolism of citrate to bicarbonate and hyperkalemia from the presence of excess extracellular potassium in stored blood. Patients with renal failure are at elevated risk for these side effects and warrant frequent pH and potassium monitoring. As the result of refrigerated blood and exposure, clinically significant hypothermia will develop in many massive transfusion patients. For patients who receive >3 to 4 U of blood, a blood warmer should be used.

Platelet Transfusion

Platelets are collected by centrifugation of fresh, whole, donated blood or by pheresis from a single donor. Generally, one pheresis unit of platelets contains five to six times the number of platelets from 1 U of donated whole blood. The primary indication to use single-donor pheresis platelets is to reduce the risk of immunization and platelet sensitization in recipients who are frequently exposed to transfusion. Although "random-donor" platelets from donated blood must be pooled or combined for most clinical uses in adults, they are more widely available than pheresis units. Platelets should not be refrigerated; they are stored up to 5 days from collection in plasma and electrolyte solutions in a volume of 250 to 350 mL. This warm storage requirement increases the risk of bacterial contamination in platelet units. In comparison to RBC units, this short storage life is more likely to place constraints on the supply and availability of platelets, particularly in smaller institutions. Platelet transfusion does not require ABO matching. Nevertheless, many clinicians select ABO-matched products to reduce the risk of immune reactions and improve the platelet survival. Rh D-negative women and girls should receive only Rh D-negative platelets, but they may receive Rh D-positive platelets in combination with Rh Ig.

There are two main indications for platelet transfusion: controlling bleeding in patients who have thrombocytopenia, and prevention of bleeding in patients with profound thrombocytopenia. Indications for platelet transfusion are related to the underlying disease process, the presence or absence of active bleeding, anticipation of invasive procedures, and platelet count. Indications for platelet transfusion are reviewed in Table 4.

In clinical practice, each unit of pooled, random-donor platelets increases the circulating platelet count by 5,000 to 10,000 cells/μL in patients with average body size. By comparison, one pheresis platelet unit may increase the platelet count by 30,000 to 60,000 cells/μL. Routine monitoring of platelet transfusion should include posttransfusion platelet count to determine transfusion responsiveness. Failure of the circulating platelet count to increase may result from destruction of the transfused platelets or consumption of the platelets at sites of injury or clot activation. Risks for ineffective platelet transfusion include ITP, presence of antiplatelet antibodies, DIC, drug-induced thrombocytopenia, and sepsis. Platelet transfusions are relatively

Table 4. *Indications for Platelet Transfusion**

Clinical Characteristics	Transfusion Trigger, cells/μL[†]
Thrombocytopenia, acute or chronic	
No active bleeding	Observation only; some authors advocate transfusion threshold of 5,000
Active bleeding present	50,000
Leukemia and hematopoietic stem-cell transplantation and patients receiving therapy for solid tumors	10,000
Surgical and invasive procedures	
Preoperative	40,000–50,000
Recent surgery or invasive procedure already performed	20,000–50,000

* Upward adjustments must be considered in the presence of severe concurrent coagulopathy or anticoagulation treatment.
† Transfuse to maintain circulating platelet count, at least.

contraindicated in patients with TTP-HUS unless the patient has severe bleeding. In general, platelet transfusions are ineffective if the cause of thrombocytopenia is enhanced destruction of circulating patients because the transfused platelets are destroyed through the same mechanism. Additionally, patients with uremia or who are receiving aspirin or clopidogrel are not likely to have significant benefit from platelet transfusion unless the medications are discontinued and the uremia is corrected.

FFP

FFP is prepared by separating plasma from single units of donated whole blood. The plasma is frozen at -18°C within 8 h of collection and has a storage life of 1 year. Each unit of FFP must be thawed immediately prior to use. Delay in transfusion after thawing results in declines in factors V and VIII. FFP should be used within 24 h of thawing. Each unit of FFP contains 250 mL of volume, which is administered in IV bolus or rapid infusion. FFP must be matched to donor ABO blood group. Use of FFP is associated with the same risks for infection and transfusion-associated acute lung injury as packed RBCs.

FFP contains all of the coagulant factors and coagulation inhibitors in normal blood. By convention, 1 mL of FFP is equivalent to 1 U of blood coagulation factor activity. Typical dosage of FFP is 10 to 15 mL/kg, which should restore coagulation factors to 25 to 30% of normal levels.[19] It has been suggested that this dosage level is inadequate and that 30 mL/kg is more likely to correct all individual coagulation factors.[20] The indications for FFP are listed in Table 5. FFP should not be used as a

Table 5. *Indications for FFP*

Replacement of individual factor deficiencies if no purified fractionated product available
Reversal of warfarin in patients with bleeding or emergent surgery
Correction of multiple simultaneous factor deficiencies
Replacement of antithrombin
Plasma replacement in TTP
Treat coagulopathy of massive transfusion
Coagulopathy of liver disease if bleeding is present
Severe DIC if bleeding is present

primary method for intravascular volume expansion. FFP also should not be used as a primary means of replacement of isolated factor deficiencies when concentrated single-factor replacement products are available. For example, recombinant factor VIII concentrate, rather than FFP, should be used preferentially in patients with hemophilia A. The decision to use FFP should be guided by clinical bedside evidence of coagulopathy and by measurements of the PT, aPTT, and other coagulation assays. Approaches to FFP transfusion based on formulas such as 2 U of FFP per 4 U of RBC transfusion are not appropriate in the majority of patients.

The effect of FFP on coagulation times and bleeding risk has been difficult to measure as the result of the large and heterogenous patient population treated with FFP and the wide variation in clinical practice. In general, higher doses of FFP than are used in most clinical settings may be required to totally correct coagulopathy. A retrospective observational study[21] described the median dose as 17 mL/kg of FFP in patients who achieved correction of INR compared with 10 mL/kg in patients who did not achieve correction of their PT-INR. Another observational trial[22] in patients with baseline INR of 1.1 to 1.85 demonstrated that the usual clinical practice of FFP transfusion resulted in normalization of PT-INR in < 1% of patients and reduced the PT-INR to half that of normal in only 15% of patients. This suggests that current practice and doses of FFP in patients with mild coagulation abnormalities are rarely effective in correcting coagulation times.

Cryoprecipitate

Cryoprecipitate is the precipitate that remains after FFP is thawed to 4°C. Cryoprecipitate contains fibrinogen, fibronectin, von Willebrand factor XIII, and factor VIII. Cryoprecipitate may be reconstituted in very low volumes (10 to 15 mL) and thus has a significant advantage over FFP in volume-overloaded patients. Each unit of cryoprecipitate contains the precipitate from the plasma of one donated blood unit. The primary indication for cryoprecipitate is replacement of fibrinogen in patients with hypofibrinogenemia caused by dilution or consumptive coagulopathy. The dose

Coagulopathies, Bleeding Disorders, and Blood Component Therapy (Thomas)

of cryoprecipitate should be titrated to maintain a target plasma level of fibrinogen at > 100 mg/dL. This usually requires 5 to 10 U of cryoprecipitate for the initial dose. Fibrinogen levels should be reassessed frequently to determine the optimal dose and dosing interval.

Correction of Thrombocytopenia and Coagulopathy for Routine Bedside Procedures

A consistent source of variation in clinical practice is the use of platelet and FFP transfusions prior to bedside procedures, including central venous catheter (CVC) placement thoracentesis and paracentesis. In general, there is limited evidence to support routine preprocedure transfusion for patients with mild elevations in PT, aPTT, or thrombocytopenia. In a cohort of 1,825 patients undergoing CVC placement, the rate of bleeding complications was 3 of 88 patients with uncorrected coagulopathy (range of platelet count, 12,000 to 46,000 cells/µL; and PT-INR, 1.1 to 1.5). There were no severe complications requiring transfusion or surgical intervention.[23] Similarly, a cohort of 76 patients with coagulopathy, thrombocytopenia, or both undergoing CVC placement had only one significant bleeding complication requiring blood product transfusion and 6.5% minor bleeding complications, which were defined as oozing from the catheter insertion site.[24] Finally, in a cohort of 40 coagulopathic liver transplant patients (average PT, 29% of control; average aPTT, 92 s; average platelet count, 47,000 cells/µL) who underwent 259 catheterizations without corrective transfusions, there were no reported serious bleeding complications.[25] For paracentesis and thoracentesis, observational data are more limited. The overall frequency of bleeding complications in a cohort of 608 consecutive patients having thoracentesis or paracentesis was 0.2%. The mildly coagulopathic group (average PT and aPTT less than twice normal and platelet count of 50,000 to 100,000 cells/µL) did not have an increased risk of bleeding complications. Patients with renal failure, however, did have higher-than-average blood loss.[26] As routine adoption of ultrasound-guided testing occurs, it is likely that the risk of bleeding complications from these bedside procedures in coagulopathic patients will decrease further. In summary, bedside line insertions, thoracentesis, and paracentesis appears to be safe without increased risk of bleeding complications in patients with mild coagulation abnormalities.

Desmopressin, Activated Factor VII, and Other Hemostatic Agents

Desmopressin is a synthetic vasopressin analog that stimulates vascular endothelial cells to release von Willebrand factor and increases plasma factor VIII:c. Desmopressin was initially established for treatment of bleeding in patients with hemophilia and von Willebrand disease. There are no data to recommend routine use of desmopressin in the general population with bleeding. There may be a limited role for desmopressin in the treatment of patients with qualitative platelet defects, such as those taking aspirin and patients with uremia.

Epsilon-aminocaproic acid and tranexamic acid inhibit the binding of plasmin to fibrin and thus inhibit fibrinolysis. As with desmopressin, there is no clinical evidence to support the routine use of these agents in the general ICU population. There is a limited role for these agents in patients with hemophilia and profound refractory thrombocytopenia who have active bleeding. The most significant side effect of epsilon-aminocaproic acid is an increased risk of thrombosis.

Recombinant activated factor VII was originally developed to provide specific factor replacement and hemostasis in patients with hemophilia and congenital factor VII deficiency. In the United States, the only US Food and Drug Administration-approved indication for the drug is for treatment of bleeding in hemophiliac patients with antibody inhibitors to coagulation factors VIII and IX. Off-label uses are well described in case report literature and have included correction of bleeding associated with trauma, intracranial hemorrhage, coagulopathy of liver disease, and reversal of warfarin-associated bleeding. The use of recombinant factor VII in these clinical scenarios is not supported by robust clinical trials. The use of recombinant-activated factor VII is associated with thrombosis and thromboembolic disease, and the appropriate dose for off-label uses has not been established.

References

1. Akca S, Haji-Michael P, de Mendonca A, et al. Time course of platelet counts in critically ill patients. Crit Care Med 2002; 30:753–756

2. Strauss R, Wehler M, Mehler K, et al. Thrombocytopenia in patients in the medical intensive care unit: bleeding prevalence, transfusion requirements, and outcome. Crit Care Med 2002; 30:1765–1771

3. Vanderschueren S, De Weerdt A, Malbrain M, et al. Thrombocytopenia and prognosis in intensive care. Crit Care Med 2000; 28:1871–1876

4. Drews RE. Critical issues in hematology: anemia, thrombocytopenia, coagulopathy, and blood product transfusions in critically ill patients. Clin Chest Med 2003; 24:607–622

5. Arepally GM, Ortel TL. Clinical practice: heparin-induced thrombocytopenia. N Engl J Med 2006; 355:809–817

6. Pene F, Vigneau C, Auburtin M, et al. Outcome of severe adult thrombotic microangiopathies in the intensive care unit. Intensive Care Med 2005; 31:71–78

7. Rock GA, Shumak KH, Buskard NA, et al; Canadian Apheresis Study Group. Comparison of plasma exchange with plasma infusion in the treatment of thrombotic thrombocytopenic purpura. N Engl J Med 1991; 325:393–397

8. Torok TJ, Holman RC, Chorba TL. Increasing mortality from thrombotic thrombocytopenic purpura in the United States: analysis of national mortality data, 1968–1991. Am J Hematol 1995; 50:84–90

9. Coppo P, Adrie C, Azoulay E, et al. Infectious diseases as a trigger in thrombotic microangiopathies in intensive care unit (ICU) patients? Intensive Care Med 2003; 29:564–569

10. Levy GG, Nichols WC, Lian EC, et al. Mutations in a member of the *ADAMTS* gene family cause thrombotic thrombocytopenic purpura. Nature 2001; 413:488–494

11. Coppo P, Bussel A, Charrier S, et al. High-dose plasma infusion versus plasma exchange as early treatment of thrombotic thrombocytopenic purpura/hemolytic-uremic syndrome. Medicine (Baltimore) 2003; 82:27–38

12. Okajima K, Sakamoto Y, Uchiba M. Heterogeneity in the incidence and clinical manifestations of disseminated intravascular coagulation: a study of 204 cases. Am J Hematol 2000; 65:215–222

13. Siegal T, Seligsohn U, Aghai E, et al. Clinical and laboratory aspects of disseminated intravascular coagulation (DIC): a study of 118 cases. Thromb Haemost 1978; 39:122–134

14. Angstwurm MW, Dempfle CE, Spannagl M. New disseminated intravascular coagulation score: a useful tool to predict mortality in comparison with Acute Physiology and Chronic Health Evaluation II and Logistic Organ Dysfunction scores [quiz 28]. Crit Care Med 2006; 34:314–320

15. Ansell J, Hirsh J, Hylek E, et al. Pharmacology and management of the vitamin K antagonists: American College of Chest Physicians Evidence-Based Clinical Practice Guidelines (8th ed.). Chest 2008; 133:160S–98S

16. Hess JR, Lawson JH. The coagulopathy of trauma versus disseminated intravascular coagulation. J Trauma 2006; 60:S12–S19

17. Cosgriff N, Moore EE, Sauaia A, et al. Predicting life-threatening coagulopathy in the massively transfused trauma patient: hypothermia and acidoses revisited. J Trauma 1997; 42:857–862

18. Malone DL, Hess JR, Fingerhut A. Massive transfusion practices around the globe and a suggestion for a common massive transfusion protocol. J Trauma 2006; 60:S91–S96

19. Lundberg GD. Practice parameter for the use of fresh-frozen plasma, cyroprecipitate, and platelets. JAMA 1994; 271:777–781

20. Chowdhury P, Saayman AG, Paulus U, et al. Efficacy of standard dose and 30 ml/kg fresh frozen plasma in correcting laboratory parameters of haemostasis in critically ill patients. Br J Haematol 2004; 125:69–73

21. Dara SI, Rana R, Afessa B, et al. Fresh frozen plasma transfusion in critically ill medical patients with coagulopathy. Crit Care Med 2005; 33:2667–2671

22. Abdel-Wahab OI, Healy B, Dzik WH. Effect of fresh-frozen plasma transfusion on prothrombin time and bleeding in patients with mild coagulation abnormalities. Transfusion 2006; 46:1279–1285

23. Mumtaz H, Williams V, Hauer-Jensen M, et al. Central venous catheter placement in patients with disorders of hemostasis. Am J Surg 2000; 180:503–506

24. Doerfler ME, Kaufman B, Goldenberg AS. Central venous catheter placement in patients with disorders of hemostasis. Chest 1996; 110:185–188

25. Foster PF, Moore LR, Sankary HN, et al. Central venous catheterization in patients with coagulopathy. Arch Surg 1992; 127:273–275

26. McVay PA, Toy PT. Lack of increased bleeding after paracentesis and thoracentesis in patients with mild coagulation abnormalities. Transfusion 1991; 31:164–171

Notes

Hemodynamic Monitoring

Jesse B. Hall, MD, FCCP

Objectives:

- Review the use of pulmonary artery catheterization
- Recognize the correlation of pressure to ventricular preload and volume
- Outline useful applications of echocardiography in the ICU

Key words: echocardiography; fluid resuscitation; hemodynamics; pulmonary artery catheter

Hemodynamic monitoring may be defined as the collection and interpretation of various parameters that inform determination of: (1) the etiology of a state of hypoperfusion and/or (2) the response of the cardiopulmonary unit to interventions such as fluid therapy, vasoactive drugs, or adjustments in positive pressure ventilation. For many patients, adequate monitoring is achieved by routine vital signs along with collection of data such as input/output, physical examination, and urine electrolytes. In other patients, invasive measurements are made, including use of arterial catheters, central venous catheters (CVC), and right heart catheters (RHC). These catheters provide for continuous transduction of pressure in either the arterial or venous circuit and sampling of blood for determination of oxygen saturation. Simultaneous determination of arterial and mixed venous blood gases also permits determination of oxygen content, oxygen delivery, oxygen consumption, arteriovenous oxygen content difference, and calculation of cardiac output by Fick determination.

The use of invasive methods of assessing hemodynamics—arterial and right heart catheters—grew during the evolution of critical care medicine despite a lack of prospective trials demonstrating efficacy and improved patient outcome. Indeed, one retrospective study suggested that use of the RHC is associated with an independent negative effect on survival. This study has been criticized largely on the basis of design—it was retrospective, and thus even reasonably sophisticated methods of case matching may have failed to control for the inevitable differences in patient status and hence prognosis that might contribute to decisions to perform invasive monitoring. However, prospective trials have been undertaken and one recent large multicenter study evaluating the use of RHC for high-risk surgical patients failed to demonstrate either a benefit or detriment to its use. It is important to note that in order for trials of invasive monitoring to demonstrate benefit, investigators must identify a patient population at risk for or exhibiting a hemodynamic state amenable to interventions that will improve outcome—monitoring alone is unlikely to confer benefit. Moreover, for many conditions—sepsis, the acute respiratory distress syndrome (ARDS)—the proper fluid and vasoactive drug interventions remain to be defined. For these conditions, trials have been designed and implemented that test not only the monitoring modality but the proper intervention as well (eg, randomizing patients with ARDS to either a RHC or CVC and then further to either a "fluid liberal" or "fluid conservative" management strategy).

Differential Diagnosis of Hypoperfused States and Bedside Assessment

A useful and readily applicable bedside algorithm at the time of resuscitation of patients with circulatory inadequacy is—is this low- or high-output hypotension? If the former, is the heart full or not? And when fluid resuscitation has occurred, is the response definitive or has low-output shock now taken on the characteristics of high-flow shock (eg, septic shock with initial hypovolemia, now fluid-resuscitated)? Often this simple algorithm succeeds in fully resuscitating the patient. If not, further information gathering from invasive monitoring and/or echocardiography is appropriate (Table 1).

Alternatives to Pulmonary Artery Catheterization

Given uncertainties concerning the benefits of invasive monitoring with the RHC, recent literature has emphasized alternative approaches. In the

Table 1. *Rapid Formulation of an Early Working Diagnosis of the Etiology of Shock*

Defining Features of Shock

Blood pressure	⇓
Heart rate	⇑
Respiratory rate	⇑
Mentation	⇓
Urine output	⇓
Arterial pH	⇓

	High Output Hypotension *Septic Shock*	*Low Cardiac Output* *Cardiogenic and Hypovolemic*
Is Cardiac Output Reduced?	No	Yes
Pulse pressure	⇑	⇓
Diastolic pressure	⇑	⇓
Extremities digits	Warm	Cool
Nailbed return	Rapid	Slow
Heart sounds	Crisp	Muffled
Temperature	⇑ or ⇓	⇔
White cell count	⇑ or ⇓	⇔
Site of infection	++	−

	Reduced Pump Function *Cardiogenic Shock*	*Reduced Venous Return* *Hypovolemic Shock*
Is the Heart Too Full?	Yes	No
Symptoms clinical context	Angina ECG	Hemorrhage dehydration
Jugular venous pressure	⇑	⇓
S$_3$, S$_4$, gallop rhythm	+++	−
Respiratory crepitations	+++	−
Chest radiograph	Large heart ⇑ upper lobe flow Pulmonary edema	Normal

What Does Not Fit?
Overlapping etiologies (septic cardiogenic, septic hypovolemic, cardiogenic hypovolemic)
Short list of other etiologies

High output *hypotension*	*High right atrial* *pressure hypotension*	*Nonresponsive* *hypovolemia*
Liver failure	Pulmonary hypertension	Adrenal insufficiency
Severe Pancreatitis	(most often pulmonary embolus)	Anaphylaxis
Trauma with significant	Right ventricular infarction	Spinal shock
SIRS	Cardiac tamponade	
Thyroid storm		
Arteriovenous fistula		
Paget's disease		

Get more information — Echocardiography, right heart catheterization

most significant recent trial evaluating resuscitation of patients with early severe sepsis and septic shock, RHC was not used but rather patients were randomized to routine care vs early goal-directed therapy (EGDT) guided by arterial blood pressure, right atrial pressure, right atrial oxygen saturation (as a surrogate of mixed venous blood saturation) and urine volume. Outcomes were improved with EGDT despite no use of RHC, suggesting the use of the cardiac output to determine the adequacy of the circulation in patients with sepsis may be less useful than the concentration of effluent blood returning from the systemic circulation.

There has also been considerable study of the use of the arterial pressure waveform alone as an indicator for the adequacy of intravascular volume and response to fluid challenge. Numerous studies have shown that responders and nonresponders to fluid challenge are not well defined by the baseline right atrial pressure or pulmonary artery occlusion pressure (Fig 1). This relates to many factors to be discussed below.

However, patients with spontaneous respirations will typically exhibit drops in right atrial pressure during inspiration related to swings in intrathoracic pressure that has been shown to

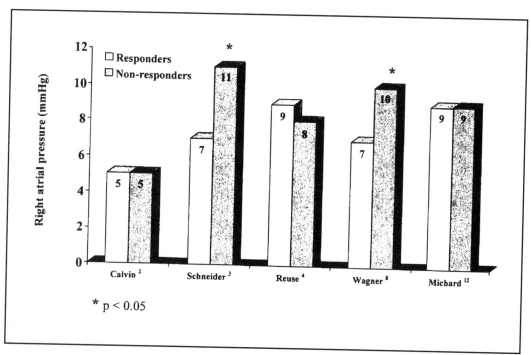

Figure 1. Mean MAP before volume expansion in responders and nonresponders.

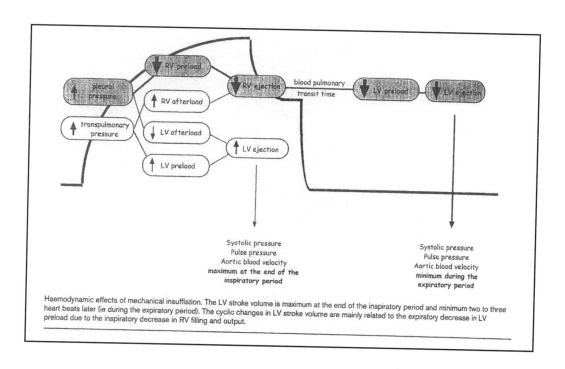

Figure 2.

correlate with relative hypovolemia and "preload reserve," making this observation useful in determining the need for further fluid resuscitation. In addition, patients undergoing mechanical ventilation often have respiratory excursion of arterial blood pressure as demonstrated below (Fig 2).

The result of these cyclical changes in tidal volume is to cause a cyclical change in stroke volume that is detectable on the arterial pressure waveform and signals the existence of hypovolemia (Fig 3).

Empiric investigation has shown that when a greater than 13% increase in the pulse pressure change between maximal (Ppmax) and minimal (Ppmin) pulse pressure exists, patients are highly likely to respond to fluid challenge:

$$\Delta PP\ (\%) = 100 \times ((Ppmax - Ppmin)/(Ppmax + Ppmin/2))$$

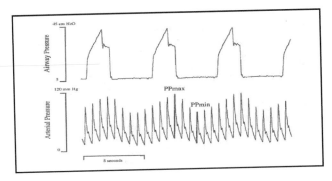

Figure 3.

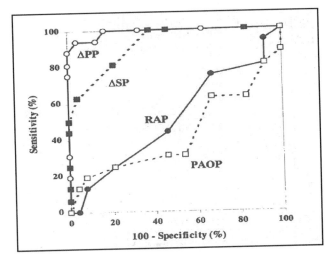

Figure 4.

The receiver operator curve for the pulse pressure variation using this threshold and other measures or cardiac preload in patients with sepsis and hypoperfusion are shown in Figure 4.

While not validated on large groups of patients, this approach is attractive and could eventually prove to be more useful than measurements of right atrial or pulmonary capillary wedge pressure.

Pulmonary Artery Catheterization

Indications and Complications

Rather than offer a list of many conditions that may require PA catheterization, the reader is guided to the statement above recommending formulation of questions concerning the etiology of hypoperfusion or the response to therapy, and answer these questions if possible with clinical data, including volume or drug challenges. When this approach is inadequate, PA catheterization is to be considered. Complications of the procedure are given in Table 2.

Table 2. *Complications of Pulmonary Artery (PA) Catheterization*

I.   Complications related to central vein cannulation
II. Complications related to insertion and use of the PA catheter
    A. Tachyarrhythmias
    B. Right bundle branch block
    C. Complete heart block (pre-existing left bundle branch block)
    D. Cardiac perforation
    E. Thrombosis and embolism
    F. Pulmonary infarction due to persistent wedging
    G. Catheter-related sepsis
    H. Pulmonary artery rupture
    I. Knotting of the catheter
    J. Endocarditis, bland and infective
    K. Pulmonic valve insufficiency
    L. Balloon fragmentation and embolization

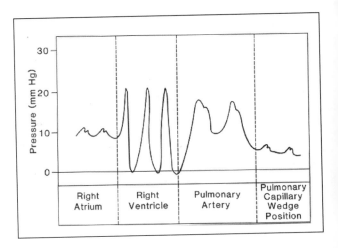

Figure 5.

Interpretation of Pressure Waveforms

Under most conditions, the waveforms obtained as the PA catheter (PAC) is advanced through the right atrium, right ventricle, and into the pulmonary artery to a wedged position are readily identified as characteristic of each segment of the circulation as it is traversed, as demonstrated in Figure 5. While waveform recognition is extremely helpful in positioning the catheter, and often makes the use of fluoroscopic techniques unnecessary, it is essential for the measurement and interpretation of waveforms displayed during PA catheterization to be correlated to the ECG tracing so that specific components of the waveform can be identified and various pitfalls in measurement of intravascular pressure can be avoided.

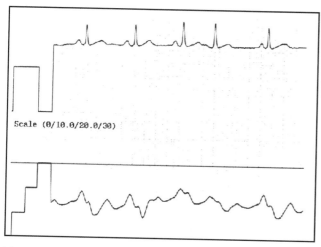

Scale (0/10.0/20.0/30)

Figure 6.

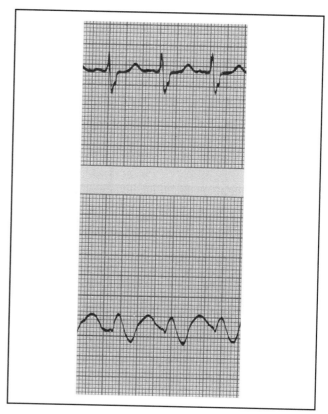

Figure 7.

The Normal Pressure Waveform: In sinus rhythm, the atrial pressure waveform is characterized by two major positive deflections (A and V waves) and two negative deflections (X and Y descents) (Fig 6). A third positive wave, the C wave, is sometimes seen. The A wave results from atrial systolic contraction and is followed by the X descent as the atria relax following contraction. The C wave results from closure of the atrioventricular valves and interrupts the X descent. After the X descent, the V (ventricular) wave is generated by passive filling of the atria during ventricular systole. Lastly, the Y descent reflects the reduction in atrial pressure as the atrioventricular valves open. In correlating these waveforms to the ECG, the first positive pressure wave to follow the P wave is the A wave. The right atrial A wave is usually seen at the beginning of the QRS complex, provided that atrioventricular conduction is normal. The peak of the right atrial V wave normally occurs simultaneously with the T wave of the ECG, provided that the Q-T interval is normal.

The pulmonary artery waveform has a systolic pressure wave and a diastolic trough. A dicrotic notch due to closure of the pulmonic valve may be seen on the terminal portion of the systolic pressure wave. Like the right atrial V wave, the PA systolic wave typically coincides with the electrical T wave. The PA diastolic pressure (Ppad) is recorded as the pressure just before the beginning of the systolic pressure wave.

The Ppw tracing contains the same sequence of waves and descents as the right atrial tracing. However, when the atrial waveform is referenced

to the ECG , the mechanical events arising in the left atrium (Ppw) will be seen later than those of the right atrium, because the left atrial pressure waves must travel back through the pulmonary vasculature and a longer length of catheter (Fig 7). Therefore, in the Ppw tracing the A wave usually appears after the QRS complex and the V wave is seen after the T wave. As such, the systolic pressure wave in the PA tracing *precedes* the V wave of the Ppw tracing. An appreciation of the latter relationship is critical when tracings are being analyzed to ensure that balloon inflation has resulted in a transition from an arterial (PA) to atrial (Ppw) waveform, and to detect the presence of a "giant" V wave in the Ppw tracing.

Common Problems Producing Erroneous Pressure Waveforms: Of the many problems causing artifact or erroneous tracings, the most commonly encountered are overdamping, catheter whip, overwedging, incomplete wedging, and Zone I catheter conditions.

Overdamping results from air bubbles within the catheter system or kinking, clotting, and fibrin deposition along the catheter course; many times these problems can be resolved by catheter flushing.

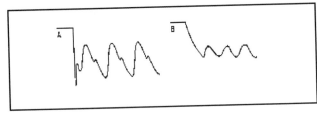

Figure 8. Rapid flush test: A) appropriately damped system; B) over damped system.

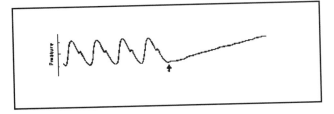

Figure 9.

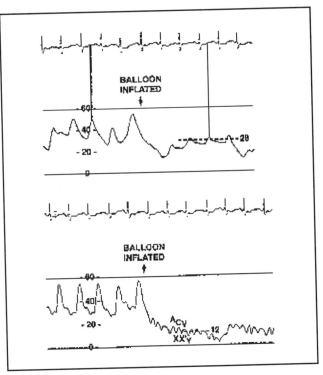

Figure 10. Incomplete wedge pressure (Ppw). *Top*: With balloon inflation, there is a decrease in pressure to a value that approximates pulmonary artery diastolic pressure (Ppad). The clinical setting (ARDS) is usually associated with a large Ppad-Ppw gradient. Review of the tracings indicates that there is a single positive wave coinciding with the electrocardiographic T wave after balloon inflation, a pattern inconsistent with a left atrial waveform. *Bottom*: Waveforms after the catheter had been retracted, the balloon inflated, and the catheter floated to a full wedge position. Now, there is a large Ppad-Ppw gradient and the tracing after balloon inflation is consistent with a left atrial waveform. The incomplete wedge tracing yielded an incorrect measurement of the wedge pressure as 28 mm Hg, substantially higher (in a very clinically relevant sense) than the true wedge pressure of approximately 12 mm Hg.

The main effect of overdamping on the pressure waveform is to artifactually lower the systolic pressure and raise the diastolic pressure with consequent effects on interpretation (Fig 8).

Catheter whip arises from cardiac contractions causing shock transients transmitted to the catheter. The results on the right ventricular or pulmonary arterial waveforms are an exaggerated diastolic pressure in some cycles, highlighting the need to avoid readings obtained by electronic systems.

Overwedging (Fig 9) is signaled by a rise in recorded pressure with balloon inflation as the balloon herniates over the catheter tip or the tip is pushed into the vessel wall with continued fluid ingress elevating the measured pressure. Overwedging requires repositioning of the catheter.

Incomplete wedging (Fig 10) and Zone I positioning of the catheter can be subtle but are important to identify since erroneous and often overestimation of Ppw occur.

Zone I conditions of the lung refer to those segments of the lung in which alveolar pressure exceeds pulmonary vascular pressure and hence there is no flow (Fig 11).

This phenomenon is uncommon when the catheter is floated into position since this typically results in Zone II or III positioning. It would be more likely to result from forceful positioning of the catheter, hypovolemia emerging after placement, or with large increases in PEEP. This condition should be considered when changes in Ppw

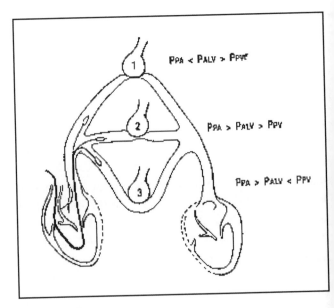

Figure 11. Lung zones.

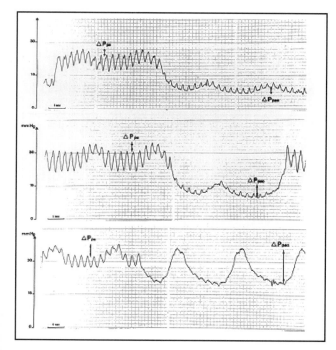

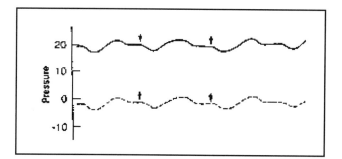

Figure 13.

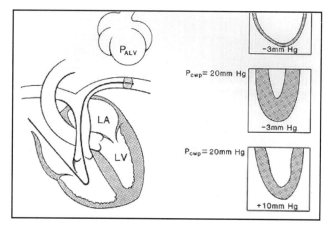

Figure 12. Pressure tracings recorded in the same patient at different levels of end-expiratory pressure-zero (ZEEP) on the *top panel*, 15 cm H_2O in the *center panel*, and 20 cm H_2O in the *bottom panel*.

Figure 14.

track PEEP changes exactly or when the excursion in pulmonary artery systolic pressures with respiration exceed those Ppw significantly (Fig 12).

The Correlation of Pressure to Ventricular Preload and Volume: The use of Ppw as a measure of left ventricular end-diastolic pressure and hence preload depends on the Ppw closely reflecting pulmonary venous, left atrial, and left ventricular pressures, that is, with minimal pressure gradient across the system. One potential confounder to interpretation of intravascular pressures is the fluctuation in intrathoracic pressure related to the respiratory cycle. The effect of varying intrathoracic pressure on the wedge (Ppw) pressure is seen in Figure 13. The top line is a Ppw tracing and the bottom in the intrapleural (Ppl) pressure. In this example the patient is receiving assisted ventilation. Arrows indicate end expiratory pressures. Negative deflections in Ppl and Ppw pressures result from inspiratory muscle activity, and subsequent positive deflections represent lung inflation by the ventilator. At end expiration, the respiratory system has returned to its relaxed state and Ppl is back to baseline (–2 cm H_2O). Transmural wedge pressure remains approximately constant throughout the ventilating cycle. Since Ppl is not usually measured clinically, it is necessary that Ppw be recorded at a point where

Ppl can be reliably estimated (*ie*, end-exhalation, assuming no expiratory muscle activity).

The correlation of pressure to volume is further complicated by a variety of conditions that cause the ventricle to be effectively stiff (diastolic dysfunction or pericardial disease) or conditions that cause juxta-cardiac pressure to rise related to positive pressure ventilation (PEEP, intrinsic PEEP [PEEPi], active expiratory effort) (Fig 14).

The effects of PEEP in conditions such as ARDS are often blunted, since the stiff lungs of these patients do not distend greatly with high ventilator pressures and hence minimal increases in juxta-cardiac pressure are encountered. However, in cases in which PEEPi exists in chronic obstructive pulmonary disease (COPD)/asthma patients undergoing mechanical ventilation, or in agitated/obstructed patients with very active expiratory muscle effort, cardiovascular effects may be large. This effect is shown in Figure 15, where the increase in blood pressure and cardiac output despite a fall in wedge pressure and esophageal pressure is shown during a brief interruption in positive pressure ventilation in a patient with COPD.

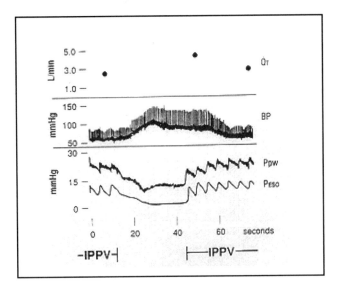

Figure 15.

This constellation of problems is best avoided by:

- Awareness of their existence
- Reading pressure tracings at end expiration
- Considering measures (sedation, ventilator adjustment, paralysis) that diminish or eliminate PEEPi
- Considering a ventilator disconnect in patients with severe airflow obstruction and PEEPi to demonstrate limitation to venous return
- Using a fluid challenge when effective "diastolic" dysfunction may be present, to determine "preload reserve"

In determining the response to a fluid challenge, it is necessary to note that a minimum of 500 mL of crystalloid is required and even then small effects on cardiac output and arterial blood pressure are typically seen. One study has suggested that the use of a drop in the right atrial pressure with respiration is a useful indicator of preload reserve.

Specific Disorders: Tricuspid regurgitation is encountered in conditions with direct valvular injury (*eg,* endocarditis) and generally in right heart failure. It is characterized by a prominent and broad V wave and a steep Y descent; the latter is often most useful for making this diagnosis (Fig 16). It is useful to note tricuspid regurgitation not only for its implications for underlying disorders but also because it will confound thermal dilution cardiac output determination.

Mitral regurgitation is characterized by a giant V wave that may confound distinction between the

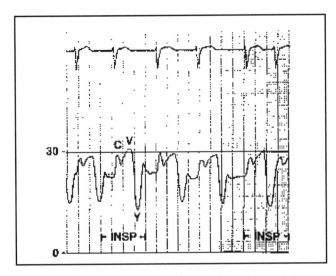

Figure 16. Giant V wave in right atrial waveform indicates tricuspid regurgitation.

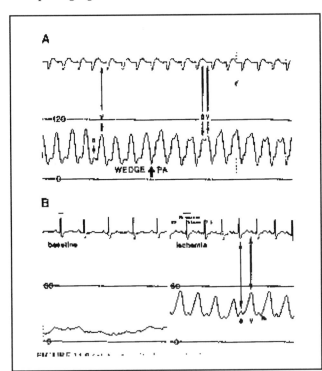

Figure 17. *A,* Acute mitral regurgitation with giant V wave in pulmonary wedge tracing. The pulmonary artery (PA) tracing has a characteristic bifid appearance due to both a PA systolic wave and the V wave. Note that the V wave occurs later in the cardiac cycle than the PA systolic wave, which is synchronous with the T wave of the electrocardiogram. *B,* Intermittent giant V wave due to ischemia of the papillary muscle. Wedge tracings are from same patient at baseline and during ischemia. Scale in mm Hg.

PA and Pwp tracings (Fig 17). Significant mitral regurgitation may be present without a giant V wave (ascribed to enlarged and compliant left atrium which does not exhibit a large pressure excursion with the additional volume) and a number of conditions can cause a giant V wave in the absence of mitral regurgitation (hypervolemia, VSD).

Right ventricular infarction is characterized by an elevated right ventricular end-diastolic pressure at initial passage of the catheter with narrow pulse pressures when there is hemodynamic compromise. This same pattern can also be present in conditions causing acute right heart failure secondary to increases in pulmonary vascular resistance (*eg*, pulmonary embolus) but in these latter conditions there will be a large PAD-Ppw gradient reflecting the increase in pulmonary vascular resistance.

Interpretation of Flows and Parameters of Oxygen Delivery

In most clinical settings, cardiac output is determined by thermal dilution. In addition to a number of technical conditions making the measurement unreliable, tricuspid regurgitation may be present and cause underestimation (usually) or overestimation (rarely) of cardiac output. Under this circumstance, determination of cardiac output by Fick may be useful.

Determination of whether a measured flow is adequate is usually best judged by peripheral parameters of perfusion (*eg*, urine volume, presence of lactic acidosis) or by the mixed venous oxygen saturation (Svo_2). Low Svo_2 (<60 %) strongly suggests inadequate oxygen delivery and anemia, hypoxemia, or inadequate cardiac output should be sought and corrected. Interpretation of a high Svo_2 in high-output states is difficult. Accordingly, the greatest utility of modified catheters which permit continuous monitoring of Svo_2 is in circumstances in which there is risk for it to be low and therapy can be directed at early recognition of this phenomenon (*eg*, postoperative cardiac surgery patients).

Echocardiography

Many of the problems of relating measured pressures to ventricular preload can be addressed by cardiac imaging by echo. In addition, this diagnostic tool is useful for identifying a host of structural abnormalities. It should be considered as an adjunct to pulmonary artery catheterization. As technology permits more continuous monitoring by transesophageal route, its use in the ICU is likely to expand.

Useful Applications of Echocardiography in the ICU

- Identification of ischemia
- Correlation of pressure to volume and identification of diastolic dysfunction
- Characterization of valve lesions, VSD, ASD
- Identification of pericardial disease
- Identification of right-left heart interactions in acute right heart failure

Selected Reading

Connors AF, Speroff T, Dawson NV, et al. The effectiveness of right heartcatheterization in the initial care of critically ill patients. JAMA 1996; 276:889–897

Fuchs RM, Heuser RR, Yin FC, et al. Limitations of pulmonary wedge V wavesin diagnosing mitral regurgitation. Am J Cardiol 1982; 49:849–854

Leatherman JW, Marini JJ. Clinical use of the pulmonary artery catheter. In:Hall JB, Schmidt GA, eds. Priciples of critical care. 2nd ed. New York, NY: McGraw Hill, 1998; 155–177

Magder S, Georgiadis G, Cheone T. Respiratory variations in right atrial pressure predict the response to fluid challenge. J Crit Care 1992; 7:76–85

Michard F, Boussat S, Chemla D, et al. Relation between respiratory changes in arterial pulse pressure and fluid responsiveness in septic patients with acute circulatory failure. Am J Respir Crit Care Med 2000; 162:134–138

Michard F, Teboul JL. Predicting fluid responsiveness in ICU patients. Chest 2002; 121:2000–2008

Michard F, Teboul JL. Using heart-lung interactions to assess fluid responsiveness during mechanical ventilation. Crit Care 2000; 4:282–289

Perret C, Tagan D, Feihl F, et al. The pulmonary artery catheter in clinical care. Oxford, England: Blackwell Science, 1996; 347

Russell JA, Phang TP. The oxygen delivery/consumption controversy: approaches to management of the critically ill. Am J Respir Crit Care Med 1994; 149:533–537

Shah KB, Rao TLK, Laughlin S, et al. A review of pulmonary artery catheterizations in 6,245 patients. Anesthesiology 1984; 61:271

Teboul JL, Besbes M, Andrivet P, et al. A bedside index assessing the reliability of pulmonary artery occlusion pressure measurements during mechanical ventilation with positive end-expiratory pressure. J Crit Care Med 1992; 7:22–29

Notes

Nutritional Support in the Critically Ill Patient

John W. Drover, MD

Objectives:

- Identify three strategies to optimize the benefits of enteral nutrition
- Identify two strategies to minimize the risk of enteral nutrition
- Identify three strategies to optimize the benefits and reduce the risks associated with parenteral nutrition
- Identify two specific nutrients that may improve the outcomes of critically ill patients

Key words: clinical practice guidelines; critical care; enteral nutrition; parenteral nutrition

In critically ill patients, malnutrition is associated with impaired immune function; impaired ventilatory drive and weakened respiratory muscles, leading to prolonged ventilatory dependence; and increased infectious morbidity and mortality. Malnutrition is prevalent in ICU patients, and has been reported as being as high as 40% and to be associated with increased morbidity and mortality.

The benefits of nutritional support in the critically ill patient include improved wound healing, a decreased catabolic response to injury, improved GI structure and function, and improved clinical outcomes, including a reduction in complication rates and length of stay, with accompanying cost savings. However, nutritional support is not without adverse effects or risks. Early enteral nutrition (EN) can be associated with high gastric residual volumes, bacterial colonization of the stomach, and an increased risk of aspiration pneumonia. Parenteral nutrition (PN) has been associated with gut mucosal atrophy, overfeeding, hyperglycemia, an increased risk of infectious complications, and increased mortality in critically ill patients. Both forms of nutritional support can increase health-care costs and the workloads of health-care providers.

A number of reviews have documented that nutritional support does influence morbidity and mortality in critically ill patients. Therefore, strategies to improve the delivery of nutritional support are relevant, and may result in decreased morbidity and mortality. Systematically developed practice guidelines that focus on these strategies will allow practitioners to make decisions about appropriate nutritional support care, and will aim at improving the quality of patient care and maximizing the efficiency with which resources are used. There have been two published sets of clinical practice guidelines[1,2] that can help the clinician make evidence-based decisions in the management of nutritional support in the critically ill patient. A rich resource associated with the practice guidelines developed in Canada is the following Web site: www.criticalcarenutrition.com.[3] This site, which is updated on a regular schedule, provides the background discussion for the recommendations as well as all the references, systematic reviews, and metaanalyses that form the basis for the recommendations. The recommendations in this article are taken from the Canadian Clinical Practice Guidelines project, and the data quoted will be from the data available on the Web site at the time of writing, unless otherwise referenced.

Goals of Nutritional Support

The goals of nutritional support are to provide (1) the macronutrient needs of the individual and (2) the specific nutrients that will improve outcome specific to the disease process. There is mounting evidence that specific nutrients may be useful in the latter context, and these will be discussed later (under specific nutrients).

Nutritional support is indicated in the critically ill patient when the benefits of that support will improve the clinically important outcomes of the patient. The rest of this treatise will be aimed at elucidating the principles that can be used to optimize the benefits and to minimize the risks of nutritional support in the critically ill patient. Specific decisions about treatment are made at the bedside, and those decisions are best made when informed by the best available evidence.

Assessing Energy Requirements

The primary focus for assessing energy requirements in the ICU is the need for the delivery of macronutrients, specifically total energy (calories) and protein delivery. In adults, the total energy needs can be estimated in several ways, which include an amount based on usual or predicted body weight. The target for goal calories in the American College of Chest Physicians recommendations[4] is 25 kcal/kg/d. The dose of energy can also be estimated using one of many equations that have been developed for this purpose. The best known one is probably the Harris-Benedict equation. If available, indirect calorimetry can be used to measure energy expenditure to define a caloric target. There have been no randomized controlled trials (RCTs) showing improved outcome with the use of this technology, and a recent study in trauma patients[5] has suggested that it does not add any information to the other strategies for estimating caloric requirements. Having estimated the total energy requirements, it is recommended that 50 to 70% of calories be delivered as carbohydrates and 15 to 30% as lipids, with a target protein dose of 1.2 to 1.5 g/kg/d.

EN

Use of EN vs PN

When considering nutritional support for critically ill patients, it is strongly recommended that EN be used over PN. When the results of 13 studies were aggregated statistically, there was no apparent difference in mortality rates across groups receiving EN or PN (relative risk [RR], 1.08; 95% confidence interval [CI], 0.70 to 1.65; p = 0.7). Compared to PN, EN was associated with a significant reduction in infectious complications (RR, 0.61; 95% CI, 0.44 to 0.84; p = 0.003). The aggregated effect of PN on infectious complications across several studies was homogeneous and resulted in a large effect size with narrow CIs. Safety, cost, and feasibility considerations favor the use of EN over PN. The subgroup analysis of the studies in which patients in the PN group

received more calories and had higher blood sugar levels than those in the EN group could not explain the higher rates of infections.

Early vs Delayed EN

When considering EN for the critically ill patient, it is recommended that EN be started with 24 to 48 h of hospital admission. There have been 11 RCTs[6–16] comparing early EN vs delayed nutrient intake (ie, delayed EN, PN, or oral diet). In all of the trials, EN was started within 24 to 48 h of resuscitation. When these studies were aggregated early EN was associated with a trend toward a reduction in mortality (RR, 0.65; 95% CI, 0.41 to 1.02; p = 0.06) when compared to delayed nutrient intake. Eight studies reported infectious complications, but only six studies[6,10–12,14,15] reported the number of patients with infections. When these were aggregated, early EN was associated with a trend toward a reduction in infectious complications (RR, 0.78; 95% CI, 0.60 to 1.01; p = 0.06) when compared to delayed nutrient intake. No differences in hospital length of stay were observed between groups. All ten studies[7–16] that reported nutritional end points showed a significant improvement in the groups receiving early EN (ie, calorie intake, protein intake, percentage of goal achieved, and better nitrogen balance achieved). There were no differences in other complications between the groups.

It is worth noting that there are inconsistent and variable definitions of early EN and delayed nutrition, and that there is considerable heterogeneity in the trial designs. Concerns have been expressed about the safety of early intragastric EN, given reports from nonrandomized trials[17,18] of increased harm experienced by patients who were fed aggressive early EN. However, given the potentially large treatment effect with respect to reduced mortality and infections, improved nutritional intake, and the minimal cost and feasibility concerns of early EN, the weight of evidence appears to favor the early use of EN.

Use of Feeding Protocols and Motility Agents

In critically ill patients who experience feeding intolerance (ie, high amounts of gastric residuals and emesis), the use of metoclopramide as a motility agent should be considered. A 2002 systematic review of the literature[19] analyzed RCTs of cisapride, metoclopramide, and erythromycin. Since then, two other RCTs[20,21] have studied the question. These data demonstrate that this class of drugs seems to have a physiologic benefit on GI motility and may improve tolerance to EN in critically ill patients. There is no demonstrated benefit on clinically important outcomes, but, given the low probability of harm, favorable feasibility, and cost considerations, it is reasonable to consider motility agents as a strategy to optimize nutritional intake. Cisapride is no longer available, and, given the concerns about emerging bacterial resistance with the use of erythromycin, metoclopramide is the preferred agent.

There is only one RCT[22] that has compared the use of a feeding protocol with higher gastric residual volume threshold (250 mL) and the routine use of metoclopramide with a feeding protocol that used a lower gastric residual volume threshold (150 mL). There was a trend toward less time taken to reach a target goal rate of feeding in the group that received the protocol with the higher residual volume threshold and prokinetics, and no harm was noted with the higher gastric residual volume threshold. There are insufficient data to make a recommendation about this issue, but, if a feeding protocol is used, this study supports the use of a higher gastric residual volume threshold and metoclopramide.

Small-Bowel Feeding vs Gastric Feeding

The Canadian clinical practice guidelines recommend the use of small-bowel feeding tubes based on the local circumstances that influence the ability to access the small bowel. If small-bowel access can be safely and easily achieved, then small-bowel feeding is recommended. In ICUs where logistic difficulties make small-bowel access more problematic, the use of small-bowel feeding should be considered for patients who are considered to be at a higher risk of complications from gastric feeding or who do not tolerate (ie, gastric residuals and emesis) gastric feeding.

There are 11 RCTs[12,23–32] that have looked at the question of small-bowel feeding vs gastric feeding in the critically ill patient. In one study by

Taylor et al,[31] only 34% of the patients achieved small-bowel access (ie, with a large number of protocol violations), and hence the metaanalysis was performed with and without this study.

The studies that reported nutritional delivery generally showed better success at meeting goal targets and reaching them sooner in patients who were fed via the small bowel. Based on the nine studies[12,23–25,27,28,30–32] that reported on infections, the metaanalysis showed that small-bowel feeding was associated with a significant reduction in infections (RR, 0.77; 95% CI, 0.60 to 1.00; p = 0.05) when compared to gastric feeding. The study by Taylor et al[31] contributes greatly to the results of this metaanalysis, and when the metaanalysis was done without the study by Taylor et al,[31] the statistical significance of the reduction in infectious outcomes with small-bowel feeding disappeared (RR, 0.83; p = 0.3). With respect to mortality, no significant differences between the groups were found (RR, 0.93; 95% CI, 0.72 to 1.20; p = 0.6).

Overall, there is a modest effect with respect to pneumonia, with wide CIs among studies that were heterogeneous. It has been expressed that the implementation of small-bowel feeding and the associated costs are institution dependent. In other words, the cost/benefit ratio would vary from institution to institution, and the recommendation needs to reflect this fact. The other considerations are improved nutritional end points and the ability to provide EN in someone who is otherwise not tolerating gastric feeding. It is hoped that there will be further information to help answer this question when a multicenter RCT that is currently enrolling patients in Australia finishes in the next few years.

The nutritional management of severe acute pancreatitis is a specific illness that should be addressed here. A recent metaanalysis[33] has demonstrated the benefit of EN compared to PN for patients with this condition, with a favorable effect on infectious complications and hospital length of stay. It is mentioned here as most of the studies to date have used small-bowel feeding for the delivery of EN in this patient group.

Body Position

Critically ill patients receiving EN should have the head of the bed elevated to a 45° angle. Where this is not possible, attempts to raise the head of the bed as much as possible should be considered. Two RCTs[34,35] have been performed addressing the question of whether semi-recumbency in critically ill patients receiving EN reduces the risk of pneumonia. One study[34] demonstrated a significant reduction in pneumonia with elevation of the head of the bed to a 45° angle, while the other study[35] failed to show any significant difference. However, patients in the latter study[35] failed to achieve the target elevation of the head of the bed. Other observational data support the association between pneumonia and the head of the bed being at a position below an angle of 30°.

EN in Combination With PN

For critically ill patients starting to receive EN, it is recommended that PN not be started at the same time as EN. In the patient who is not tolerating adequate EN, there are insufficient data to put forward a recommendation about when PN should be initiated. Practitioners will have to weigh the safety and benefits of initiating PN in patients who are not tolerating EN on an individual case-by-case basis. PN should not be started in critically ill patients until all strategies designed to maximize EN delivery (eg, the use of small-bowel feeding tubes and motility agents) have been attempted.

There are five RCTs[36-40] that have compared a strategy of combined EN and PN (started at the same time) to EN alone in critically ill patients. All five studies reported on mortality, and the aggregated results demonstrated a trend toward an increased mortality associated with the use of combination EN and PN (RR, 1.27; 95% CI, 0.82 to 1.94; p = 0.3). When a subgroup analysis was done comparing the trials that overfed to those that did not, there was no difference in effect. Supplemental PN was not associated with a higher incidence of infections (RR, 1.14; 95% CI, 0.66 to 1.96; p = 0.6), and had no effect on hospital length of stay or on the number of ventilator days.

It is important to note that these data pertain to patients with an intact GI tract, not to those who have an absolute indication for PN. When aggregated statistically, the studies that initiated PN at the same time as starting EN suggest a trend toward harm. The increase in mortality seen in the patients receiving combination EN and PN could not be explained by overfeeding. Given the probability of harm and the excess costs associated with the addition of PN when initiating EN, this practice is not recommended. However, there is an absence of data from randomized trials related to patients not tolerating adequate amounts of EN and when PN should be used in combination in this scenario. It would be reasonable to consider this method of nutritional support when strategies to optimize enteral feeding have been unsuccessful over a period of 5 days.

PN

Use of PN vs Standard Care in Patients With an Intact GI Tract

In critically ill patients with an intact GI tract, the routine use of PN is not recommended. [41]In a metaanalysis of PN vs standard care in critically ill and surgical patients, 6 of 26 studies included patients that would routinely be admitted to the ICU as part of their management. Two of these trials evaluated the use of combination EN and PN, and hence were excluded from this current analysis and incorporated into the previous section ("EN in Combination With PN"). In the only study[42] that reported the number of patients with infectious complications, PN was associated with an increase in infectious complications (4.0% vs 14.0%, respectively; p = 0.36).

In critically ill patients, the current aggregated results suggest no effect on mortality except that PN may be associated with an increase in complications and length of hospital stay. Given the concerns about the possibility of harm and the higher cost associated with PN when compared to standard treatment, its use in patients with an intact GI tract is not recommended. An intact GI tract excludes patients in whom PN would be life-sustaining, such as patients with short bowel syndrome, a perforated gut, or a high-output enteric fistula.

Hypocaloric PN

In critically ill patients who are not malnourished or are tolerating some EN, or when PN is indicated for short-term use (ie, <10 days), hypocaloric PN should be considered. There are insufficient data to make recommendations about the use of hypocaloric PN in the following patients: those requiring long-term PN (*ie*, >10 days); obese critically ill patients; and malnourished critically ill patients. Practitioners will have to weigh the safety and benefits of hypocaloric PN on an individual case-by-case basis in these latter patient populations.

Only two small RCTs have evaluated the effect of hypocaloric feeding in critically ill patients. To achieve a hypocaloric dose of PN, Choban et al[43] reduced both carbohydrates and lipids in obese critically ill patients, while McCowen et al[44] withheld lipids in a heterogeneous group of patients, including critically ill patients. Only one study[44] reported infectious complications, and in that study hypocaloric feeding was associated with a trend toward a reduction in infectious complications (p = 0.2). There were no significant differences in mortality or length of hospital stay between groups in either study.

The recommendation related to hypocaloric PN is in the context of an earlier recommendation that EN be used preferentially to PN and that strategies to maximize EN be utilized prior to initiating PN. The issue of hypocaloric PN is only relevant to those patients tolerating some (inadequate) EN where practitioners are, on a case-by-case basis deliberating about adding PN (see sections on "Use of EN vs PN" and "EN in combination With PN"). There is not a consistent definition of the term *hypocaloric PN* among the studies included, and hypocaloric PN could be achieved either by withholding lipids or reducing the carbohydrate load. Hypocaloric PN may be equivalent to standard PN with respect to cost and feasibility. However, given that all of the other signals related to PN suggest that PN is associated with no benefit or possibly harm in critically ill patients, despite the weak evidence available and equivocal cost considerations, minimizing the dose of PN should be the norm; stronger evidence to justify increased dosing of PN is needed. Although concerns regarding hypocaloric nutrition and essential fatty acid deficiency are probably minimal for those patients tolerating some EN and requiring short-term PN (*ie*, <10 days), this cannot be extrapolated to those who have an

absolute contraindication to EN and need PN for a longer duration.

Use of Lipids

In critically ill patients who are not malnourished and are tolerating some EN, or when PN is indicated for short-term use (*ie*, <10 days), withholding lipids high in soybean oil should be considered. There are insufficient data to make a recommendation about withholding lipids high in soybean oil in critically ill patients who are malnourished or in those requiring long-term PN (*ie*, >10 days). Practitioners will have to weigh the safety and benefits of withholding lipids high in soybean oil on an individual case-by-case basis in these latter patient populations.

There have been two RCTs[44,45] that have compared the use of lipids to no lipids in PN. These studies demonstrated no effect of withholding lipids on mortality (RR, 1.29; 95% CI, 0.16 to 10.7; p = 0.8). A significant reduction in pneumonia (48% vs 73%, respectively; p = 0.05), catheter-related sepsis (19% vs 43%, respectively; p = 0.04), and a significantly shorter stay in both the ICU (18 vs 29 days, respectively; p = 0.02) and the hospital (27 vs 39 days, respectively; p = 0.03) were observed in trauma patients not receiving lipids compared to those receiving lipids.[45] In the study by McCowen et al,[44] the group that received no lipids (the hypocaloric group) showed a trend toward a reduction in infections (29% vs 53%, respectively; p = 0.2). Combining these two studies, the metaanalysis showed a significant reduction in infections in the group that received no lipids (RR, 0.63; 95% CI, 0.42 to 0.93; p = 0.02).

The large reduction in infectious complications associated with withholding lipids may be influenced by the reduction in calories. However, the small reduction in calories is unlikely to explain such a large reduction in infectious complications, particularly when there is such supportive experimental data that lipids cause immune dysfunction. While the concerns regarding withholding lipids (*ie*, hypocaloric nutrition and essential fatty acid deficiency) are probably minimal for those patients tolerating some EN and requiring short-term PN (*ie*, <10 days), this cannot be extrapolated to those patients who have an absolute contraindication to EN and need PN

Specific Nutrients

Glutamine

The use of enteral glutamine should be considered in burn and trauma patients. There are insufficient data to support the routine use of enteral glutamine in other critically ill patients. There have been seven RCTs[46–52] that have studied the effect of glutamine on outcome, but only two studies[46,47] in select populations of burn and trauma patients have shown a favorable effect on infectious complications. Other studies[48,50] have not been able to demonstrate a benefit in heterogeneous ICU patients.

When PN is prescribed for critically ill patients, parenteral supplementation with glutamine, where available, is recommended. There are insufficient data to generate recommendations for the use of parenteral glutamine in patients receiving EN. There have been nine RCTs[53–62] aggregated that have addressed the issue of parenteral glutamine in association with PN. When aggregated in a metaanalysis, glutamine is associated with a favorable effect on mortality (RR, 0.67; 95% CI, 0.48 to 0.92; p = 0.01) and a trend toward reduced infectious complications (RR, 0.75; 95% CI, 0.54 to 1.04; p = 0.08).

Supplemental Antioxidant Nutrients

The use of supplemental parenteral selenium alone or in combination with other antioxidant nutrients and supplementation with trace elements and vitamins should be considered in critically ill patients. There have been >20 RCTs that have studied this question with different combinations of nutrients. For those who want to read more about the topic, I would suggest a systematic review that was published in 2005.[63] There is mounting evidence that these micronutrients have a favorable effect on mortality. The strongest evidence to date supports the use of selenium alone, but these agents act synergistically to reduce oxidative stress; combining them has biological plausibility.

It is anticipated that there will be further data to answer this question with more certainty in the next few years as a large multicenter RCT, known as the Reducing Deaths due to Oxidative Stress (or REDOXS) trial (sponsored by the Canadian Critical Care Trials Group), evaluating the use of glutamine, selenium, and other antioxidants is underway.

Fish Oils

The use of an enteral formula that contains fish oils, borage oils, and antioxidants (ie, vitamin C, vitamin E, beta carotene, and taurine) is recommended for patients with ARDS. When the data from three industry-sponsored RCTs are combined in a metaanalysis, the use of the combined formulation was associated with a significant reduction in mortality (RR, 0.63; 95% CI, 0.48 to 0.84; p = 0.002). The use of the enteral formula was also associated with a reduction in ventilator days and a trend toward a reduction in ICU length of stay. Currently, only one formula (Oxepa; Abbott Laboratories; Abbott Park, IL) has been evaluated in this manner. The acquisition costs of this product are higher than those of most standard enteral formulations, and, since the effect of the fish oils cannot be distinguished from the effects of the borage oils and antioxidants, this recommendation pertains to the combination product and not to fish oils generally.

Arginine

Diets supplemented with arginine and other select nutrients are not recommended for use in critically ill patients. There have been 21 RCTs in critically patients that form the basis for this recommendation, and this specifically excludes the studies that have been performed using elective surgery patients. Discussion of the use of this type of enteral formula in surgical patients would form a completely different topic that is not addressed in this article. The aggregated results from the studies in critically ill patients show no improvement in infectious complications or mortality. Some studies and a subgroup analysis suggest possible harm in patients with sepsis.

Glycemic Control

In critically ill surgical patients receiving nutritional support, intensive insulin therapy to tightly control blood sugars at levels between 4.4 and 6.6 mmol/L should be considered. In all critically ill patients, avoiding hyperglycemia (ie, blood glucose level, >10 mmol/L) by minimizing IV dextrose and using insulin administration when necessary is recommended.

Of the three RCTs performed, two were with surgical patients[64,65] and only one was with medical patients.[66] In the 2001 study by van den Berge et al,[65] patients started therapy by receiving a glucose load (200 to 300 g/d) and then advanced to receive PN, combined PN/EN, or EN 24 h after hospital admission. Grey et al[64] compared strict insulin therapy (target blood sugar range, 4.4 to 6.6 mmol/L) vs standard insulin therapy (target blood sugar range, 10 to 12 mmol/L) in surgical critically ill patients requiring treatment for hyperglycemia (blood sugar level, >7.7 mmol/L). In the 2006 study by van den Berghe et al in medical patients,[66] the target range for blood sugars was the same as that for the earlier study by the same authors (in 2001); the calories received from EN was similar in both groups.

All three studies reported on hospital mortality, and only two reported ICU mortality. When the data from the three trials were aggregated, intensive insulin therapy was associated with a significant reduction in hospital mortality (RR, 0.79; 95% CI, 0.59 to 1.07; $p = 0.13$; I^2 interclass correlation, 55% [suggesting moderate heterogeneity]). When a sensitivity analysis was performed on studies in surgical patients (excluding the one trial involving medical patients[66]), intensive insulin therapy was associated with a significant reduction in hospital mortality (RR, 0.65; 95% CI, 0.48 to 0.89; $p = 0.007$ [no heterogeneity present]). In the one study of medical patients,[22] a significant increase in mortality was noted in the subgroup of patients who stayed in the ICU for <3 days and received intensive insulin therapy (56 of 433 vs 42 of 433 patients, respectively; $p = 0.05$). However, there were no significant differences in ICU mortality rate (46% vs 67%, respectively; $p = 0.1$) or hospital mortality rate (62% vs 73%, respectively; $p = 0.4$) among patients who had hypoglycemia in the intensive insulin therapy group when compared to conventional

therapy. Intensive insulin therapy was associated with a trend toward a reduction in infectious complications compared to conventional insulin therapy in critically ill surgical patients (RR, 0.68; 95% CI, 0.41 to 1.11; $p = 0.12$).

The two studies by van den Berghe et al[20,22] have high internal validity, strong effect size, and narrow CIs. However, there is concern that the blood sugar levels were elevated by the early excessive use of parenteral glucose administration and the high use of PN. This limits the applicability of the results to other units that do not manage their nutritional support in that manner. These studies and other observational data have highlighted the detrimental effects of hyperglycemia on the outcome of critically ill patients. Although responding with treatment to blood sugar levels of >10 mmol/L (ie, 180 g/dL) is recommended based on these data, it is not yet clear what the optimal level of blood sugar control is for a heterogeneous group of critically ill patients. Ongoing trials will provide more information regarding the optimal insulin therapy in critically ill patients. One such trial is the Normoglycaemia in Intensive Care Evaluation and Survival Using Glucose Algorithm Regulation (or NICE-SUGAR) study that is jointly sponsored by the Australia and New Zealand Intensive Care Society and the Canadian Critical Care Trials Group.

Conclusion

Appropriately delivered nutritional support can improve the outcomes of critically ill patients. It is recommended that the mainstay of this support be through the enteral route (in patients with an intact GI tract) with strategies used to optimize the benefits and minimize the risks. These strategies include the following: (1) early initiation of enteral feeding; (2) the use of feeding protocols and motility agents; (3) the use of small-bowel feeding; and (4) the provision of care with the patient in the semirecumbent position. When initiating enteral feeding, PN should not be started simultaneously but could be considered if strategies to deliver EN are unsuccessful. Hyperglycemia should be avoided by minimizing the use of IV glucose and using IV insulin.

When using PN, consideration should be given to the time of initiation, and strategies to optimize benefits and minimize risks. These strategies are as follows: (1) consideration of limiting the dose of calories used; and (2) avoidance of the use of lipids high in soybean oil. Specific nutrients that may be used to optimize outcomes for critically ill patients include the following: (1) fish oils, borage oils, and antioxidants for ARDS patients; (2) glutamine; and (3) selenium and other antioxidants.

ACKNOWLEDGMENT: I would like to thank my colleagues, Dr. Daren Heyland and Rupinder Dhaliwal, who have been instrumental in the development of the Canadian Clinical Practice Guidelines for the Critically Ill.

References

1. Kreymann KG, Berger MM, Deutz NE, et al. ESPEN guidelines on enteral nutrition: intensive care. Clin Nutr 2006; 25:210–223

2. Heyland DK, Dhaliwal R, Drover JW, et al. Clinical practice guidelines for nutrition support in the adult critically ill patient. JPEN J Parenter Enteral Nutr 2003; 27:355–373

3. Critical Care Connections. Clinical practice guidelines. Available at: http://www.criticalcarenutrition.com. Accessed April 2, 2007

4. Cerra FB, Benitez MR, Blackburn GL, et al. Applied nutrition in ICU patients: a consensus statement of the American College of Chest Physicians. Chest 1997; 111:769–778

5. Davis KA, Kinn T, Esposito TJ, et al. Nutritional gain versus financial gain: the role of metabolic carts in the surgical ICU. J Trauma 2006; 61:1436–1440

6. Moore EE, Jones TN. Benefits of immediate jejunostomy feeding after major abdominal trauma—a prospective, randomized study. J Trauma 1986; 26:874–881

7. Chiarelli A, Enzi G, Casadei A, et al. Very early nutrition supplementation in burned patients. Am J Clin Nutr 1990; 51:1035–1039

8. Eyer SD, Micon LT, Konstantinides FN, et al. Early enteral feeding does not attenuate metabolic response after blunt trauma. J Trauma 1993; 34:639–644

9. Chuntrasakul C, Siltharm S, Chinswangwatanakul V, et al. Early nutritional support in severe traumatic patients. J Med Assoc Thai 1996; 79:21–26

10. Singh G, Ram RP, Khanna SK. Early postoperative enteral feeding in patients with nontraumatic intestinal perforation and peritonitis. J Am Coll Surg 1998; 187:142–146

11. Kompan L, Kremzar B, Gadzijev E, et al. Effects of early enteral nutrition on intestinal permeability and the development of multiple organ failure after multiple injury. Intensive Care Med 1999; 25:157–161

12. Minard G, Kudsk KA, Melton S, et al. Early versus delayed feeding with an immune-enhancing diet in patients with severe head injuries. J Parenter Enteral Nutr 2000; 24:145–149

13. Pupelis G, Selga G, Austrums E, et al. Jejunal feeding, even when instituted late, improves outcomes in patients with severe pancreatitis and peritonitis. Nutrition 2001; 17:91–94

14. Peck MD, Kessler M, Cairns BA, et al. Early enteral nutrition does not decrease hypermetabolism associated with burn injury. J Trauma 2004; 57:1143–1148

15. Malhotra A, Mathur AK, Gupta S, et al. Early enteral nutrition after surgical treatment of gut perforations: a prospective randomised study. J Postgrad Med 2004; 50:102–106

16. Dvorak MF, Noonan VK, Belanger L, et al. Early versus late enteral feeding in patients with acute cervical spinal cord injury: a pilot study. Spine 2004; 29:E175–E180

17. Mentec H, Dupont H, Bocchetti M, et al. Upper digestive intolerance during enteral nutrition in critically ill patients: frequency, risk factors, and complications. Crit Care Med 2001; 29:1955–1961

18. Ibrahim EH, Mehringer L, Prentice D, et al. Early versus late enteral feeding of mechanically ventilated patients: results of a clinical trial. JPEN J Parenter Enteral Nutr 2002; 26:174–181

19. Booth CM, Heyland DK, Paterson WG. Gastrointestinal promotility drugs in the critical care setting: a systematic review of the evidence. Crit Care Med 2002; 30:1429–1435

20. Yavagal DR, Karnad DR, Oak JL, et al. Metoclopramide for preventing pneumonia in critically ill patients receiving enteral tube feeding: a randomized controlled trial. Crit Care Med 2000; 28:1408–1411

21. Berne JD, Norwood SH, McAuley CE, et al. Erythromycin reduces delayed gastric emptying in critically ill trauma patients: a randomized, controlled trial. J Trauma 2002; 53:422–425

22. Pinilla JC, Samphire J, Arnold C, et al. Comparison of gastrointestinal tolerance to two enteral feeding protocols in critically ill patients: a

Nutritional Support in the Critically Ill Patient (Drover)

prospective, randomized controlled trial. JPEN J Parenter Enteral Nutr 2001; 25:81–86

23. Kortbeek JB, Haigh PI, Doig C. Duodenal versus gastric feeding in ventilated blunt trauma patients: a randomized controlled trial. J Trauma 1999; 46: 992–996

24. Davies AR, Froomes PR, French CJ, et al. Randomized comparison of nasojejunal and nasogastric feeding in critically ill patients. Crit Care Med 2002; 30:586–590

25. Montecalvo MA, Steger KA, Farber HW, et al. Nutritional outcome and pneumonia in critical care patients randomized to gastric versus jejunal tube feedings. The Critical Care Research Team. Crit Care Med 1992; 20:1377–1387

26. Esparza J, Boivin MA, Hartshorne MF, et al. Equal aspiration rates in gastrically and transpylorically fed critically ill patients. Intensive Care Med 2001; 27:660–664

27. Neumann DA, DeLegge MH. Gastric versus small-bowel tube feeding in the intensive care unit: a prospective comparison of efficacy. Crit Care Med 2002; 30:1436–1438

28. Kearns PJ, Chin D, Mueller L, et al. The incidence of ventilator-associated pneumonia and success in nutrient delivery with gastric versus small intestinal feeding: a randomized clinical trial. Crit Care Med 2000; 28:1742–1746

29. Boivin MA, Levy H. Gastric feeding with erythromycin is equivalent to transpyloric feeding in the critically ill. Crit Care Med 2001; 29:1916–1919

30. Montejo JC, Grau T, Acosta J, et al. Multicenter, prospective, randomized, single-blind study comparing the efficacy and gastrointestinal complications of early jejunal feeding with early gastric feeding in critically ill patients. Crit Care Med 2002; 30:796–800

31. Taylor SJ, Fettes SB, Jewkes C, et al. Prospective, randomized, controlled trial to determine the effect of early enhanced enteral nutrition on clinical outcome in mechanically ventilated patients suffering head injury. Crit Care Med 1999; 27:2525–2531

32. Day L, Stotts NA, Frankfurt A, et al. Gastric versus duodenal feeding in patients with neurological disease: a pilot study. J Neurosci Nurs 155; 33: 148–149

33. McClave SA, Chang WK, Dhaliwal R, et al. Nutrition support in acute pancreatitis: a systematic review of the literature. JPEN J Parenter Enteral Nutr 2006; 30:143–156

34. Drakulovic MB, Torres A, Bauer TT, et al. Supine body position as a risk factor for nosocomial pneumonia in mechanically ventilated patients: a randomised trial. Lancet 1999; 354:1851–1858

35. van Nieuwenhoven CA, Vandenbroucke-Grauls C, van Tiel FH, et al. Feasibility and effects of the semirecumbent position to prevent ventilator-associated pneumonia: a randomized study. Crit Care Med 2006; 34:396–402

36. Dunham CM, Frankenfield D, Belzberg H, et al. Gut failure-predictor of or contributor to mortality in mechanically ventilated blunt trauma patients? J Trauma 1994; 37:30–34

37. Herndon DN, Barrow RE, Stein M, et al. Increased mortality with intravenous supplemental feeding in severely burned patients. J Burn Care Rehabil 1989; 10:309–313

38. Herndon DN, Stein MD, Rutan TC, et al. Failure of TPN supplementation to improve liver function, immunity, and mortality in thermally injured patients. J Trauma 1987; 27:195–204

39. Chiarelli AG, Ferrarello S, Piccioli A, et al. Total enteral nutrition versus mixed enteral and parenteral nutrition in patients at an intensive care unit. Minerva Anestesiol 1996; 62:1–7

40. Bauer P, Charpentier C, Bouchet C, et al. Parenteral with enteral nutrition in the critically ill. Intensive Care Med 2000; 26:893–900

41. Heyland DK, MacDonald S, Keefe L, et al. Total parenteral nutrition in the critically ill patient: a meta-analysis. JAMA 1998; 280:2013–2019

42. Sax HC, Warner BW, Talamini MA, et al. Early total parenteral nutrition in acute pancreatitis: lack of beneficial effects. Am J Surg 1987; 153:117–124

43. Choban PS, Burge JC, Scales D, et al. Hypoenergetic nutrition support in hospitalized obese patients: a simplified method for clinical application. Am J Clin Nutr 1997; 66:546–550

44. McCowen KC, Friel C, Sternberg J, et al. Hypocaloric total parenteral nutrition: effectiveness in prevention of hyperglycemia and infectious complications: a randomized clinical trial. Crit Care Med 2000; 28:3606–3611

45. Battistella FD, Widergren JT, Anderson JT, et al. A prospective, randomized trial of intravenous fat emulsion administration in trauma victims requiring total parenteral nutrition. J Trauma 1997; 43:52–60

46. Houdijk AP, Rijnsburger ER, Jansen J, et al. Randomised trial of glutamine-enriched enteral

nutrition on infectious morbidity in patients with multiple trauma. Lancet 1998; 352:772–776

47. Zhou YP, Jiang ZM, Sun YH, et al. The effect of supplemental enteral glutamine on plasma levels, gut function, and outcome in severe burns: a randomized, double-blind, controlled clinical trial. J Parenter Enteral Nutr 2003; 27:241–245

48. Jones C, Palmer TE, Griffiths RD, et al. Randomized clinical outcome study of critically ill patients given glutamine-supplemented enteral nutrition. [see comment]. Nutrition 1999; 15:108–115

49. Brantley S, Pierce J. Effects of enteral glutamine on trauma patients. Nutr Clin Pract 2000; 15:S13

50. Hall JC, Dobb G, Hall J, et al. A prospective randomized trial of enteral glutamine in critical illness. Intensive Care Med 2003; 29:1710–1716

51. Garrel D, Patenaude J, Nedelec B, et al. Decreased mortality and infectious morbidity in adult burn patients given enteral glutamine supplements: a prospective, controlled, randomized clinical trial [see Comment]. Crit Care Med 2003; 31:2444–2449

52. Peng X, Yan H, You Z, et al. Effects of enteral supplementation with glutamine granules on intestinal mucosal barrier function in severe burned patients. Burns 2004; 30:135–139

53. Dechelotte P, Hasselmann M, Cynober L, et al. L-alanyl-L-glutamine dipeptide-supplemented total parenteral nutrition reduces infectious complications and glucose intolerance in critically ill patients: the French controlled, randomized, double-blind, multicenter study [see Comment]. Crit Care Med 2006; 34:598–604

54. Griffiths RD, Jones C, Palmer TE, et al. Six-month outcome of critically ill patients given glutamine-supplemented parenteral nutrition. Nutrition 1997; 13:295–302

55. Griffiths RD, Allen KD, Andrews FJ, et al. Infection, multiple organ failure, and survival in the intensive care unit: influence of glutamine-supplemented parenteral nutrition on acquired infection. Nutrition 2002; 18:546–552

56. Powell-Tuck J, Jamieson CP, Bettany GE, et al. A double blind, randomised, controlled trial of glutamine supplementation in parenteral nutrition [see Comment]. Gut 1999; 45:82–88

57. Wischmeyer PE, Lynch J, Liedel J, et al. Glutamine administration reduces Gram-negative bacteremia in severely burned patients: a prospective, randomized, double-blind trial versus isonitrogenous control. Crit Care Med 2001; 29:2075–2080

58. Goeters C, Wenn A, Mertes N, et al. Parenteral L-alanyl-L-glutamine improves 6-month outcome in critically ill patients [see Comment]. Crit Care Med 2002; 30:2032–2037

59. Fuentes-Orozco C, naya-Prado R, Gonzalez-Ojeda A, et al. L-alanyl-L-glutamine-supplemented parenteral nutrition improves infectious morbidity in secondary peritonitis. Clin Nutr 2004; 23:13–21

60. Zhou YP, Jiang ZM, Sun YH, et al. The effects of supplemental glutamine dipeptide on gut integrity and clinical outcomes after major escharectomy in severe burns: a randomized, double blind, controlled clinical trial. Clin Nutr Suppl 2004; 1:55–60

61. Ziegler TR, Fernandez-Estivariz C, Griffith DP, et al. Parenteral nutrition supplemented with alanyl-glutamine dipeptide decreases infectious morbidity and improves organ function in critically ill post-operative patients: results of a double-blind, randomized, controlled pilot study. JPEN J Parenter Enteral Nutr 2004; 28(S):11

62. Xian-Li H, Qing-jiu M, Jian-guo L, et al. Effect of total parenteral nutrition TPN. with and without glutamine dipeptide supplementation on outcome in severe acute pancreatitis (SAP). Clin Nutr Suppl 2004; 1:43–47

63. Heyland D, Dhaliwal R, Suchner U, et al. Antioxidant nutrients: a systematic review of trace elements and vitamins in the critically ill patient. Intensive Care Med 2005; 31:327–337

64. Grey NJ, Perdrizet GA, Grey NJ, et al. Reduction of nosocomial infections in the surgical intensive-care unit by strict glycemic control. Endocr Pract 2004; 10(suppl):46–52

65. van den Berghe G, Wouters P, Weekers F, et al. Intensive insulin therapy in the critically ill patients. N Engl J Med 2001; 345:1359–1367

66. van den Berghe G, Wilmer A, Milants I, et al. Intensive insulin therapy in mixed medical/surgical intensive care units: benefit versus harm. Diabetes 2006; 55:3151–3159

Acid-Base Disorders

Gregory A. Schmidt, MD, FCCP

Objectives:

- Describe the effects of acidemia and alkalemia in critically ill patients, especially regarding hemodynamic consequences
- Present a structured approach to analyzing acid-base disorders
- Discuss the differential diagnoses of the four fundamental acid-base derangements
- Discuss the treatment of acid-base disorders and provide clinical recommendations

Key words: acidemia; acidosis; alkalemia; alkalosis; bicarbonate; lactic acidosis; permissive hypercapnia; tromethamine

---

Disturbances of acid-base equilibrium occur in a wide variety of critical illnesses and are among the most commonly encountered disorders in the ICU. These derangements are often signaled by commonly obtained screening tests, such as arterial (or venous) blood gas analyses or electrolyte determinations. In addition to reflecting the seriousness of the underlying disease, disturbances in H^+ concentration have important physiologic effects.

A blood pH less than normal is called *acidemia*; the underlying process causing acidemia is called *acidosis*. Similarly, the terms *alkalemia* and *alkalosis* refer to elevated pH and the underlying process, respectively. While acidosis and alkalosis may coexist, there can be only one resulting pH. Therefore, acidemia and alkalemia are mutually exclusive conditions.

The approach to acid-base derangements should emphasize a search for the cause, rather than an immediate attempt to normalize the pH. Many disorders are mild and do not require treatment. Furthermore, treatment may be more detrimental than the acid-base disorder itself. Generally more important than a specific treatment is a full consideration of the possible underlying pathologic states. This may facilitate a directed intervention that will benefit the patient more than normalization of the pH would.

Approach to Acid-Base Disturbances

This discussion will generally follow the more widely accepted "bicarbonate-based" approach to understanding acid-base disturbances, although a superior method, developed by Peter Stewart, is available.[1,2] The Stewart method identifies the following true determinants of the pH: the strong ion difference (SID); the total concentration of weak acids (Atot); and the Pco_2. Using any method, diagnosing disorders of acid-base homeostasis in the ICU can be challenging. Many critically ill patients have combinations of disorders. In addition, patients admitted to the ICU often have pre-existing disturbances (*eg*, respiratory acidosis in patients with COPD and metabolic alkalosis in patients receiving diuretics) that must be taken into account when one is evaluating subsequent changes.

A Stepwise, Conventional Approach

Step 1: Do the numbers make sense? Use the Henderson equation, as follows: $[H^+] = 24 \times Pco_2/HCO_3$. If this equation is not true, there is an error in at least one of the numbers.

Step 2: Determine whether acidemia (pH <7.36) or alkalemia (pH >7.44) is present. In patients with mixed disorders, the pH may be in the normal range, but the bicarbonate level, the Pco_2, or the anion gap will signal the presence of an acid-base disturbance).

Step 3: Is the primary disturbance metabolic or respiratory? That is, does any change in the Pco_2 account for the direction of the change in pH?

Step 4: Is there appropriate compensation for the primary disturbance? See Table 1.

Step 5: Is the anion gap elevated? If so, is the change in the anion gap almost equal to the change in HCO_3^-? If not, there is an additional non-anion gap acidosis or a metabolic alkalosis.

Step 6: Put it all together: what is the most likely diagnosis?

Table 1. *Appropriate Compensation in Simple Acid-Base Disorders*

Acid-Base Disorder	Compensation
Metabolic acidosis	$Pco_2 = (1.5 \times HCO_3^-) + 8 \pm 2$
Metabolic alkalosis	$Pco_2 = (0.7 \times HCO_3^-) + 21 \pm 1.5^*$
Respiratory acidosis	Acute: $HCO_3^- = ([Pco_2 - 40]/10) + 24$
	Chronic: $HCO_3^- = ([Pco_2 - 40]/3) + 24$
Respiratory alkalosis	Acute: $HCO_3^- = ([40 - Pco_2]/5) + 24$
	Chronic: $HCO_3^- = ([40 - Pco_2]/2) + 24$

*For a bicarbonate (HCO_3^-) level >40 mEq/L, the formula to be used is $Pco_2 = (0.75 \times HCO_3^-) + 19 \pm 7.5$.

Physiologic Effects of Alkalemia and Acidemia

The effects of alkalemia and acidemia are difficult to discern because any physiologic consequences in patients may be obscured or modified by the severe illness causing the acid-base disorder. For example, a patient with lactic acidosis due to sepsis may have severe hypotension and depressed left ventricular systolic function. It is possible that the acidemia is the basis for circulatory failure but it is also possible (even likely, in this example) that some other consequence of sepsis underlies the hypotension. In an individual patient, it may be difficult to know how much trouble the acidemia is causing, if any. Even treatment with alkalinizing drugs or dialysis typically does not clarify the situation since these interventions have additional, nonhydrogen ion, actions that may account for clinically recognized effects.

Alkalemia appears to increase myocardial contractility, at least to a pH of 7.7. Some animals exhibit spontaneous ventricular fibrillation at pH levels >7.8. There are reports of alkalemic patients with atrial and ventricular arrhythmias who were refractory to treatment until the alkalemia was corrected. Respiratory alkalosis lowers BP and calculated systemic vascular resistance. Most vascular beds demonstrate vasodilation, but vasoconstriction predominates in the cerebral circulation. Cerebral blood flow falls maximally, to 50% of basal flow, at a Pco_2 of 20 mm Hg; this effect has been utilized to acutely lower intracranial pressure, but the effect lasts only 6 h. Both respiratory and metabolic alkalemia can lead to seizures. Alkalemia can also cause coronary artery spasm with ECG evidence of ischemia. The clinical effect of alkalemia-induced changes in oxygen delivery is small, but in patients with ongoing tissue hypoxia the increased hemoglobin oxygen affinity may be detrimental and clinically significant.

Acidemia causes stimulation of the sympathetic-adrenal axis. In patients with severe acidemia, this effect is countered by a depressed responsiveness of adrenergic receptors to circulating catecholamines. The net effect on ventricular performance, heart rhythm, and vascular tone depends on the relative effects of these competing influences. For example, mild acidemia causes increased cardiac output, a response that can be prevented by β-adrenergic blockade. Severe acidemia typically causes a decrease in cardiac output and vasodilation despite sympathetic stimulation. Clinically, no increase in arrhythmias is seen in patients with respiratory acidemia during permissive hypercapnia, except that attributable to hypoxia. Once ventricular fibrillation is established, acidemia has little or no effect on the success of conversion to sinus rhythm.

Acute respiratory acidemia causes marked increases in cerebral blood flow. When Pco_2 is >70 mm Hg, loss of consciousness and seizures can occur. This is likely due to an abrupt lowering of intracellular pH rather than to any effect of CO_2 *per se*. The encephalopathy of acute-on-chronic respiratory failure is poorly understood, but may include elements of intracellular acidosis, hypoxia, and endogenous neuropeptide secretion. Thus, the term *CO_2 narcosis*, which implies a direct effect of CO_2, is a misnomer.

Acute hypercapnia causes the depression of diaphragmatic contractility and a decrease in endurance time. This effect may contribute to the downward spiral of respiratory failure in patients with short-term CO_2 retention.

During intentional hypoventilation, as practiced in patients with status asthmaticus or ARDS, hypercapnia has been tolerated quite well. No significant impact on systemic vascular resistance, pulmonary vascular resistance, cardiac output, or systemic oxygen delivery has been seen.[3] There are several cautions, however. Patients are generally carefully chosen so as to have no increased intracranial pressure or cardiac ischemia; the inspired gas must be enriched with oxygen to prevent hypoxemia, and patients should be well sedated.[4] Alkalinizing medications are generally

Acid-Base Disorders (Schmidt)

not administered during episodes of permissive hypercapnia.

Respiratory Acidosis

Respiratory acidosis is characterized by a primary increase in the arterial Pco_2 and a compensatory rise in the bicarbonate concentration. Respiratory acidosis represents ventilatory failure or disordered central control of ventilation, the pathophysiology, etiology, and treatment of which have been described elsewhere. In mechanically ventilated patients with hypercapnia, it is important to consider the consequences of attempting to raise the minute ventilation. In many patients, normalizing the Pco_2 comes at the cost of alveolar overdistention (volutrauma) or exacerbation of auto-positive end-expiratory pressure. The point here is that normalizing the Pco_2 comes at a cost; that cost is in the form of volutrauma, frank barotraumas, or hypotension. The experience with permissive hypercapnia for patients with ARDS or status asthmaticus,[5] in which hypercapnia and acidemia are tolerated in order to avoid alveolar overdistention, has changed the perspective of many clinicians about the adverse impact of acidemia. In sedated and ventilated patients with ARDS, rapid intentional hypoventilation (*ie*, pH falling from 7.40 to 7.26 in 30 to 60 min) lowered systemic vascular resistance while cardiac output rose. Mean systemic arterial pressure and pulmonary vascular resistance were unchanged. Furthermore, in many studies[5a] of patients undergoing permissive hypercapnia, a pH of well below 7.2 was tolerated well. The feared consequences of acidemia, projected from the experience with patients having lactic acidosis (and, usually, concomitant sepsis), failed to materialize. With data now available for many patients who have been permissively hypoventilated, the systemic hemodynamic effects are quite small even as the pH falls to 7.15, with the typical patient experiencing no change or small increases in cardiac output and BP. Patients whose pH falls far below 7.0 are fewer in number, so firm conclusions cannot be drawn, but they similarly tolerate their acidemia. The current practice of permissive hypercapnia does not generally include an attempt to alkalinize the blood to compensate for respiratory acidosis. When the ventilator is used to correct respiratory acidosis, the end-inspiratory plateau pressure and auto-positive end-expiratory pressure should be monitored routinely to detect any adverse effects of ventilation.

Metabolic Acidosis

Metabolic acidosis is characterized by a primary decrease in bicarbonate concentration and a compensatory reduction in the Pco_2. The etiologies of metabolic acidosis are divided into those that cause an increase in the anion gap and those associated with a normal anion gap (called *hyperchloremic acidosis*). The *anion gap* is the difference between measured cations and measured anions, defined as $[Na^+] - [Cl^-] - [HCO_3^-]$, with a normal value traditionally defined as 8 to 14 mEq/L. The majority of unmeasured anions normally is accounted for by plasma proteins, primarily albumin. The remainder consists of phosphate, sulfates, lactate, and other organic anions. Seventy percent of patients with an anion gap >20 mEq/L will have an identifiable organic anion, as will virtually all of those with an anion gap >30 mEq/L. However, significant lactic acidosis can be present despite a normal measured anion gap, typically due to the hypoalbuminemia of critical illness.

Normal-anion-gap acidosis occurs from the loss of bicarbonate (through the kidneys or through the gut) or from the addition of an acid with chloride as the accompanying anion. The most common cause of normal-anion-gap metabolic acidosis in the ICU is diarrhea; in the absence of diarrhea, renal tubular acidosis is likely. The causes of renal tubular acidosis encountered in the ICU are listed in Table 2. The other causes of normal-anion-gap acidosis are usually obvious from the medical history and medication list. The etiologies of normal-anion-gap metabolic acidosis are listed in Table 3. The etiologies of increased-anion-gap metabolic acidosis are given in Table 4.

Ketoacidosis

Ketoacidosis occurs when free fatty acids are overproduced and preferentially shunted to form ketones, typically in states of low insulin and increased glucagon. Diabetic ketoacidosis is a common reason for ICU admission and is easily diagnosed from glucose and ketone measurements.

Table 2. *Etiologies of Renal Tubular Acidosis in the ICU**

RTA	Etiologies
Proximal	Primary renal disease
	Nephrotic syndrome
	Systemic diseases
	Amyloidosis
	Multiple myeloma
	Systemic lupus erythematosus
	Drugs and toxins
	Heavy metal toxicity
	Carbonic anhydrase inhibitors
Type I distal	Primary renal disease
	Obstructive uropathy
	Renal transplant rejection
	Nephrocalcinosis
	Pyelonephritis
	Allergic interstitial nephritis
	Systemic diseases
	Cirrhosis
	Multiple myeloma
	Sickle cell disease
	Amyloidosis
	Systemic lupus erythematosus
	Drugs and toxins
	Amphotericin
	Lithium
	Analgesic abuse
Type IV distal	Primary renal disease
	Obstructive uropathy
	Hyporeninemia
	Systemic diseases
	Diabetes mellitus
	Addison disease
	Sickle cell disease
	Drugs and toxins
	Spironolactone
	Triamterene
	Amiloride
	Pentamidine

*RTA = renal tubular acidosis.

Table 4. *Etiologies of Increased-Anion-Gap Metabolic Acidosis*

Etiologies	Anion
Ketoacidosis (diabetic, alcoholic, or starvation)	Acetoacetate, β-hydroxybutyrate
Lactic acidosis	Lactate
Uremia	Phosphates, sulfates, organic anions
Toxins	
Ethylene glycol	Glycolate, lactate
Methanol	Formate, lactate
Salicylate	Salicylate, lactate, organic anions
Paraldehyde	Unknown

Treatment involves rehydration, insulin administration, and attention to electrolyte disturbances. Alcoholic ketoacidosis (AKA) generally occurs after binge drinking in alcoholics who have no food intake and vomit repeatedly. AKA is characterized by a normal or slightly elevated serum glucose level with increased ketones. Because of the altered redox state of the liver, many of the ketones in patients with AKA occur in the form of β-hydroxybutyrate, which is not measured by some tests (Ketostix or Acetest; Bayer Diagnostics; Tarrytown, NY). Specific enzymatic testing is necessary to detect β-hydroxybutyrate. Rehydration and provision of glucose are generally sufficient therapy for AKA, although insulin administration may be useful in some patients. Alkali therapy is not useful in the treatment of ketoacidosis.

Toxins

Toxin ingestion is an uncommon but important cause of increased-anion-gap acidosis. Any patient who presents with an anion-gap acidosis that is not explained by tests for ketones and

Table 3. *Etiologies of Normal-Anion-Gap Metabolic Acidosis*

Etiologies	Description
GI loss of bicarbonate	Diarrhea; urinary diversion; small bowel, pancreatic, or bile drainage (fistulas, surgical drains); and cholestyramine
Renal loss of bicarbonate (or bicarbonate equivalent)	Renal tubular acidosis; recovery phase of diabetic ketoacidosis; renal insufficiency; and posthypocapneic
Acidifying substances	HCl; NH_4Cl; arginine HCl; lysine HCl; $CaCl_2$ or $MgCl_2$ (oral); and sulfur

Acid-Base Disorders (Schmidt)

lactate should be suspected of having ingested a toxin. However, it should also be remembered that lactic acidosis can occur with toxin ingestion, so an increased lactate level does not rule out an acidosis from toxins. Often, the laboratory diagnosis of toxin ingestion is slow; thus, the diagnosis must be suspected, and clinical clues sought, prior to laboratory confirmation. Specific tests must be ordered, as methanol and ethylene glycol are not included in a routine toxicology screen. Salicylate intoxication is the most common of these ingestions, and patients often present with mixed respiratory alkalosis and metabolic acidosis, which can be an important diagnostic clue.

The toxic effects of ethylene glycol and methanol are mediated by metabolites (glycolate in the case of ethylene glycol, and formaldehyde and formate in the case of methanol). The osmolal gap, which is the difference between the measured osmolality and that calculated from the formula osm = $2[Na^+] + [glucose]/18 + [BUN]/2.8 + [ethanol]/4.6$, is increased above its normal value of <10 mosmol/L. The osmolal gap may lack sensitivity, however, and its value as a screening test has been questioned. The loss of retinal sheen or even frank papilledema seen with methanol poisoning and the characteristic urinary oxalate crystals seen with methylene glycol poisoning can be helpful diagnostically. Fomepizole, an inhibitor of alcohol dehydrogenase, is safe and effective in the treatment of ethylene glycol and methanol poisoning.[6]

The identification of the anion associated with an increased-anion-gap acidosis in the ICU is not as precise as it might seem from the relatively short list of possibilities. In some cases of acidosis, either no anion is found or the rise in anions accounts for only a fraction of the rise in the anion gap; the identity of the offending anion, or anions, in these circumstances has not been determined.

Lactic Acidosis

Lactic acidosis, commonly defined as a lactate level of >5 mmol/L with an arterial pH of <7.35, is the most common and most important metabolic acidosis encountered in the ICU. The acidemia serves as a marker for a diverse group of serious underlying conditions and has important prognostic implications. The etiologies of lactic acidosis are numerous and are listed in Table 5.

Table 5. *Etiologies of Lactic Acidosis**

Increased oxygen consumption
  Strenuous exercise
  Grand mal seizure
  Neuroleptic malignant syndrome
  Severe asthma
  Pheochromocytoma
Decreased oxygen delivery
  Decreased cardiac output
    Hypovolemia
    Cardiogenic shock (including pericardial and
      pulmonary vascular disease)
  Decreased arterial oxygen content
    Profound anemia
    Severe hypoxemia
  Regional ischemia (mesentery or extremity)
Alterations in cellular metabolism
  Sepsis
  Diabetes mellitus, hypoglycemia
  Thiamine deficiency
  Severe alkalemia
  Malignancy
  Mitochondrial myopathies
  AIDS
Toxins and drugs
  Carbon monoxide
  Ethanol, methanol
  Biguanides (eg, metformin)
  Ethylene glycol, propylene glycol
  Salicylates
  Isoniazid
  Streptozocin, nalidixic acid
  Cyanide, nitroprusside
  Papaverine
  Acetaminophen
  Ritodrine
  Terbutaline
  Fructose, sorbitol, xylitol
  Epinephrine, norepinephrine, cocaine
  Zidovudine and other HAARTs
  Kombucha tea
  Propofol
Congenital
  Glucose-6-phosphatase deficiency
  Fructose-1,6-diphosphatase deficiency
  Pyruvate carboxylase deficiency
  Pyruvate-dehydrogenase deficiency
  Oxidative phosphorylation defects
Decreased lactate clearance
  Fulminant hepatic failure
d-Lactate
  Short-gut syndrome
  Antibiotic-induced

*HAART = highly active antiretroviral drug.

Most cases of lactic acidosis encountered in the ICU occur secondarily to a handful of processes; shock is the most common cause, with hypoxia, seizures, regional ischemia (ie, mesenteric or in an extremity), and toxin exposure accounting for a majority of the remaining cases.

Sepsis is a common cause of lactic acidosis in patients in the ICU, but the mechanism is still debated. The belief that the lactic acidosis of sepsis is caused by anaerobic metabolism has come under question based on several lines of evidence. If cellular oxygen lack were the basis of lactic acid production, the lactate/pyruvate ratio should be elevated, a finding that is absent in resuscitated septic patients. Furthermore, when the adequacy of cellular oxygenation has been assayed by various methods, it has been found to be adequate. Pathologic supply dependence, a finding that was often interpreted to support tissue hypoxia, now appears to be an artifact of mathematical coupling, at least regarding this phenomenon at the whole-body level. No dependence of oxygen consumption on oxygen delivery can be found when each is measured by independent means. Additionally, various methods of boosting oxygen delivery fail to lower lactate levels in resuscitated septic patients. Finally, in an animal model of sepsis and lactic acidosis, hypoxic challenge failed to worsen lactic acidosis. Possible alternate mechanisms include hypermetabolism-induced protein catabolism, leading to increased circulating levels of alanine, pyruvate, and lactate (consistent with the normal lactate/pyruvate ratio); regional (ie, gut) production of lactate, possibly due to local hypoxia; mitochondrial dysfunction; and many others.

Alkalinizing Therapies

Use of therapy with alkalinizing solutions to normalize arterial hydrogen ion concentration ($[H^+]$) has as its rationale that the correction of the acid-base disorder will improve clinical outcome. While the use of sodium bicarbonate or other alkalinizing solutions has been established by this empiric approach, there is limited and often conflicting experimental evidence to justify this practice. Alkali therapies may either improve or worsen clinically relevant end points such as

arterial $[H^+]$, P_{CO_2}, lactate concentration, SID, or cardiac output. The variability in the effects of alkali therapy has contributed to a wide range of clinical practices and expert recommendations regarding these treatments.

Physiologic Rationale

The underlying rationale for the administration of bicarbonate or alkalinizing solutions to patients with acidemia can be summarized within the framework of the following four related clinical hypotheses: (1) an elevation in arterial $[H^+]$ in and of itself contributes to the observed pathology (eg, organ dysfunction, hemodynamic instability, or death); (2) administering alkali IV will lower the arterial $[H^+]$ level; (3) lowering the arterial $[H^+]$ level will mitigate pathology or reduce the risk of deterioration; and (4) the benefits of alkali administration outweigh any adverse effects. The physiologic rationale for the use of alkali therapy depends on the validity of these four main hypotheses.

Arterial $[H^+]$, Organ Dysfunction, and Cell Viability

Investigations using isolated cardiac preparations, whole-animal models, and human tissue have consistently demonstrated depressed myocardial contractility when the $[H^+]$ level is raised. However, the overall effect of increased extracellular $[H^+]$ on cellular function depends on a large number of variables, which limits generalizations about these effects. For example, in the myocardium as well as other organ systems, the end result of increased extracellular $[H^+]$ levels on intracellular $[H^+]$ and cellular function is related to the disease state producing the acidosis, the organ and cell type in question, catecholamine response, intracellular energy stores, and other extracellular conditions such as oxygen tension and the concentrations of sodium, chloride, and lactate. Furthermore, it is likely that diseases that cause acidosis (eg, sepsis) also produce profound changes in cellular energy metabolism and local microcirculatory regulation, which contribute to organ dysfunction and confound our understanding of the effect of increased $[H^+]$. Thus, it is little surprise that in experimental whole-animal preparations, acidosis causes a wide range of myocardial consequences, as follows: no change in contractility; a marginal decrease in contractility; or a transient increase in contractility followed by a decrease (despite controlled heart rate, preload, and afterload).

In contrast to early assumptions that elevated [H$^+$] levels are surely harmful, many protective or beneficial effects have also been described. In a wide variety of cell preparations and experimental conditions, raising extracellular [H$^+$] levels has been shown to protect cells against the effects of hypoxia and energy depletion. Furthermore, acidosis limits myocardial infarction size, stroke volume, hepatocyte death, and lung damage in models of ischemia-reperfusion injury. Many potential salutary effects of acidemia have been described with regard to inflammation, free radical generation, and regulation of gene expression to suppress injury pathways. In conclusion, it is not clear that the association of acidemia with organ dysfunction or cell death is causal.

Effect of Alkalinizing Therapy on Arterial [H$^+$]

Bicarbonate is not one of the fundamental determinants of the acid-base state. Rather, the independent determinants of the blood [H$^+$] are the SID, Atot, and the Paco$_2$. Sodium bicarbonate and other alkalinizing solutions affect arterial [H$^+$] by changing these quantities. The administration of sodium bicarbonate increases the SID because sodium is a strong cation (while $^-$HCO$_3$ is not a strong anion) but at the same time raises Paco$_2$. The net effect of the increase in SID, which tends to lower [H$^+$], and the increase in Paco$_2$, which tends to raise the [H$^+$] level, may be to counteract each other (ie, no change in [H$^+$] level) or to raise or lower the [H$^+$] level. The impact in an individual patient depends on other factors such as ventilatory response and the patient's ability to exhale the generated CO$_2$. Thus, while most clinical studies have demonstrated that bicarbonate will lower [H$^+$] in acidemic conditions, the effect is modest and in some instances (most notably during lung-protective ventilation) [H$^+$] may remain constant or even rise after bicarbonate infusion.

Effect of Alkalinizing Therapy on Critical Organ Function

There are several alkalinizing treatments that have been evaluated for clinical use including sodium bicarbonate, dichloroacetate, carbicarb and tromethamine (ie, tris-hydroxymethyl aminomethane [THAM]). Sodium bicarbonate administered in animal models of lactic acidosis, hemorrhagic shock, and respiratory acidosis has consistently demonstrated improvements in arterial [H$^+$] levels but no significant effects on myocardial function or hemodynamic parameters. Two clinical trials[7,8] of sodium bicarbonate in patients with lactic acidosis failed to demonstrate any significant hemodynamic effects following the administration of a bicarbonate dose of 1 to 2 mmol/kg body weight. Animal studies in dogs and one clinical study[8a] in humans with intraoperative metabolic acidosis have demonstrated the negative effects of bicarbonate administration on myocardial contractility and cardiac function. In comparison to therapy with saline or dextrose solutions, bicarbonate therapy in other clinical situations, including neonatal resuscitation and cardiopulmonary resuscitation, has no consistent benefit on hemodynamic end points. Therapy with bicarbonate solution also has not been shown to confer any significant benefit over therapy with saline and dextrose solutions on metabolic recovery in patients with diabetic ketoacidosis. Finally, despite the inclusion of options for bicarbonate treatment in patients with permissive hypercapnia and low-tidal-volume ventilation protocols in the ARDS, there are data[9] to suggest that arterial [H$^+$] levels may actually rise after bicarbonate therapy in this group.

THAM is a weak base that is excreted in urine after protonation. Thus, the effect of THAM on [H$^+$] levels does not depend on respiratory function to excrete CO$_2$, as is the case with sodium bicarbonate. THAM has shown favorable effects on the normalization of [H$^+$] levels and improvement in myocardial contractility in an animal heart model.[9a] Small clinical trials[9] in patients with metabolic acidosis, ARDS, or acute lung injury have demonstrated improvements in [H$^+$] level, no change or decreases in arterial Pco$_2$, and improvements in myocardial contractility after THAM administration. It is unknown whether these physiologic effects confer a clinical benefit.

Potential Adverse Effects of Alkalinizing Therapy

When treating patients with unproved medications, safety concerns are paramount. Alkalinizing therapies have generally been subjected to little scrutiny in this regard, perhaps because we fully expect most of our severely acidemic patients who have been treated in this way to die. Animal and human data have both shown the potential for decreased cardiac function and cardiac output. Other potential adverse effects of these treatments may result from effects on $Paco_2$, sodium concentration, ionized calcium level, and intravascular volume. Of particular concern is the generation of carbon dioxide by bicarbonate infusion. Although the rise in arterial Pco_2 is modest in most patients and the carbon dioxide will generally be excreted with time, there may be greater effects on intracellular Pco_2 (and, therefore, on intracellular $[H^+]$). Such effects on many tissues have been shown in both animal and human studies, although it is not clear that any of these are clinically meaningful. Other adverse effects of bicarbonate treatment for acidosis include hypernatremia, hyperosmolality, hypervolemia, increases in lactate concentration, decreases in ionized calcium concentration, and heightened risk of cerebral edema. The reported adverse effects of THAM include hypoglycemia, hyperkalemia, extravasation-related skin necrosis, and (in neonates) hepatic necrosis.

Clinical Approach to Alkalinizing Therapy

The complexity and diversity of acid-base disorders in critically ill patients, combined with the lack of definitive evidence of benefit in human clinical trials, has produced significant variability in the use of alkali therapy. A survey of nephrology and pulmonary/critical care training directors has confirmed the absence of a standard approach to treatment recommendations for the treatment of acute metabolic acidosis. Surveys of the published literature including systematic reviews and metaanalyses have demonstrated controversy and the absence of consistent recommendations.

Given the absence of clinical data that demonstrate improvements in mortality, length of stay, or other clinical outcome variables, the decision to use alkali therapy remains empiric and cannot be directly supported by robust experimental data. Clinical decision making for or against alkali therapy thus should depend on (1) treating the underlying condition, (2) identifying subsets of patients who may be harmed by treatment or are very likely to benefit from treatment, and (3) monitoring the impact of treatment.

Treat the Underlying Condition

Patients with lactic acidosis as the result of hypoxemia, hypoperfusion, or sepsis, especially those who are hemodynamically unstable despite vasoactive drug infusions, are commonly considered for bicarbonate or other alkalinizing therapy. There is no published, clinical experimental evidence that has demonstrated an improvement in hemodynamic parameters, vasopressor requirements, or clinical outcome when bicarbonate is administered to these patients. On the other hand, effective resuscitation both repairs acidosis and improves outcome. Effort should be directed primarily to the timely administration of antibiotics, the early initiation of hemodynamic monitoring, intravascular volume repletion, lung-protective mechanical ventilation, and prophylaxis for common intensive care complications, including pneumonia, deep venous thrombosis, gastric ulceration, and skin breakdown.

Identify Patients Likely To Benefit From or Be Harmed by Alkali Therapy

The specific populations of critically ill patients who must be identified for alkali therapy include those who are most likely to benefit from treatment and those who are most likely to be harmed by treatment. For unstable patients with septic lactic acidosis, clinicians should exhaust all effective treatment strategies before considering salvage therapy with alkali. It is important that alkali therapy not interfere with or distract from proven interventions. Lacking data on effectiveness, we discourage the clinical use of alkalinizing treatments, no matter the degree of acidemia. Nevertheless, since clinical studies are lacking in scope, we recognize that some intensivists will choose to administer bicarbonate or provide other treatment, but we emphasize that doses and regimens of therapy lack any evidentiary basis. Furthermore, even the calculations of doses based on, for example, the volume of bicarbonate distribution, rely on outmoded concepts of acid-base physiology.

Monitor the Effects of Alkali Treatment

Given the diversity in both the diseases and the patients with metabolic acidosis who may be considered for alkali treatment, no uniform recommendations on therapeutic end points can be made. These decisions will depend on the underlying disease state, the comorbid conditions, and the available treatment options. THAM may not be consistently available or routinely supplied by hospital pharmacies. If the clinician determines that the patient is likely to benefit from alkalinizing therapy, a rational framework for treatment decisions should include careful attention to physiologic parameters that can be frequently and easily measured. The clinician should actively determine the primary variables that will function as indicators of therapeutic effect (eg, global perfusion, work of breathing, or stability of cardiac rhythm) and the frequency of clinical monitoring. Therapeutic monitoring variables should include arterial [H^+] level; $Paco_2$; hemodynamic status; intravascular volume; patient-ventilator interaction; and concentrations of serum sodium, calcium, and potassium. Further clinical studies will be necessary to resolve uncertain aspects of alkalinizing therapy such as dosage calculations, bolus or continuous dosing regimens, and meaningful end points such as the target [H^+] level.

The decision about whether to use bicarbonate is a difficult one. It is the choice between (1) a long-standing but unproven therapy with potential deleterious effects and (2) reliance on limited studies; neither is an entirely satisfactory choice. The debate will most likely continue until additional trials of bicarbonate therapy are conducted. With respect to the primary rationale for bicarbonate use (improvement in cardiovascular function), bicarbonate has shown no benefit. Because of the lack of data supporting bicarbonate use in human beings and the arguments reviewed above, I do not recommend the use of bicarbonate in patients with lactic acidosis, regardless of the pH.[10] This recommendation has been supported by the Surviving Sepsis Campaign.[11]

Metabolic Alkalosis

Metabolic alkalosis is characterized by a primary increase in the bicarbonate concentration and a compensatory increase in the Pco_2. The fact that patients will hypoventilate to compensate for metabolic alkalosis, even unto hypoxemia, is often not fully appreciated.[12] For metabolic alkalosis to persist, there must be both a process that elevates serum bicarbonate concentration (generally, gastric or renal loss) and a stimulus for renal bicarbonate reabsorption (typically, hypovolemia, hypokalemia, or mineralocorticoid excess). The major causes of metabolic alkalosis in the ICU (ie, vomiting, nasogastric suction, diuretics, corticosteroids, and the overventilation of patients with long-term increases in bicarbonate levels) are obvious, when present, from a patient's medical history and medication list. A careful search of all substances administered to the patient is needed to disclose the administration of compounds, such as citrate with blood products and acetate in parenteral nutrition, that can raise the bicarbonate level. If the etiology is not clear, a trial of volume and chloride replacement, as well as the correction of hypokalemia, can be attempted. If this does not effect an improvement in alkalosis, a search for increased mineralocorticoids may be warranted. The etiologies of metabolic alkalosis are listed in Table 6.

In patients who require continued diuresis but exhibit rising bicarbonate levels, acetazolamide can be used to reduce the bicarbonate level. When the rapid correction of severe alkalosis is desired, hemodialysis can be performed or hydrochloric acid can be infused (a 0.1N to 0.2N solution infused into a central vein at 20 to 50 mEq/h with arterial pH monitored every hour).

Respiratory Alkalosis

Respiratory alkalosis is characterized by a primary reduction in the arterial Pco_2. Respiratory alkalosis is very common in patients in the ICU, and its causes range from benign (simple anxiety) to life-threatening (sepsis or pulmonary embolism).

Table 6. *Etiologies of Metabolic Alkalosis*

Chloride-responsive
  Renal H$^+$ loss
    Diuretic therapy
    Post-hypercapnia
    Penicillin, ampicillin, carbenicillin therapy
  GI H$^+$ losses
    Vomiting, nasogastric suction
    Villous adenoma, congenital chloridorrhea
    Watery diarrhea-hypokalemia-achlorhydria syndrome
      (VIPoma, pancreatic cholera)
  Alkali administration
    Bicarbonate
    Citrate in blood products
    Acetate in total parenteral nutrition
    Nonabsorbable alkali (Mg[OH]$_2$, Al[OH]$_3$) and
      exchange resins
Chloride-resistant
  Increased mineralocorticoid activity
    Primary aldosteronism
    Cushing syndrome
    Drugs with mineralocorticoid activity
  Profound hypokalemia
  Refeeding
  Bartter syndrome
  Parathyroid disease
  Hypercalcemia

Table 7. *Etiologies of Respiratory Alkalosis*

Hypoxia
  High-altitude
  Pulmonary disease
  Decreased fraction of inspired oxygen
  Profound anemia
Increased CNS respiratory drive
  Anxiety, pain, and voluntary hyperventilation
  CNS disease (cerebrovascular accident, tumor,
    infection, trauma)
  Fever, sepsis, and endotoxin
  Drugs (salicylates, catecholamines, progesterone,
    analeptics, doxapram)
  Hyperthyroidism
  Liver disease
  Pregnancy, progesterone
  Epinephrine
  Exercise
Pulmonary disorders
  Pneumonia
  Pulmonary embolism
  Restrictive lung disease
  Pulmonary edema
  Bronchospasm
  Pleural effusion
  Pneumothorax
  Mechanical ventilation

Distinguishing those episodes of respiratory alkalosis that are manifestations of serious disease requires a thorough clinical review. The etiologies of respiratory alkalosis are listed in Table 7.

The primary treatment for respiratory alkalosis is of the underlying cause of the hyperventilation. The alkalemia itself generally does not require treatment. In patients in whom severe alkalemia is present (generally, when respiratory alkalosis is superimposed on metabolic alkalosis), sedation may be necessary. In patients with sepsis, in whom a significant portion of cardiac output can go to the respiratory muscles, intubation and muscle relaxation are occasionally used to control hyperventilation and redirect blood flow.

Annotated References

1. Stewart PA. How to understand acid-base: a quantitative acid-base primer for biology and medicine. New York, NY: Elsevier, 1981
   This outstanding text, now out of print, develops acid-base medicine from the ground up, replacing the unwieldy "bicarbonate-based" approach with a more accurate and computationally amenable method. Describes the determinants of the pH: the SID; the Atot; and the PCO_2.

2. Fencl V, Jabor A, Kazda A, et al. Diagnosis of metabolic acid-base disturbances in critically ill patients. Am J Respir Crit Care Med 2000; 162:2246–2251
   Compared two commonly used diagnostic approaches, one relying on plasma bicarbonate concentration and "anion gap" and the other on "base excess," with Stewart's approach[1] for their value in detecting complex metabolic acid-base disturbances. Of 152 patients, one sixth had normal base excess and plasma bicarbonate levels. In a great majority of these apparently normal samples, the Stewart method detected the simultaneous presence of acidifying and alkalinizing disturbances, many of them grave. The almost ubiquitous hypoalbuminemia confounded the interpretation of acid-base data when the customary approaches were applied.

3. Thorens J-B, Jolliet P, Ritz M, et al. Effects of rapid permissive hypercapnia on hemodynamics, gas exchange, and oxygen transport and consumption during mechanical ventilation for the acute respiratory distress syndrome. Intensive Care Med 1996; 22:182–191
   Describes the hemodynamic effects of acute respiratory acidosis in patients with ARDS, showing that permissive hypercapnia is well tolerated.

4. Feihl F, Perret C. Permissive hypercapnia: how permissive should we be? Am J Respir Crit Care Med 1994; 150:1722–1737

Commentary regarding the potential risks of permissive hypercapnia.

5. Tuxen DV, Williams TJ, Scheinkestel CD, et al. Use of a measurement of pulmonary hyperinflation to control the level of mechanical ventilation in patients with acute severe asthma. Am Rev Respir Dis 1992; 146:1136–1142

Key study validating the approach of intentionally hypoventilating patients with status asthmaticus to avoid the consequences of barotrauma.

5a. Thorens J-B, Jolliet P, Ritz M, et al. Effects of rapid permissive hypercapnia on hemodynamics, gas exchange, and oxygen transport and consumption during mechanical ventilation for the acute respiratory distress syndrome. Intensive Care Med 1996; 22:182–191

Eleven sedated and ventilated ARDS patients were hypoventilated (Pco_2 from 40 to 59 mm Hg) while hemodynamic indices were measured. Respiratory acidosis was well tolerated, blood pressure was unchanged, and cardiac index and oxygen delivery rose.

6. Brent J, McMartin K, Phillips S, et al. Fomepizole for the treatment of methanol poisoning. N Engl J Med 2001; 344:424–429

Clinical trial confirming the efficacy of an inhibitor of alcohol dehydrogenase in patients with methanol poisoning.

7. Cooper DJ, Walley KR, Wiggs BR, et al. Bicarbonate does not improve hemodynamics in critically ill patients who have lactic acidosis: a prospective controlled clinical study. Ann Intern Med 1990; 112:492–498

Well-controlled study in patients with septic lactic acidosis, almost all of whom were receiving catecholamines, directly addressing the role of bicarbonate therapy in these patients. These investigators showed that bicarbonate was no different from control with respect to any relevant hemodynamic parameter, despite the known lack of responsiveness to catecholamine therapy during acidemia.

8. Mathieu D, Neviere R, Billard V, et al. Effects of bicarbonate therapy on hemodynamics and tissue oxygenation in patients with lactic acidosis: a prospective, controlled clinical study. Crit Care Med 1991; 19:1352–1356

Another study demonstrating the lack of efficacy of bicarbonate with regard to any hemodynamic benefit.

8a. Mark NH, Leung JM, Arieff AI, et al. Safety of low-dose intraoperative bicarbonate therapy: a prospective, double-blind, randomized study. The Study of Perioperative Ischemia (SPI) Research Group. Crit Care Med 1993; 21:659–665

Forty subjects with coronary artery disease undergoing major surgery who developed very mild acidosis (pH 7.36) were given low-dose sodium bicarbonate or saline. Bicarbonate raised pH, serum bicarbonate concentration, and Pco_2, while lowering cardiac output.

9. Kallet RH, Jasmer RM, Luce JM, et al. The treatment of acidosis in acute lung injury with tris-hydroxymethyl aminomethane (THAM). Am J Respir Crit Care Med 2000; 161:1149–1153

Patients who received mechanical ventilation for acute lung injury who also had significant metabolic acidosis were given THAM. Arterial pH rose and Pco_2 fell, which is in contrast to the effects of sodium bicarbonate (which lowered the pH and raised the Pco_2).

9a. Sirieix D, Delayance S, Paris M, et al. Tris-hydroxymethyl aminomethane and sodium bicarbonate to buffer metabolic acidosis in an isolated heart model. Am J Respir Crit Care Med 1997; 155:957–963

Using an isolated heart preparation, ventricular contractility and relaxation were depressed during acidosis (pH 7.0). Sodium bicarbonate initially worsened these parameters, then slightly improved them, while THAM improved both contractility and relaxation.

10. Forsythe SM, Schmidt GA. Sodium bicarbonate for the treatment of lactic acidosis. Chest 2000; 117:260–267

Critically reviews the clinical and laboratory data regarding bicarbonate therapy for metabolic acidosis, concluding that bicarbonate should not be given routinely for lactic acidosis, no matter what the pH.

11. Cariou A, Vinsonneau C, Dhainaut J-F. Adjunctive therapies in sepsis: an evidence-based review. Crit Care Med 2004; 32(suppl):S562–S570

Critical literature review of adjunctive therapies for patients with sepsis carried out by critical care and infectious disease experts representing 11 international organizations. This article reviews the evidence regarding glycemic control, renal replacement, and correction of metabolic acidosis. Bicarbonate should not be given (grade C). For those with a pH <7.15, the recommendation is uncertain (grade E).

12. Javaheri S, Kazemi H. Metabolic alkalosis and hypoventilation in humans. Am Rev Respir Dis 1987; 136:1011–1016

Study of patients with metabolic alkalosis showing that compensatory respiratory acidosis is a predictable response, even when the Po_2 falls significantly.

Notes

Issues in Postoperative Management: Postoperative Pain Management and Intensive Glycemic Control

Michael A. Gropper, MD, PhD, FCCP

Objectives:

- Understand the implications of pain management practices in critically ill patients
- Review the pharmacodynamics and pharmacokinetics of commonly used opiates
- Understand the use of intrathecal and epidural opiates and local anesthetics
- Understand the importance of the stress response and glycemic control in perioperative patients

Key words: epidural analgesia; glycemic control; insulin; opiates; pain; stress response

---

As intensive care therapies have evolved, there is now greater understanding as to the importance of pain management. Failure to control pain may have deleterious effects. Fortunately, because of the development of better analgesics and sedatives and better methods of drug delivery, significant advances have been made in our ability to address these issues.

Consensus recommendations to guide analgesic and sedative therapy in the ICU were published in 1995 and then revised in 2002; however, substantial variability in practice still exists. The reasons for this disparity are multifold, but the most important reasons are that (1) no single depth of sedation or single sedative agent is appropriate for every patient and every situation encountered in the ICU, and (2) we still lack reliable methods for measuring pain and anxiety. As discussed in the chapter entitled, "Issues in Sedation, Paralytic Agents, and Airway Management," excessive analgesic or sedative administration may result in significant morbidity, and possibly mortality.

Theoretically, the choice of the ideal drug should be based on pharmacokinetic and pharmacodynamic properties, the cost of therapy (including the drug and the required delivery apparatus), and the cost of treating side effects, but the critically ill often have systemic illnesses, multiple organ failure, and hemodynamic instability, which limit drug choices. This chapter will discuss complications from inadequate and excessive pain and sedation therapy, the assessment of pain and sedation, pharmacokinetic and pharmacodynamic properties of analgesics and sedatives used in critical care practice, and some recent practice guidelines on the use of analgesics and anxiolytics in the ICU.

Complications From Pain and Anxiety

Undertreated pain results in many physiologic responses that are associated with poor outcomes.[1] Stimulation of the autonomic nervous system and the release of humoral factors such as catecholamines, cortisol, glucagon, leukotrienes, prostaglandins, vasopressin, and β-endorphins following injury, sepsis, or surgery are known as the stress response. This activation of the sympathetic nervous system increases heart rate, BP, and myocardial oxygen consumption, which can lead to myocardial ischemia or infarction.[2] The altered hormonal milieu can lead to hypercoagulability due to increased levels of factor VIII and fibrinogen-platelet activity and the inhibition of fibrinolysis.[3] The stress hormones also produce insulin resistance, increased metabolic rate, and protein catabolism. Immunosuppression is common because of a reduction in the number and function of lymphocytes and granulocytes.[4] Previously, the stress response was considered a homeostatic mechanism that was beneficial, but more recent data have shown that this response may be detrimental in part. Many studies[5-8] have shown that the adequate treatment of pain can decrease the magnitude of these changes that occur following surgery and thereby decrease some postoperative complications.

The ICU environment can lead to psychological difficulties as well. Of the patients discharged from the ICU, 40% recall having pain and 55% recall having anxiety during their stay in the ICU.[9] Patients who have received mechanical ventilation, been sedated, and paralyzed have reported experiencing hallucinations, delusions, and altered sense of reality.[10] Although some procedures can be explained to the patient in order to help alleviate anxiety, unfortunately not all patients who require procedures during the acute illness are in a state receptive to reasoning. These experiences lead to the development of posttraumatic stress syndromes in some patients after their stay in the ICU.[11] For these patients, effective therapy for anxiety and pain can reduce some of the emotional suffering and decrease the incidence of postoperative neurosis.[12] By the same token, excessive usage of sedatives can prolong mechanical ventilation and may increase the risk of delirium, especially in older patients.

Assessment of Pain and Anxiety

Pain and anxiety are intrinsically subjective. They are difficult to standardize and monitor from one care provider to another unless a standard is developed for assessing and monitoring these states. This is what makes the management of sedation in critically ill patients one of the more challenging areas of ICU care.

For pain, the most widely used scale is the visual analog scale, in which patients point to a point on a horizontal line that is a representation of the spectrum of pain from "no pain" to "the worst pain I've ever had." The scale is simplistic and has a high degree of reliability and validity,[13] but ignores other dimensions such as the qualitative aspects of pain. Not all critically ill patients can use this scale because of the severity of their illnesses. Sometimes, bedside nurses have to use behavioral signs such as facial expressions, movement, or posturing, or physiologic signs such as tachycardia, hypertension, or tachypnea. Unfortunately, none of these methods are exact. They depend on the cultural interpretation of pain, and often the type of illness and use of other drugs can alter the hemodynamic parameters.

Monitoring sedation is also inexact, and a true "gold standard" has not been established. The Glasgow Coma Scale is widely used for the assessment of level of consciousness, but validity is established only in patients with neurologic deficits in the acute setting. A scale that may be more applicable to the medical-surgical ICU is the 6-point Ramsay Scale.[14] The Ramsay Scale is a numerical scale of motor responsiveness based on increasing depth of sedation. Most comparative studies have used the Ramsay Scale, but it also has drawbacks. Because it is based on motor response, the scale has to be modified for patients receiving muscle relaxants, and, like the assessment of pain, there is no consensus as to what represents an adequate level of sedation in an individual patient. Other scales include the Sedation-Agitation Scale and the Motor Activity Assessment Scale, but all have similar drawbacks. On the horizon, the bispectral index (BIS) of the EEG is known to provide information about the interaction between cortical and subcortical regions.[15,16] The BIS, which is based on a score between 0 and 100, is an index of the level of consciousness.[17] It is more often used in the operating room as an index of the degree of the depth of general anesthesia, to prevent awareness. Recently, attempts have been made to extend the use of BIS into the ICU, but preliminary reports have been conflicting because of muscle-based electrical activity or metabolic or structural abnormalities of the brain in ICU patients.[18,19] Additional studies are required to validate this technique in ICU patients, but the theoretical benefits of a noninvasive monitor of cerebral function are plausible. To date, however, no data have been able to show that BIS monitoring when used to assess depth of sedation significantly alters patient outcomes in the ICU.[20] Because of the lack of evidence, the routine use of this device was not recommended by the new clinical practice guidelines.[21]

Analgesics

Pain in the critically ill is best treated with a pure opioid agonist. The commonly available opiates all work at the μ-receptor, so the choice of which agent to use should be based on pharmacokinetic characteristics. In a recent clinical guideline,[21] the recommended choices have been narrowed to morphine, fentanyl, and hydromorphone. The use of meperidine, nonsteroidal antiinflammatory drugs (NSAIDs), and mixed opioid agonist-antagonist agents are discouraged because of potential side effects, but their use will not be discussed here. However, drugs such as methadone, a long-acting opioid that can be administered parenterally or enterally, and ketamine, a sedative drug with analgesic qualities, will be discussed at the end of this section because they do have specific advantages in the ICU patient and can be used for the difficult-to-sedate patient.

Morphine

Recommended as the first-line opioid for use in the ICU, morphine, because of its water solubility, has a delayed peak effect when compared with the more lipid-soluble opioids such as fentanyl (30 min vs 4 min, respectively). Morphine administration leads to venodilation and decreases heart rate through sympatholysis and direct effects at the sinoatrial node.[22] The primary side effect is its propensity to cause respiratory depression. Other side effects include sedation, nausea, ileus, and spasm of the sphincter of Oddi. The primary nonreceptor-based side effect from morphine is histamine release, causing hypotension, tachycardia, and possibly bronchospasm in susceptible patients. Morphine has an elimination half-life of 2 to 4 h. It does have an active metabolite, morphine-6-glucuronide, that may accumulate and cause excessive sedation in patients with renal failure.[23]

Fentanyl

Fentanyl is the preferred analgesic agent for critically ill patients with hemodynamic instability or those with a morphine allergy. Fentanyl is a synthetic opioid that is 80 to 100 times more potent than morphine. Fentanyl has opioid receptor-based side effects that are similar to morphine, but it does not release histamine. Fentanyl causes only minor hemodynamic changes and does not affect the inotropic state of the heart. Virtually all hemodynamic variables, including cardiac output and systemic and pulmonary vascular resistance, are unchanged after large doses of fentanyl.[24] The rapid administration of large doses may be associated with bradycardia and chest wall rigidity.

Because of the lipid solubility of fentanyl, the duration of action with small doses is short because of redistribution from the brain to other tissues. This is an example of a context-sensitive half-life. Larger cumulative doses become dependent on elimination as opposed to redistribution. The duration of action lengthens and becomes similar to morphine because the elimination half-lives of the drugs are similar. The pharmacokinetics of fentanyl are not significantly altered in the presence of liver or kidney dysfunction.[25] Fentanyl metabolites may accumulate, but they are largely inactive and nontoxic, and the terminal elimination half-life of fentanyl is based on release from tissue stores rather than hepatic elimination.[26] Only with severe hepatic dysfunction and high-dose fentanyl will altered pharmacokinetics be observed.

Hydromorphone

Recommended as an acceptable alternative to morphine, hydromorphone is a semisynthetic opioid that is five times more potent than morphine. Time to onset and duration of action are similar to those of morphine. Hydromorphone has minimal hemodynamic effects and does not result in histamine release. Studies[27] also have shown that pruritus, sedation, and nausea and vomiting may occur less often with hydromorphone than with morphine, so it can be a good alternative, especially in patients who are unable to tolerate morphine.

Like morphine, hydromorphone is metabolized by conjugation with glucuronide, but it also undergoes reduction via a nicotinamide adenine dinucleotide phosphate reductase to two active metabolites. The metabolites have greater analgesic activity than the parent compound but are in such small amounts that they are probably insignificant except in the presence of renal failure or large doses over a prolonged time, when their levels may accumulate to toxic levels.[28]

Methadone

Methadone is a synthetic opioid agent with morphine-like properties that can be administered enterally and parenterally. It is much longer acting than morphine and has a similar receptor-associated side effect profile, but it is less sedating. The oral bioavailability is three times greater than the bioavailability of oral morphine.[29] Methadone has had a negative stigma given its association with drug abuse and opioid detoxification, and its long half-life makes titratability very difficult for most ICU patients. Although methadone is not the drug of choice for an acutely ill patient whose hospital course is rapidly changing, it is a good alternative for the patient who has a long recovery ahead and an anticipated prolonged ventilatory wean. Often, once things are stable, transition from fentanyl or morphine infusions to methadone administered via the feeding tube can help simplify care regimens and decrease dependence on infusions.

Methadone, unlike morphine, lacks active metabolites.[30] It is metabolized in the liver, and a small portion of it is eliminated in the kidney. Nonrenal routes eliminate 60%, so ketamine does not accumulate in patients with renal failure.[29]

Ketamine

Ketamine, a phencyclidine compound, is an IV anesthetic that has analgesic properties. It works via the N-methyl-D-aspartate receptor as well as the μ-receptor.[31] Traditionally, its primary use in the ICU has been during short procedures with intense pain such as dressing changes and wound debridement in burn patients. An advantage of ketamine is that it causes minimal respiratory depression.

Ketamine increases BP, heart rate, and cardiac output by causing the release of catecholamines.[32] Patients who have been critically ill for a prolonged period may have exhausted their catecholamine stores and may exhibit the myocardial depressant effects of ketamine.[33]

Subhypnotic doses of ketamine infusions have been used for patients who are very difficult to sedate with narcotic and benzodiazepine infusions.[34] These low-dose ketamine infusions (<5 μg/kg/min) do not seem to be associated with the usual side effects of ketamine such as hypertension, tachycardia, increased intracranial pressure, excessive secretions, and vivid dreams and hallucinations (termed *emergence reactions*).[34] Tolerance is known to develop with prolonged use of larger bolus doses but has not been observed at lower dosages due to limited experience. Because of its potential adverse side effects, ketamine is not recommended for routine sedation of the critically ill patient, but it can be helpful for more difficult situations. Ketamine also has bronchodilatory effects, which could

be beneficial during the intubation of asthmatic patients.[35] Ketamine also may be useful as an adjunct in opiate-tolerant patients.

Postoperative Pain and Pain Relief

Several investigations[36,36a] (although not all) in experimental animals and in patients have documented that preemptive analgesia improves the quality of postoperative pain management. Preemptive analgesia can decrease the sensitization of the CNS that would ordinarily amplify subsequent nociceptive input (termed *windup*); preemptive analgesia requires the administration of local anesthesia or other pain medication prior to the development of pain.[36] Patients who have more severe pain preoperatively will require larger quantities of pain medication perioperatively than patients who deny pain or have infrequent pain preoperatively.[37]

The choices for pharmacologic postoperative pain relief therapy for hospitalized patients include the following: the administration of NSAIDs, including cyclooxygenase-2 inhibitors,[38] and the administration of narcotic or narcoticlike medications parentally into the epidural space or into the cerebrospinal fluid. The administration of NSAIDs can decrease the total dose of narcotic medication required for postoperative pain control; there are no significant data that cyclooxygenase-2 inhibitors provide a major advantage over traditional NSAIDs.[38] Moreover, NSAIDs should not be administered to patients with renal insufficiency, a history of ulcer disease, or bleeding tendencies. Therefore, patients who have undergone craniotomies or major vascular surgery are not considered good candidates for these medications.

The intrathecal administration of narcotics is not as popular as the administration of these medications into the epidural space because of the duration of the analgesia and the respiratory depression and headaches that can be associated with this procedure.[39] Usually, only one dose of intrathecal opioid is administered; duration of pain relief is a problem for some patients. After the administration of 0.5 to 1.0 mg of intrathecal morphine, 15 to 22 h of analgesia have been reported.[39,40] Nonetheless, intrathecal opioids are now used for perioperative analgesia for cardiac, vascular, and hip arthroplasty surgeries, and patients receive parenteral narcotics if the spinal narcotic is insufficient for pain relief.

Another reason intrathecal opioids have been underused is the fear of respiratory depression. The incidence of this event in one report[41] was 3% of 6,000 patients (180 patients) who had received intrathecal preservative-free morphine, 0.2 to 0.8 mg, plus 25 µg of fentanyl; none of the patients required intubation, and all of the patients responded to naloxone infusions without reversal of their analgesia. Pruritus (37% incidence) and nausea and vomiting (25% incidence) occurred at the same frequency that is seen after the administration of parenteral or epidural opioids.[42] (Pruritus should be treated with naloxone rather than diphenhydramine hydrogen chloride, as the pruritus is not histamine mediated.) Finally, there is a fear of severe postdural puncture headaches that can require an epidural blood patch for relief. This complication and therapy occurred in 0.37% of 6,000 patients who received intrathecal opioids.[42] However, the investigators admitted that intrathecal opioids were not offered to patients who had a history of frequent headaches. In addition, the use of "pencil-point" spinal needles can significantly reduce the incidence of postdural puncture headaches.

The administration of epidural opioids is associated with complications similar to those of the intrathecal administration of opioids. The incidence of dural puncture with epidurals ranges between 0.16% and 1.3%, and the incidence of headache in the group of patients who had a puncture is between 16% and 86%.[43,44] A unique complication to the epidural approach is the formation of epidural hematomas. The incidence of epidural hematomas appears to be very rare unless the patient is anticoagulated or has a coagulation disorder.[45] There have been epidural hematomas reported in patients who have received low-molecular-weight heparin and then had epidural catheters placed.[45] There have been three separate national advisory panels on this issue; there is now a warning in all packages of low-molecular-weight heparins. Because of these reports, guidelines have been generated; the practice at the University of California, San Francisco is that epidural catheters not be placed for 12 h after the last dose of low-molecular-weight heparin.[45] Close communication is required among the anesthesiologist, surgeon, and postoperative pain management physicians.

Local anesthetics and narcotics are often administered in combination via epidural catheters because investigations[40,44] have documented improved perioperative outcomes with this technique, including improved pulmonary function, decreased pulmonary complications, and decreased sedation. Similarly, the administration of local anesthetics via an epidural catheter appears to reduce postoperative ileus, reduce the requirements of systemic opioids, and decrease the duration of hospitalization after abdominal surgeries.[40,44] The local anesthetic appears to be the important agent in achieving these outcome benefits. However, as local anesthetics have significant hemodynamic side effects that depend on the extent of the neural blockade and can cause motor blockade, which precludes postoperative ambulation, small doses of local anesthetic are administered in combination with opioids via the epidural catheters to obtain pain relief and minor nerve blockade, and to produce minimal side effects from both agents. For example, a solution of 0.05% ropivacaine (a new local anesthetic that causes less motor blockade than bupivacaine) and 1 µg/mL of fentanyl has been administered at 8 mL/h via an epidural catheter, and postoperative patients obtained optimal pain relief without motor blockade.[46] Note that patients are allowed to ambulate only with assistance when they are receiving these agents, and specific orders are required regarding additional pain medication.

Perioperative Glycemic Control

Critically ill patients are frequently hyperglycemic. The metabolic response to critical illness includes stimulation of the hypothalamic-pituitary-adrenal axis, resulting in increased growth hormone and prolactin levels. Growth hormone levels are high early in the course of critical illness and then typically become quite low. Takala et al[47] demonstrated that growth hormone administered to patients with prolonged critical illness resulted in increased mortality when compared with placebo. Cortisol levels are usually increased, and these endocrine changes result in hyperglycemia. Catecholamines, both endogenous and exogenous, also contribute to the hyperglycemia of critical illness. Whereas previous practice had been to treat only marked hyperglycemia (eg, >200 mg/dL), recent evidence suggests that control should be much more rigorous.

van den Berghe and colleagues[48] performed a prospective, randomized trial of intensive insulin therapy in critically ill patients, most of whom had undergone cardiac surgery. The intervention group received an insulin infusion to maintain serum glucose concentration between 80 and 100 mg/dL, whereas the control group blood glucose concentration was maintained between 180 and 200 mg/dL. The ICU mortality rate was decreased in the treatment group from 8 to 4.6% (p < 0.04). In addition to the mortality rate reduction, the patients with insulin infusion had fewer infections, decreased transfusion requirements, and a shorter duration of mechanical ventilation. The mechanism for this outcome is unclear. Possibilities include both the avoidance of hyperglycemia and a therapeutic effect of insulin. Can the results of this study be extrapolated to other critically ill patients? Unlike the other studies discussed, the patients in this study did not require a diagnosis of sepsis to be enrolled. It is possible that because of a longer length of stay, these patients may obtain even greater benefit. This hypothesis, however, must be tested prospectively.

A prospective, observational study[42] examined the effects of glucose control in 523 patients admitted to a single surgical ICU. In this trial, the primary determinant of a bad outcome was hyperglycemia, rather than hypoinsulinemia. That is, lower mortality was associated with glycemic control, rather than a protective effect of insulin administration. Indeed, increased insulin dosing was associated with increased mortality across all ranges of glycemia. These data suggest that keeping the blood glucose concentration below 140 mg/dL may provide a similar survival benefit as the "tighter" range of 80 to 110 mg/dL used by van den Berghe et al.[48]

Implementation of strict glucose control protocols is difficult, and the consequences of severe hypoglycemia are devastating. For example, implementation of a similar protocol in our 24-bed medical-surgical ICU required extensive nurse and physician training. Whereas tight control may not be feasible in settings other than the ICU, more attention needs to be paid to perioperative glycemic control. A follow-up study by van den Berghe et al[49] in medical ICU patients was unable to replicate their robust findings in surgical ICU patients. Mortality rate was not reduced with glycemic control; however, in patients with ICU stays >3 days, there was still significant benefit. Two more recent studies have added additional doubt to the efficacy of intensive insulin therapy. Brunkhorst et al[50] performed a multicenter randomized trial comparing intensive insulin therapy with more conservative treatment of hyperglycemia. The trial was terminated early because of episodes of severe hypoglycemia associated with insulin administration. The definitive trial, termed *NICE SUGAR*, was recently published in the *New England Journal of Medicine*.[51] This was also a randomized, controlled trial, enrolling >6,000 patients. Unlike the previous study, NICE SUGAR demonstrated increased mortality rate in patients receiving intensive insulin therapy.

References

1. Lewis KS, Whipple JK, Michael KA, et al. Effect of analgesic treatment on the physiological consequences of acute pain. Am J Hosp Pharm 1994; 51:1539–1554
2. Mangano DT, Siliciano D, Hollenberg M, et al. Postoperative myocardial ischemia: therapeutic trials using intensive analgesia following surgery. Anesthesiology 1992; 76:342–353
3. Britton BJ, Hawkey C, Wood WG, et al. Stress: a significant factor in venous thrombosis? Br J Surg 1974; 61:814–820
4. Slade MS, Greenberg LJ, Yunis EJ, et al. Integrated immune response to standard major surgical trauma in normal patients. Surg Forum 1974; 25:425–427
5. Swinamer DL, Phang PT, Jones RL, et al. Effect of routine administration of analgesia on energy expenditure in critically ill patients. Chest 1988 Jan; 93:4–10
6. Moller IW, Dinesen K, Sondergard S, et al. Effect of patient-controlled analgesia on plasma catecholamine, cortisol and glucose concentrations after cholecystectomy. Br J Anaesth 1988; 61:160–164
7. Modig L, Borg T, Bagge L, et al. Role of extradural and of general anesthesia in fibrinolysis and coagulation after total hip replacement. Br J Anaesth 1983; 55:625–629

8. Salomaki TE, Leppaluto J, Laitinen JO, et al. Epidural versus intravenous fentanyl for reducing hormonal, metabolic and physiologic responses after thoracotomy. Anesthesiology 1993; 79:672–679

9. Jones C, Macmillan RR, Griffiths RD. Providing psychological support for patients after critical illness. Clin Intensive Care 1994; 5:176–179

10. Parker M, Schubert W, Shelhamer J, et al. Perceptions of a critically ill patient experiencing therapeutic paralysis in an ICU. Crit Care Med 1984; 12:69–71

11. Stoll C, Haller M, Briegel J, et al. Health-related quality of life in long-term survivors after treatment with extracorporeal membrane oxygenation (ECMO) for the acute respiratory distress syndrome (ARDS). Anaesthesist 1998; 47:24–29

12. Bond M. Psychological and psychiatric aspects of pain. Anaesthesia 1978; 33:355–361

13. Chapman CR, Casey KL, Dubner R, et al. Pain measurement: an overview. Pain 1985; 22:1–31

14. Ramsay MA, Savege TM, Simpson BR, et al. Controlled sedation with alphaxalone-alphadolone. BMJ 1974; 2:656–659

15. Shapiro BA. Bispectral index: better information for sedation in the intensive care unit? Crit Care Med 1999; 27:1663–1664

16. Glass PS, Bloom M, Kearse L, et al. Bispectral analysis measures sedation and memory effects of propofol, midazolam, isoflurane, and alfentanil in healthy volunteers. Anesthesiology 1997; 86:836–847

17. Liu J, Singh H, White PF. Electroencephalographic bispectral index correlates with intraoperative recall and depth of propofol-induced sedation. Anesth Analg 1997; 84:185–189

18. Shah N, Clack S, Chea F, et al. Does bispectral index of EEG correlate with Ramsay sedation score in ICU patients? [abstract] Anesthesiology 1996; 85:A469

19. Frenzel D, Greim C, Sommer C, et al. Is the bispectral index appropriate for monitoring the sedation level of mechanically ventilated surgical ICU patients? Intensive Care Med 2002; 28:178–183

20. De Deyne C, Struys M, Decruyenaere J, et al. Use of continuous bispectral EEG monitoring to assess depth of sedation in ICU patients. Intensive Care Med 1998; 24:1294–1298

21. Jacobi J, Fraser G, Coursin D, et al. Clinical practice guidelines for the sustained use of sedatives and analgesics in the critically ill adult. Crit Care Med 2002; 30:119–141

22. Hsu HO, Hickey RF, Forbes AR. Morphine decreases peripheral vascular resistance and increases capacitance in man. Anesthesiology 1979; 50:98–102

23. Osborne R, Joel S, Slevin M. Morphine intoxication in renal failure; the role of morphine-6-glucuronide. Br Med J (Clin Res Ed) 1986; 293:1101

24. Stanley T, Webster L. Anesthetic requirements and cardiovascular effects of fentanyl-oxygen and fentanyl-diazepam-oxygen anesthesia in man. Anesth Analg 1978; 57:411–416

25. Bodenham A, Shelly MP, Park GR. The altered pharmacokinetics and pharmacodynamics of drugs commonly used in critically ill patients. Clin Pharmacokinet 1988; 14:347–373

26. Haberer J, Schoeffler P, Courderc E, et al. Fentanyl pharmacokinetics in anaesthetized patients with cirrhosis. Br J Anaesth 1982; 54:1267–1270

27. Sarhill N, Walsh D, Nelson KA. Hydromorphone: pharmacology and clinical applications in cancer patients. Support Care Cancer 2001; 9:84–96

28. Zheng M, McErlane KM, Ong MC. Hydromorphone metabolites: isolation and identification from pooled urine samples of a cancer patient. Xenobiotica 2002; 32:427–439

29. Davis MP, Walsh D. Methadone for relief of cancer pain: a review of pharmacokinetics, pharmacodynamics, drug interactions and protocols of administration. Support Care Cancer 2001; 9:73–83

30. Felder C, Uehlinger C, Baumann P, et al. Oral and intravenous methadone use: some clinical and pharmacokinetic aspects. Drug Alcohol Depend 1999; 55:137–143

31. Irifune M, Shimizu T, Nomoto M, et al. Ketamine-induced anesthesia involves the N-methyl-D-aspartate receptor-channel complex in mice. Brain Res 1992; 596:1–9

32. Gooding J, Dimick A, Tavakoli M, et al. A physiologic analysis of cardiopulmonary responses to ketamine anesthesia in noncardiac patients. Anesth Analg 1977; 56:813-816

33. Waxman K, Shoemaker W, Lippmann M. Cardiovascular effects of anesthetic induction with ketamine. Anesth Analg 1980; 59:355–358

34. Joachimsson PO, Hedstrand U, Eklund A. Low-dose ketamine infusion for analgesia during postoperative ventilator treatment. Acta Anaesthesiol Scand 1986; 30:697–702

35. Corssen G, Gutierrez J, Reves J, et al. Ketamine in the anesthetic management of asthmatic patients. Anesth Analg 1972; 51:588–596

36. Gottschalk A, Smith DS, Jobes DR, et al. Preemptive epidural analgesia and recovery from radical prostatectomy: a randomized controlled trial. JAMA 1998; 279:1076–1082

36a. Dahl JB, Møiniche S. Pre-emptive analgesia.Br Med Bull 2004 Dec 13; 71:13–27

37. Slappendel R, Weber EW, Bugter ML, et al. The intensity of preoperative pain is directly correlated with the amount of morphine needed for postoperative analgesia. Anesth Analg 1999; 88:146–148

38. Gilron I, Milne B, Hong M. Cyclooxygenase-2 inhibitors in postoperative pain management: current evidence and future directions. Anesthesiology 2003; 99:1198–1208

39. Gwirtz KH, Young JV, Byers RS, et al. The safety and efficacy of intrathecal opioid analgesia for acute postoperative pain: seven years' experience with 5969 surgical patients at Indiana University Hospital. Anesth Analg 1999; 88:599–604

40. Peyton PJ, Myles PS, Silbert BS, et al. Perioperative epidural analgesia and outcome after major abdominal surgery in high-risk patients. Anesth Analg 2003; 96:548–554

41. Bates JJ, Foss JF, Murphy DB. Are peripheral opioid antagonists the solution to opioid side effects? Anesth Analg 2004; 98:116–122

42. Finney SJ, Zekveld C, Elia A, et al. Glucose control and mortality in critically ill patients. JAMA 2003; 290:2041–2047

43. Peyton PJ, Rigg JA, Jamrozik K, et al. The MASTER Trial has successfully addressed requirements of protocols for large trials. Anesth Analg 2003; 97:922–923

44. Rigg JR, Jamrozik K, Myles PS, et al. Epidural anaesthesia and analgesia and outcome of major surgery: a randomised trial. Lancet 2002; 359:1276–1282

45. Horlocker TT, Wedel DJ. Spinal and epidural blockade and perioperative low molecular weight heparin: smooth sailing on the Titanic. Anesth Analg 1998; 86:1153–1156

46. Liu SS, Moore JM, Luo AM, et al. Comparison of three solutions of ropivacaine/fentanyl for postoperative patient-controlled epidural analgesia. Anesthesiology 1999; 90:727–733

47. Takala J, Ruokonen E, Webster NR, et al. Increased mortality associated with growth hormone treatment in critically ill adults. N Engl J Med 1999; 341:7857–7892

48. van den Berghe G, Wouters P, Weekers F, et al. Intensive insulin therapy in the critically ill patients. N Engl J Med 2001; 345:1359–1367

49. van den Berghe G, Wilmer A, Hermans G, et al. Intensive insulin therapy in the medical ICU. N Engl J Med 2006; 354:449–461

50. Brunkhorst FM, Engel C, Bloos F, et al. Intensive insulin therapy and pentastarch resuscitation in severe sepsis. N Engl J Med 2008; 358:125–139

51. The NICE-SUGAR Study Investigators. Intensive versus conventional glucose control in critically ill patients. N Engl J Med 2009; 360:1283–1297

Seizures, Stroke, and Other Neurologic Emergencies

Thomas P. Bleck, MD, FCCP

Objectives:

- Improve the recognition, differential diagnosis, and management of seizures occurring in critically ill patients
- Understand the pharmacology and application of newer anticonvulsant drugs in the ICU
- Recognize and manage status epilepticus
- Understand the special diagnostic and management issues of refractory status epilepticus
- Improve recognition of patients with acute subarachnoid hemorrhage
- Recognize and manage the major CNS complications of subarachnoid hemorrhage
- Recognize the common systemic complications of subarachnoid hemorrhage
- Review the role of the critical care service in the management of stroke
- Briefly review other neurologic emergencies in the ICU setting

Key words: brain abscess; diazepam; encephalitis; Guillain-Barré syndrome; herpes simplex; ketamine; lorazepam; meningitis; myasthenia gravis; neurogenic respiratory failure; nonconvulsive status epilepticus; polymerase chain reaction; propofol; recombinant tissue-plasminogen activator; seizure; status epilepticus; stroke; subarachnoid hemorrhage

Seizures

Seizures complicate about 3% of adult ICU admissions for nonneurologic conditions. The medical and economic impact of these seizures confers importance on them out of proportion to their incidence. A seizure is often the first indication of a CNS complication; thus, their rapid etiologic diagnosis is mandatory. In addition, because epilepsy affects 2% of the population, patients with preexisting seizures occasionally enter the ICU for other problems. Because the initial treatment of these patients is the province of the intensivist, he or she must be familiar with seizure management as it affects the critically ill patient. Patients developing status epilepticus (SE) will often require the care of a critical care specialist in addition to a neurologist.

Seizures have been recognized at least since hippocratic times, their relatively high rate of occurrence in critically ill patients has only recently been recognized. Seizures complicating critical care treatments (*eg*, lidocaine) are also a recent phenomenon. Early attempts at treatment included bromide,[1] morphine,[2] and ice applications. Barbiturates were first employed in 1912, and phenytoin in the 1937.[3] Paraldehyde was popular in the next decades.[4] More recently, emphasis has shifted to the benzodiazepines, which were pioneered in the 1960s.[5]

Epidemiology

Limited data are available on the epidemiology of seizures the ICU. A 10-year retrospective study of all ICU patients with seizures at the Mayo Clinic found 7 patients per 1,000 ICU admissions.[6] Our 2-year prospective study of medical ICU patients identified 35 with seizures per 1,000 admissions.[7] These studies are not exactly comparable, as the patient populations and methods of detection differed. Seizures are probably even more frequent in pediatric ICUs.

Certain ICU patients are at higher risk for seizures, but the degree of that increase has not been quantified. Renal failure or an altered blood-brain barrier increases the seizure likelihood for patients receiving imipenem-cilastatin, but other patients receiving this antibiotic [or γ-aminobutyric acid (GABA) antagonists like penicillin] are also at risk. Transplant recipients, especially receiving cyclosporine, are also at increased risk, as are those who rapidly become hypo-osmolar from any etiology. Nonketotic hyperglycemia patients have an unusual predisposition toward partial seizures and partial SE.

Incidence estimates for generalized convulsive SE (GCSE) in the United States vary from 50,000 cases/yr[8] to 250,000 cases/yr.[9] Some portion of this difference derives from different definitions; the latter estimate represents the only population-based data available, however, and may be more accurate. Mortality estimates similarly vary from 1 to 2% in the former study to 22% in the latter. This disagreement follows from a conceptual discordance: the smaller number describes mortality that the authors directly attributed to SE, while the larger figure estimates the overall mortality rate, even though the cause of death was frequently the underlying disease rather than SE itself. For example, the study by DeLorenzo et al[9] included SE due to anoxia in its SE mortality estimate. In many of the reports surveyed in the earlier review, such patients would not have been counted.

Many risk factors emerged from the Richmond study. SE lasting >1 h carried a mortality of 32%, compared with 2.7% for a duration <1 h. SE caused by anoxia resulted in 70% mortality in adults, but <10% in children. The commonest cause of SE in adults was stroke, followed by withdrawal from antiepileptic drug therapy; cryptogenic SE; and SE related to alcohol withdrawal, anoxia, and metabolic disorders. Systemic infection was the commonest cause of childhood SE, followed by congenital anomalies, anoxia, metabolic problems, anticonvulsant withdrawal, CNS infections, and trauma.

The data in Table 1, based on 20 years of experience at the San Francisco General Hospital,[10–12] are of interest because almost all patients with SE in the city of San Francisco who begin to seize outside of a hospital are transported there. About 10% of epilepsy patients present with SE,[13] and nearly 20% of seizure patients experience an episode of SE within 5 years of their first seizure.[9]

Classification

The most frequently used classification schema is that of the International League Against Epilepsy[14] (Table 2). This allows classification based on clinical criteria without inferring etiology. *Simple partial seizures* start focally in the cerebral cortex, without invading other structures. The patient is aware throughout the episode, and appears otherwise unchanged. Bilateral limbic dysfunction produces a *complex partial seizure*; awareness and ability to interact are diminished (but may not be completely abolished). *Automatisms* (movements that the patient makes without awareness) may occur. *Secondary generalization* results from invasion of the other hemisphere or subcortical structures.

Primary generalized seizures arise from the cerebral cortex and diencephalon at the same time; no focal phenomena are visible, and consciousness is lost at the onset. *Absence seizures* are frequently

Table 1. *Etiologies of SE at the San Francisco General Hospital**

Etiology	1970–1980 (%) (n = 98)		1980–1989 (%) (n = 152)	
	Prior Seizures	No Prior Seizures	Prior Seizures	No Prior Seizures
Ethanol-related	11	4	25	12
Anticonvulsant noncompliance	27	0	41	0
Drug toxicity	0	10	5	10
Refractory epilepsy	—	—	8	0
CNS infection[†]	0	4	2	10
Trauma	1	2	2	6
Tumor	0	4	2	7
Metabolic[†]	3	5	2	4
Stroke[†]	4	11	2	5
Anoxia[†]	0	4	0	6
Other	11	5	3	5

*Data from Lowenstein and Alldredge.[11]
[†]Indicates conditions most likely to result in ICU admission.

Table 2. *International Classification of Epileptic Seizures**

  I. Partial seizures (seizures beginning locally)
   A. Simple partial seizures (SPS)—consciousness not impaired
     1. With motor symptoms
     2. With somatosensory or special sensory symptoms
     3. With autonomic symptoms
     4. With psychic symptoms
   B. Complex partial seizures—with impairment of consciousness
     1. Beginning as SPS and progressing to impairment of consciousness
       a. Without automatisms
       b. With automatisms
     2. With impairment of consciousness at onset
       a. With no other features
       b. With features of SPS
       c. With automatisms
   C. Partial seizures (simple or complex), secondarily generalized
 II. Primary generalized seizures (bilaterally symmetric, without localized onset)
   A. Absence seizures
     1. True absence (*petit mal*)
     2. Atypical absence
   B. Myoclonic seizures
   C. Clonic seizures
   D. Tonic seizures
   E. Tonic-clonic seizures (grand mal; generalized tonic-clonic)
   F. Atonic seizures
III. Unclassified seizures

*Adapted from Bleck.[16]

confined to childhood, consisting of the abrupt onset of a blank stare, usually lasting 5 to 15 s, from which the patient abruptly returns to normal. Atypical absence occurs in children with the Lennox-Gastaut syndrome. *Myoclonic seizures* start with brief synchronous jerking without initially altered consciousness, followed by a generalized convulsion. They frequently occur in the genetic epilepsies; in the ICU, they commonly follow anoxia or metabolic disturbances.[15] *Tonic-clonic seizures* start with tonic extension and evolve to bilaterally synchronous clonus, and conclude with a postictal phase. Clinical judgment is required to apply this system in the ICU. In patients whose consciousness has already been altered by drugs, hypotension, sepsis, or intracranial pathology, the nature of their partial seizures may be difficult to classify.

SE is classified by a similar system, altered to match observable clinical phenomena (Table 3).[16] *Generalized convulsive SE* (GCSE) is the commonest type encountered in the ICU, and poses the greatest risk to the patient. It may either be primarily generalized, as in the drug-intoxicated patient, or secondarily generalized, as in the brain abscess patient in whom GCSE develops. *Nonconvulsive SE* (NCSE) in the ICU frequently follows partially treated GCSE. Some use the term for all SE involving altered consciousness without convulsive movements; this blurs the distinctions among absence SE, partially treated GCSE, and *complex partial SE* (CPSE), which have different etiologies and treatments. *Epilepsia partialis continua* (a special form of partial SE in which repetitive movements affect a small area of the body) sometimes lasts for months or years.

Pathogenesis and Pathophysiology

The reported "causes" of SE can be divided into predispositions and precipitants. *Predispositions* are static conditions increasing the likelihood of SE in the presence of a precipitant. *Precipitants* are events that can produce SE in most, if not all, people, but tend to affect those with predispositions at lesser degrees of severity (*eg*, barbiturate withdrawal). The causes and effects of SE at the cellular, brain, and systemic levels are interrelated, but their individual analysis is useful for understanding them and their therapeutic implications. Longer SE durations produce more profound alterations with an increasing likelihood of permanence, and of becoming refractory to treatment. The processes involved in a single seizure and the transition to SE have recently been reviewed.[17]

The ionic events of a seizure follow the opening of ion channels coupled to excitatory amino acid (EAA) receptors. From the standpoint of the intensivist, three channels are particularly important because their activation may raise intracellular free calcium to toxic concentrations: alpha-amino-3-hydroxy-5-methyl-4-isoxazolepropionate (AMPA) channels, N-methyl-D-aspartate (NMDA) channels, and metabotropic channels. These EAA systems are crucial for learning and memory. Many drugs affect these systems but are too toxic for chronic use. The deleterious consequences of SE, and the brief period for which such agents would be needed, suggest that they may have a role in SE. Counterregulatory ionic events are triggered by the epileptiform discharge as well, such as the activation of inhibitory interneurons, which suppress excited neurons via GABA-A synapses.

The cellular effects of excessive EAA channel activity include (1) generating toxic concentrations of intracellular free calcium; (2) activating autolytic enzyme systems; (3) producing oxygen

Table 3. *Clinical Classification of Status Epilepticus**

I. Generalized seizures
  A. Generalized convulsive SE (GCSE)
    1. Primary generalized SE
      a. Tonic-clonic SE
      b. Myoclonic SE
      c. Clonic-tonic-clonic SE
    2. Secondarily generalized SE
      a. Partial seizure with secondary
        generalization
      b. Tonic SE
  B. Nonconvulsive SE (NCSE)
    1. Absence SE (*petit mal* status)
    2. Atypical absence SE
      (*eg*, in the Lennox-Gastaut syndrome)
    3. Atonic SE
    4. NCSE as a sequel of partially treated GCSE
II. Partial SE
  A. Simple partial SE
    1. Typical
    2. Epilepsia partialis continua
  B. Complex partial SE (CPSE)
III. Neonatal SE

*Adapted from Lothman.[17]

free radicals; (4) generating nitric oxide, which both enhances subsequent excitation and serves as a toxin; (5) phosphorylating enzyme and receptor systems, making seizures likely; and (6) increasing intracellular osmolality, producing neuronal swelling. If adenosine triphosphate production fails, membrane ion exchange ceases, and the neuron swells further. These events produce the neuronal damage associated with SE.

Many other biophysical and biochemical alterations occur during and after SE. The intense neuronal activity activates immediate-early genes and produces heat shock proteins, providing indications of the deleterious effects of SE and insight into the mechanisms of neuronal protection.[18] Wasterlain's group has summarized mechanisms by which SE damages the nervous system.[19] Absence SE is an exception among these conditions; it consists of rhythmically increased inhibition and does not produce clinical or pathologic abnormalities.

The mechanisms that terminate seizure activity are poorly understood. The leading candidates are inhibitory mechanisms, primarily GABAergic neuronal systems. Clinical observation supports the contention that human SE frequently follows withdrawal from GABA agonists (eg, benzodiazepines).

The electrical phenomena of SE at the whole brain level, as seen in the scalp EEG, reflect the seizure type that initiates SE, eg, absence SE begins with a 3-Hz wave-and-spike pattern. During SE, there is slowing of this rhythm, but the wave-and-spike characteristic remains. GCSE goes through a sequence of electrographic changes (Table 4).[20] The initial discharge becomes less well formed, implying that neuronal firing is losing synchrony. The sustained depolarizations that characterize SE alter the extracellular milieu, most importantly by raising extracellular potassium. The excess potassium ejected during SE exceeds the buffering ability of astrocytes. Raising extracellular potassium potentiates more seizures.

The increased cellular activity of SE elevates demand for oxygen and glucose, and blood flow initially increases. After about 20 min, however, energy supplies become exhausted. This causes local catabolism to support ion pumps (attempting to restore the internal milieu). This is a major cause of epileptic brain damage.

The brain contains systems to terminate seizure activity; GABAergic interneurons and inhibitory thalamic neurons are both important.

SE produces neuropathology even in patients who are paralyzed, ventilated, and maintained at normal temperature and blood pressure. The hippocampus, a crucial area for memory, contains the most susceptible neurons, but other regions are also vulnerable. In addition to damaging the CNS, GCSE produces life-threatening, systemic effects.[21] Systemic and pulmonary arterial pressures rise dramatically at seizure onset. Epinephrine and cortisol prompt further elevations and also produce hyperglycemia. Muscular work raises blood lactate. Breathing suffers from both airway obstruction and abnormal diaphragmatic contractions. CO_2 excretion falls while its production increases markedly. Muscular work accelerates heat production; skin blood flow falls concomitantly, sometimes raising core temperature dangerously.

After about 20 min, motor activity begins to diminish, and ventilation usually improves. Body temperature may rise further, however.

Table 4. *Electrographic-Clinical Correlations in GCSE**

Stage	Typical Clinical Manifestations	Electroencephalographic Features
1	Tonic-clonic convulsions; hypertension and hyperglycemia common	Discrete seizures with interictal slowing
2	Low- or medium-amplitude clonic activity, with rare convulsions	Waxing and waning of ictal discharges
3	Slight, but frequent, clonic activity, often confined to the eyes, face, or hands	Continuous ictal discharges
4	Rare episodes of slight clonic activity; hypotension and hypoglycemia become manifest	Continuous ictal discharges punctuated by flat periods
5	Coma without other manifestations of seizure activity	Periodic epileptiform discharges on a flat background

*Data from Treiman.[20]

Seizures, Stroke, and Other Neurologic Emergencies (Bleck)

Hyperglycemia diminishes; after 1 h, gluconeogenesis can fail, producing hypoglycemia. GCSE patients often aspirate oral or gastric contents, producing pneumonia. Rhabdomyolysis is common, and may lead to renal failure. Compression fractures, joint dislocations, and tendon avulsions are other sequelae.

Clinical Manifestations

Three problems occur in seizure recognition: (1) complex partial seizures in the setting of impaired awareness; (2) seizures in patients receiving pharmacologic paralysis; and (3) misinterpretation of other abnormal movements as seizures. ICU patients often have depressed consciousness in the absence of seizures, as a result of their disease, its complications (such as septic encephalopathy[22]), or drugs. A further decline in alertness may reflect a seizure; an EEG is required to diagnose one.

Patients receiving neuromuscular junction (NMJ) blocking agents do not manifest the usual signs of seizures. Because most such patients receive sedation with GABA agonists, the likelihood of seizures is small. Autonomic signs of seizures (hypertension, tachycardia, pupillary dilation) may also be the effects of pain or the response to inadequate sedation. Hence, in patients manifesting these findings who have a potential for seizures (eg, intracranial pathology), an EEG should be performed. The actual incidence of this problem is unknown.

Abnormal movements can occur in patients with metabolic disturbances or anoxia. Some can be distinguished from seizures by observation, but if doubt about their nature persists, an EEG should be performed. Psychiatric disturbances in the ICU occasionally resemble complex partial seizures. Prolonged EEG monitoring may be required if the problem is intermittent.

Manifestations of SE: The manifestations of SE depend on the type and, for partial SE, the cortical area of abnormality. Table 3 depicts the types of SE encountered. This focuses on those seen most in the ICU.

Primary GCSE begins as tonic extension of the trunk and extremities without preceding focal activity. No aura is reported and consciousness is immediately lost. After several seconds of tonic extension, the extremities start to vibrate, quickly giving way to clonic (rhythmic) extension of the extremities. This phase wanes in intensity over a few minutes. The patient may then repeat the cycle of tonus followed by clonic movements, or continue to have intermittent bursts of clonic activity without recovery. Less common forms of GCSE are *myoclonic SE* (bursts of myoclonic jerks increasing in intensity, leading to a convulsion) and *clonic-tonic-clonic SE* (clonic activity precedes the first tonic contraction). Myoclonic SE is usually seen in patients with anoxic encephalopathy or metabolic disturbances.

Secondarily generalized SE begins with a partial seizure and progresses to a convulsion. The initial focal clinical activity may be overlooked. This seizure type implies a structural lesion, so care must be taken to elicit evidence of lateralized movements.

Of the several forms of generalized *NCSE*, the one of greatest importance to intensivists is NCSE as a sequel of inadequately treated GCSE. When a patient with GCSE is treated with anticonvulsants (often in inadequate doses), visible convulsive activity may stop while the electrochemical seizure continues. Patients begin to awaken within 15 to 20 min after the successful termination of SE; many regain consciousness much faster. Patients who do not start to awaken after 20 min should be assumed to have entered NCSE. Careful observation may disclose slight clonic activity. NCSE is an extremely dangerous problem because the destructive effects of SE continue even without obvious motor activity. NCSE demands emergent treatment *under EEG monitoring* to prevent further cerebral damage, because there are no clinical criteria to indicate when therapy is effective.

Partial SE in ICU patients often follows a stroke or occurs with rapidly expanding brain masses. Clonic motor activity is most easily recognized, but the seizure takes on the characteristics of adjacent functional tissue. Therefore, somatosensory or special sensory manifestations occur, and the ICU patient may be unable to report such symptoms. Aphasic SE occurs when a seizure begins in a language area, and may resemble a stroke. *Epilepsia partialis continua* involves repetitive movements confined to a small region of the body. It may be seen with nonketotic hyperglycemia or with focal brain disease; anticonvulsant treatment is seldom useful. CPSE presents with diminished awareness. The diagnosis often comes as a surprise when an EEG is obtained.

Diagnostic Approach

When an ICU patient seizes, one has a natural tendency to try to stop the event. This leads to both diagnostic obscuration and iatrogenic complication. Beyond protecting the patient from harm, very little can be done rapidly enough to influence the course of the seizure. Padded tongue blades or similar items should not be placed in the mouth; they are more likely to obstruct the airway than to preserve it. Most patients stop seizing before any medication can reach the brain in an effective concentration.

Observation is the most important activity during a single seizure. This is the time to collect evidence of a partial onset, in order to implicate structural brain disease. The postictal examination is similarly valuable; language, motor, sensory, or reflex abnormalities after an apparently generalized seizure are evidence In the ICU patient, several potential seizure etiologies must be investigated. Drugs are a major cause of ICU seizures, especially in the setting of diminished renal or hepatic function, or when the blood-brain barrier is breached. Drug withdrawal is also a frequent offender. While ethanol withdrawal is common, discontinuing any hypnosedative agent may prompt convulsions 1 to 3 days later. A recent report suggests that narcotic withdrawal may produce seizures in the critically ill.[9]

The physical examination should emphasize the areas listed for the postictal examination. Evidence of cardiovascular disease or systemic infection should be sought, and the skin and fundi closely examined.

Illicit drug screening should be performed on patients with unexplained seizures. Cocaine is becoming a major cause of seizures.[23] Electrolytes and serum osmolality should also be measured. However, hypocalcemia rarely causes seizures beyond the neonatal period; its discovery must not end the diagnostic work-up. Hypomagnesemia has an equally unwarranted reputation as the cause of seizures in malnourished alcoholic patients.

The need for imaging studies in these patients has been an area of uncertainty. A prospective study of neurologic complications in medical ICU patients determined that 38 of 61 patients (62%) had a vascular, infectious, or neoplastic explanation for their fits. Hence, CT or MRI should be performed on most ICU patients with new seizures. Hypoglycemia and nonketotic hyperglycemia can produce seizures, and such patients might be treated for metabolic disturbances and observed if they lack other evidence of focal disease. With current technology, there are almost no patients who cannot undergo CT scanning. While MRI is preferable in most situations, the magnetic field precludes infusion pumps and other metallic devices. Whether to administer contrast for a CT depends on the clinical setting and on the appearance of the plain scan.

The EEG is a vital diagnostic tool for the seizure patient. Partial seizures usually have EEG abnormalities that begin in the area of cortex producing the seizures. Primary generalized seizures appear to start over the entire cortex simultaneously. Postictal slowing or depressed amplitude provide clues to the focal etiology of the seizures, and epileptiform activity helps to classify the type of seizure and guide treatment. In patients who do not begin to awaken soon after seizures have apparently been controlled, an emergent EEG is necessary to exclude NCSE.

Considering the etiologies of seizures in the ICU setting, patients who need cerebrospinal fluid (CSF) analysis usually require a CT scan first. When CNS infection is suspected, empiric antibiotic treatment should be started while these studies are being performed.

In contrast to the patient with a single seizure or a few seizures, the SE patient requires concomitant diagnostic and therapeutic efforts. Although 20 min of continuous or recurrent seizure activity usually define SE, one does not stand by waiting for this period to start treatment. Because most seizures stop within 2 to 3 min, it is reasonable to treat after 5 min of continuous seizure activity, or after the second or third seizure occurring without recovery between the spells.

GCSE can rarely be confused with decerebrate posturing, but observation usually makes the distinction straightforward. Tetanus patients are awake during their spasms, and flex their arms rather than extending them as seizure patients do.[18]

Seizures, Stroke, and Other Neurologic Emergencies (Bleck)

Treatment for SE should not be delayed to obtain an EEG. A variety of findings may be present on the EEG, depending on the type of SE and its duration (Table 4). CPSE patients often lack such organized discharges of GCSE, but instead have waxing and waning rhythmic activity in one or several head regions. A diagnostic trial of an IV benzodiazepine is often necessary to diagnose CPSE. Patients developing refractory SE or having seizures during NMJ blockade require continuous EEG monitoring.

Management Approach

Deciding to administer anticonvulsants to an ICU patient who experiences one seizure or a few seizures requires a provisional etiology, estimation of the recurrence likelihood, and recognition of the utility and limitations of anticonvulsants. For example, seizures during ethanol withdrawal do not indicate a need for chronic treatment, and giving phenytoin will not prevent more withdrawal convulsions. The patient may need prophylaxis against delirium tremens, but the few seizures themselves seldom require treatment. Patients who experience convulsions during barbiturate or benzodiazepine withdrawal, in contrast, should usually receive short-term treatment with lorazepam to prevent SE. Seizures related to drugs or metabolic disorders should also be treated briefly but not chronically.

The ICU patient with CNS disease who has even one seizure should usually start chronic anticonvulsant therapy, with review of this decision before discharge. Initiating this treatment after the first unprovoked seizure helps prevent subsequent epilepsy.[24] Starting after the first seizure in a critically ill patient at risk for seizure recurrence may be even more important, especially in conditions that would be seriously complicated by a convulsion. In the ICU setting, phenytoin is frequently selected for ease of administration and lack of sedation. The hypotension and arrhythmias that may complicate rapid administration can usually be prevented by slowing the infusion to <25 mg/min. Because of the rare occurrence of third-degree AV block, an external pacemaker should be available when patients with conduction abnormalities receive IV phenytoin. Fosphenytoin is safer to administer from an extravasation standpoint, but still carries risks of hypotension and arrhythmias. The phenytoin concentration should be kept in the "therapeutic" range of 10 to 20 µg/mL unless further seizures occur; the level may then be increased until signs of toxicity occur. Failure to prevent seizures at a concentration of 25 µg/mL is usually an indication to add phenobarbital.

Phenytoin is usually 90% protein-bound. Patients with renal dysfunction have lower total phenytoin levels at a given dose because the drug is displaced from binding sites, but the unbound level is not affected. Thus, renal failure patients, and perhaps others who are receiving highly protein-bound drugs (which compete for binding), may benefit from free-phenytoin level determination. Only the free fraction is metabolized, so the dose is not altered with changing renal function. The clearance half-time with normal liver function varies from about 12 to 20 h (IV form) to >24 h (extended-release capsules), so a new steady-state serum concentration occurs in 3 to 6 days. Phenytoin need not be given more frequently than every 12 h. Hepatic dysfunction mandates decreasing the maintenance dose.

Hypersensitivity is the major adverse effect of concern to the intensivist. This may manifest itself solely as fever, but commonly includes rash and eosinophilia. Adverse reactions to phenytoin and other anticonvulsants have been reviewed.[25]

Phenobarbital remains a useful anticonvulsant for those intolerant to phenytoin, or who have persistent seizures after adequate phenytoin. The target for phenobarbital in the ICU should be 20 to 40 µg/mL. Hepatic and renal dysfunction alter phenobarbital metabolism. Because its usual clearance half-time is about 96 h, give maintenance doses of this agent once a day. A steady-state level takes about 3 weeks to be established. Sedation is the major adverse effect; allergy occurs rarely.

Carbamazepine is seldom started in the ICU because its insolubility precludes parenteral formulation. Oral loading in conscious patients may produce coma lasting several days. This drug causes hyponatremia in patients receiving it chronically.

Management Issues in Acute Repetitive (Serial) Seizures

Despite the near-certainty that acute repetitive seizures not meeting a definition of SE must occur more frequently than SE itself, and that many cases of SE emerge from such a state, there has been little study of the issue of treatment. Although the use of IV benzodiazepines has become common in many inpatient settings, the choice of drug and the appropriate dose are uncertain. Many clinicians use IV diazepam, perhaps based more on tradition than pharmacokinetics. The anticonvulsant effect of a single dose of diazepam is very brief (about 20 min), while that of lorazepam is much longer (4 h or longer). Because the risk of serious adverse effects (eg, respiratory depression) is potentially greater for diazepam, lorazepam may represent a better choice.[26] If a shorter-acting agent is desired for diagnostic purposes when the diagnosis of a seizure is uncertain, midazolam may be a better choice. The role of other agents, such as intranasal or buccal midazolam or IV valproate, remain to be determined.[27]

Outside of the hospital setting, there is reasonably good evidence that rectal diazepam is effective and safe in the management of serial seizures, especially in children, at a dose of 0.2 to 0.5 mg/kg, with the dose repeated as necessary according to an age-based protocol.[28]

Management Issues in SE

Once the decision is made to treat the patient for SE, considerations for therapy should proceed on four fronts simultaneously (Table 5): (1) termination of SE; (2) prevention of seizure recurrence once SE is terminated; (3) management of potential precipitating causes for SE; and (4) management of the complications of SE and of underlying conditions.[29]

There is an implicit assumption here that the forms of SE that can produce neuronal damage should be terminated as rapidly as is safely possible. While there is no direct proof of this contention in humans, it appears to be the most reasonable approach.

The intensity of treatment for SE should reflect the risk that the patient experiences from the SE and its etiology. For example, GCSE puts the patient at risk for a panoply of neurologic, cardiac, respiratory, renal, hepatic, and orthopedic disorders, and should be terminated as rapidly one can safely accomplish the task, even if

such termination requires the full support of a critical care unit. Typical absence SE, in contrast, probably poses a risk to the patient only if it occurs during a potentially dangerous activity (eg, driving an automobile), and initial attempts at its termination probably should not include agents likely to profoundly depress respiration and blood pressure. Treatment of CPSE, in which the risk of neurologic sequelae is considerable, should probably be similar to that recommended for GCSE. Simple partial SE appears to pose less risk to the patient than CPSE, and furthermore, attempts at therapy along the lines recommended for GCSE seldom result in prolonged seizure control. Therefore, therapy for simple partial SE is often pursued with somewhat less vigor that GCSE or CPSE.

The following recommendations were developed for patients in GCSE. There is very limited evidence regarding the optimal therapy for other types of SE. Because of the life-threatening nature of GCSE, and of the risks associated with its treatment, physicians caring for these patients must be constantly vigilant for respiratory and cardiovascular compromise, which may develop abruptly. Thus, neurologists and others caring for these patients should be adept at basic aspects of airway and blood pressure management. During the termination of SE, the patient should be constantly attended by personnel who can effectively perform bag-valve-mask ventilation, and plans for the rapid endotracheal intubation of such patients should be devised before intubation becomes necessary.

Termination of SE: The linchpin of treatment for SE is the rapid, safe termination of ictal activity. Numerous treatment modalities are available for this goal, and until recently there were few data to guide a decision among the various possible choices. The publication of the Veterans' Affairs (VA) cooperative trial allows a much greater degree of rational choice, and raises many new questions for study.[30]

Within the VA trial, patients were divided into the categories of "overt" and "subtle" SE. All patients were believed to have GCSE, which could be either primarily or secondarily generalized; the distinction between overt and subtle depended on the intensity of the clinically viewed convulsive activity. The subtle-SE patients were much

Seizures, Stroke, and Other Neurologic Emergencies (Bleck)

Table 5. *Suggested Management Protocol for Status Epilepticus*

I. Establish an airway. Whether to perform endotracheal intubation emergently depends primarily on the safety with which the airway can be maintained during the control of SE. Should NMJ blockade be needed, one must assume that the patient is still in SE despite the appearance of relaxation, unless EEG monitoring is available to demonstrate the actual state of brain function. Use a nondepolarizing agent (eg, vecuronium).

II. Determine the blood pressure. If the patient is hypotensive, begin volume replacement and/or vasoactive agents as clinically indicated. GCSE patients who present with hypotension will usually require admission to a critical care unit. (Hypertension should not be treated until SE is controlled, as terminating SE will usually substantially correct it, and many of the agents used to terminate SE can produce hypotension).

III. Rapidly determine the blood glucose. Unless the patient is known to be normo- or hyperglycemic, administer dextrose (1 mg/kg) and thiamine (1 mg/kg).

IV. Terminate SE. We recommend the following sequence:

    A. Lorazepam, 0.1 mg/kg at 0.04 mg/kg/min. This drug should be diluted in an equal volume of the solution being used for IV infusion, as it is quite viscous. Most adult patients who will respond will do so by a total dose of 8 mg. The latency of effect is debated, but lack of response after 5 min should be considered a failure.

    B. If SE persists after lorazepam, begin phenytoin, 20 mg/kg at 0.3 mg/kg/min. If the patient tolerates this infusion rate, it may be increased to a maximum of 50 mg/min. Alternatively, administer fosphenytoin at the same dose, but at a rate of up to 150 mg/min. Hypotension and arrhythmias are the major concern. Many investigators believe that an additional 5-mg/kg dose of phenytoin or fosphenytoin should be administered before advancing to the next line of therapy.

    C. If SE persists, administer either midazolam or propofol. Midazolam can be given with a loading dose of 0.2 mg/kg, followed by an infusion of 0.1 to 2.0 mg/kg/h to achieve seizure control (as determined by EEG monitoring). Propofol can be given with a loading dose of 1 to 3 mg/kg, followed by an infusion of 1 to 15 mg/kg/h. We routinely intubate patients at this stage if this has not already been accomplished. Patients reaching this stage should be treated in a critical care unit.

    D. Should the patient not be controlled with propofol or midazolam, administer pentobarbital 12 mg/kg at 0.2 to 0.4 mg/kg/min as tolerated, followed by an infusion of 0.25 to 2.0 mg/kg/h as determined by EEG monitoring (with a goal of seizure suppression). Most patients will require systemic and pulmonary arterial catheterization, with fluid and vasoactive therapy as indicated to maintain blood pressure.

    E. Ketamine (1 mg/kg, followed by 10 to 50 μg/kg/min) is a potent NMDA antagonist[48] with intrinsic sympathomimetic properties that may be useful in patients who have become refractory to GABA-A agonists.

V. Prevent recurrence of SE. The choice of drugs depends greatly on the etiology of SE and the patient's medical and social situation. In general, patients not previously receiving anticonvulsants whose SE is easily controlled often respond well to chronic treatment with phenytoin or carbamazepine. In contrast, others (eg, patients with acute encephalitis) will require two or three anticonvulsants at "toxic" levels (eg, phenobarbital at greater than 100 μg/mL) to be weaned from midazolam or pentobarbital, and may still have occasional seizures.

VI. Treat complications.

    A. Rhabdomyolysis should be treated with a vigorous saline diuresis to prevent acute renal failure; urinary alkalinization may be a useful adjunct.

    B. Hyperthermia usually remits rapidly after termination of SE. External cooling usually suffices if the core temperature remains elevated. In rare instances, cool peritoneal lavage or extracorporeal blood cooling may be required. High-dose pentobarbital generally produces poikilothermia.

    C. The treatment of cerebral edema secondary to SE has not been well studied. When substantial edema is present, one should suspect that SE and cerebral edema are both manifestations of the same underlying condition. Hyperventilation and mannitol may be valuable if edema is life-threatening. Edema due to SE is vasogenic, so steroids may be useful as well.

---

more likely to have a serious underlying medical condition, and in general responded poorly to therapy. This discussion will concentrate on the overt-SE patients, because their results underlie the treatment paradigm developed herein.

In the study, 384 patients with overt SE were randomly divided into four treatment arms, which were chosen based on a survey of North American neurologists prior to the study's inception. These arms were (1) lorazepam, 0.1 mg/kg; (2) diazepam, 0.15 mg/kg, followed by phenytoin, 18 mg/kg; (3) phenytoin alone, 18 mg/kg; and (4) phenobarbital, 15 mg/kg. Successful treatment required both clinical and EEG termination of seizures within 20 min of the start of therapy, with noseizure recurrence within 60 min of the start of therapy. Patients in whom the first treatment failed received a second, and if necessary, a third study drug. These latter choices were not randomized, as this would have resulted in some patients

Table 6. *Treatment Results for First Agents in the VA Cooperative Study**

Agent	Overt SE Success Rate (%)	Subtle SE Success Rate (%)
Lorazepam	64.9	17.9
Phenobarbital	58.2	24.2
Diazepam/phenytoin	55.8	8.3
Phenytoin alone	43.6	7.7

*Data from Treiman and colleagues.[30]

receiving two loading doses of phenytoin, but the treating physician remained blinded to the treatments being given.

The overall success rates for patients whose diagnosis of overt SE was confirmed by subsequent review of clinical and EEG data are presented in Table 6. The results for patients with subtle SE are included for reference. Treatment with lorazepam demonstrated a statistically significant advantage over phenytoin (p = 0.002); there were no significant differences among the other agents. This differs from the intention-to-treat analysis, which showed similar trends but did not find a statistically significant difference among the treatment arms.

The results of this study may be compared with those of Leppik and colleagues,[31] who found lorazepam to be successful in about 85% of cases. However, this study used only clinical cessation of seizures as the criterion of success; preliminary data from the VA trial indicates that 20% of patients in whom SE appears to have been terminated actually remain in electrographic SE.

Preliminary analysis of the results of subsequent treatments in patients who did not respond to the first-line agents indicates that the aggregate response rate to the second-line drug regimen was 7.0%, and to the third-line treatment, 2.3% (Treiman DM; personal communication; 1998). These results call into question the common practice of using three conventional agents (eg, lorazepam, phenytoin, and phenobarbital) in the management of SE before using a more definitive approach.

Based on these results and the experience of many workers in the field, we recommend that treatment for GCSE begin with a single dose of lorazepam, 0.1 mg/kg. The limited data available

do not suggest that administration of further conventional doses of lorazepam will be useful.[31] The drug should be administered after dilution with an equal volume of the IV solution through which it will be administered. If this fails to control SE within 5 to 7 min, a second agent should be chosen. The results of the VA trial suggest that a second conventional agent is unlikely to be successful. At this time, however, we still recommend the use of phenytoin (or fosphenytoin), 20 mg/kg, as the second drug. This approach carries the advantage that if it is effective, the patient may not require endotracheal intubation and extended critical care. However, it may delay the eventual termination of SE by more definitive treatment.

The introduction of the phenytoin prodrug fosphenytoin as a safer way of rapidly achieving an effective serum phenytoin concentration may prompt some reconsideration of the way in which this drug is used.[32] At its maximal rate of administration (150 mg phenytoin equivalent/min), and its 7-min half-time of conversion to phenytoin, a free-phenytoin level of about 2 μg/mL can be achieved with fosphenytoin in about 15 min, as opposed to about 25 min for phenytoin itself. Whether this greater speed of administration will produce a higher rate of SE control remains to be demonstrated. It is clear that fosphenytoin administration is safer, in that the risk of hypotension may be somewhat less, and the adverse effects of extravasation are nil with the newer drug. The much greater cost of fosphenytoin has discouraged many from using it, although pharmacoeconomic simulations suggest that its use may be cost-effective.[33]

Valproate is available in an IV form; its role in the termination of SE remains to be defined. Experimental data suggest that a serum valproate concentration of 250 μg/mL or greater may be necessary to control secondarily generalized SE.[34] We have limited experience using doses of 60 to 70 mg/kg to obtain such a concentration in patients, and have found the drug effective on occasion in situations where in was necessary to avoid the risks of hypotension and respiratory depression associated with other treatment modalities. However, more information is required before the role of this agent in SE becomes clear.

Patients who continue in SE after lorazepam and phenytoin have traditionally been treated

Seizures, Stroke, and Other Neurologic Emergencies (Bleck)

with conventional doses of phenobarbital, but the results of the VA study suggest that this is very unlikely to result in the rapid termination of SE. At this point, we consider SE to be refractory, and go on to one of the more definitive forms of treatment.[35] These treatment modalities are very likely to result in termination of SE, but are also carry higher risks of respiratory depression, hypotension, and secondary complications such as infection. Patients who are to undergo one of these definitive therapies should be in a critical care unit and be endotracheally intubated if this has not yet been accomplished.

Discussion of the entire range of proposed definitive treatments for SE is beyond the scope of this paper. Three categories will be considered: high-dose barbiturates, high-dose benzodiazepines, and propofol.

It is our contention that patients reaching this stage in the treatment of SE should undergo continuous EEG monitoring. The technologic aspects of continuous EEG monitoring have been reviewed elsewhere.[36] What the goal regarding the activity on the EEG should be remains a matter of debate. There is no prospectively collected evidence that a burst-suppression EEG pattern is required for, or is efficacious for, the termination of SE. Many patients can achieve complete seizure control with a background of continuous slow activity, and do not thereby incur the greater risks associated with the higher doses of medication required to achieve a burst-suppression pattern. Conversely, a few patients will continue to have frequent seizures that emerge out of a burst-suppression background, and presumably need even higher doses of medication, which may result in very long periods of suppression or even a "flat" EEG. Without continuous EEG monitoring, one must rely on occasional samples of the EEG, which are thus associated with risks of under- and overtreatment.

Most of the published experience with high-dose barbiturates involves pentobarbital, although some of the earlier investigators used thiopental, and a few reports discuss phenobarbital. There are few data regarding efficacy rates and adverse effects of these drugs. Thiopental is the most rapidly acting of these drugs, but may produce more hypotension. Pentobarbital has emerged as one of the standard choices for refractory SE. A loading dose of 5 to 12 mg/kg is usually given IV, followed by an infusion of the drug at a dose chosen to achieve the desired effect on the EEG; this is usually in the range of 1 to 10 mg/kg/h. We usually increase the infusion rate, along with an additional 3- to 5-mg/kg loading dose, when a seizure occurs; almost all seizures at this stage of treatment are electrographic, probably as a consequence of the medications suppressing clinical seizure activity (twitchless electrical activity), and perhaps also as a consequence of the prolonged duration of SE by the time definitive treatment has commenced. After 12 h free of seizures, the pentobarbital infusion rate is decreased by 50%. If seizures recur, the patient again receives the smaller loading dose, and the infusion rate is raised to obtain another 12-h seizure-free period. Other medications (eg, phenytoin) are continued. Many patients reaching this point will require substantial maintenance anticonvulsant treatment in order to be weaned from the pentobarbital; we commonly maintain the serum phenytoin concentration in excess of 20 µg/mL, and load with phenobarbital to achieve a concentration in excess of 40 µg/mL (often, 100 µg/mL or an even higher concentration is required to successfully wean severely refractory patients, such as those with encephalitis, from their pentobarbital infusions). High doses of barbiturates are potently immunosuppressive, indicating extra care to avoid nosocomial infection and aggressive treatment if infection is suspected.

High-dose benzodiazepine strategies for SE usually employ either midazolam or lorazepam. Midazolam has the advantages of rapid onset of activity and greater water solubility, avoiding the problem of metabolic acidosis from the propylene glycol vehicle of the other benzodiazepines and the barbiturates. Its major disadvantage is tachyphylaxis; over 24 to 48 h, the dose of the drug must often be increased several-fold in order to maintain seizure control. A loading dose of 0.2 mg/kg is followed by an infusion of 0.1 to 2.0 mg/kg/h, titrated to produce seizure suppression by continuous EEG monitoring.[37] High-dose lorazepam, used in doses of up to 9 mg/h, was the subject of a report by Labar and colleagues.[38]

Propofol is a pharmacologically unique GABA-A agonist that may also have other mechanisms of anticonvulsant action. Soon after its introduction as a general anesthetic agent, concerns about a potential proconvulsant effect arose;

this apparently represented myoclonus rather than seizure activity. At the doses used to control SE, it has a very potent anticonvulsant action. A loading dose of 3 to 5 mg/kg is frequently administered, followed by an infusion of 1 to 15 mg/kg/h,[39] titrated to EEG seizure suppression. After 12 h of seizure suppression, we taper the dose as outlined above for pentobarbital. There is evidence that rapid discontinuation of propofol can induce withdrawal seizures.

In our experience, propofol is more likely than midazolam to provide rapid control of refractory SE, exhibits less tachyphylaxis than midazolam, and produces less hypotension than pentobarbital for an equivalent degree of seizure control.[40] However, a recent retrospective analysis of our patients suggests that those with APACHE (acute physiology and chronic health evaluation) II scores >20 may have better survival when treatment is started with midazolam.[41] There are few data addressing the immunosuppressive effects of the benzodiazepines or propofol[42]; clinically, these drugs appear associated with fewer nosocomial infections than high-dose pentobarbital. Although it is difficult to determine functionally equivalent doses of these agents because of differing rates of tachyphylaxis, in our institution the patient charge for midazolam appears to be about 10 times that for pentobarbital, and propofol about 2.5 times that for pentobarbital.

Many other agents have been employed for the control of refractory SE.[43] The information above represents a distillation of our experience; the available published data are inadequate to support more definite treatment recommendations.

Prevention of Seizure Recurrence Once SE Is Terminated: Once SE is controlled, attention turns to preventing its recurrence. The best regimen for an individual patient will depend on the cause of the patient's seizures and any previous history of anticonvulsant therapy. For example, a patient developing SE in the course of ethanol withdrawal may not need anticonvulsant therapy once the withdrawal phenomena have run their course. SE following changes in a previously effective anticonvulsant regimen will often mandate a return to the former successful mode of treatment. In contrast, patients with a new, ongoing epileptogenic stimulus (*eg*, encephalitis) may require

extraordinarily high serum concentrations of anticonvulsant drugs to control their seizures as therapy for refractory SE is decreased.

Management of the Complications of SE and of Underlying Conditions: The major systemic complications of GCSE include rhabdomyolysis and hyperthermia. Patients presenting with GCSE should be screened at presentation for myoglobinuria (most effectively by a dipstick evaluation of the urine for occult blood; the reagent will react with myoglobin as well as hemoglobin, and if the reaction is present, a microscopic examination will determine whether red blood cells are present) and elevation of serum creatine kinase (CK). If myoglobinuria is present, or if the CK concentration is >10 times the upper limit of normal, one should consider instituting a saline diuresis as well as urinary alkalinization.

If the patient's core temperature exceeds 40°C, the patient should be cooled. The techniques available for managing hyperthermic patients have been reviewed elsewhere.[44]

Cerebral edema may complicate SE. Vasogenic edema may develop as a consequence of the seizures themselves, and the underlying cause of SE may also produce either vasogenic or cytotoxic edema. The management of secondary cerebral edema with increased intracranial pressure (ICP) depends on the etiology; edema due solely to seizures rarely causes problems with ICP.

Prognosis

Wijdicks and Sharbrough[6] report that 34% of patients experiencing a seizure died during that hospitalization. Our prospective study of neurologic complications in medical ICU patients found that having even one seizure if in the unit for a nonneurologic reason doubled in-hospital mortality.[7] This effect on prognosis primarily reflected the etiology of the seizure.

Three major factors determine outcome in SE: the type of SE, its etiology, and its duration. GCSE has the worst prognosis for neurologic recovery; in contrast, myoclonic SE that follows an anoxic episode carries a very poor prognosis for survival. CPSE can produce limbic system damage, usually manifested as a memory disturbance. Most studies of outcome concentrate on GCSE mortality. Hauser,[8] summarizing data available in 1990, suggested that mortality rates vary from 1 to 53%. Those studies attempting to distinguish mortality due to SE from that of the underlying disease have attributed mortality rates of 1 to 7% to SE and 2 to 25% to its cause. Population-based studies in Richmond, VA showed the mortality of SE lasting >1 h was increased 10-fold over SE lasting <1 h. Etiologies associated with increased mortality included anoxia, intracranial hemorrhages, tumors, infections, and trauma.

Limited data are available concerning the functional abilities of GCSE survivors, and none reliably permit a distinction between the effects of SE and of its etiologies. One review concluded that intellectual ability declined as a consequence of SE.[45] Survivors of SE frequently seem to have memory and behavioral disorders out of proportion to structural damage produced by the etiology of their seizures. A wealth of experimental data support this observation, arguing strongly for rapid and effective control of SE. Case reports of severe memory deficits following prolonged CPSE have also been published.[46] Whether treatment of SE reduces the risk of subsequent epilepsy remains uncertain. Recent experimental studies indicate that SE lowers the threshold for subsequent seizures.[47]

Subarachnoid Hemorrhage

The management of patients with acute aneurysmal subarachnoid hemorrhage (SAH) has changed substantially in the past two decades. Previously, patients were typically put on bed rest for 2 weeks, until the periods of maximal risk for rebleeding and vasospasm had passed; if they survived, they were then given the option of surgical treatment. Current management strategies recognize (1) improvements in surgical technique that make early, definitive obliteration of the aneurysm more feasible and safer; (2) the consequent ability to use induced hypertension and hypervolemia to treat cerebral vasospasm; (3) the introduction of nitrendipine-class calcium channel blockers to relieve or ameliorate the effects of vasospasm; (4) the development of interventional neuroradiologic techniques (eg, angioplasty and intra-arterial papaverine infusion) to treat symptomatic vasospasm; (5) the use of ventricular drainage to treat communicating hydrocephalus; and (6) the introduction in several countries, although not in North America, of a free-radical scavenger that appears to improve outcome in patients who present with high-grade SAH.

Future directions in the medical management of patients following SAH will probably depend primarily on the ability to recognize and manage cerebral vasospasm before it becomes symptomatic and before it produces cerebral infarction.

Epidemiology

The principal medical complications of aneurysmal SAH include rebleeding, cerebral vasospasm, and volume and osmolar disturbances. The risk of rebleeding from unsecured aneurysms varies with time after the initial hemorrhage: about 4% on the first postbleed day and about 1.5% per day up to day 28.[49] The mortality associated with rebleeding after the diagnosis of SAH exceeds 75%.[50] This complication is more frequent in patients with higher grades of SAH, in women, and in those with systolic blood pressures exceeding 170 mm Hg.[51] Cerebral vasospasm produces symptoms in up to 45% of patients,[52] but is noted angiographically in another 25% who appear asymptomatic.[53] Vasospasm usually starts to occur between postbleed days 4 and 6; the risk of its development is minimal after day 14. Volume and osmolar disturbances are reported in about 30% of patients.[54]

A number of other complications occur in this group of patients that are less directly related to the SAH itself.[52] Life-threatening cardiac arrhythmias are found 5%, with less ominous rhythm disturbances in 30%. Pulmonary edema is diagnosed in 23%, with 6% experiencing a severe form. Some degree of hepatic dysfunction is noted in 24% of patients, predominantly mild elevation of transaminase levels without symptoms; 4% experience severe hepatic dysfunction. Many of these patients are probably manifesting hepatic toxicity from anticonvulsants or other medications. Thrombocytopenia is reported in 4% of patients, usually related to sepsis or medications. Renal dysfunction is seen in 7%, but rarely requires dialysis.

Although this paper deals primarily with aneurysmal SAH, there are other causes of SAH, and their epidemiology is different. SAH following rupture of an arteriovenous malformation tends to occur at a younger age, with a peak incidence in the mid-20s. Traumatic SAH is a common accompaniment of severe head trauma, occurring in 15 to 40% of patients with severe head trauma. The incidence of the major complications of SAH in these patients appears to be lower than in patients with aneurysmal SAH, but data are scarce. After arteriovenous malformation rupture, the time course of angiographically diagnosable vasospasm is similar to that seen in aneurysmal SAH patients; it is usually asymptomatic,[55] except in rare cases.[56] The significance of vasospasm related to traumatic SAH continues to be debated, but in one series, 7 of 29 patients with large amounts of subarachnoid blood (detected by CT scanning) developed symptomatic vasospasm (detected angiographically) with subsequent infarction.[57] In patients with penetrating head trauma, the incidence (detected by transcranial Doppler [TCD] flow velocity measurements) may be as high as 40%.[58]

Pathophysiology

Rebleeding: Rebleeding of an aneurysm prior to its obliteration presumably reflects further leakage of blood at the site of the initial rupture. The tendency for this to occur appears to increase with arterial hypertension, which increases the stress on the aneurysm wall and the clot that occludes the original rupture site. Lowering the pressure in the subarachnoid space (*eg*, by lumbar puncture, or by allowing a ventriculostomy system to have a low pop-off pressure) similarly increases the pressure gradient across the aneurysm wall. Whether these procedures actually increase the risk of rebleeding is uncertain, and this theoretical concern does not militate against performing diagnostic lumbar punctures if needed either to prove the diagnosis of SAH or to exclude meningitis. Systemic factors that alter the balance between thrombosis and fibrinolysis (*eg*, disseminated intravascular coagulation) would presumably affect the risk of rebleeding as well.

Cerebral Vasospasm: Vasospasm appears to be a two-stage process, with an initial vasoconstrictive phase followed by a proliferative arteriopathy, associated with smooth-muscle-cell necrosis and fibrosis of the arterial wall.[59,60] Vasospasm appears to depend primarily on the presence of erythrocytes in the subarachnoid space,[61] but why it occurs more frequently and more symptomatically after aneurysmal SAH than after SAH due to other causes remains unexplained. The list of potential mediators contributing to the development of vasospasm is substantial, but the vasoconstrictor peptide endothelin-1 appears to be one of the most important.[62] Endothelin antagonists are promising experimental agents for the prevention and treatment of this condition.[63]

The maximal risk for vasospasm occurs from day 4 through day 14 after SAH, although about 10% of patients may have some angiographic signs of vasospasm at the time of the initial angiogram.[64]

The risk of developing vasospasm is related to the amount of blood in the subarachnoid space. Fisher and colleagues[65] reported that patients with thick subarachnoid clots were much more likely to develop vasospasm than those without such clots. Antifibrinolytic agents (*eg*, ε-aminocaproic acid, tranexamic acid) used to prevent rebleeding raise the risk of symptomatic vasospasm and delayed ischemic deficits,[66] but whether there is an actual increase in the rate of vasospasm, or an increase in the rate of occlusion of already spastic vessels, is uncertain.

Hyperglycemia probably worsens outcome in stroke patients,[67] and therefore presumably in SAH patients developing delayed ischemia. Plasma glucose concentrations exceeding 120 mg/dL in the first postbleed week are associated with poor outcome.[68] All of these studies suffer from the confounding effect of severity of illness on intrinsic plasma glucose regulation, but they do suggest that maintenance of normoglycemia is a reasonable goal.

Volume and Osmolar Disturbances: Although earlier studies attributed the hyponatremia and hypo-osmolality occurring after SAH to the syndrome of inappropriate antidiuretic hormone secretion (SIADH),[69] most investigators now believe that these disturbances are the result of cerebral salt wasting.[70] The pathophysiology of this condition remains to be completely elucidated, but probably begins with the release of atrial, brain, and C-type natriuretic factors from the brain.[71] These peptides produce isotonic volume loss by their renal effects, resulting in hypovolemia. This hypovolemic state then prompts an appropriate antidiuretic hormone response, causing a fall in free water clearance and thereby producing hyponatremia and hypo-osmolality. Hypovolemia appears to increase the risk of cerebral infarction (delayed ischemic deficits) in patients with vasospasm, and should therefore be prevented with prophylactic volume replacement.[72]

Physical signs of hypovolemia are rare in SAH patients, who are usually kept flat in bed, and in whom a putative increase in adrenal catecholamine secretion and increased sympathetic nervous system activity often produce hypertension. Overly vigorous treatment of this hypertension after the aneurysm is secured appears to worsen outcome.[73]

Seizures: Following SAH, patients may experience any of four patterns of seizures. About 6% of patients appear to suffer a seizure at the time of the hemorrhage,[74] although the distinction between a generalized convulsion and an episode of decerebrate posturing may be difficult to establish from the reports of nonmedical observers. Postoperative seizures occur in about 1.5% of SAH patients despite anticonvulsant prophylaxis (usually phenytoin).[75] Patients developing delayed ischemia from vasospasm may seize following reperfusion by angioplasty.[76] Late seizures occur in about 3% of patients over several years of follow-up.[75]

SAH patients are somewhat more likely to have a seizure at the time of presentation than are patients with other types of stroke.[77]

The mechanisms producing seizures in SAH patients are uncertain. Patients in whom aneurysmal rupture produces a concomitant intracerebral hematoma probably have a direct epileptogenic stimulus. Irritation from the aneurysm clipping appears to account for some postoperative seizures. Reperfusion injury accounts for a small percentage.[76] Late seizures may reflect the epileptogenic effects of iron on the cerebral cortex.[78]

Cardiovascular Complications: Cardiac arrhythmias and ECG signs of ischemia are frequent in SAH patients.[79] In one series, all 61 patients had at least one such abnormal finding.[80] The most serious of such problems is the development of ventricular tachycardia, typically of the *torsades de pointes* form.[81]

ECG changes resembling acute myocardial infarction, and elevation of the MB isoenzyme of CK (and, by inference, elevation of troponins)

occur without evidence of coronary arterial occlusion. About 10% of patients will have an ECG suggesting acute myocardial infarction during the first 3 days post-SAH.[82] In one study, elevation of CK was associated with left ventricular wall motion abnormalities.[83] Histopathologically, these findings correspond to myocardial contraction band necrosis, which resembles the cardiomyopathic changes associated with pheochromocytomas.

Pulmonary edema occurring in SAH patients may be either cardiogenic or noncardiogenic in origin. Some patients have echocardiographic evidence of left ventricular dysfunction at the time their pulmonary edema is severe.[84] However, the majority of SAH patients have a defect in pulmonary gas exchange in the absence of evidence of cardiac dysfunction or aspiration, suggesting that neurogenic pulmonary edema is responsible.[85] This probably occurs as the consequence of a neurally mediated increase in extravascular lung water.[86]

CNS Infection: Excepting cases of ruptured mycotic aneurysms, CNS infections in SAH patients are almost always iatrogenic, either from organisms introduced during aneurysm clipping or, much more commonly, from ventriculostomy systems that become colonized with bacteria.

Other Infectious Complications: The non-CNS infectious complications of SAH patients vary with the severity of their illness. Patients remaining in Hunt and Hess grades 1 and 2 do not seem to be at particular risk for aspiration and may not need urinary catheters, feeding tubes, or central venous lines, which are the proximate causes of many ICU infections. Higher-grade patients are susceptible to the typical infectious complications of critical care. The contribution of corticosteroids in decreasing resistance to infection in these patients is unquantified. SAH patients in the trials of tirilazad mesylate,[87] a steroid free-radical scavenger without glucocorticoid effects, were not given glucocorticoids either before or after procedures to secure their aneurysms; they did not appear to suffer ICP problems. Although this question has not been formally tested, it raises the possibility that routine dexamethasone administration may not be necessary in this population. Withholding this agent would be expected to decrease both infectious and metabolic complications in these patients.

Higher-grade patients may need feeding tubes for nutritional support, or larger-bore gastric tubes should an ileus develop. Placing these tubes via the nasal route appears to increase the risk of nosocomial sinusitis, and probably of pneumonia as well.[88]

Deep Venous Thrombosis and Pulmonary Embolism: SAH patients are at risk for the development of deep venous thromboses and subsequent pulmonary embolism by virtue of immobilization. Whether the use of antifibrinolytic agents increases the risk of deep venous thrombosis has long been debated; the use of these agents for 2 weeks in patients undergoing late aneurysm surgery probably does increase these risks.[89] Brief use of these agents to decrease the risk of rebleeding prior to early surgery probably carries a lower risk.[90] Although the concentration of circulating fibrinogen complexes is increased in SAH patients (and other stroke patients) compared with controls,[91] the role of this finding in the genesis of venous thrombosis remains speculative.

Nutrition

Although standard critical care practice emphasizes the early institution of nutritional support to maintain muscle mass and gut integrity, the importance of nutritional support for SAH patients remains unproven. Starvation prior to experimental ischemia may result in a shift to the metabolism of fuels other than glucose, even in the brain, and potentially result in an improved outcome after delayed ischemia.[92] However, the balance between risks and benefits of this approach remains to be established. SAH patients are markedly catabolic, and may have a defect in the utilization of amino acids[93]; the mechanism of this defect is unknown.

Management

The higher-grade SAH patient may require all of the skills a critical care team can muster. The sickest of these patients can still attain a good functional outcome despite what appear to be overwhelming difficulties. Thus, attention to all of the details of care in these patients is essential. Guidelines for the care of SAH patients have recently been published by the American Heart Association[94] and the Canadian Neurosurgical Society.[95]

Rebleeding: Although aneurysm obliteration is the most important method of preventing rebleeding, antihypertensive drugs and antifibrinolytic agents may be valuable prior to surgery or interventional radiologic approaches. Preoperative blood pressures are typically elevated; we strive to maintain systolic pressures below 150 mm Hg and mean arterial pressures below 100 mm Hg in these patients. Nimodipine, which is used to try to prevent delayed ischemic deficits, often lowers the blood pressure to a modest degree. Labetolol (Table 7), which has both α- and β-adrenergic blocking effects when given IV, is commonly the first drug employed for blood pressure control. Hydralazine is also commonly used, although there is a theoretical concern about the use of pure vasodilators in preoperative SAH patients (increasing pulse pressure may increase stress on the aneurysm wall). Enalaprilat may be useful for patients who do not respond to these

Table 7. *Selected Drugs Useful in the Management of SAH Patients*

Agent	Dose	Comments
Enalaprilat	0.625 to 1.25 mg q6h	May decrease renal plasma flow and raise creatinine
Esmolol	250 to 500 µg/kg, then 50 to 200 µg/kg/min	May produce congestive heart failure
Hydralazine	10 to 20 mg q3-4h	Theoretical risk of increasing shear forces
Labetolol	10 mg q10min, up to 300 mg	Oral form lacks significant β-adrenergic blocking effect
Nicardipine	0.075 to 0.15 mg/kg/h	May produce congestive heart failure
Nimodipine	60 mg q4h for 14 to 21 days	Duration of therapy uncertain
Nitroprusside	0.25 to 10 µg/kg/min	Rarely necessary
Phenytoin	15 to 20 mg/kg loading dose, then 5 to 8 mg/kg/day maintenance (q12h for suspension, q24h for Dilantin* capsules	Duration of therapy uncertain; maintain serum concentration between 10 and 20 µg/mL. Hold tube feeding 1 h before and after dose.

*Dilantin; Parke-Davis; Morris Plains, NJ.

agents. We tend to avoid nitrates because of the potential for increased ICP, but rarely nitroprusside may be the only effective drug. Pain relief with acetaminophen, codeine, or fentanyl is often necessary, and is frequently helpful in lowering blood pressure as well.

Postoperatively, the blood pressure may be allowed to rise to higher levels. Patients at risk for vasospasm may require higher blood pressures for adequate cerebral perfusion. In patients with more than one aneurysm, the risk of producing a new SAH from a previously unruptured aneurysm appears to be small (but not absent[96]) during the first few postbleed weeks.

Cerebral Vasospasm: Delayed ischemic deficits from vasospasm have emerged as the major cause of morbidity and mortality in patients undergoing early aneurysm obliteration. Management approaches attempt to prevent both spasm and its consequences, although it is not clear that any of the currently used techniques actually prevent vasospasm. Rather, most attempt to preserve either perfusion or neuronal survival in areas affected by vasospasm.

Vasospasm is definitively diagnosed angiographically, although spasm in vessels below the resolution of angiography probably occurs in patients whose symptoms suggest vasospasm. The initial symptom of vasospasm is typically decreased interaction with the unit staff and the patient's family and visitors. The patient may then progress to an abulic state, or appear to have bilateral frontal lobe dysfunction. The etiology of these symptoms is uncertain, as they do not appear to depend on the location of the aneurysm, the localization of subarachnoid blood, or the development of complications such as hydrocephalus. At this point, the TCD velocity measurements are usually elevated (*eg*, mean velocities >120 cm/s). Xenon-CT blood flow studies suggest that TCD may underestimate the incidence and severity of vasospasm.[97] Lateralized motor findings suggest the development of delayed ischemic lesions.

Nimodipine, a voltage-sensitive calcium channel blocker, was introduced with the expectation that it would prevent vasospasm. Angiographic studies did not confirm this effect, at least in vessels visible by radiologic techniques, but clinical trials did confirm its utility in improving outcome.[98] Nicardipine, a related agent, does appear to

decrease angiographically diagnosed vasospasm.[99] The outcome of patients treated with nicardipine did not differ statistically from that in patients receiving placebo, but the placebo patients received rescue hypertensive-hypervolemic therapy (HHT) more frequently.

Volume replacement and expansion, usually practiced by attempts to maintain either a fixed, relatively high saline solution intake (*eg*, 3 to 6 L/d of normal or mildly hypertonic saline solution) or a positive fluid balance, is relatively standard in centers caring for SAH patients. While this usually prevents volume contraction due to cerebral salt wasting, it is unlikely that it prevents vasospasm *per se*. However, it appears to be very useful in preventing or decreasing the extent of symptomatic vasospasm and delayed ischemic deficits.

The free-radical scavenger tirilazad may be effective in improving outcome in SAH patients, primarily those in higher grades. A European-Australian trial showed efficacy at a dose of 6 mg/kg/d only in men,[100] presumably because the drug is more rapidly metabolized in women. A parallel North American trial did not achieve a statistically significant result.[87] This appears at least in part to reflect a higher percentage of North American patients receiving phenytoin, which accelerates the metabolism of tirilazad.[101] Higher-dose trials have been concluded, but the results have not yet been published. This agent has been licensed for SAH in men in 13 countries. The drug has poor blood-brain barrier penetration; more lipophilic derivatives have been synthesized,[102] and await clinical trials.

Treatment for Vasospasm: Two approaches are currently used for the management of vasospasm. The first is volume expansion, usually accompanied by induced hypertension (by means of HHT).[103] Although some consider hemodilution (to hemoglobin concentrations between 10 and 11 *g*/dL) to be part of this treatment as well, in the hope that decreasing blood viscosity will improve perfusion, this is the least consistently practiced part of this approach. HHT has not been subjected to a randomized clinical trial, and substantial debate persists regarding its utility.[104,105] If it is to be employed, careful patient monitoring is necessary, involving an arterial line and either a central venous line or, preferably, a pulmonary artery catheter to guide vasopressor and volume management. Angiographic confirmation of the diagnosis of vasospasm is usually obtained before instituting vasopressor therapy.

Because SAH patients appear to have low thresholds for the development of hydrostatic pulmonary edema, we try to maintain the pulmonary capillary wedge pressure (PCWP) between 15 and 18 mm Hg. In some patients, this volume expansion alone is adequate to produce an increase in cardiac index and mean arterial pressure. What mixture of colloid and crystalloid to use for volume expansion in this setting is the subject of endless debate and absent data. If the patient's examination does not improve, we next raise the mean arterial pressure using phenylephrine, dopamine, norepinephrine, epinephrine, or a combination of phenylephrine and dobutamine, as suggested by the patient's heart rate, the cardiac index produced, and evidence of ectopy, cardiac ischemia, or renal dysfunction. None of these medications has a proven advantage over the others in this setting, and each case provides individual challenges. Hypertensive encephalopathy can apparently complicate overly vigorous therapy.[106]

The second approach to vasospasm patient management involves interventional radiologic techniques, either angioplasty or papaverine infusion.[107] We use both hemodynamic and radiologic techniques. Intraventricular infusion of nitroprusside may be useful in the future.[108]

Volume and Osmolar Disturbances: Volume deficits are prevented or corrected as discussed above. If SAH patients receive adequate saline solution replacement, hypo-osmolality is an infrequent occurrence.

Evaluation of the SAH patient whose laboratory results indicate a low serum sodium concentration requires both clinical and laboratory evaluation. Prior to intervention, serum and urine osmolality measurements should be obtained. This will prevent the inadvertent treatment of the patient for hypo-osmolality when the real problem is, for example, a factitious hyponatremia due to hyperglycemia or pseudohyponatremia from hyperlipidemia. Truly hypo-osmolar SAH patients require careful thought, rather than just salt administration. Unless the patient has developed pulmonary edema or other signs suggesting congestive heart failure, one should not assume that hyponatremia is due to combined salt and water excess. The likely occurrence of cerebral salt wasting favors a diagnosis of salt loss with water retention. Osmolality measurements will usually indicate that the patient's urine is inappropriately concentrated for a patient with hypotonic serum. While this combination may suggest SIADH in many circumstances, this condition should rarely be diagnosed during the first 2 weeks postbleed. Attempts to treat the patient with volume restriction will likely lead to greater problems with delayed ischemic deficits. One potentially useful biochemical assay is the serum uric acid level, which tends to be low in SIADH but normal in cerebral salt wasting.

Management of hypo-osmolar states depends critically on their rate of development.[109] Rapidly developing (*eg*, over hours) hypo-osmolality produces neuronal swelling, and is associated with elevated ICP and seizures. More slowly developing (over days) hypo-osmolality is accompanied by solute shifts out of neurons, which prevent ICP increases and are unlikely to produce seizures; the patient may become confused, lethargic, and weak, but seldom experiences any life-threatening complications from the osmolality itself. However, these are the patients at risk for central and extrapontine myelinolysis if their osmolalities are raised too rapidly.

Patients who became rapidly hypo-osmolar may be treated with small doses of hypertonic saline solution (*eg*, 100 mL of 3N) to begin correcting this problem. They usually respond quickly with lower ICP and resolution of seizures. Those who became hypo-osmolar more slowly must be corrected more slowly; a goal of 6 mOsm/L/day increases appears safe. Because these patients should not be allowed to become volume-depleted, this is best performed by replacement of their urine output and insensible loss by mildly hypertonic solutions, or, in patients receiving enteral feeding, addition of salt to their food. Attempts to decrease the urine osmolality with loop diuretics are seldom sufficiently successful to be useful.

Cardiovascular Complications: Prevention of electrolyte disturbances and magnesium replacement are probably useful for the prevention of arrhythmias. α- and β-adrenergic blockade may decrease or prevent myocardial contraction band necrosis, but this has not been tested.

Cardiac arrhythmias in SAH are seldom life-threatening. Sinus tachycardia and other supraventricular tachycardias should lead to a reassessment of electrolytes, volume status, pain control, infection, and endocrine (especially thyroid) function. Depending on the arrhythmia and its hemodynamic consequences, treatment with adenosine, calcium antagonists, β-blocking agents, or digoxin may be indicated. Ventricular arrhythmias frequently reflect adrenergic drug administration (eg, dopamine) or electrolyte disorders; alternatively, they may represent signs of myocardial ischemia. If possible, dopamine-induced rhythm disorders indicate switching to another agent. Lidocaine or procainamide may be required if runs of ventricular tachycardia appear. *Torsades de pointes* may respond to supplemental magnesium, or may require overdrive pacing.

SAH patients with heart failure who develop signs suggesting vasospasm will usually require pulmonary artery catheterization for volume and hemodynamic management.

CNS Infection: Infection is a major problem for SAH patients, because fever may increase the degree of damage produced by delayed ischemia. Another problem is the diagnosis of the etiology of fever in these patients. A preliminary analysis in our unit suggests that about 20% of SAH patients experience fever without evidence of infection on retrospective review, suggesting that they have developed "central fever."[110] These patients frequently receive antibiotics, putting them at risk for drug reactions and increasing expense, because it is difficult to prove that they do not have an infection. Drug-induced fevers are a major problem in all ICU patients, and SAH patients are no exception. Commonly implicated drugs include phenytoin, antibiotics, and, less frequently, agents such as histamine$_2$-antagonists and stool softeners.

Whether patients with ventriculostomies or lumbar drains should receive antibiotic prophylaxis is an open question. If prophylaxis is to be given, a cephalosporin with activity against *Staphylococcus aureus* (eg, cefazolin) is probably the most reasonable choice. Activity against coagulase-negative staphylococci does not seem important; nor do the brain or CSF penetration characteristics of the drug. A risk-benefit analysis suggests that ventriculostomy catheters probably should be changed every 5 days.[111]

Treatment of ventriculostomy infections should be based initially on a Gram stain of CSF. If staphylococcal infection is suspected, initial treatment with vancomycin is appropriate pending culture and sensitivity results. Patients with Gram-negative rods in the CSF should receive either a cephalosporin with antipseudomonal activity (eg, cefepime) or meropenem until microbiologic results are available. If the CSF contains increasing numbers of white cells but the Gram stain is negative, a combination of vancomycin and either meropenem or cefepime seems reasonable, although some of these patients will have an aseptic postoperative meningitis.

Other Infectious Complications: The question of routine changes of central venous catheters and pulmonary artery catheters is beyond the scope of this discussion. Whatever local practices control these policies for other critically ill patients should apply to SAH patients.

We attempt to place all tracheal and gastric tubes through the mouth, rather than the nose, to decrease the incidence of sinusitis.[112]

Seizures: Because seizures in patients with unsecured aneurysms may promote rebleeding, it is a common, although by no means universal, practice to administer anticonvulsants to SAH patients.

The standard agent for prophylaxis in North America is phenytoin. Fosphenytoin, a water-soluble prodrug, is safer to administer IV, and may be given IM if necessary. An adequate loading dose should be given.

Should seizures occur in an SAH patient, one should obtain a CT scan to look for new intracranial pathology. At the same time, one should give an additional dose of phenytoin to raise the serum concentration. If seizures recur, and the phenytoin has been pushed to the point of symptomatic toxicity (in the responsive patient) or a level of about 24 μg/mL (in patients with impaired ability to respond), adding either phenobarbital or carbamazepine have been standard approaches. The recent introductions of gabapentin and an IV form of valproate increase the number of therapeutic options. This choice must be individualized.

Phenytoin is frequently implicated as a cause of drug-induced fever. When a rash and fever appear in a patient taking this drug, it is typically discontinued. Because of its long half-life, several days will elapse before it is cleared from the patient. Substitution of another anticonvulsant (*eg*, gabapentin) without sedative effects and without cross-sensitivity is a reasonable approach. Suspected allergy is the only circumstance in which most anticonvulsants should be stopped abruptly.

Deep Venous Thrombosis and Pulmonary Embolism: Before securing the aneurysm, many physicians are reluctant to give prophylactic doses of heparin, and instead rely on sequential compression devices to prevent deep venous thrombosis. These devices are effective in many circumstances, but have not been formally tested in SAH patients. Interestingly, sequential compression devices accelerate *in vitro* measurements of fibrinolysis,[113] and part of their effectiveness probably stems from this mechanism. We continue to use these devices for prophylaxis in bed-bound patients after the aneurysm has been secured.

Deep venous thrombosis or pulmonary embolism in patients with either unsecured aneurysms or fresh craniotomies pose difficult management problems. Our approach is usually to place an inferior vena cava filter, and not to give anticoagulant therapy until at least 1 week after surgery. The filter is generally held to be safer than immediate anticoagulation.[114]

Nutrition and GI Bleeding Prophylaxis: Despite strongly held opinions, there are few data on which to base recommendations for nutrition in SAH patients. In view of the likely deleterious effect of hyperglycemia on outcome after delayed ischemia, whatever nutritional approach is taken should include frequent measurements of blood glucose, and probably its tight control. So-called "trophic" feeding, in which a small volume (*eg*, 5 mL/h) of an enteral nutrition formula is constantly infused via a gastric or jejunal feeding tube, may maintain the structure of the intestinal villi and help to prevent both bacterial translocation and the subsequent incidence of diarrhea when full feedings are instituted.

If patients are npo, some form of prophylaxis against GI bleeding seems reasonable. Clinically important GI bleeding occurs in up to 6% of SAH patients.[115] Histamine$_2$-blocking agents such as ranitidine or nizatidine are commonly used. These agents are occasionally associated with neutropenia or thrombocytopenia; in this circumstance,

sucralfate or omeprazole may be substituted. The use of nonsteroidal anti-inflammatory agents appears to increase the risk of GI bleeding; we routinely administer misoprostol with these agents. Once patients are fully fed, these prophylactic agents may no longer be necessary.

When feedings begin, patients frequently develop diarrhea. Because a large percentage of patients are receiving antibiotics, the possibility of antibiotic-induced *Clostridium difficile* infection must be considered. After sending specimens for fecal leukocyte, cytotoxin, and *C difficile* cultures, we use kaolin and pectin to attempt to decrease the diarrhea. Some patients appear to have diarrhea induced by sorbitol, used in many solutions of drugs for tube administration.

Intracerebral Hemorrhage

The major causes of intracerebral hemorrhage (ICH) include chronic hypertension, coagulation disturbances, and underlying vascular lesions. Hypertensive ICH occurs where small penetrating arteries arise from large arterial trunks. There is reasonable evidence demonstrating that it is safe to acutely lower blood pressure in an attempt to decrease hematoma formation, but it is not known whether this is useful. A recent phase II study of recombinant factor VIIa shows that it will limit hematoma growth and improve functional outcome; a phase III study is in progress.[115a] This has only been studied in patients without coagulation disturbances.

Stroke

Stroke is the most common neurologic cause for hospital admission in the United States. About 80% of strokes are ischemic, with the remainder divided between intracerebral hemorrhage and SAH. The incidence of stroke is declining, coincident with and probably in part reflecting improvement in the treatment of hypertension. The association of stroke with hypertension, particularly intracerebral hemorrhage, has been slightly overstated in the past (blood pressures were often measured when the patient presented with the stroke, rather than seeking a documented history of hypertension; the same is true of many studies of hyperglycemia in stroke). Other risk factors include diabetes, cardiac disease, previous cerebrovascular disease (transient ischemic attack or stroke), age, sex, lipid disorders, excessive ethanol ingestion, elevated hematocrit, elevated fibrinogen, and cigarette smoking. Smoking is the most powerful risk factor for aneurysmal SAH. In younger patients (usually defined as those <55 years old), one should consider abnormalities of antithrombin III, protein S, protein C, or antiphospholipid antibodies. Young stroke patients with marfanoid habitus should be worked up for homocysteinuria; the heterozygous state is associated with stroke, and many patients respond to pyridoxine treatment.

The intensivist most commonly encounters potential stroke patients in the settings of (1) suspected carotid artery disease, and (2) cardiac disturbances that are potentially emboligenic. Patients with *asymptomatic* carotid bruits have approximately a 2% annual risk of stroke, but the side of the bruit does not predict the side of the stroke. There are no data on which to base the selection of patients for further work-up. I tend to start an aspirin regimen (80 to 325 mg/d) in these people, but not investigate them further. If studies (noninvasive or angiographic) have already been obtained, I would *consider* endarterectomy for *otherwise healthy* patients who have >70% stenosis or a large area of ulceration. The common practice of "prophylactic" endarterectomy before other vascular surgical procedures lacks validation; from the poor data available, the risk of stroke related to such procedures does not seem to exceed the risks related to endarterectomy itself. The results of the Asymptomatic Carotid Artery Stenosis (ACAS) trial suggest that men with asymptomatic carotid stenosis of >70% derive greater benefit from carotid endarteractomy than from medical therapy alone. Endarterectomy of the vertebral arteries and angioplasty of any cerebral vessel remain experimental techniques.

About 30% of untreated patients with new-onset transient ischemic attacks will suffer a stroke in the next 2 years. If the patient has 70 to 99% stenosis in the relevant carotid artery, endarterectomy reduces the risk of stroke or death to about 10%. Patients not appropriate candidates for surgery should probably receive ticlopidine 250 mg bid (with appropriate monitoring of the WBC count); this drug appears effective in both men and women (aspirin has not been universally efficacious in women).

If a cardiac source of embolism is suspected, anticoagulation with warfarin is usually indicated. For patients with nonvalvular atrial fibrillation, a prothrombin time of 1.3 to 1.7 times control (or an international normalized ratio of about 3.0; should be >2.0 and <5.0) is probably adequate and has few side effects (in three recent studies of prophylaxis, minor bleeding was more common in the warfarin groups than in the control group, but intracerebral hemorrhage or other major bleeding was not). One study suggested that aspirin also reduced stroke rates; it could be used in patients who are poor risks for warfarin. In patients with suspected embolism from other cardiac disorders (*eg*, cardiomyopathies, left ventricular aneurysms), low-dose warfarin has not been well studied. The aortic arch is a hitherto underrecognized source of emboli; management of this condition remains to be established.

Transesophageal echocardiography can detect clots and other lesions that escape detection by transthoracic echocardiography. In some series, the rate of detection of cardiac lesions is so high that their significance is uncertain.

In patients 6 h or more into acute ischemic stroke, no treatment has been proven useful. Heparin may be indicated to prevent subsequent embolic strokes, but does not affect either a completed stroke or so-called stroke-in-evolution. If the patient is to receive anticoagulant therapy because of a suspected source of embolism, some investigators feel that patients with large infarcts should not be given anticoagulants for several days because of a presumed risk of hemorrhage into the infarct. Other data suggest that the greatest risk of re-embolization occurs in the first few days after the initial stroke, which argues for early anticoagulation of this group. I favor the latter approach.

Patients who follow a stuttering course may benefit from induced hypertension to improve flow through stenotic vessels until collateral vessels can open. Spontaneous hypertension in these patients should be considered a compensatory response, and should not be treated in the first few poststroke days unless evidence of end-organ damage develops. We avoid treating blood pressure unless the *mean* pressure exceeds 160 mm Hg.

After the patient has stabilized neurologically, a course of chronic antihypertensive treatment can be instituted.

The role of hyperglycemia in worsening stroke outcome seems established, but no studies have been done to determine whether tight control of blood sugar will improve prognosis.

The National Institute of Neurological Disorders and Stroke rt-PA Stroke Study Group (NINDS) trial[116] showed that thrombolysis was safe and effective if performed within 3 h of stroke onset (this does not mean 3 h after waking up with a new stroke; the time of stroke onset must be known). The recombinant tissue-plasminogen activator dose in this study was 0.9 mg/kg, with 10% of the dose as a bolus and the remainder over 1 h. The treated patients had a very significant improvement in functional outcome. There were more intracerebral hemorrhages in the treated group, but their mortality was actually lower (this did not reach statistical significance).

Patients who develop serious increases in ICP during the first 3 to 4 days poststroke are at risk for herniation and death. The earliest sign is usually diminished consciousness, often followed by an ipsilateral third-nerve palsy. Corticosteroids do not decrease the cytotoxic edema associated with strokes, and should not be used (unless the cause of the stroke is vasculitic). Although the routine use of hyperventilation in stroke patients is not indicated, this technique is appropriate to prevent herniation. Mannitol can also be used. If more drastic therapy is contemplated (eg, high-dose barbiturates), an ICP monitor should be inserted. We now use hemicraniectomy to reduce ICP in these patients, with surprisingly good functional outcomes; this has not become the standard of care. Experimental results suggest that the skull should be removed before swelling occurs, in order to protect the cortex from loss of pial collaterals.

Intracerebral hemorrhage produces much more rapid rises in ICP because of the volume of the hematoma. The major concerns for the internist are (1) exclusion or treatment of a bleeding diathesis, which should always be considered, and (2) management of ICP. Although the edema around an intracerebral hemorrhage is vasogenic, it does not respond to steroids. Three controlled studies have documented poorer outcome in steroid-treated patients, owing to the side effects of the steroids. In older patients, especially those with more than one episode of hemorrhage and without a history of hypertension, amyloid angiopathy becomes a diagnostic consideration (about 15% of all intracerebral hemorrhages). In younger patients, intracerebral hemorrhage related to sympathomimetic agents (including cocaine) is becoming an increasingly frequent problem.

Although neurogenic pulmonary edema may occur in any acute intracranial condition, SAH patients seem particularly prone to it; about 40% of our SAH patients have some degree of oxygenation difficulty not explained by other conditions. In neurogenic pulmonary edema, the PCWP is normal, and the edema fluid has a high protein content; this reflects the presumed pathogenic mechanism of pulmonary venoconstriction. One must then attempt to balance the need to expand volume in patients with the need to keep their lungs dry. We tend to keep the PCWP around 10 mm Hg, and use vasopressors to improve cerebral perfusion if necessary.

Nervous System Infections

Meningitis

The consensus of opinion seems to favor presumptive treatment for suspected meningitis in any situation in which lumbar puncture (LP) is delayed. This includes even delays to obtain CT scans, because the commonest causes of meningitis in adults (pneumococcal and meningococcal) can kill the patient while waiting for the scan. I believe that patients who are alert and have normal fundi and neurologic exams can undergo LP without scanning, because the possibility of a patient in that setting herniating soon after LP is infinitesimally small, but presumptive treatment is clearly more important than intellectual purity. With the increasing prevalence of penicillin-resistant pneumococci, cefotaxime (2 g q4h) or ceftriaxone (2 g q12h) should be used for empiric therapy. A few pneumococci with significant resistance to third-generation cephalosporins have emerged, prompting some to add vancomycin until results of sensitivity testing are available. Cefuroxime is inferior to these third-generation cephalosporins and should no longer be used.

Because ampicillin-resistant *Haemophilus influenzae* infections are common, children should also receive the third-generation agents. Chloramphenicol is often recommended for truly penicillin-allergic (*eg*, anaphylactic) patients, although clinical failures have been reported in patients with penicillin-resistant pneumococci. In most cases, the initial dose of antibiotics will not sterilize the CSF within 30 to 60 min; even if this occurs, testing for bacterial antigens will reveal the etiology in the majority of cases. Blood cultures should be obtained before antibiotics are given. Further treatment decisions can be made based on the Gram stain and antigen results. If listeriosis is suspected (immune-compromised host, or negative Gram stain and bacterial antigen tests), ampicillin or sulfamethoxazole-trimethoprim should be added until an organism is isolated or blood and CSF cultures have been negative for at least 3 days. Because of its epileptogenic effects, imipenem should usually be avoided in CNS infections.

In infants and children, pretreatment with steroids (dexamethasone, 0.15 mg/kg q6h for 4 days) appears to decrease neurologic dysfunction after recovery from meningitis (predominantly that due to *H influenzae*). This is presumed to reflect a decrease in inflammation from lysis of organisms, with the subsequent host elaboration of tumor necrosis factor and other inflammatory mediators. The use of steroids in adult meningitides remains controversial, but does not appear to be deleterious in the few patients so far studied. I think that the evidence favors its use in adults as well, but this is still debated. A recent study in children suggests that 2 days of dexamethasone is as useful as 4 days. The issue is clouded when vancomycin is used for potential penicillin-resistant pneumococci, because steroids may decrease vancomycin penetration into the CSF (this is debated in humans).

Increased ICP in meningitis patients is treated as described above. Cerebral edema in children appears to respond to steroids; it is probably appropriate to treat adults in the same fashion if elevated ICP is a problem. Hyponatremia is common, and may exacerbate vasogenic cerebral edema; it usually responds to fluid restriction. Whether this increases the rate of cerebral venous thrombosis is not clear. However, it is important not to let the cerebral perfusion pressure fall below about 60 mm Hg; this is more important that fluid restriction. Seizures are initially managed with benzodiazepines and phenytoin; the treatment of SE is covered above.

Encephalitis

As in meningitis, the weight of expert opinion is shifting (albeit more slowly) to the "shoot first and ask questions later" approach. When encephalitis is suspected, acyclovir (10 to 15 mg/kg q8h) is begun while the work-up is in progress; adequate hydration is necessary to prevent renal toxicity. The most sensitive test is CSF–polymerase chain reaction; MRI with gadolinium is second, with EEG third. Even though brain biopsy has a low rate of complications (3%, most of which are minor), the relative safety of acyclovir has encouraged many physicians to treat presumptively, and perform a biopsy only in patients who do not respond or in whom the work-up raises the possibility of another diagnosis. The commonly quoted list of "treatable disorders that mimic herpes simplex encephalitis" from the National Institute of Allergy and Infectious Diseases cooperative studies is not relevant in the MRI era. Seizures and elevated ICP are common.

Brain Abscess

Unless there is a strong suspicion of the etiology of a brain abscess (*eg*, the patient had a proven bacteremia prior to developing the abscess), empiric treatment for suspected brain abscess should include a third-generation cephalosporin, vancomycin, and metronidazole. Vancomycin is probably adequate treatment for Listeria, but if there is a reason to suspect this organism, one usually adds ampicillin or sulfamethoxazole-trimethoprim. Although some surgeons have tried to avoid aspiration, biopsy, or resection of these patients on the grounds that empiric medical treatment seems effective, this contention is based on small numbers of patients. Furthermore, it is often difficult to be certain that a particular lesion is an abscess and not a high-grade astrocytoma. Surgery also offers some direct relief of ICP problems. For these reasons, I recommend early aspiration of suspected abscesses, with possible later debulking or resection.

Neurogenic Respiratory Failure

Myasthenia Gravis

Although the standard teaching about myasthenia gravis stresses fatigability with exercise, this is rarely what brings the patient to medical attention. The usual complaints are diplopia, ptosis, difficulty with speech and secretions, proximal limb weakness, and ventilatory dysfunction. The condition preferentially affects young women and older men. There is overrepresentation of human leukocyte antigen-A1 (HLA-A1), HLA-B8, and HLA-DRw3 (another instance in which HLA testing is not clinically useful). This is a true autoimmune disease, in which antibodies directed at myoid cells in the thymus [which express acetylcholine receptors (AChR)] attack the NMJ. There is a greater than expected incidence of other autoimmune diseases, including systemic lupus erythematosus, Sjögren's syndrome, polymyositis, and autoimmune thyroid disease. About 70% of patients have thymic hyperplasia, and 15% have thymomas. Anti-AChR antibodies are present in most patients with generalized myasthenia, and about 60% of those with ocular myasthenia. Antistriated muscle antibodies are a marker for thymoma.

Diagnostic studies include the edrophonium test (for which change in ptosis is the only truly objective bedside parameter to follow), measurement of anti-AChR antibodies, electromyography with repetitive stimulation, and chest CT to evaluate the thymus. Patients with generalized myasthenia who are developing ventilatory failure should be followed with vital capacity and negative inspiratory force (maximal inspiratory pressure) measurements; hypercapnia is a late finding. We usually intubate and ventilate patients when the vital capacity falls below about 12 mL/kg; some will require intubation because of upper airway problems but not need mechanical ventilation. Sometimes we will permit hypercapnia if the upper airway is intact and the patient is in the ICU. Edrophonium testing to distinguish myasthenic crisis from cholinergic crisis (too much anticholinesterase) is dangerous and should rarely be performed.

Treatment includes anticholinesterases (pyridostigmine), immunosuppressives (steroids, azathioprine, cyclophosphamide, some times cyclosporine), and thymectomy. Plasma exchange or IVIg can be dramatically effective, but each is only a short-term measure, primarily used for patients in crisis or to prepare them for thymectomy. Patients with purely ocular symptoms and normal thymic size on CT can be treated with anticholinesterases alone, but most other patients should be treated for the progressive autoimmune disease they have.

A large number of drugs have been reported to exacerbate myasthenia. The most important ones to remember are aminoglycosides, macrolides, lidocaine, propranolol, and quinidine. The effects of neuromuscular blocking agents is usually quite prolonged. Steroids often worsen the weakness before the patient improves.

Other Conditions

Respiratory failure due to diseases of the nervous system is predominantly hypercapnic, except in the case of neurogenic pulmonary edema. The diagnosis of neuromuscular respiratory failure is usually straightforward if one considers it as a possibility. Many of these conditions will be apparent at presentation, but on occasion a diagnosis of amyotrophic lateral sclerosis is made only when the patient has difficulty weaning from the ventilator. Critical illness polyneuropathy is a relatively recently described entity in which critically ill patients (most of whom have been septic) cannot be weaned from mechanical ventilation. Electromyographic studies show an axonal neuropathy; the prognosis for eventual recovery is very good, but these patients commonly require 4 to 6 months of mechanical ventilation.

Roelofs and coworkers,[117] Zochodne and colleagues,[118] and others described a unique peripheral neuropathy in patients who fail to wean from mechanical ventilation after an episode of critical illness, usually involving bacteremia. In a prospective study, Witt and colleagues[119] identified 43 patients with sepsis and multiple organ failure; electrophysiologic studies revealed sensorimotor axonal neuropathy in 70% of these patients, and 15 (35%) experienced difficulty in weaning from ventilatory support after improvement in their underlying conditions. Such patients display limb weakness on examination, with diminished or absent deep tendon reflexes. In the study by Witt and colleagues,[119] 23 of the patients (53%) survived; although all of the neuropathic patients improved, three with very severe neuropathy made incomplete recoveries. The authors suggested that the decrements in peripheral nerve function were related to hyperglycemia and hypoalbuminemia. They speculated that the likely etiologies of this neuropathy include the metabolic stresses that accompany sepsis, as well as the microcirculatory abnormalities. A study of other neurologic causes of failure to wean from ventilatory support has been reported, and emphasizes the high frequency of neuromuscular diseases in ICU patients with respiratory failure.[120] Interestingly, in general ICU patients, failure to wean from a neurologic cause carries a better prognosis than does similar failure due to a pulmonary cause.[121]

Patients who have flaccid paralysis after the use of NMJ blockers have received considerable attention in recent years. One group, with a relatively brief duration of paralysis, represents patients who have accumulated large amounts of these agents and take days to clear them. A second group, most commonly including asthmatics and other patients treated with steroids in addition to NMJ blockade, appears to have a myopathy, and the patients may take a very long time to recover. While earlier reports emphasized a relationship with the steroid-based NMJ-blocking drugs, this condition has been seen with atracurium as well.

Plasmapheresis is well established as a treatment for acute idiopathic polyneuritis (Guillain-Barré syndrome) if it is started in the first 2 weeks after onset. Usually, five treatments are given over 10 days. Ventilatory support is initiated as described above for myasthenia gravis. Autonomic instability may appear in the second week of the illness, and has become a leading cause of death. Thus, patients need careful observation until they are clearly improving. IVIg is also commonly used for both acute idiopathic polyneuritis and myasthenia gravis.

Neuroleptic Malignant Syndrome

The neuroleptic malignant syndrome (NMS) was recognized in the late 1950s.[122] It occurs in <1% of patients exposed to these agents, but may be more frequent in patients requiring higher than normal doses or multiple agents.[123] Although some agents have been more frequently associated with NMS than others (most prominently haloperidol, fluphenazine, and the thioxanthines), it has been reported with almost every neuroleptic agent and mixed dopamine-serotonin agents. Long-acting forms of haloperidol may result in more cases in the next several years. It may also occur in parkinsonian patients from whom either dopaminergic agonists or anticholinergic agents are abruptly withdrawn,[124] although the epidemiology of this problem is uncertain. Early studies cite a mortality rate of up to 20%,[123] although more recent work suggests approximately 4% to be correct.[125]

The condition appears to stem from central dopaminergic blockade in the majority of cases;[126] the few reports of parkinsonian patients who develop the condition when dopaminergic therapy is terminated suggest that lack of dopamine effect alone, rather than some other effect on the receptor, is necessary and sufficient to produce NMS. Drugs with stronger D_2-receptor antagonist effects are more likely to produce NMS. A patient with a mutation in the D_2 receptor has been reported.[127] Dopaminergic blockade may also affect thermoregulation by altering the hypothalamic set-point for temperature.

Most cases occur within a few weeks of either a dosage increase or, less commonly, the start of neuroleptic treatment.[128] Reported predispositions include strenuous exercise, dehydration, other CNS disorders, and the use of fluphenazine decanoate.[129] States of diminished osmolality may contribute to the pathogenesis of NMS.[130]

The major diagnostic findings of NMS include fever, severe rigidity (usually, but not always, accompanied by tremor), obtundation, and autonomic dysfunction (diaphoresis, pallor, unstable blood pressure, tachycardia, tachypnea, and pulmonary congestion).[131] Kurlan and colleagues[128] reviewed 52 published cases, summarized in Table 8.

NMS patients typically have a mild to marked leukocytosis.[132] The combination of sustained muscular contraction and immobility predisposes these patients to rhabdomyolysis; in combination with volume depletion, this often produces acute renal failure. The differential diagnosis of rhabdomyolysis in association with acute CNS dysfunction is extensive; Table 9 is adapted from the review by Bertorini.[44]

Table 8. *Clinical Findings in NMS**

Feature	% Affected
Systemic findings	
Fever	100
Tachycardia	79
Diaphoresis	60
Labile blood pressure	54
Tachypnea	25
Movement-related findings	98
Tremor	56
Dystonia	33[†]
Chorea	15
Other neurologic findings	
Dysphagia	40
Akinetic mutism	38
Stupor	27
Coma	27

*Data from Kurlan and colleagues.[128]
†Includes 6% with oculogyric crises.

Other common systemic complications include disseminated intravascular coagulation and pulmonary embolism. Thrombocytopenia has recently been reported.[133]

The major differential diagnostic concerns are malignant hyperthermia (MH), the serotonin syndrome, and lethal catatonia.

Once NMS is suspected, neuroleptic drugs should be withdrawn and the patient adequately hydrated. Whether to administer dopaminergic agonists (*eg*, bromocriptine) or a direct muscle relaxant[134] (dantrolene) remains the subject of debate. Dantrolene relaxes muscle contraction by decreasing Ca^{2+} release from the sarcoplasmic reticulum. Electroconvulsive therapy has also been proposed as a treatment,[135] blurring the distinction between NMS and lethal catatonia. Neuroleptic medications should not be resumed for at least 2 weeks because of the risk of recurrence.[136]

Malignant Hyperthermia

MH was recognized as an anesthetic complication in the 1960s.[137] It is an autosomal-dominant disorder that most typically follows exposure to anesthetic agents. A porcine model and several clinical studies have implicated abnormally high levels of Ca^{2+} release from a sarcoplasmic calcium channel (also known as the ryanodine receptor). This results in Ca^{2+}-induced Ca^{2+} release, which lowers the threshold for sustained muscle

Table 9. *Differential Diagnosis of Rhabdomyolysis in Association With Acute CNS Dysfunction**

Myofiber Metabolic Exhaustion
  Seizures
  Delirium
  Tetanus
  Strychnine intoxication
  Extremes of environmental temperature
  Malignant hyperthermia
  Neuroleptic malignant syndrome
  Diabetic ketoacidosis
  Electric shock
Infectious Myositides
  Influenza
  HIV
  Toxic shock
  Clostridial myonecrosis (*Clostridium perfringens* bacteremia)
Toxins and Abused Drugs
  Alcohol
  Cocaine and other central stimulants
  LSD
  Narcotics
  Phencyclidine
  Envenomations (wasps, bees, spiders, snakes, etc)
  Medications
  Salicylate overdose
  Theophylline
  Lithium
Fluid and Electrolyte Disturbances
  Hyperosmolar states
  Hypo-osmolar states
  Severe hypophosphatemia
  Trauma

Adapted from Bertorini.[44]

contracture.[138] (Most human cases are associated with a defect on chromosome 19, although a few cases are not associated with the defined ryanodine-receptor abnormality.[139]) The drugs that induce MH do so by triggering this Ca^{2+} release; the sustained contraction produced by Ca^{2+} release causes excessive oxygen consumption and heat production. High-energy phosphate stores are quickly depleted, resulting in failure of Ca^{2+} reuptake. As in other cells, sustained excessive elevation of free intracellular Ca^{2+} produces membrane lysis, and consequently myoglobin leaks from muscle cells.

MH begins with muscle contraction (classically, although not always, in the masseters) in response to a triggering agent (Table 10).

In a typical anesthetic-induced case, a rise in end-tidal CO_2 often signifies MH onset.[140] Quickly thereafter, rapidly rising temperature, metabolic acidosis, hypoxemia, and cardiac

Table 10. *Triggering Agents in Malignant Hyperthermia*

Recognized Agents

Inhalational anesthetics	Desflurane
	Enflurane
	Halothane (most common)
	Isoflurane
	Sevoflurane
Depolarizing NMJ blockers	Decamethonium
	Succinylcholine (most common)
	Suxamethonium

Possible Agents
Calcium
Catecholamines
Ketamine
Monoamine oxidase inhibitors
Phenothiazines
Potassium

"Safe Agents"
Barbiturates
β-Blockers
Benzodiazepines
Local anesthetics
Nitrous oxide
Nondepolarizing NMJ blockers
Propofol

arrhythmias may follow. The combination of muscle breakdown and acidosis results in hyperkalemia. On rare occasions, the condition may not arise until after the operation is over, or may occur in other situations of metabolic stress, such as exercise.

A personal or appropriate family history of anesthetic complications is usually sufficient reason to suspect MH, and to consider *in vitro* muscle testing where it is available. A muscle biopsy specimen (obtained under local anesthesia) is electrically stimulated during exposure to varying concentrations of caffeine or halothane. Patients with other muscle diseases, such as central core disease, dystrophinopathies, and several others, may be at risk for MH-like reactions. Muscle biopsies from MH patients are frequently abnormal, but not specifically so.[44]

The major management issues in MH involve termination of exposure to the triggering agent and the use of dantrolene.

Serotonin Syndrome

In 1955, a patient died after taking a combination of iproniazid and meperidine.[141] By 1960, the serotonin syndrome (SS) was well described.[142] Most patients with SS are receiving more than one serotonergic agent (or a monoamine oxidase inhibitor, raising extracellular serotonin concentrations), although overdoses of single agents may trigger the syndrome.[143] The newer reversible monoamine oxidase inhibitors, such as moclobemide, may be less likely to precipitate SS[144] but are not devoid of this potential.[145] SS resembles NMS, but is frequently associated with myoclonus, and less frequently involves muscle rigidity.[146] Autonomic instability is common in both conditions.[147] The duration of SS is usually shorter than that of NMS. A case of SS also involving stroke in a young patient suggests that the spectrum of this disorder may involve precipitation of complicated migraine.[148] Treatment is supportive.

Lethal Catatonia

Lethal catatonia was described by Stauder in 1934, almost half a decade before the introduction of neuroleptic agents. The presentation of lethal catatonia is essentially indistinguishable from NMS, although published case reports of the two syndromes indicate differences in mode of onset, signs and symptoms, and outcome.[149] Lethal catatonia often begins with extreme psychotic excitement, which leads to fever, exhaustion, and death. In contrast, NMS begins with severe muscle rigidity. Lethal catatonia may require neuroleptic treatment, although electroconvulsive therapy is more commonly employed. Occasional reports of cases "requiring" treatment with both electroconvulsive therapy and dantrolene serve to blur the distinction between lethal catatonia and NMS.[150] The underlying pathophysiology of lethal catatonia remains unknown.

References

1. Wilks S. Bromide and iodide of potassium in epilepsy. Med Times Gaz (Lond) 1861; 2:635–636
2. Gowers WR. Epilepsy and other chronic convulsive diseases: their causes, symptoms, and treatment. London, UK: J. and A. Churchill, 1881
3. Bleck TP, Klawans HL. Mechanisms of epilepsy and anticonvulsant action. In: Klawans HL, Goetz CG, Tanner CM, eds. Textbook of clinical neuropharmacology. New York, NY: Raven Press, 1992; 23–30

4. Weschler IS. Intravenous injection of paraldehyde for control of convulsions. JAMA 1940; 114:2198

5. Gastaut H, Naquet R, Poiré R, et al. Treatment of status epilepticus with diazepam (Valium). Epilepsia 1965; 6:167–182

6. Wijdicks EFM, Sharbrough FW. New-onset seizures in critically ill patients. Neurology 1993; 43:1042–1044

7. Bleck TP, Smith MC, Pierre-Louis JC, et al. Neurologic complications of critical medical illnesses. Crit Care Med 1993; 21:98–103

8. Hauser WA. Status epilepticus: epidemiologic considerations. Neurology 1990; 40(suppl 2):9–13

9. DeLorenzo RJ, Towne AR, Pellock JM, et al. Status epilepticus in children, adults, and the elderly. Epilepsia 1992; 33(suppl 4):S15–S25

10. Aminoff MJ, Simon RP. Status epilepticus: causes, clinical features and consequences in 98 patients. Am J Med 1980; 69:657–666

11. Lowenstein DH, Alldredge BK. Status epilepticus in an urban public hospital in the 1980s. Neurology 1993; 42:483–488

12. Bleck TP. Status epilepticus. University Reports on Epilepsy 1992; 1:1–7

13. Ettinger AB, Shinnar S. New-onset seizures in an elderly hospitalized population. Neurology 1993; 43:489–492

14. Proposal for revised clinical and electroencephalographic classification of epileptic seizures: from the Commission on Classification and Terminology of the International League Against Epilepsy. Epilepsia 1981; 22:489–501

15. Bleck TP. Metabolic encephalopathy. In: Weiner WJ, ed. Emergent and urgent neurology. Philadelphia, PA: Lippincott, 1991; 27–57

16. Bleck TP. Status epilepticus. In: Klawans HL, Goetz CG, Tanner CM, eds. Textbook of clinical neuropharmacology. 2nd ed. New York, NY: Raven Press, 1992; 65–73

17. Lothman EW. The biochemical basis and pathophysiology of status epilepticus. Neurology 1990; 40(suppl 2):13–23

18. Lowenstein DH, Simon RP, Sharp FR. The pattern of 72-kDa heat shock protein-like immunoreactivity in the rat brain following fluothyl-induced status epilepticus. Brain Res 1990; 531:173–182

19. Wasterlain CG, Fujikawa DG, Penix L, et al. Pathophysiological mechanisms of brain damage from status epilepticus. Epilepsia 1993; 34(suppl 1):S37–S53

20. Treiman DM. Generalized convulsive status epilepticus in the adult. Epilepsia 1993; 34(suppl 1) S2–S11

21. Walton NY. Systemic effects of generalized convulsive status epilepticus. Epilepsia 1993; 34 (suppl 1):S54–S58

22. Bolton CF, Young GB, Zochodne DW. The neurologic complications of sepsis. Ann Neurol 1993; 33:94–100

23. Rowbotham MC; Lowenstein DH. Neurologic complications of cocaine use. Annu Rev Med 1990; 41:417–422

24. Randomized clinical trial of the efficacy of antiepileptic drugs in reducing the risk of relapse after a first unprovoked tonic-clonic seizure: First Seizure Trial Group (FIR.S.T. Group). Neurology 1993; 43:478–483

25. Smith MC, Bleck TP. Toxicity of anticonvulsants. In: Klawans HL, Goetz CG, Tanner CM, eds. Textbook of clinical neuropharmacology. 2nd ed. New York, NY: Raven Press, 1992; 45–64

26. Mitchell WG. Status epilepticus and acute repetitive seizures in children, adolescents, and young adults: etiology, outcome, and treatment. Epilepsia 1996; 37(suppl 1):S74–S80

27. Bebin EM. Additional modalities for treating acute seizures in children: overview. J Child Neurol 1998; 13(suppl 1):S23–S26

28. Dreifuss FE, Rosman NP, Cloyd JC, et al. A comparison of rectal diazepam gel and placebo for acute repetitive seizures. N Engl J Med 1998; 338: 1869–1875

29. Chang CWJ, Bleck TP. Status epilepticus. Neurol Clin 1995; 13:529–548

30. Treiman DM, Meyers PD, Walton NY, et al. A comparison of four treatments for generalized convulsive status epilepticus: Veterans Affairs Status Epilepticus Cooperative Study Group. N Engl J Med 1998; 339:792–798

31. Leppik IE, Derivan AT, Homan RW, et al. Double-blind study of lorazepam and diazepam in status epilepticus. JAMA 1983; 249:1452–1454

32. Bebin M, Bleck TP. New anticonvulsant drugs. Drugs 1994; 48:153–171

33. Graves N. Pharmacoeconomic considerations in treatment options for acute seizures. J Child Neurol 1998; 13(suppl 1):S27–S29

34. Walton NY, Treiman DM. Valproic acid treatment of experimental status epilepticus. Epilepsy Res 1992; 12:199–205

35. Bleck TP. Refractory status epilepticus in 2001. Arch Neurol 2002; 59:188–189

36. Bleck TP. Electroencephalographic monitoring. In: Tobin MR, ed. Principles and practice of intensive care monitoring. New York, NY: McGraw Hill, 1998; 1035–1046

37. Kumar A, Bleck TP. Intravenous midazolam for the treatment of refractory status epilepticus. Crit Care Med 1992; 20:483–488

38. Labar DR, Ali A, Root J. High-dose intravenous lorazepam for the treatment of refractory status epilepticus. Neurology 1994; 44:1400–1403

39. Stecker MM, Kramer TH, Raps EC, et al. Treatment of refractory status epilepticus with propofol: clinical and pharmacokinetic findings. Epilepsia 1998; 39:18–26

40. Huff JS, Bleck TP. Propofol in the treatment of refractory status epilepticus. Acad Emerg Med 1996; 3:179

41. Prasad A, Worrall BB, Bertram EB, et al. Propofol and midazolam in the treatment of refractory status epilepticus. Epilepsia 2001; 42:380–386

42. Galley HF, Dubbels AM, Webster NR. The effect of midazolam and propofol on interleukin-8 from human polymorphonuclear leukocytes. Anesth Analg 1998; 86:1289–1293

43. Weise KL, Bleck TP. Status epilepticus in children and adults. Crit Care Clin 1997; 14:629–646

44. Bertorini TE. Myoglobinuria, malignant hyperthermia, neuroleptic malignant syndrome and serotonin syndrome. Neurol Clin 1997; 15:649–671

45. Dodrill CB, Wilensky AJ. Intellectual impairment as an outcome of status epilepticus. Neurology 1990; 40(suppl 2):23–27

46. Treiman DM, Delgado-Escueta AV. Complex partial status epilepticus. Adv Neurol 1983; 34:69–81

47. Lothman EW, Bertram EH. Epileptogenic effects of status epilepticus. Epilepsia 1993; 34(suppl 1): S59–S70

48. Borris DJ, Bertram EH, Kapur J. Ketamine controls prolonged status epilepticus. Epilepsy Res 2000; 42:117–122

49. Kassell NF, Torner JC. Aneurysmal rebleeding: a preliminary report from the Cooperative Aneurysm Study. Neurosurgery 1983; 13:479–481

50. Nishioka H, Torner JC, Graf CJ, et al. Cooperative study of intracranial aneurysms and subarachnoid hemorrhage: a long-term prognostic study. II. Ruptured intracranial aneurysms managed conservatively. Arch Neurol 1984; 41:1142–1146

51. Torner JC, Kassell NF, Wallace RB, et al. Preoperative prognostic factors for rebleeding and survival in aneurysm patients receiving antifibrinolytic therapy: a report of the cooperative aneurysm study. Neurosurgery 1981; 9:506–513

52. Solenski NJ, Haley EC Jr, Kassell NF, et al. Medical complications of aneurysmal subarachnoid hemorrhage: a report of the multicenter, cooperative aneurysm study. Crit Care Med 1995:23:1007–1017

53. Biller J, Godersky JC, Adams HP Jr. Management of aneurysmal subarachnoid hemorrhage. Stroke 1988; 19:1300–1305

54. Hasan D, Wijdicks EF, Vermeulen M. Hyponatremia is associated with cerebral ischemia in patients with aneurysmal subarachnoid hemorrhage. Ann Neurol 1990; 27:106–108

55. von Holst H, Ericson K, Haberbeck-Modesto M, et al. Angiographic investigation of cerebral vasospasm in subarachnoid haemorrhage due to arteriovenous malformation. Acta Neurochir (Wien) 1988; 94:129–132

56. Kothbauer K, Schroth G, Seiler RW, et al. Severe symptomatic vasospasm after rupture of an arteriovenous malformation. AJNR Am J Neuroradiol 1995; 16:1073–1075

57. Taneda M, Kataoka K, Akai F, et al. Traumatic subarachnoid hemorrhage as a predictable indicator of delayed ischemic symptoms. J Neurosurg 1996; 84:762–768

58. Kordestani RK, Counelis GJ. McBride DQ, et al. Cerebral arterial spasm after penetrating craniocerebral gunshot wounds: transcranial Doppler and cerebral blood flow findings. Neurosurgery 1997; 41:351–359

59. Macdonald RL, Weir B. Cerebral vasospasm: prevention and treatment. In: Batjer HH, ed. Cerebrovascular disease. Philadelphia, PA: Lippincott-Raven, 1997; 1111–1121

60. Vorkapic P, Bevan JA, Bevan RD. Longitudinal *in vivo* and in vitro time-course study of chronic cerebrovasospasm in the rabbit basilar artery. Neurosurg Rev 1991; 14:215–219

61. Macdonald RL, Weir BKA. A review of hemoglobin and the pathogenesis of cerebral vasospasm. Stroke 1991; 22:971–982

62. Pluta RM, Boock RJ, Afshar JK, et al. Source and cause of endothelin-1 release into cerebrospinal fluid after subarachnoid hemorrhage. J Neurosurg 1997; 87:287–293

63. Kwan AL, Bavbek M, Jeng AY, et al. Prevention and reversal of cerebral vasospasm by an endothelin-converting enzyme inhibitor, CGS 26303, in an experimental model of subarachnoid hemorrhage. J Neurosurg 1997; 87:281–286

64. Qureshi AI, Sung GY, Suri MA, et al. Prognostic value and determinants of ultraearly angiographic vasospasm after aneurysmal subarachnoid hemorrhage. Neurosurgery 1999; 44:967–973

65. Fisher CM, Kistler JP, Davis JM. Relation of cerebral vasospasm to subarachnoid hemorrhage visualized by computerized tomographic scanning. Neurosurgery 1980; 6:1–9

66. Haley EC Jr, Torner JC, Kassell NF. Antifibrinolytic therapy and cerebral vasospasm. Neurosurg Clin N Am 1990; 1:349–356

67. Wass CT, Lanier WL. Glucose modulation of ischemic brain injury: review and clinical recommendations. Mayo Clin Proc 1996; 71:801–812

68. Lanzino G, Kassell NF, Germanson T, et al. Plasma glucose levels and outcome after aneurysmal subarachnoid hemorrhage. J Neurosurg 1993; 79:885–891

69. Doczi T, Bende J, Huszka E, et al. Syndrome of inappropriate secretion of antidiuretic hormone after subarachnoid hemorrhage. Neurosurgery 1981; 9:394–397

70. Harringan MR. Cerebral salt wasting syndrome: a review. Neurosurgery 1996; 38:152–160

71. Wijdicks EF, Schievink WI, Burnett JC Jr. Natriuretic peptide system and endothelin in aneurysmal subarachnoid hemorrhage. J Neurosurg 1997; 87:275–280

72. Wijdicks EF, Vermeulen M, ten Haaf JA, et al. Volume depletion and natriuresis in patients with a ruptured intracranial aneurysm. Ann Neurol 1985; 18:211–216

73. Hasan D, Vermeulen M, Wijdicks EF, et al. Effect of fluid intake and antihypertensive treatment on cerebral ischemia after subarachnoid hemorrhage. Stroke 1989; 20:1511–1515

74. Pinto AN, Canhao P Ferro JM. Seizures at the onset of subarachnoid haemorrhage. J Neurol 1996; 243:161–164

75. Baker CJ, Prestigiacomo CJ, Solomon RA. Short-term perioperative anticonvulsant prophylaxis for the surgical treatment of low-risk patients with intracranial aneurysms. Neurosurgery 1995; 37:863–870

76. Schoser BG, Heesen C, Eckert B, et al. Cerebral hyperperfusion injury after percutaneous transluminal angioplasty of extracranial arteries. J Neurol 1997; 244:101–104

77. Talavera JO, Wacher NH, Laredo F, et al. Predictive value of signs and symptoms in the diagnosis of subarachnoid hemorrhage among stroke patients. Arch Med Res 1996; 27:353–357

78. Kabuto H, Yokoi I, Habu H, et al. Reduction in nitric oxide synthase activity with development of an epileptogenic focus induced by ferric chloride in the rat brain. Epilepsy Res 1996; 25:65–68

79. Lanzino G, Kongable G, Kassell N. Electrographic abnormalities after nontraumatic subarachnoid hemorrhage. J Neurosurg Anesth 1994; 6:156–162

80. Brouwers PJ, Wijdicks EF, Hasan D, et al. Serial electrocardiographic recording in aneurysmal subarachnoid hemorrhage. Stroke 1989; 20:1162–1167

81. Provencio JJ, Bleck TP. Cardiovascular disorders related to neurologic and neurosurgical emergencies. In: Cruz J, ed. Neurologic and neurosurgical emergencies. Philadelphia, PA: WB Saunders, 1997; 39–50

82. Zaroff JG, Rordorf GA, Newell JB, et al. Cardiac outcome in patients with subarachnoid hemorrhage and electrocardiographic abnormalities. Neurosurgery 1999; 44:34–39

83. Mayer SA, Lin J, Homma S, et al. Myocardial injury and left ventricular performance after subarachnoid hemorrhage. Stroke 1999; 30:780–786

84. Mayer SA. LiMandri G. Sherman D, et al. Electrocardiographic markers of abnormal left ventricular wall motion in acute subarachnoid hemorrhage. J Neurosurg 1995; 83:889–896

85. Vespa P, Bleck TP, Brock DG, et al. Impaired oxygenation after acute aneurysmal subarachnoid hemorrhage [abstract]. Neurology 1994; 44(suppl 1):A344

86. Touho H, Karasawa J, Shishido H, et al. Neurogenic pulmonary edema in the acute stage of hemorrhagic cerebrovascular disease. Neurosurgery 1989; 25:762–768

87. Haley EC Jr, Kassell NF, Apperson-Hansen C, et al. A randomized, double-blind, vehicle-controlled trial of tirilazad mesylate in patients with aneurysmal subarachnoid hemorrhage: a cooperative study in North America. J Neurosurg 1997; 86:467–474

88. Rouby JJ, Laurent P, Gosnach M, et al. Risk factors and clinical relevance of nosocomial maxillary sinusitis in the critically ill. Am J Respir Crit Care Med 1994; 150:776–783

89. Sundt TM Jr, Kobayashi S, Fode NC, et al. Results and complications of surgical management of 809 intracranial aneurysms in 722 cases: related and unrelated to grade of patient, type of aneurysm, and timing of surgery. J Neurosurg 1982; 56: 753–765

90. Leipzig TJ, Redelman K, Horner TG. Reducing the risk of rebleeding before early aneurysm surgery: a possible role for antifibrinolytic therapy. J Neurosurg 1997; 86:220–225

91. Fletcher AP, Alkjaersig N, Davies A, et al. Blood coagulation and plasma fibrinolytic enzyme system pathophysiology in stroke. Stroke 1976; 7: 337–348

92. Kirsch JR, D'Alecy LG. Effect of altered availability of energy-yielding substrates upon survival from hypoxia in mice. Stroke 1979; 10:288–291

93. Hersio K, Vapalahti M, Kari A, et al. Impaired utilization of exogenous amino acids after surgery for subarachnoid haemorrhage. Acta Neurochir (Wien) 1990; 106:13–17

94. Mayberg MR, Batjer HH, Dacey R, et al. Guidelines for the management of aneurysmal subarachnoid hemorrhage: a statement for healthcare professionals from a special writing group of the Stroke Council, American Heart Association. Stroke 1994; 25:2315–2328

95. Findlay JM. Current management of aneurysmal subarachnoid hemorrhage guidelines from the Canadian Neurosurgical Society. Can J Neurol Sci 1997; 24:161–170

96. Levy M, Giannotta S. Cardiac performance indices during hypervolemic therapy for cerebral vasospasm. J Neurosurg 1991; 75:27–31

97. Clyde BL, Resnick DK, Yonas H, et al. The relationship of blood velocity as measured by transcranial doppler ultrasonography to cerebral blood flow as determined by stable xenon computed tomographic studies after aneurysmal subarachnoid hemorrhage. Neurosurgery 1996; 38:896–904

98. Adams HP Jr. Calcium antagonists in the management of patients with aneurysmal subarachnoid hemorrhage: a review. Angiology 1990; 41 (11 pt 2):1010–1016

99. Haley EC Jr, Kassell NF, Torner JC. A randomized trial of nicardipine in subarachnoid hemorrhage: angiographic and transcranial Doppler ultrasound results; a report of the Cooperative Aneurysm Study. J Neurosurg 1993; 78:548–553

100. Kassell NF, Haley EC Jr, Apperson-Hansen C, et al. Randomized, double-blind, vehicle-controlled trial of tirilazad mesylate in patients with aneurysmal subarachnoid hemorrhage: a cooperative study in Europe, Australia, and New Zealand. J Neurosurg 1996; 84:221–228

101. Fleishaker JC, Fiedler-Kelly J, Grasela TH. Population phamacokinetics of tirilazad: effects of weight, gender, concomitant phenytoin, and subarachnoid hemorrhage. Pharm Res 1999; 16:575–583

102. Hall ED, Andrus PK, Smith SL, et al. Pyrrolopyrimidines: novel brain-penetrating antioxidants with neuroprotective activity in brain injury and ischemia models. J Pharmacol Exp Ther 1997; 281:895–904

103. Kassell NF, Peerless SJ, Durward QJ, et al. Treatment of ischemic deficits from vasospasm with intravascular volume expansion and induced arterial hypertension. Neurosurgery 1982; 11:337–343

104. Oropello JM, Weiner L, Benjamin E. Hypertensive, hypervolemic, hemodilutional therapy for aneurysmal subarachnoid hemorrhage: is it efficacious? No. Crit Care Clin 1996; 12:709–730

105. Ullman JS, Bederson JB. Hypertensive, hypervolemic, hemodilutional therapy for aneurysmal subarachnoid hemorrhage: is it efficacious? Yes. Crit Care Clin 1996; 12:697–707

106. Amin-Hanjani S, Schwartz RB, Sathi S, et al. Hypertensive encephalopathy as a complication of hyperdynamic therapy for vasospasm: report of two cases. Neurosurgery 1999; 44:1113–1116

107. Firlik KS, Kaufmann AM, Firlik AD, et al. Intra-arterial papaverine for the treatment of cerebral vasospasm following aneurysmal subarachnoid hemorrhage. Surg Neurol 1999; 51:66–74

108. Thomas JE, Rosenwasser RH. Reversal of severe cerebral vasospasm in three patients after aneurysmal subarachnoid hemorrhage: initial observations regarding the use of intraventricular sodium nitroprusside in humans. Neurosurgery 1999; 44:48–57

109. Bleck TP. Metabolic encephalopathy. In: Weiner WJ, Shulman LM, eds. Emergent and urgent neurology. 2nd ed. Philadelphia, PA: Lippincott, 1999; 223–253

110. Bleck TP, Henson S. Sources of fever in patients after surgery for aneurysmal subarachnoid hemorrhage. Crit Care Med 1992; 20(suppl):S31

111. Paramore CG, Turner DA. Relative risks of ventriculostomy infection and morbidity. Acta Neurochir (Wien) 1994; 127:79–84

112. Deutschman CS, Wilton PB, Sinow J, et al. Paranasal sinusitis: a common complication of nasotracheal intubation in neurosurgical patients. Neurosurgery 1985; 17:296–299

113. Jacobs DG, Piotrowski JJ, Hoppensteadt DA, et al. Hemodynamic and fibrinolytic consequences of intermittent pneumatic compression: preliminary results. J Trauma 1996; 40:710–716

114. Swann KW, Black PM, Baker MF. Management of symptomatic deep venous thrombosis and pulmonary embolism on a neurosurgical service. J Neurosurg 1986; 64:563–567

115. Takaku A, Tanaka S, Mori T, et al. Postoperative complications in 1,000 cases of intracranial aneurysms. Surg Neurol 1979; 12:137–144

115a. Mayer SA, Brun NC, Begtrup K, et al. Recombinant activated factor VII for acute intracerebral hemorrage. N Engl J Med 2005; 352:777–785

116. Tissue plasminogen activator for acute ischemic stroke: The National Institute of Neurological Disorders and Stroke rt-PA Stroke Study Group. N Engl J Med 1995; 333:1581–1587

117. Roelofs RI, Cerra F, Bielka N, et al. Prolonged respiratory insufficiency due to acute motor neuropathy: a new syndrome. Neurology 1983; 33(suppl 2):240

118. Zochodne W, Bolton CF, Wells GA, et al. Critical illness polyneuropathy: a complication of sepsis and multiple organ failure. Brain 1987; 110:819–842

119. Witt NJ, Zochodne DW, Bolton CF, et al. Peripheral nerve function in sepsis and multiple organ failure. Chest 1991; 99:176–184

120. Spitzer AR, Giancarlo T, Maher L, et al. Neuromuscular causes of prolonged ventilator dependency. Muscle Nerve 1992; 15:682–686

121. Kelly BJ, Luce JM. The diagnosis and management of neuromuscular diseases causing respiratory failure. Chest 1991; 99:1485–1494

122. Preston J. Central nervous system reaction to small doses of tranquilizers: report of one death. American Practitoner and Digest of Treatment 1959; 10:627–630

123. Caroff SN, Mann SC. The neuroleptic malignant syndrome. J Clin Psychiatr 1908; 41:79–83

124. Keyser DL, Rodnitzky RL. Neuroleptic malignant syndrome in Parkinson's disease after withdrawal or alteration of dopaminergic therapy. Arch Intern Med 1977; 86:794–796

125. Addonizio G, Susman VL, Roth SD. Neuroleptic malignant syndrome: review and analysis of 115 cases. Biol Psychiatr 1987; 22:1004–1020

126. Henderson VM, Wooten GF. Neuroleptic malignant syndrome: a pathogenetic role for dopamine receptor blockade? Neurology 1981; 31:132–137

127. Ram A, Cao Q, Keck PE Jr, et al. Structural change in dopamine D_2 receptor gene in a patient with neuroleptic malignant syndrome. Am J Med Genet 1995; 60:228–230

128. Kurlan R, Hamill R, Shoulson I. Neuroleptic malignant syndrome. Clin Neuropharmacol 1984; 7:109–120

129. Guzé BH, Baxter LR. Neuroleptic malignant syndrome. N Engl J Med 1985; 313:163–166

130. Wedzicha JA, Hoffbrand BI. Neuroleptic malignant syndrome and hyponatraemia. Lancet 1984; 1:963

131. Weiner WJ, Lang AE. Movement disorders: a comprehensive survey. Mount Kisco, NY: Futura Publishing Co, 1989; 617

132. Keyser DL, Rodnitzky RL. Neuroleptic malignant syndrome in Parkinson's disease after withdrawal or alteration of dopaminergic therapy. Arch Intern Med 1991; 151:794-796

133. Ray JG. Neuroleptic malignant syndrome associated with severe thrombocytopenia. J Intern Med 1997; 241:245–247

134. Buckley PF, Hutchinson M. Neuroleptic malignant syndrome. J Neurol Neurosurg Psychiatr 1995; 58:271–278

135. Addonizio G, Susman VL. ECT as a treatment alternative for patients with symptoms of neuroleptic malignant syndrome. J Clin Psychiatry 1987; 48:102–105

136. Susman VL, Addonizio G. Recurrence of neuroleptic malignant syndrome. J Nerv Ment Dis 1988; 176:234–241

137. Denborough MA, Lovell RRH. Anaesthetic deaths in a family. Lancet 1960; 2:45–46

138. El-Hayek R, Yano M, Antonui B, et al. Altered E-C coupling in trials isolated from malignant hyperthermia-susceptible porcine muscle. Am J Physiol 1995; 268(6 pt 1):C1831

139. Gronert GA, Mott J, Lee J. Aetiology of malignant hyperthermia. Br J Anaesth 1988; 60:253–260

140. Struebing VL. Differential diagnosis of malignant hyperthermia: a case report. AANA J 1995; 63: 455–460

141. Mitchell RS. Fatal toxic encephalitis occurring during iproniazid therapy in pulmonary tuberculosis. Ann Intern Med 1955; 42:417–419

142. Oates JA, Sjoerdsma A. Neurotoxic effects of tryptophan in patients receiving a monoamine oxidase inhibitor. Neurology 1960:10:1076–1080

143. Kolecki P. Isolated venlafaxine-induced serotonin syndrome. J Emerg Med 1997; 15:491–493

144. Hilton SE, Maradit H, Moller HJ. Serotonin syndrome and drug combinations: focus on MAOI and RIMA. Eur Arch Psychiatry Clin Neurosci 1997; 247:113–119

145. Singer PP, Jones GR. An uncommon fatality due to moclobemide and paroxetine. J Anal Toxicol 1997; 21:518–520

146. Kam PC, Chang GW. Selective serotonin reuptake inhibitors: pharmacology and clinical implications in anaesthesia and critical care medicine. Anaesthesia 1997; 52:982–988

147. Halman M, Goldbloom DS. Fluoxetine and neuroleptic malignant syndrome. Biol Psychiatry 1990; 28:518–522

148. Molaie M. Serotonin syndrome presenting with migrainelike stroke. Headache 1997; 37: 519–521

149. Castillo E, Rubin RT, Holsboer-Trachsler E. Clinical differentiation between lethal catatonia and neuroleptic malignant syndrome. Am J Psychiatry 1989; 146:324–328

150. Nolen WA, Zwaan WA. Treatment of lethal catatonia with electroconvulsive therapy and dantrolene sodium: a case report. Acta Psychiatr Scand 1990; 82:90–92

Notes

Resuscitation: Cooling, Drugs, and Fluids

Brian K. Gehlbach, MD

Objectives:

- Discuss fluid resuscitation in septic shock
- Discuss the use of focused assessment with sonography for trauma in the trauma patient
- Highlight key aspects of the 2005 Advanced Cardiac Life Support guidelines for cardiac arrest
- Review the use of therapeutic hypothermia following cardiac arrest
- Review the approach to prognostication following cardiac arrest

Key words: cardiac arrest; induced hypothermia; resuscitation; septic shock; trauma

Fluid Resuscitation in Septic Shock

Identifying Preload Reserve

In 2001, Rivers et al[1] reported the results of a randomized, controlled trial comparing usual care with an early, "goal-directed therapy" (EGDT) approach to the resuscitation of patients with severe sepsis and septic shock. Patients in the usual care group received conventional resuscitation and were transferred to beds in the ICUs as they became available. In contrast, the EGDT group received its initial treatment in the emergency department according to an algorithm designed to achieve four goals within the first 6 h of resuscitation: a central venous pressure (CVP) of 8 to 12 mm Hg, a mean arterial pressure of ≥ 65 mm Hg and ≤ 90 mm Hg, a central venous saturation of $\geq 70\%$, and a urine output of ≥ 0.5 mL/kg/h. Depending on the situation, patients received fluids (crystalloid or colloid), vasoactive drugs (including inotropes), and/or packed RBCs in order to achieve these goals. Patients in the EGDT group had a significant reduction in in-hospital mortality (30.5% vs 46.5%) when compared with the usual care group.

Although this study raises many questions—are these "goals" the best ones for this group of patients? How long should these goals be targeted?

Which conditions or situations should prompt the selection of different therapeutic goals? Which specific therapies are helpful? It is likely the case that patients who received EGDT had better outcomes, at least in part, because they received more vigorous volume resuscitation—nearly 5 L within the first 6 h, vs approximately 3.5 L in the control group. This study highlights the importance of restoring an adequate intravascular volume for the patient with septic shock, in whom functional hypovolemia due to venodilation and increased capillary permeability may be profound.

When a clinician decides to administer fluid to a patient with septic shock, the intent is generally to increase the cardiac output, and commonly the BP as well. When such a patient responds to a fluid bolus with an increase in cardiac output, the patient is said to have preload reserve. Although the study by Rivers et al[1] demonstrates the importance of urgently resuscitating the patient with septic shock, experienced clinicians recognize that a CVP target of 8 to 12 mm Hg may not be appropriate for all patients. Some patients with a CVP in this range will still have preload reserve, and other patients will not. This is because "static" measurements like the CVP and the pulmonary capillary wedge pressure are poor predictors of fluid responsiveness, not only because vigorous respiratory efforts (eg, abdominal muscle recruitment during the exhalation of a patient with COPD) can confound interpretation of the pressure tracing, but also because such values are poor surrogates for preload in critically ill patients.

When preload reserve cannot be accurately identified, the patient may receive either too little or too much fluid, both of which are likely harmful to the patient. Given the limitations of static measurements of preload reserve, other approaches have been developed. These "dynamic" indices of preload reserve, such as respiratory changes in arterial pulse pressure, exploit the fact that the heart and great vessels reside within a chamber—the thorax—in which the pressure changes with respiration, whether the patient is breathing spontaneously or receiving positive pressure ventilation. These pressure changes affect right and left ventricular preload in a cyclical manner. Empirical data suggest that the presence of preload reserve can be inferred from the physiologic responses to these changes.

For instance, in a small study by Magder et al[2] performed in spontaneously breathing patients, an inspiratory fall in the CVP of >1 mm Hg indicated preload reserve. Why might this be? In the spontaneously breathing patient, inspiration reduces pleural pressure and, consequently, right atrial pressure. This increases the driving pressure for venous return and thereby increases right ventricular preload. In the patient who is hypovolemic (or even euvolemic, which is the normal condition), the fall in right atrial pressure caused by inspiration is not "overcome" by the resulting increase in venous return and cardiac filling. If a fluid bolus is administered to such a patient, the cardiac output will rise.

In patients receiving mechanical ventilation for septic shock, the change in arterial pulse pressure with mechanical insufflation may be used to diagnose preload reserve.[3] In patients receiving mechanical ventilation, the left ventricular stroke volume, and therefore the arterial pulse pressure, is greatest at the end of the inspiratory period and least during the expiratory period two to three beats later. The reasons for this are as follows. Pressurization of the thorax with insufflation increases both the pleural and the transpulmonary pressure, reducing right ventricular preload and increasing right ventricular afterload accordingly. Simultaneously, the increase in pleural pressure and transpulmonary pressure cause a decrease in left ventricular afterload and an increase in left ventricular preload, respectively. Thus, the net effect of mechanical insufflation is to (1) increase left ventricular ejection, and (2) reduce right ventricular ejection, thereby reducing left ventricular preload several beats later during expiration. Passive expiration has the opposite effects on the right and left ventricles. Accordingly, the pulse pressure is greatest during mechanical insufflation and least during expiration. These differences are exaggerated when the patient is hypovolemic and has a reduced driving pressure for venous return.

Michard et al[3] assessed preload reserve in a cohort of patients receiving mechanical ventilation for septic shock. All patients were sedated and passive while on ventilatory support, and receiving a tidal volume of ≥ 8 mL/kg. A change in pulse pressure of $\geq 13\%$ predicted preload reserve (in this case, an increase in cardiac index by at least 15% with volume expansion) with a sensitivity of 94% and a specificity of 96%.

$$\Delta Pp\ (\%) = \frac{(Ppmax - Ppmin)}{(Ppmax + Ppmin)/2} \times 100$$

where Pp = pulse pressure, Ppmax = maximal pulse pressure, and Ppmin = minimum pulse pressure.

It is important to note that just because a patient *has* preload reserve does not mean that the patient *needs* more preload (or a higher cardiac output). You and I both have preload reserve, and yet probably do not need volume expansion at the present time. Additionally, it is important to note that the sensitivity of this technique is likely reduced somewhat at lower tidal volumes. Finally, and importantly, active respiratory efforts and arrhythmias should preclude the use of this technique. Table 1 presents a summary of important caveats regarding the use of arterial pulse pressure variation as a guide to fluid resuscitation.

Colloid vs Crystalloid

Although the colloid vs crystalloid debate continues, to date there is no convincing evidence that colloids are superior to crystalloids in the resuscitation of critically ill patients. In fact, harmful effects have been detected from some colloids (*eg*, 10% pentastarch) and in some settings (*eg*, the use of albumin in traumatic brain injury). There

Table 1. *Important Caveats for the Use of Respiratory Changes in Arterial Pulse Pressure To Guide Volume Resuscitation*

May be less sensitive when low tidal volume ventilation is used

Typically requires deep sedation (inaccurate if patient is not passive)

Arrhythmias invalidate use

Does not answer the question of whether the patient *needs* an increased preload and/or cardiac output

Resuscitation: Cooling, Drugs, and Fluids (Gehlbach)

are somewhat more data supporting the use of colloids in certain other clinical settings; for instance, the use of albumin for patients undergoing large-volume paracentesis. For patients in septic shock, however, it is the author's opinion that there is no advantage to the use of colloids over crystalloids.

Guidelines for Resuscitating the Patient With Septic Shock

1. Establish a mechanism and/or team to identify and urgently resuscitate patients with septic shock.
2. Volume expansion with crystalloid is usually indicated. Frequently, between 4 and 6 L are required. Fluid responsiveness may be assessed by examining CVP variation with breathing (in the spontaneously breathing patient), or arterial pulse pressure variation (in the patient receiving mechanical ventilation). Alternatively, fluids may be administered to achieve a goal CVP of 8 to 12 mm Hg.
3. Adequacy of perfusion may be judged by clinical criteria—mentation, urine output, peripheral extremity warmth, capillary refill, and BP—and by achieving a goal central venous saturation of >70%. These targets should be achieved within 6 h of patient presentation.
4. Transfusion of packed RBCs to achieve a hemoglobin level of ≥ 10 g/dL can be considered in the early hours of resuscitation if the central venous oxygen saturation is <70% despite adequate fluid resuscitation;
5. Treatment of hypotension despite adequate intravascular volume:
   a. If the cardiac output and/or central venous saturation is low, the presence of cardiac dysfunction should be considered, and echocardiography is indicated. Dobutamine (as with left ventricular or global dysfunction) or norepinephrine (as with right ventricular failure) may be useful.
   b. If the cardiac output and/or central venous saturation are judged to be adequate, vasopressors such as norepinephrine or vasopressin should be administered.
6. In many patients, intubation and mechanical ventilation will be required. This therapy

may be particularly useful when the targets of EGDT are unable to be achieved despite volume expansion, and when the work of breathing is elevated.

Focused Assessment With Sonography for Trauma

Focused assessment with sonography for trauma, otherwise known as FAST, examines the trauma patient for evidence of free fluid. Four areas are examined: the perihepatic and hepatorenal space, the perisplenic space, the pelvis, and the pericardium. FAST has supplanted diagnostic peritoneal lavage in some settings and in some circumstances. This technique has obvious advantages, being fast, noninvasive, and repeatable. Perhaps not surprisingly, however, the technique is highly operator dependent. It also provides limited information regarding the nature and extent of the patient's injuries, and is imperfectly sensitive in diagnosing solid organ injury, for which CT is superior.

FAST is therefore suitable as a "first-look" technology used as an adjunct to the Advanced Trauma Life Support primary survey. Used in this way, FAST may facilitate early operative intervention. A negative result from the FAST examination should not provide false reassurance, however, when the suspicion for solid organ injury is high. A summary of this approach is provided here.

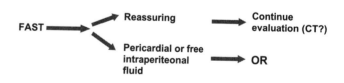

Cardiac Arrest: A Brief Review of Advanced Cardiac Life Support Guidelines

A comprehensive review of the Advanced Cardiac Life Support guidelines is beyond the scope of this review. Hopefully, many of you will have undergone recent recertification, or had occasion to use these guidelines recently in the care of patients. Following is a brief review of some of the major changes and points of emphasis highlighted in the 2005 guidelines.

1. Coronary perfusion pressure is a major determinant of survival after cardiac arrest, and it falls quickly when chest compressions stop! Data supporting this concept prompted the following recommendations:

   - A 30:2 ratio of compressions to breaths for all ages (except newborns)
   - Push hard and push fast (100 times per min) with adequate recoil and minimal interruptions
   - Minimize interruptions in chest compressions:

     Five cycles of cardiopulmonary resuscitation (CPR) between rhythm checks.
     CPR is resumed after shock for 2 min prior to rhythm check.

2. Too much breathing can be a bad thing. Excessive bagging raises pleural pressure and therefore diminishes venous return, while an obsessive focus on placing an artificial airway may hinder chest compressions. Therefore:

   - Intubation is a low priority if mask ventilation is deemed effective.
   - A 30:2 compression to ventilation ratio is appropriate prior to placing an artificial airway.
   - Once an advanced airway is placed, asynchronous ventilation at 8 to 10 breaths/min is recommended.

3. Administer fewer shocks, ideally with a biphasic defibrillator. Biphasic defibrillators are highly effective at restoring sinus rhythm when the heart is susceptible to defibrillation. If the heart is not susceptible to defibrillation, further shocks are not likely to be successful and the time spent on these shocks may dramatically reduce the efficacy of chest compressions. Therefore:

   - For ventricular fibrillation/pulseless ventricular tachycardia, administer one shock followed immediately by CPR (instead of three stacked shocks as in previous guidelines).

   Biphasic defibrillator: 200 J
   Monophasic defibrillator: 360 J

After Cardiac Arrest: Therapeutic Hypothermia

The available evidence suggests that survivors of cardiac arrest have better long-term neurologic outcomes if they are treated with mild therapeutic hypothermia. Accordingly, in the 2005 Advanced Cardiac Life Support guidelines, this strategy is given a class IIA recommendation for the unconscious adult patient with return of spontaneous circulation following out-of-hospital ventricular fibrillation arrest, and a class IIB recommendation for the unconscious adult patient with return of spontaneous circulation after non-ventricular fibrillation arrest or following an in-hospital arrest.

Although it appropriate to not "cool" patients who have significant bradycardia or active bleeding, it is the author's opinion that many patients who may benefit from this therapy are frequently not considered for it. It is true that instituting this therapy in an unstable patient can be challenging, particularly if the collective experience of the treating clinicians is low. Because of this, institutions may benefit from the creation of a therapeutic hypothermia protocol. Ideally, this protocol would also include training and/or orientation sessions and the identification of content experts available for consultation when necessary. Major elements of a therapeutic hypothermia protocol are listed in Table 2.

Prognostication After Cardiac Arrest

Intensivists are frequently asked to help predict the neurologic outcome of comatose survivors of a cardiac arrest. The approach to such patients commonly involves a combination of

Table 2. *Key Elements of Therapeutic Hypothermia*

Exclude patients with active bleeding or significant bradycardia
Target 32°C–34°C for 12–24 h
Hypothermia may be achieved with the use of endovascular cooling devices, cooled fluids, or external techniques such as cooling blankets and ice packs
Sedatives, ± paralytics ± meperidine (to prevent shivering) usually needed
Monitor metabolites and heart rate, observe for bleeding
Slow rewarming (over 6–8 h)

Resuscitation: Cooling, Drugs, and Fluids (Gehlbach)

clinical assessment and focused neurodiagnostic testing. An understanding of potential confounders in prognostication, as well as the limitations of currently available approaches, is critical for the practicing intensivist.

Potential Confounders in Prognostication

A number of medical conditions and treatments may confound prognostication, either by contributing to the patient's coma or by interfering with the various methods available for examining the brain. These confounders include organ dysfunction, metabolic derangements, shock, sepsis, sedatives and other medications, and, importantly, hypothermia! It is unclear exactly how the approach to prognostication should be modified for the patient who has been treated with therapeutic hypothermia. At a minimum, however, it seems appropriate to not begin "counting days" after arrest until after the patient has been rewarmed and any residual sedatives, narcotics, and/or muscle relaxants have been completely eliminated.

Clinical Evaluation

It is important to note that the circumstances of the arrest, including the duration of the arrest and the initial rhythm, are not adequately predictive of neurologic outcome as to be clinically useful. In contrast, the clinical findings that are most predictive of a poor long-term neurologic outcome include:

- Absent pupillary or corneal reflexes at day +3 after arrest
- Absent or extensor motor responses at day +3 after arrest
- True myoclonus status epilepticus within the first day after a primary circulatory arrest

Imaging

The role of brain imaging in prognostication is not clearly defined. Although findings compatible with anoxic brain injury and/or edema may be evident on brain scans, the prognostic value of such findings is unclear at the present time. MRI is considerably more sensitive than CT at demonstrating subtle abnormalities and may hold more promise in prognostication, but even fewer studies examining the utility of this modality postcardiac arrest have been performed.

Neurophysiologic Testing

EEG is commonly performed postarrest in order to exclude nonconvulsive status epilepticus as a cause of coma and to provide some limited prognostic information. It is important to note that the EEG literature is hampered by the use of different classification schemes and variable recording intervals after arrest. In addition, it is important to remember that the EEG is affected by sedatives and coexisting illnesses (for instance, sepsis or metabolic encephalopathy) and that it may evolve in the days following cardiac arrest. Thus, although helpful in excluding seizures and providing some limited prognostic information, EEG findings alone lack sufficient specificity to accurately predict prognosis.

Somatosensory evoked potentials are electrical potentials triggered by a stimulus applied to a peripheral nerve and generated by various components of the ascending sensory pathway. Potentials can be measured at the peripheral nerve, nerve root, spinal cord, subcortical brain structures, and the sensory cortex. The latter includes, among others, the N20 component. Bilateral absence of the N20 component of the median nerve somatosensory evoked potential on day 1 to 3 after arrest, *when present*, almost universally predicts a poor outcome.

Other Tests

A number of biochemical markers have been investigated. The most helpful is a marker called serum neuron-specific enolase. A neuron-specific enolase value of >33 μg/L at day 1 to 3 is highly predictive of a poor outcome.

An Approach to Prognostication

A practice parameter for prognostication following cardiac arrest was published in *Neurology* in 2006.[4] The decision algorithm does not attempt to incorporate therapeutic hypothermia. As mentioned previously, it is the author's opinion that patients treated with this approach should be given more time for evaluation.

References

1. Rivers E, Nguyen B, Havstad S, et al, for the Early Goal-Directed Therapy Collaborative Group. Early goal-directed therapy in the treatment of severe sepsis and septic shock. N Engl J Med 2001; 345:1368–1377
2. Magder S, Georgiadis G, Cheone T. Respiratory variations in right atrial pressure predict the response to fluid challenge. J Crit Care 1992; 7:76–85
3. Michard F, Boussat S, Chemla D, et al. Relation between respiratory changes in arterial pulse pressure and fluid responsiveness in septic patients with acute circulatory failure. Am J Respir Crit Care Med 2000; 162:134–138
4. Wijdicks EFM, Hijdra A, Young GB, et al. Practice parameter: prediction of outcome in comatose survivors after cardiopulmonary resuscitation (an evidence-based review). Report of the Quality Standards Subcommittee of the American Academy of Neurology. Neurology 2006; 67:203–210

Additional Reading

Diamond LM. Cardiopulmonary resuscitation and acute cardiovascular life support: a protocol review of the updated guidelines. Crit Care Clin 2007; 23:873–880

Geocadin RG, Koenig MA, Jia X, et al. Management of brain injury after resuscitation from cardiac arrest. Neurol Clin 2008; 26:487–506

Koenig MA, Kaplan PW, Thakor NV. Clinical neurophysiologic monitoring and brain injury from cardiac arrest. Neurol Clin 2006; 24:89–106

Korner M, Krotz MM, Degenhart C, et al. Current role of emergency US in patients with major trauma. Radiographics 2008; 28:225–244

Magder S. Central venous pressure: a useful but not so simple measurement. Crit Care Med 2006; 34:2224–2227

Pinsky MR. Hemodynamic evaluation and monitoring in the ICU. Chest 2007; 132:2020–2029

Puttgen HA, Geocadin R. Predicting neurological outcome following cardiac arrest. J Neurol Sci 2007; 261:108–117

The SAFE Study Investigators. A comparison of albumin and saline for fluid resuscitation in the intensive care unit. N Engl J Med 2004; 350:2247–2256

The SAFE Study Investigators. Saline or albumin for fluid resuscitation in patients with traumatic brain injury. N Engl J Med 2007; 357:874–884

Tiainen M, Kovala TT, Takkunen OS, et al. Somatosensory and brainstem auditory evoked potentials in cardiac arrest patients treated with hypothermia. Crit Care Med 2005; 33:1736–1740

Issues in Sedation, Paralytic Agents, and Airway Management

Michael A. Gropper, MD, PhD, FCCP

Objectives:

- Review the indications for sedative and paralytic agents and methods of administration of these agents in the ICU
- Review the pharmacokinetics and pharmacodynamics of sedative and paralytic agents
- Review techniques of airway management

Key words: assessment; cisatracurium; etomidate; fentanyl; ketamine; morphine; propofol; rocuronium; sedation; sedation interruption; vecuronium

Sedation of Critically Ill Patients

Publications from the late 1980s suggested that approximately one-half of all patients in the ICU described their period of mechanical ventilation as unpleasant and stressful, and that their time requiring mechanical ventilation was associated with fear, agony, and panic. In the late 1990s and more recently, publications have suggested that there is an association between the administration of large quantities of sedative agents in the ICU and the development of posttraumatic stress disorders and memory problems in the recipients.[1] Furthermore, there have now been investigations that have documented undesirable outcomes associated with the administration of large quantities of sedatives. These outcomes include delayed weaning from mechanical ventilation, significantly prolonged length of stays in the ICU and in the hospital,[2,3] significantly increased acquisition of CT scans for patients because of depressed mental function,[3] and an increased incidence of nosocomial pneumonia in patients receiving sedation and paralytic agents.[4] More recently, it has been suggested that excessive sedation has even been shown to result in increased mortality.[5] Therefore, the present-day conundrum is how to appropriately sedate patients in the ICU to prevent their fear and anxiety, and which agents to use.

Assessment of Sedation

There is no consensus as to what level of sedation is optimal for patients in the ICU; most likely, the optimal level of sedation will vary depending on the underlying physical and mental problems of each patient and the level of movement that is safe for the patient. An investigation[6] documented that the more severely ill a patient is in the ICU, the less the patients remember about their ICU experience. The more severely ill patients tend to receive more sedation because they require mechanical ventilation for more prolonged periods, and there is some question whether their illness and their medicines may affect short-term memory.[6] More is being discovered about the effects of sedatives on cognition, memory, and learning; precise goals may eventually be possible (ie, anxiolysis without decreased cognition). Furthermore, we may be able to achieve some anxiolysis with nonpharmacologic interventions; relaxation tapes, warm milk, and herbal tea were shown to be useful in the treatment of hospitalized elderly patients because the administration of these adjunctive "therapies" decreased the need for sedation and decreased the incidence of delirium.[7]

Despite the lack of consensus and our incomplete knowledge, sedation should be administered only after an assessment of the patient is done. Thus, some quantitative assessment of a patient's anxiety should be made before the administration of medication; the patient then should be reassessed after receiving the drug. The most common assessment tool used is the Ramsay scale (Table 1). The Ramsay scale is a 6-point scale that describes the patient as anxious and agitated (+3) to unresponsive (level -3). The scale includes an assessment of movement; thus, that the administration of neuromuscular blockade would preclude the use of this assessment tool. Titration of sedative agents to these scoring systems allows continuous assessment of the appropriate amount of sedative

Table 1. *Sedation-Agitation Scale*

Score	Description
1	Patient anxious and agitated, or restless, or both
2	Patient cooperative, oriented, and tranquil
3	Patient responds to commands only
4	Brisk response to a light glabellar tap or loud auditory stimulus
5	Sluggish response to a light glabellar tap or loud auditory stimulus
6	No response to a light glabellar tap or loud auditory stimulus

agent. Targeted sedation will minimize the tendency to oversedate critically ill patients.

Narcotics and Sedative-Hypnotic Agents

All the sedative-hypnotic agents used for sedation or to optimize airway management have a depressant effect on BP and cardiac function. The effects vary depending on the patient's age,[8] underlying medical problems, and cardiovascular stability. Furthermore, when drugs are used in combination, their effects can be synergistic. This potentiation of effects can be beneficial, as when analgesic effects are intensified; however, combinations of drugs may also potentiate respiratory depression and cardiovascular instability. Therefore, the decision to administer a sedative-hypnotic agent must first address whether the patient is stable enough to tolerate such a medication and, if so, what dose the patient will tolerate.

Patients who do not tolerate the cardiac depressant effects of sedative-hypnotics include patients who are in shock, bleeding, severely volume depleted, or who have inadequate cardiac function. Patients who have experienced a cardiac arrest or are very hypotensive should not be administered normal doses of sedative-hypnotic agents because the drugs will hinder cardiac function. Conversely, analgesics should not be withheld if BP can be supported with volume resuscitation and low doses of inotropes or vasopressors. Aging affects the pharmacokinetics and pharmacodynamics of the sedative-hypnotic agents; furthermore, the sensitivity of the elderly brain to sedative-hypnotic agents appears to be increased.[8] Sedative-hypnotic agents are also associated with confusion and delirium in the elderly (see chapter entitled "Pain, Delirium, and Ischemia in the Perioperative Period").

Liver disease affects the metabolism of drugs in many ways, and is difficult to predict. In severe cirrhosis (associated with altered clotting times, ascites, and encephalopathy), elimination half-lives of drugs are increased and drug clearance is reduced. These results suggest that smaller doses of drugs should be administered, and should be administered less frequently.[8,9] Metabolism of drugs that undergo glucuronidation (*ie*, lorazepam, oxazepam) appear to be relatively unaffected by liver disease. Drugs that are metabolized by phase I oxidative pathways (*ie*, diazepam and chlordiazepoxide) are affected by acute and chronic liver disease.[10] Nonetheless, morphine, which undergoes glucuronidation, is associated with an increased half-life and decreased clearance in patients with end-stage, decompensated liver disease.[10] Titration of sedatives to a scoring scale should simplify the complex pharmacology of drug administration in patients with hepatic and renal dysfunction.

A retrospective examination of the medical records of 28 patients who required >7 days of intensive care documented the occurrence of withdrawal symptoms and signs (restlessness, irritability, nausea, cramps, muscle aches, dysphoria, insomnia, myoclonus, delirium, sweating, tachycardia, vomiting, diarrhea, hypertension, fever, seizure, or tachypnea) in 9 of these patients.[11] The patients had to have three or more signs, or three or more symptoms, to be considered as having withdrawal. These patients received several-fold higher doses of analgesic and sedative-hypnotic medications than the patients who did not experience withdrawal symptoms.[11] The patients who did not experience withdrawal received an average daily doses of fentanyl equivalent to 1.4 mg/d and lorazepam equivalent to 11.1 mg/d. The patients who experienced withdrawal were significantly more likely to have received neuromuscular blocking agents. Increased doses of narcotics and sedatives might have been administered to ensure that patients were not paralyzed and awake. The patients who experienced withdrawal symptoms were also significantly younger than those who did not experience symptoms; the younger patients may be more prone to tolerance of opioids and sedatives, or the younger patients may have been more likely to survive. The authors recommended the following: (1) weaning the doses of the drugs by 5 to 10% per day; (2) that drugs might be weaned even more slowly if both opioids and benzodiazepines are being weaned; and (3) that long-acting oral agents could be administered, which can be weaned outside the ICU.[11] For example, oral methadone provides an efficient method for opiate weaning.

Continuous Infusions

The clearance of a sedative drug is affected by the duration of the infusion of the drug. Both midazolam and lorazepam become longer-acting drugs when they are administered as continuous infusions.[12] Patients also rapidly become tolerant to benzodiazepines when these agents are administered frequently.[12] Nevertheless, continuous infusion can minimize hemodynamic instability associated with analgesic and sedative administration. A reasonable target is for approximately 50% of the total analgesic or sedative dose to be administered as a continuous infusion, with the balance as needed. The term *context-sensitive half-life* refers to the changes in drug elimination that occur as a function of duration of infusion.

Assessment of Pain

The treatment of pain is not only compassionate, but it is now mandated by The Joint Commission. Pain associated with procedures should be treated with analgesics. Chronic pain may require therapy other than opioids, as most patients who have been treated for chronic pain are tolerant to narcotics.

Increased concentrations of morphine are found to develop in elderly patients when compared with younger patients given the same dose, and the morphine plasma concentration persists for longer intervals, suggesting decreased clearance. Therefore, smaller doses of morphine should be used in elderly patients.

Morphine administration is associated with hypotension; doses of 1 to 4 mg/kg IV are commonly associated with hypotension, but hypotension has been reported with doses of 5 mg IV.[10] The faster the rate of administration, the more pronounced the hypotension seen; morphine can also be associated with histamine release, and morphine causes arterial and venous dilation that potentiates hypotension. Finally, morphine can slow the heart rate, probably by its stimulation of the vagus nerve and its depressant effects on the sinoatrial node. These hemodynamic effects are magnified when pain levels, and therefore circulating catecholamines, are increased. Continuous infusion, by preventing development of pain, may minimize hypotension.

Fentanyl

Fentanyl is 50 to 100 times more potent than morphine (fentanyl has greater affinity for the μ opiate receptor), so that the usual IV doses are 50 to 100 μg, depending on the condition of the patient. As fentanyl is very lipid soluble (40 times more lipid soluble than morphine), it penetrates the CNS quickly and leaves it quickly, and therefore has a very rapid onset of action and a short duration of action (Table 2). The onset of action of fentanyl is within 30 s, and its peak effect is within

Table 2. *Pharmacokinetics and Pharmacodynamics of Opioid Agents**

Drug	Lipid Solubility	Half-life, h	Onset of Action, min	Peak Effect, min	Duration of Action, h
Morphine	Low	2–3	5	20–30	2–7
Fentanyl	High	4–10	1–2	5–15	0.5–1
Meperidine	Moderate	5–8	5	20–60	2–4
Hydromorphone	Low	2.5–3	10–15	15–30	2–4

*Volles and McGory.[10]

5 to 15 min.[10,13] The liver metabolizes fentanyl, and the kidney eliminates inactive metabolites. Decreased liver perfusion can decrease the clearance of fentanyl. When fentanyl is administered as a continuous infusion, the terminal half-life of the drug is 16 h; prolonged effects seen after infusions or repeated bolus injections of fentanyl occur because of the large amounts of the drug, which accumulate in the fatty tissues and then have to be metabolized by the liver.

Fentanyl is similar to morphine in that fentanyl concentrations are higher in elderly patients, apparently due to decreased clearance of the drug. Fentanyl is more potent in the elderly in that loss of consciousness occurs with smaller doses. Chest wall rigidity may occur with rapid administration of large doses of fentanyl.[13-15]

Fentanyl administration infrequently causes hypotension; however, it can cause hypotension by causing bradycardia and decreased sympathetic tone.[13,14] Patients who are maintaining their BP by an increase in sympathetic tone can become hypotensive with the administration of fentanyl.[13,16] The rate of administration appears to affect the development of bradycardia; when fentanyl is administered rapidly, bradycardia develops more frequently.[13–16]

Remifentanil

Remifentanil is an ultrashort-acting narcotic with potency that is similar to that of fentanyl. Remifentanil penetrates the blood-brain barrier within 1 min, and its blood concentration decreases 50% by 6 min after a 1-min infusion and 80% by 15 min.[17] The novel aspect of remifentanil is its rapid hydrolysis by circulating and tissue nonspecific esterases (the (β-adrenergic blocker esmolol is metabolized by similar enzymatic machinery). Unlike fentanyl, there does not appear to be a cumulative effect seen with longer infusions because of this unique metabolism. Organ dysfunction does not appear to alter the metabolism of this drug.[17] The clearance of remifentanil is reduced by about 25% in the elderly, according to the product information.

This drug produces respiratory depression, hypotension, bradycardia, and hypertonus of skeletal muscle; the rigidity produced by this drug can make ventilation by mask difficult or impossible. The administration of propofol or a paralytic agent prior to the administration of remifentanil can attenuate the skeletal rigidity seen with the drug. In studies in which fentanyl, 1 μg/kg IV, was compared with remifentanil, 0.5 to 1 μg/kg IV, hypotension occurred somewhat more often with fentanyl.[16,18] Peak hemodynamic effects of remifentanil are seen within 3 to 5 min after the administration of a single bolus, and hemodynamic effects are dose dependent.

It has been shown that when large doses of remifentanil are administered intraoperatively, acute opioid tolerance develops. Tolerance occurs more quickly in response to shorter-acting narcotics such as remifentanil and alfentanil. In fact, profound tolerance can be documented after 90 min of remifentanil administration to volunteers. However, it also appears that the administration of large doses of opioids can also produce delayed hyperalgesia, suggesting a central sensitization that reduces the threshold to receptive fields. In support of this, the administration of N-methyl-D-aspartate receptor antagonists before the administration of large doses of opioids can block the hyperalgesia that can be induced by heroin or fentanyl. Because of its potency and short half-life, this agent is complex to use, and is usually reserved for intraoperative use.

Etomidate

Etomidate exists as two isomers, but only the + isomer is active; etomidate is R-(+)-ethyl-l-(α-methylbenzyl)-lH-imidazole-5-carboxylate. It is formulated as a 2 mg/mL solution in 35% propylene glycol. The propylene glycol is irritating to veins, and etomidate should not be mixed with other IV solutions. Etomidate had been used in critical care units throughout the world because of its characteristics, including its minimal hemodynamic effects, minimal respiratory depression, and cerebral protective effects. However, etomidate causes a dose-dependent, temporary, and reversible inhibition of steroid synthesis after a single dose or after an infusion. Other side effects that discourage its use include nausea and vomiting due to activation of the nausea center (concurrent administration of fentanyl increases the incidence), pain on injection, superficial thrombophlebitis 48 to 72 h after injection, and myoclonus. Etomidate appears to enhance the neuromuscular blockade of nondepolarizing paralytic agents.[15] Nonetheless, etomidate continues to be used as it causes minimal hemodynamic perturbations when small doses are administered.

The liver metabolizes etomidate, and its main metabolites are inactive. Doses of etomidate that have been used are 0.2 to 0.6 mg/kg; this dose can be decreased if narcotics and/or benzodiazepines are also administered. After 0.3 mg/kg, the effect is seen within the time that it takes the drug to circulate to the brain; redistribution is the mechanism that terminates the effects of a bolus of etomidate. Hepatic dysfunction does not appear to alter the rapid recovery from the hypnotic effects of etomidate.[15,19] The elimination half-life of the drug is 2.9 to 5.3 h.[15] In the elderly, the elimination clearance and volume of the central compartment are both decreased, causing a higher blood concentration from a given dose.[19]

Etomidate affects transmission at γ-aminobutyric acid-a receptors and may increase the number of γ-aminobutyric acid-a receptors.[13] Etomidate causes hypnosis and does not have analgesic activity. Etomidate has minimal effects on ventilation; in fact, etomidate can produce a brief period of hyperventilation, which can be followed by apnea.[15,19] Hiccups and coughing may also be seen after etomidate administration. After the administration of 0.3 mg/kg of etomidate to patients, there is almost no change in heart rate, mean arterial pressure, mean pulmonary artery pressure, central venous pressure, stroke volume, or cardiac index.[15,19] Etomidate does not affect the sympathetic nervous system or baroreceptor function. Because of the potential for adrenal suppression with etomidate, it should not be used in repeated doses or as a continuous infusion. In addition, adrenal axis testing results will be abnormal in patients who have recently received etomidate. However, it is a desirable agent for use in brief procedures such as endotracheal intubation.

Propofol

Propofol is a short-acting sedative-hypnotic widely used for sedation and general anesthesia. Propofol, 2,6,-diisopropylphenol, is formulated as a 1% aqueous emulsion, containing 10% soybean oil, 2.25% glycerol, and 1.2% egg phosphatide.[20] Ethylenediaminetetraacetic acid has recently been added to propofol in an attempt to discourage bacterial growth; propofol has been found to be the drug most frequently contaminated by bacteria. An ampule of the drug should only be used for one patient; great care should be taken when the drug is used for infusions so that bacterial contamination does not occur.

The effects of propofol, 2 mg/kg, are seen within the time it takes for the drug to circulate to the brain. The duration of the hypnosis is 5 to 10 min after a bolus injection; redistribution and elimination terminates the effects of propofol. Propofol has no analgesic activity but has some antiemetic properties. The clearance of propofol cannot be explained by hepatic clearance alone; there appear to be extrahepatic sites of elimination. The clearance of propofol is extremely rapid, and the recovery from propofol remains rapid even after prolonged infusions.[15] The pharmacokinetics of propofol in patients age ≥ 65 years old reveal that the elimination clearance is slower, but that plasma concentrations appear similar to those of younger patients.[19]

Propofol causes dose-dependent hypotension that is very similar or somewhat greater than the hypotension produced by the administration of thiopental. Propofol causes vasodilation and myocardial depression.[20] The hypotensive effects of this drug can be exaggerated in elderly patients and in patients who have poor cardiac function or hypovolemia.[15,20] Propofol causes respiratory depression; initially, an increase in respiratory rate is seen for about 30 s and then apnea occurs. Airway reflexes are depressed, and propofol prophylactically attenuates induced bronchoconstriction by depression of neurally induced bronchoconstriction.[15,21] Propofol does not affect resting airway tone, nor has it been used in asthmatic patients to treat acute bronchoconstriction.[20,21] The dosing of propofol should be adjusted to take into account volume status and cardiac function when used for either intubation or sedation. Side effects produced by propofol include intense dreams and disinhibition, dystonic or choreiform movements, pain at the injection site, phlebitis, hyperlipidemia, and pancreatitis.

Ketamine

Ketamine, a phencyclidine derivative, is unique among the IV agents in that it causes analgesia as well as amnesia. The drug does not necessarily cause a loss of consciousness, but the patient is not aware; the drug appears to cause a dissociative state by electrophysiologic inhibition of the thalamocortical pathways and stimulation of the limbic system.[21-23] The drug is a racemic mixture of two optical enantiomers; the S(+) ketamine has approximately four-fold-greater affinity at phencyclidine binding sites on the N-methyl-d-aspartate receptor than does the R(−) ketamine. The S(+) ketamine appears to allow the use of significantly smaller doses, faster recovery, and possibly fewer side effects. The compound is available for use in Europe.[21-23]

Doses of ketamine, 0.1 to 0.5 mg/kg, have analgesic action and can be used before the onset of pain for effective preemptive analgesia. Ketamine has an elimination half-life of 3 h. Recovery from an induction dose (0.5 to 1.5 mg/kg) is from redistribution from its receptor. Ketamine causes amnesia, altered short-term memory, decreased ability to concentrate, altered cognitive performance, nightmares, nausea, and vomiting. Thus, it is common practice to administer small doses of benzodiazepine with ketamine; this practice does prolong recovery from ketamine, but usually eliminates these adverse effects.

Ketamine directly stimulates the autonomic nervous system, releases catecholamines and steroids, and causes tachycardia and increases BP. If a patient cannot release catecholamines (ie, is critically ill or has autonomic nervous system blockade), then ketamine administration can cause vasodilation and myocardial depression.[21-23] Data regarding ketamine in the elderly are lacking; the emergence phenomena and dysphoria ketamine causes may be difficult for the elderly, particularly if the baseline mental status is not normal.[21-23]

Ketamine is a useful agent for patients with reactive airway disease in that it attenuates neurally induced bronchoconstriction.[21] It also has a small direct effect on smooth muscle activation; however, it is unclear whether it can be used to improve asthma attacks. Ketamine administration will decrease the neurally induced bronchoconstriction that occurs with airway manipulation during intubation.

Midazolam

Midazolam is a water-soluble benzodiazepine that has the notable property of causing antegrade amnesia in conscious patients. Midazolam has an elimination half-life of 2.7 h (compared with 46.6 h for diazepam).[15,19] In the elderly, the elimination half-life is longer and elimination clearance decreases.[15,19] Drug effects are terminated by redistribution, suggesting that pharmacodynamic changes in the elderly cause the prolonged effects seen in this age group.[15,19]

After doses of 0.05 to 0.2 mg/kg of midazolam IV, tidal volumes will decrease by 40%, but minute ventilation remains unchanged. However, after slightly larger doses, apnea is seen. When opioids and midazolam are administered together, respiratory depression is assured, as midazolam decreases tidal volume and the opioids will decrease the respiratory rate. More prolonged and more profound respiratory depression has been noted in patients with chronic obstructive airways disease and in patients with altered respiratory drives.[15,19]

Midazolam causes more hypotension than etomidate; when administered to patients with normal cardiovascular function, small decreases in BP and increases in heart rate are seen. When midazolam was administered to patients who had valvular heart disease, some impairment of cardiac function was seen; when it was used for cardiac catheterization in patients with coronary artery disease, these patients experienced approximately a 15% decrease in their mean arterial pressures.[15,19] When patients have significant cardiac dysfunction or are hypovolemic, midazolam will depress cardiovascular function and has been associated with fatalities.

Unlike propofol, ketamine, or etomidate, midazolam will take longer for its peak effect on the CNS. The drug takes approximately 5 min to achieve its peak effect; recovery of normal central nervous function takes about 20 min after one dose.[15,19] However, in the elderly, prolonged amnesia even during the recovery period may occur.

Midazolam and the other benzodiazepines, except for lorazepam or temazepam, have been noted to interact with protease inhibitors, including ritonavir, indinavir, nelfinavir, and saquinavir. The interaction involves the inhibition of P-450-3A enzyme that metabolizes many of the benzodiazepines. Therefore, the levels of the benzodiazepines can be increased and cause prolonged amnesia and sedation.[24] There is now a warning on protease inhibitor labels to avoid the administration of these benzodiazepines to patients who are receiving protease inhibitors. The warning also exists for meperidine, fentanyl, codeine, and hydromorphone, levels of which are also increased by the protease inhibitors.[24]

Dexmedetomidine

Dexmedetomidine, an α_2-adrenoreceptor agonist, is a newer sedative drug that is being introduced for use in the ICU. It binds α_2-agonist receptors eight times more avidly than clonidine and is shorter acting.[25] Beneficial properties include marked sedation with only mild reductions in minute ventilation, reduced hemodynamic response to intubation and extubation, attenuated stress response to surgery, and potentiation of analgesics.[26] A prospective, randomized study[27] reported that ICU patients who received dexmedetomidine required significantly less additional sedative or analgesic medication than did the control patients. In 1999, dexmedetomidine was approved by the US Food and Drug Administration for short-term (<24 h) infusion as a sedative agent in critically ill patients. Clinical trials are underway to determine safety and efficacy for periods >24 h. Patients sedated with dexmedetomidine appear tranquil while being readily arousable and interactive when stimulated.[25]

Adverse effects of etomidate include hypertension, followed by hypotension and bradycardia from inhibition of sympathetic activity in the CNS.[28] Because of this, boluses may not be tolerated as well as maintenance infusions in critically ill patients. Elimination may be prolonged in the presence of hepatic dysfunction, but additional data will be necessary to determine whether this drug can be used in patients with renal or hepatic failure.[28]

Choosing the Optimal Sedative

Two studies have suggested that benzodiazepines may not be beneficial for long-term sedation. The MENDS trial[29] was a multicenter, randomized, controlled trial comparing sedation with dexmedetomidine to sedation with lorazepam. Sedation with dexmedetomidine resulted in more days alive without delirium or coma, along with improved sedation targeting. There was also a trend toward reduced mortality in patients receiving dexmedetomidine. In a more recent study, Riker et al[30] compared midazolam to dexmedetomidine for sedation of critically ill patients. Although they found that midazolam and dexmedetomidine resulted in a similar quality of sedation, dexmedetomidine-treated patients spent less time receiving ventilation, experienced less delirium, and had less hypotension. Patients receiving dexmedetomidine did have a higher incidence of bradycardia.

Neuromuscular Alterations in Critically Ill Patients

A variety of neuromuscular alterations have now been described in critically ill patients. Critical illness polyneuropathy (CIP) is the most frequent acute polyneuropathy in this population. Risk factors for CIP include parenteral nutrition, autoimmune disorders, steroid use, use of muscle relaxants (pancuronium or vecuronium), hyperglycemia, hyperosmolality, and catecholamine use.[31] Intensive insulin therapy in critically ill patients was found to reduce the incidence of CIP by 44%.[32] Mortality was found to be up to 3.5 times higher for patients with CIP vs patients without CIP.[31]

The data suggest that CIP will develop in 58% of patients who remain in the ICU for >1 week, and in 82% of patients with sepsis and multiorgan failure. CIP is associated with persistent ataxia, muscle weakness, and paralysis in survivors of critical illness.[33] CIP is an acute axonal polyneuropathy; affected nerves have a reduced number of fibers so that the amplitude of nerve action potentials are reduced while the nerve conduction velocity is normal. Latency and conduction velocity are unchanged. Sensory and motor nerves are typically involved, but pure motor and pure sensory forms have been described. Deep tendon reflexes are decreased or absent. Creatine kinase levels can be normal or slightly increased. Diaphragmatic denervation may play a role in ventilator dependency.[34]

Critical illness myopathy (CIM) is a primary myopathy, and it appears to be as frequent as CIP. To differentiate between CIP and CIM, the patient needs electromyographic evaluation. Muscle biopsies are usually required to confirm CIM. Muscle biopsies should be considered in patients with normal sensory neurography, low motor amplitudes, and little spontaneous activity for the degree of weakness, findings typical of myopathies.[31] CIM encompasses a spectrum of disease, including acute necrotizing myopathy to evidence of intact muscle. Direct stimulation of muscle fibers is now being used, instead of and in addition to muscle biopsies, to confirm the diagnosis of CIM when there is an absolute reduction in direct muscle stimulation below critical values.[35] In patients with sepsis and systemic inflammatory response syndrome, patients frequently have both CIP and CIM.[31]

An algorithm has been created to simplify the differential diagnosis of weakness in critically ill patients.[31] Steroids are associated with a thick-filament myopathy. The steroid components of the muscle relaxants pancuronium and vecuronium have been suggested as a cause of necrotizing myopathy.[31]

Introduction to Muscle Relaxants

Muscle relaxants are used for several purposes, including facilitating endotracheal intubation, facilitating mechanical ventilation, reducing elevated intracranial pressure, reducing work of breathing, reducing spasms associated with tetanus, and reducing movement associated with status epilepticus.[36] Short-term use is considered <2 days because complications have rarely been reported with administration for <2 days.[36] Complications associated with muscle relaxants include anaphylaxis, hyperkalemia associated with succinylcholine administration (seen in patients with burns, neurologic injury, muscle trauma, long-term immobilization, or elevated serum potassium), inadequate ventilation of paralyzed patients, inadequate analgesia and sedation of paralyzed patients, and persistent weakness after long-term use.[36,37]

Most investigations have not found neuromuscular blocking agents to be associated with CIP.[31] Persistent weakness occurs in about 20% of patients who receive muscle relaxants for >6 days and in up to 70% of patients who are receiving steroids as well as receiving muscle relaxants.[36] Risk factors for prolonged weakness include vecuronium in female patients who have renal failure, high-dose steroids, and >2-day duration of relaxant administration and administration of high doses of muscle relaxants.

There appear to be several etiologies to the persistent weakness. The persistent weakness may be due to persistent paralysis. Vecuronium has an active metabolite, 3-desacetyl vecuronium, which persists particularly in female patients with renal failure. Pancuronium and pipecuronium also form these metabolites. Therefore, these drugs should not be administered long term to patients who have renal failure.

A myopathic syndrome characterized by flaccid paralysis, increased creatine kinase, and myonecrosis appears to develop in patients receiving corticosteroids and who receive long-term therapy with muscle relaxants; these patients recover after many months. Plasma creatine kinase concentrations appear to increase when the myopathy develops; therefore, serum creatine kinase should be monitored in patients receiving corticosteroids who are receiving muscle relaxants. All muscle relaxants have been associated with this syndrome.

A motor neuropathy has been reported after the administration of vecuronium, pancuronium, or atracurium. The neuropathy affects all extremities, is associated with absent tendon reflexes, and can be accompanied by muscle wasting. This syndrome also takes months to resolve. Another syndrome consisting of persistent motor weakness but with preservation of sensory function has been reported in patients receiving pancuronium, vecuronium, or metocurine. These patients do not have normal neuromuscular transmission, and their symptoms also take months to resolve.

Patients do become tolerant to the effects of the muscle relaxants. The tolerance can develop within 24 to 48 h and appears to be due to up-regulation of acetylcholine receptors secondary to chronic denervation. One method to decrease the incidence of tolerance is to minimize the amount of muscle relaxant administered; the drug should only be administered for a defined

Issues in Sedation, Paralytic Agents, and Airway Management (Gropper)

clinical outcome. The only reason to monitor the train-of-four method is to document that complete block is not obtained because the presence of a train-of-four response does not ensure that persistent weakness will not occur. In addition, train-of-four monitoring can help ensure that an overdose is not administered.

Comparison of Muscle Relaxants

For rapid tracheal intubation, either succinylcholine or rocuronium (Table 3) should be administered. Succinylcholine only lasts for 5 to 10 min, which may be helpful if there is concern that the patient's trachea cannot be intubated. Succinylcholine has several significant side effects, including hyperkalemia, bradycardia, junctional arrhythmias, ventricular arrhythmias, masseter spasm, and muscle pains. Rocuronium is a nondepolarizing muscle relaxant that has a fast onset.

Unlike succinylcholine, however, paralysis will persist for up to 90 min; thus, mask ventilation and/or tracheal intubation must be successful. Succinylcholine should not be used in patients with hyperkalemia, or in patients with burns, massive trauma, or denervation injuries such as paraplegia or quadriplegia. In these patients, acetylcholine receptors are up-regulated; hyperkalemia will be exaggerated and may result in cardiac arrest.

Vecuronium has active metabolites that have been associated with persistent weakness, particularly in female patients with renal failure. Rocuronium does not have active metabolites. Atracurium and cisatracurium are used because their duration of action is not affected by liver or kidney disease. The duration of action of cisatracurium is as long as, if not longer than, that of rocuronium. All muscle relaxants have been associated with allergic reactions. In fact, muscle relaxants are the leading cause of perioperative anaphylaxis (succinylcholine is associated with 48% of the cases).[37] A recent report of cisatracurium-induced anaphylaxis documented that cardiovascular collapse can be the only sign of the allergic reaction.[37]

An important advance in reversal of neuromuscular blockade is the imminent availability of sugammadex. This is a novel agent that specifically binds rocuronium.

Airway Management

When one needs to emergently secure an airway, there are certain principles to remember: oxygenation even without removal of carbon dioxide can be lifesaving, and the complete inability to oxygenate will cause brain damage within 3 to 5 min. Therefore, as long as a needle can be placed in the trachea and oxygen can be administered, the patient can be kept alive until a surgical

Table 3. *Properties of Muscle Relaxants Used in the ICU**

Drug	Initial Dose,[†] mg/kg	Duration,[‡] min	Cost Factor[§]	Advantages	Complications
Pancuronium	0.07–0.1	60–120	1	Inexpensive	Tachycardia; active metabolite
Vecuronium	0.1	30–45	20	CVS stability	Active metabolite
Atracurium	0.05	30–45	20	Reliable recovery	Histamine release; active metabolite
Rocuronium	0.6–1.2	30–90	20	Rapid onset	None
Cisatracurium	0.1–0.2	30–90	10	Reliable recovery	Slow onset; active metabolite
Mivacurium	0.2	10–20	N/A	Short duration	Histamine release; metabolites
Succinylcholine	1–2	5–10	N/A	Fast onset; fast recovery	Hyperkalemia; dysrhythmia

* CVS = cardiovascular system; N/A = not recommended for long-term use. Reproduced with permission from Caldwell and Miller.[36]

[†] For tracheal intubation.

[‡] Time from intubation dose until first train-of-four response might return.

[§] Numbers are multiples of the cost of pancuronium, which is ~$10/d.

airway can be obtained. Percutaneous kits are available to perform emergency cricothyroidotomies; the operator must be able to complete the procedure in <3 min, and preferably the procedure should be completed within 1 min.

If a patient is not actively vomiting or otherwise soiling the airway, mask ventilation should be attempted. Successful mask ventilation can require two or more hands, and an oral and/or nasal airway. Mask ventilation is all that is required if aspiration is not a risk and the operator is not expert at tracheal intubation. The complications of mask ventilation include damage to the eyes, insufflation of the stomach, and possible regurgitation.

Intubation of the trachea can be done via conventional laryngoscopy; this procedure requires practice. A laryngeal mask can be placed at the patient's glottic opening by pushing it into the patient's mouth and down the pharynx; proper placement of the laryngeal mask may require less practice and training than conventional laryngoscopy. The laryngeal mask does not protect against aspiration but has been used in patients whose tracheas cannot be intubated using conventional laryngoscopy. Operators with expertise in tracheal intubation may encounter patients in whom conventional laryngoscopy is unsuccessful. An algorithm is then followed; depending on the status of the patient, either the procedure is aborted or a surgical airway is obtained (Fig 1).[38]

Situations in which conventional laryngoscopy may be difficult include restriction of the oral airway, reduced pharyngeal space, noncompliant submandibular tissue, limited atlantooccipital extension, and partial airway obstruction. Small mouth openings are encountered in patients who have temporomandibular joint disease, scarring near the mouth, congenital and surgical deformities, large tongues, and diseased teeth. The pharyngeal space can be decreased by edema and by masses. The submandibular tissue can be altered by infection (Ludwig angina), by scarring as from burns, by surgery, by radiation, and by cancer. Patients who cannot extend their necks include patients in a halo jacket, those with ankylosing spondylitis, cervical disk disease, or cervical spinal injuries. Airway obstruction occurs when there is epiglottitis, pedunculated

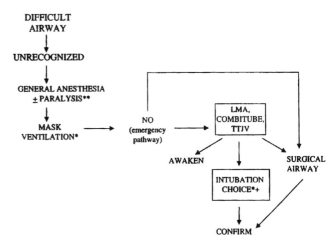

Figure 1. Difficult airway algorithm. Reproduced with permission from Benumof JL. Laryngeal mask airway and the ASA difficult airway algorithm. Anesthesiology 1996; 84:687-688
*Always consider calling for help (*eg*, technical, medical, surgical) when difficulty with mask ventilation and/or tracheal intubation is encountered.
**Consider the need to preserve spontaneous ventilation.
+Nonsurgical tracheal intubation choices of laryngoscopy with a rigid laryngoscope blade (many types), blind orotracheal or nasotracheal technique, fiberoptic/stylet technique, retrograde technique, illuminating stylet, rigid bronchoscope, percutaneous dilational tracheal entry. See Reference 38 for a complete discussion of these tracheal intubation choices.

tumors and cysts in the airways, large tonsils, mediastinal and subcutaneous emphysema, or edema is present. In these patients, the safest approach is nasal or oral fiberoptic bronchoscopic intubation while the patient maintains spontaneous ventilation.

A number of devices have been developed to help with intubation of the difficult airway. These devices include the LMA Fastrach, (LMA North America; San Diego, CA) and GlideScope (Verathon Inc; Bothwell, WA). All of these devices allow intubation of the trachea without direct visualization of the vocal cords.[39]

References

1. Nelson BJ, Weinert CR, Bury CL, et al. Intensive care unit drug use and subsequent quality of life in acute lung injury patients. Crit Care Med 2000; 28:3626–3630
2. Brook AD, Ahrens TS, Schaiff R, et al. Effect of a nursing-implemented sedation protocol on the duration of mechanical ventilation. Crit Care Med 1999; 27:2609–2615

3. Kress JP, Pohlman AS, O'Connor MF, et al. Daily interruption of sedative infusions in critically ill patients undergoing mechanical ventilation. N Engl J Med 2000; 342:1471–1477

4. Cook DJ, Walter SD, Cook RJ, et al. Incidence of and risk factors for ventilator-associated pneumonia in critically ill patients. Ann Intern Med 1998; 129:433–440

5. Girard TD, Kress JP, Fuchs BD, et al. Efficacy and safety of a paired sedation and ventilator weaning protocol for mechanically ventilated patients in intensive care (Awakening and Breathing Controlled Trial): a randomised controlled trial. Lancet 2008; 371:126–134

6. Rotondi AJ, Chelluri L, Sirio C, et al. Patients' recollections of stressful experiences while receiving prolonged mechanical ventilation in an intensive care unit. Crit Care Med 2002; 30:746–752

7. Inouye SK, Bogardus ST Jr, Charpentier PA, et al. A multicomponent intervention to prevent delirium in hospitalized older patients. N Engl J Med 1999; 340:669–676

8. Silverstein J, Bloom H, Cassel C. Geriatrics and anesthesia. Clin Anesthesiol 1999; 17:8–12

9. Cammarano W, Wiener-Kronish J. Analgesics, tranquilizers, and sedatives. In: Brown D, ed. Cardiac intensive care. Philadelphia, PA: WB Saunders, 1998; 591–602

10. Volles DF, McGory R. Pharmacokinetic considerations. Crit Care Clin 1999; 15:55–75

11. Cammarano WB, Pittet JF, Weitz S, et al. Acute withdrawal syndrome related to the administration of analgesic and sedative medications in adult intensive care unit patients. Crit Care Med 1998; 26:676–684

12. Lowson SM, Sawh S. Adjuncts to analgesia: sedation and neuromuscular blockade. Crit Care Clin1999; 15:119–141, vii

13. Bailey P, Stanley T. Intravenous opioid anesthetics. In: Miller R, ed. Anesthesia (vol 1). New York, NY: Churchill Livingstone, 1994; 291–388

14. Ornstein E, Matteo R. Effects of opioids. In: McLeskey C, ed. Geriatric anesthesiology. Baltimore, MD: Williams & Wilkins, 1997; 249–260

15. Reves J, Glass P, Lubarsky D. Nonbarbiturate intra venous anesthetics. In: Miller R, ed. Anesthesiology (vol 1). New York, NY: Churchill Livingstone, 1994; 291–388

16. Peng PW, Sandler AN. A review of the use of fentanyl analgesia in the management of acute pain in adults. Anesthesiology 1999; 90:576–599

17. Egan TD, Lemmens HJ, Fiset P, et al. The pharmacokinetics of the new short-acting opioid remifentanil (GI87084B) in healthy adult male volunteers. Anesthesiology 1993; 79:881–892

18. Song D, Whitten CW, White PF. Use of remifentanil during anesthetic induction: a comparison with fentanyl in the ambulatory setting. Anesth Analg 1999; 88:734–736

19. Fragen R. Effects of barbiturates, benzodiazpines, and other intravenous agents. In: McLeskey C, ed. Geriatric anesthesiology. Baltimore, MD: Williams & Wilkins, 1997; 249–260

20. Smith I, White PF, Nathanson M, et al. Propofol: an update on its clinical use. Anesthesiology 1994; 81:1005–1043

21. Brown RH, Wagner EM. Mechanisms of bronchoprotection by anesthetic induction agents: propofol versus ketamine. Anesthesiology 1999; 90:822–828

22. Eames WO, Rooke GA, Wu RS, et al. Comparison of the effects of etomidate, propofol, and thiopental on respiratory resistance after tracheal intubation. Anesthesiology 1996; 84:1307–1311

23. Kohrs R, Durieux ME. Ketamine: teaching an old drug new tricks. Anesth Analg 1998; 87:1186-1193

24. Flexner C. HIV-protease inhibitors. N Engl J Med 1998; 338:1281–1292

25. Coursin D, Coursin D, Maccioli G. Dexmedetomidine. Curr Opin Crit Care 2001; 7:221–226

26. Scheinin B, Lindgren L, Randell T, et al. Dexmedetomidine attenuates sympathoadrenal responses to tracheal intubation and reduces the need for thiopentone and perioperative fentanyl. Br J Anaesth 1992; 68:126–131

27. Venn R, Bradshaw C, Spencer R, et al. Preliminary UK experience of dexmedetomidine, a novel agent for postoperative sedation in the intensive care unit. Anesthesia 1999; 54:1136–1142

28. Bhana N, Goa KL, McClellan KJ. Dexmedetomidine. Drugs 2000; 59:263–268

29. Pandharipande PP, Pun BT, Herr DL, et al. Effect of sedation with dexmedetomidine vs lorazepam on acute brain dysfunction in mechanically ventilated patients. JAMA 2007; 298:2644–2653

30. Riker RR, Shehabi Y, Bokesch PM et al. Dexmedetomidine vs midazolam for sedation of critically ill patients. JAMA 2009; 301:489–499

31. van Mook WN, Hulsewe-Evers RP. Critical illness polyneuropathy. Curr Opin Crit Care 2002; 8:302–310

32. van den Berghe G, Wouters P, Weekers F, et al. Intensive insulin therapy in the critically ill patients. N Engl J Med 2001; 345:1359–1367

33. Garnacho-Montero J, Madrazo-Osuna J, Garcia-Garmendia JL, et al. Critical illness polyneuropathy: risk factors and clinical consequences: a cohort study in septic patients. Intensive Care Med 2001; 27:1288–1296

34. Leijten FS, De Weerd AW, Poortvliet DC, et al. Critical illness polyneuropathy in multiple organ dysfunction syndrome and weaning from the ventilator. Intensive Care Med 1996; 22:856–861

35. Bednarik J, Lukas Z, Vondracek P. Critical illness polyneuromyopathy: the electrophysiological components of a complex entity. Intensive Care Med 2003; 29:1505–1514

36. Caldwell J, Miller R. A review of muscle relaxants and their use in the intensive care unit. Hosp Physician 1996; 32:11–24

37. Toh KW, Deacock SJ, Fawcett WJ. Severe anaphylactic reaction to cisatracurium. Anesth Analg 1999; 88:462–464

38. Benumof JL. Laryngeal mask airway and the ASA difficult airway algorithm. Anesthesiology 1996; 84:686–669

39. Walz JM, Zayaruzny M, Heard SO. Airway management in critical illness. Chest 2007; 131:608–620

Issues in Sedation, Paralytic Agents, and Airway Management (Gropper)

Severe Pneumonia

Michael S. Niederman, MD, FCCP

Objectives:

- Define the epidemiology of community-acquired pneumonia (CAP) and risk factors for mortality
- Discuss the common etiologic pathogens and therapy of severe CAP, including the impact of atypical pathogens and penicillin-resistant pneumococcus
- Describe the pathogenesis and bacteriology of ventilator-associated pneumonia (VAP)
- Outline therapies and prevention strategies for VAP

Key words: adequate therapy; antibiotic therapy; community-acquired; drug-resistant pneumococcus; health-care-associated pneumonia; methicillin-resistant *Staphylococcus aureus*; multidrug-resistant pathogens; nosocomial; pneumonia

Pneumonia is the seventh-leading cause of death in the United States and the number one cause of death from infectious diseases. The patient with pneumonia is managed in the ICU when severe forms of community-acquired pneumonia (CAP) are present, or when a life-threatening nosocomial pneumonia develops in a hospitalized. A newly defined entity, health-care-associated pneumonia (HCAP), is considered a form of nosocomial pneumonia that arises in patients who have been in contact with environments (nursing homes, hemodialysis centers) that expose them to the multidrug-resistant bacteria that are present in the hospital. Patients in these situations frequently develop severe pneumonia.[1,2] In the ICU, almost 90% of episodes of nosocomial pneumonia occur in patients who are receiving mechanical ventilation for other reasons, and this is termed *ventilator-associated pneumonia* (VAP). The elderly account for a disproportionate number of critically ill patients with all forms of pneumonia, often because they commonly have comorbid illness that predisposes them to more severe forms of infection, and their short- and long-term mortality rates are higher than that of younger patients.[3] In all forms of severe pneumonia, antibiotic resistance is an increasing problem, especially among pneumococci in CAP, and with *Pseudomonas aeruginosa*, Acinetobacter spp, extended-spectrum β-lactamase producing Gram-negative organisms, and methicillin-resistant *Staphylococcus aureus* (MRSA) in VAP, CAP, and HCAP.[1,2] Although patients with HIV infection and those with other immunocompromising diseases commonly develop pneumonia, the approach to managing these patients is very specific and different from that used in immunocompetent patients. These populations are not discussed here. Pneumonia remains a controversial illness because of difficulties in diagnosis and in establishing an etiologic pathogen. A number of studies[2,4,5] have focused on whether a more precise and accurate bacteriologic definition of pneumonia would lead to improved patient outcome, with some recent studies focusing on this issue.

Definitions of Severe Pneumonia, Risk Factors, and Prognosis

Among patients with CAP admitted to the hospital, 10 to 20% require care in the ICU, and the rates are higher in elderly patients.[6,7] There is no uniform definition of severe pneumonia, but patients who need ICU care are often those with either respiratory failure (hypoxemic or hypercarbic), requiring mechanical ventilation or noninvasive ventilation, septic shock, or other clinical features of serious illness such as respiratory rate ≥ 30/min, systolic BP ≤ 90 mm Hg, or diastolic BP ≤ 60 mm Hg, multilobar infiltrates, Pao_2/fraction of inspired oxygen ratio < 250, confusion, or destabilization of another serious medical problem.[1,8] In patients with severe CAP, the expected mortality rate for those admitted to the ICU is 35 to 40%, but higher rates have been observed if the majority of patients admitted to the ICU are receiving mechanical ventilation, implying that the prognosis is worse if ICU care is first provided late in the course of illness.[9] In the United Kingdom, 59% of patients with CAP in the ICU were admitted within the first 2 days of hospital stay, and the mortality rate was lowest (46%) in those admitted within the first 2 days, compared with those admitted later in the course of hospital illness.[9] Based on a number of studies,[6,7,10] a reasonable benchmark is that about 60% of all ICU CAP patients will be receiving mechanical ventilation at the time of admission.

Among those with VAP, mortality rates can be as high as 50 to 70%, and case-control studies[11] have documented mortality directly attributable to the presence of pneumonia. Antibiotic-resistant organisms may add to the mortality of VAP, generally because these organisms are often not anticipated, and when present are often initially treated with ineffective antibiotic regimens.[12] HCAP is a form of nosocomial pneumonia that includes patients with pneumonia developing at any time during their hospital stay (including on admission) who have been exposed to the drug-resistant bacteria present in the health-care environment. This includes any patient with a history of hospitalization in the past 3 months, admission from a long-term care facility, need for dialysis or home infusion therapy, home wound care, or antibiotic therapy in the past 3 months.[2,13] Although not all patients with HCAP are at risk for multidrug-resistant (MDR) pathogens, those with multiple risk factors should be considered as potentially infected with these organisms. Risk factors, in addition to severe illness, include poor functional status, recent hospitalization, recent antibiotic therapy, and immune suppression.

Risk Factors for Severe Forms of CAP

Most patients with severe CAP (45 to 65%) have coexisting illnesses, and there is an increased likelihood that patients who are chronically ill will develop a complicated pneumonic illness[1,14] (Table 1). The most common chronic illnesses in these patients are respiratory disease such as COPD, cardiovascular disease, and diabetes mellitus. In addition, certain habits such as cigarette smoking and alcohol abuse are common in those with severe CAP, and cigarette smoking has been identified as a risk factor for bacteremic pneumococcal infection.[15] Other common illnesses in those with CAP include malignancy and neurologic illness (including seizures). Milder forms of pneumonia may be more severe on presentation if patients have not received antibiotic therapy prior to hospital admission. In addition, genetic

Table 1. *Risk Factors for Developing Severe CAP*

Advanced age (> 65 yr)
Comorbid illness
    Chronic respiratory illness (including COPD), cardiovascular disease, diabetes mellitus, neurologic illness, renal insufficiency, malignancy
Cigarette smoking (risk for pneumococcal bacteremia)
Alcohol abuse
Absence of antibiotic therapy prior to hospitalization
Failure to contain infection to its initial site of entry
    Immune suppression
    Genetic polymorphisms in the immune response

differences in the immune response may predispose certain individuals to more severe forms of infection and adverse outcomes, and may be reflected by a family history of severe pneumonia or adverse outcomes from infection.[16]

Risk Factors for Mortality From CAP

In a metaanalysis[17] of 33,148 patients with CAP, the overall mortality rate was 13.7%, but those admitted to the ICU had a mortality rate of 36.5%. Eleven prognostic factors were significantly associated with different odds ratios (ORs) for mortality: male sex (OR, 1.3), pleuritic chest pain (OR, 0.5), hypothermia (OR, 5.0), systolic hypotension (OR, 4.8), tachypnea (OR, 2.9), diabetes mellitus (OR, 1.3), neoplastic disease (OR, 2.8), neurologic disease (OR, 4.6), bacteremia (OR, 2.8), leukopenia (OR, 2.5), and multilobar infiltrates (OR, 3.1). In other studies,[1] the clinical features that predict a poor outcome (Table 2) include advanced age (> 65 years), preexisting chronic illness of any type, the absence of fever on admission, respiratory rate ≥ 30/ min, diastolic or systolic hypotension, elevated BUN (> 19.6 mg/dL), profound leukopenia or leukocytosis, inadequate antibiotic therapy, need for mechanical ventilation, hypoalbuminemia, and the presence of certain high-risk organisms (type III pneumococcus, *S aureus*, Gram-negative bacilli, aspiration organisms, or postobstructive pneumonia). Other studies[8–20] have found that when CAP patients have a delay in the initiation of appropriate antibiotic therapy of more than 4 h, mortality is increased.[1]

Prognostic scoring approaches have been applied to predict mortality in CAP patients,

Severe Pneumonia (Niederman)

Table 2. *Risk Factors for a Poor Outcome From CAP*

Patient-related factors

    Male sex

    Absence of pleuritic chest pain

    Nonclassic clinical presentation (nonrespiratory
       presentation)

    Neoplastic illness

    Neurologic illness

    Age >65 yr

    Family history of severe pneumonia or death from sepsis

Abnormal physical findings

    Respiratory rate >30/min on admission

    Systolic (<90 mm Hg) or diastolic (<60 mm Hg)
       hypotension

    Tachycardia (>125/min)

    High fever (>40°C) or afebrile

    Confusion

    Hypothermia (<36°C)

Laboratory abnormalities

    BUN >19.6 mg/dL

    Leukocytosis or leukopenia

    Multilobar radiographic abnormalities

    Rapidly progressive radiographic abnormalities during
       therapy

    Bacteremia

    Hyponatremia (<130 mmol/L)

    Thrombocytopenia (<100,000/mm³)

    Leukopenia (<4,000 cells/mm³)

    Multiple-organ failure

    Respiratory failure

    Hypoalbuminemia

    Arterial pH <7.35

    Pleural effusion

Pathogen-related factors

    High-risk organisms

    Type III pneumococcus, *S aureus*, Gram-negative bacilli
       (including *P aeruginosa*), aspiration organisms, SARS

    Possibly high levels of penicillin resistance (minimum
       inhibitory concentration of at least 4 mg/L) in pneu-
       mococcus

Therapy-related factors

    Delay in initial antibiotic therapy (more than 4–6 h)

    Initial therapy with inappropriate antibiotic therapy

    Failure to have a clinical response to empiric therapy
       within 72 h

and two prominent systems are the pneumonia severity index (PSI) and a modification of the British Thoracic Society rule, referred to as *CURB-65*.[8,21–24] The PSI is a complex scoring system that places patients into one of five risk groups for death, based on age, and the presence of male sex, comorbid illness, and certain laboratory and physical findings. This tool is good for predicting mortality, but it heavily weights age and comorbidity, and does not account for the social needs of patients, so it may not help to define the optimal site of care for a given patient. The CURB-65 approach assesses the presence of confusion, elevated BUN, respiratory rate ≥30/min, low BP (either systolic ≤90 mm Hg or diastolic ≤60 mm Hg) and whether the patient is at least 65 years old. If three of these five criteria are present, the predicted mortality rate is >20%.[22,23]

The PSI approach divides patients into five groups with different risks of death and suggests that outpatient care be given for classes I and II, admission for classes IV and V, and individualized decision for class III. The system heavily weights age and comorbid illness. In a large prospective study, the rule was successful in increasing the number of low-risk patients who were discharged compared with situations when the rule was not used; however, the admission decision remains an "art of medicine" decision that cannot easily be determined by a rule. The Pneumonia Outcomes Research Team (PORT) criteria are not able to discriminate which patients need ICU admission, because in one study 27% of all patients admitted to the ICU fell into risk classes I to III. In an ICU population, the rule could predict mortality, even though it could not define need for ICU care. In another study,[8] as many as 37% of those admitted to the ICU are in PSI classes I to III, pointing out that risk for death (which PSI can measure) is not always the same as need for intensive care. Conversely, patients in higher PSI classes do not always need ICU care if they fall into these high mortality risk groups because of advanced age and comorbid illness in the absence of physiologic findings of severe pneumonia.

Neither of the current prognostic scoring systems is ideal by itself for defining the need for ICU care, and both can be regarded only as providing decision support information that must be supplemented by clinical assessment and judgment. In addition, the two scoring approaches should be viewed as being complementary to one another.[24] Ewig et al[25] have examined the 10 criteria in the 1993 American Thoracic Society guidelines to define severe CAP. They found that need for ICU was defined by the presence of two of three minor criteria (systolic BP ≤90, multilobar disease, Pao$_2$/fraction of inspired oxygen ratio ≤250), or one of two major criteria (need for mechanical ventilation or septic shock). Based on these observations, the 2001 American Thoracic Society guidelines for CAP recommend that severe CAP could be defined on the basis of the presence of these features.[1] In the newest guidelines for CAP published in 2007, other criteria for severity have been added, including leukopenia (<4,000 cells/mL), thrombocytopenia (<100,000/mL), and hypothermia (<36°C).[1]

Another approach to defining the presence of severe CAP is to try to predict which patients will need intensive respiratory or vasopressor support using a tool referred to as *SMART-COP*.[24] The acronym "SMART COP" refers to systolic BP <90 mm Hg, multilobar infiltrates, albumin <3.5 g/dL, respiratory rate elevation (>25 for those age <50 years, and >30 for those age >50 years), tachycardia (>125 beats/min), confusion, low oxygen (<70 mm Hg if age <50 years or <60 mm Hg if age >50 years), and arterial pH <7.35. The abnormalities in systolic BP, oxygenation, and arterial pH each received 2 points, while the five other criteria received 1 point each; and with this system, the need for intensive respiratory or vasopressor support was predicted by a SMART COP score of at least 3 points. Using this cutoff, the sensitivity for need for intensive respiratory or vasopressor support was 92.3% and the specificity 62.3%, with a positive and negative predictive value of 22% and 98.6%, respectively. The PSI and CURB-65 did not perform as well overall.[24]

Other investigators have shown that the use of early and effective empiric therapy can improve survival in the setting of severe CAP, particularly if therapy is given within 4 to 6 h of arrival to the hospital, and if therapy is effective.[1,19,20] In the setting of severe CAP, the earlier that therapy is administered the better, and mortality is increased for each hour of delay in initiating therapy in the setting of septic shock due to CAP. Ineffective initial empiric therapy was a potent predictor of death, being associated with a 60% mortality rate, compared with an 11% mortality rate for those who received initial effective therapy.[10] Similarly, in other studies[26,27] of CAP, the use of a combination of a β-lactam and a macrolide antibiotic was associated with a lower mortality rate than if other therapies were given.

Among patients with severe CAP, another important prognostic finding is clinical evolution, as reflected by radiographic progression during therapy.[6] The elderly with CAP often have a higher risk of dying than other populations, and in one series,[28] the mortality rate of nursing home-acquired pneumonia was 32% compared with a mortality rate of 14% in other patients with CAP. One factor that may explain this finding is that older patients often have atypical clinical presentations of pneumonia, which may lead to a diagnosis being made at a later, more advanced stage of illness, resulting in an increased risk of death.[29]

Risk Factors for VAP

Mechanical ventilation (for >2 days) is the most important risk factor for nosocomial pneumonia, but other identified risks include age >60 years; malnutrition (serum albumin <2.2 g/dL); acute lung injury (ARDS); coma; burns; recent abdominal or thoracic surgery; multiple-organ failure; transfusion of >4 U of blood; transport from the ICU; prior antibiotic therapy; elevation of gastric pH (by antacids or histamine type-2 blocking agents); large-volume aspiration; use of a nasogastric tube (rather than a tube placed in the jejunum or a tube inserted through the mouth); use of inadequate endotracheal tube cuff pressure; prolonged sedation and paralysis; maintaining patients in the supine position in bed; use of total parenteral nutrition feeding rather than enteral feeding; and repeated reintubation.[2] When a patient is receiving mechanical ventilation, the risk of pneumonia is greatest in the first 5 days (3% per day), and declines thereafter to a risk of 2% per day for days 6 to 10, and to a rate of 1% per day or lower after this.[30] Noninvasive ventilation for respiratory failure is associated with a much lower risk of pneumonia than endotracheal intubation. The relation between pneumonia and ARDS is particularly interesting because not only can a variety of CAPs serve as a cause of ARDS, but secondary nosocomial pneumonia is the most common infection acquired by patients with established ARDS.[31-33] However, it has been shown that when pneumonia develops in patients with ARDS, it is generally a late event, occurring after at least 7 days of mechanical ventilation.[32]

Risk Factors for Mortality From VAP

The factor associated with the greatest impact on attributable mortality is the accuracy and timeliness of initial antibiotic therapy. Use of the wrong therapy or delays in the initiation of therapy are the most important predictors of VAP mortality.[11,12,34] Initial appropriate therapy (using an agent to which the etiologic pathogen is sensitive) can reduce mortality, but administration of correct therapy at a later date, after initially incorrect therapy, may not effectively reduce mortality.[34] The benefit of accurate empiric therapy may not apply to all patients but may be greatest for those infected with *P aeruginosa* or *S aureus*[35] and for those without the most severe degree of multiple-organ dysfunction at the time of therapy.[36] Even using the correct therapy may not reduce mortality if it is not given in adequate doses and if the therapy does not reach the site of infection. Closely related to appropriateness of initial therapy is the ability to decrease the number and/or spectrum of antimicrobial therapy once culture data become available, referred to as *de-escalation*. Several recent studies[37,38] have demonstrated that the use of de-escalation is associated with lower mortality compared with escalation or compared with a strategy of making no effort to reduce antibiotic therapy.

The choice of how to administer a specific agent can also affect outcome, and one study[39] of MRSA VAP found that the mortality rate with intermittent infusion of vancomycin was twice as high as when this agent was administered by continuous infusion. Other risk factors for mortality include prolonged duration of ventilation, coma on admission, creatinine level >1.5 mg/dL, and transfer from another ward to the ICU, the presence of certain high-risk pathogens (particularly an antibiotic-resistant organism such as *P aeruginosa*, Acinetobacter spp, or *S aureus*), bilateral radiographic abnormalities, age >60 years, ultimately fatal underlying condition, shock, prior antibiotic therapy, multiple system organ failure, nonsurgical primary diagnosis, or a rising APACHE (acute physiology and chronic health evaluation) score during pneumonia therapy (Table 3).[2,40]

Superinfection, as opposed to a primary nosocomial pneumonia, is a particularly ominous finding. Rello et al[41] observed that patients with

Table 3. *Risk Factors for Mortality From Nosocomial Pneumonia*

Physiologic findings
  Respiratory failure
  Coma on admission
  Multiple system organ failure
  Acute physiology and chronic health evaluation II score rising to >20 at 72 h after diagnosis

Laboratory findings
  Creatinine level >1.5 mg/dL
  Gram-negative pneumonia, especially *Pseudomonas* or *Acinetobacter* infection
  Infection with any drug-resistant pathogen
  Bilateral radiographic abnormalities
  Fungal pneumonia
  Polymicrobial infection

Historical data
  Prior antibiotic therapy
  Age >60 yr
  Underlying fatal illness
  Prolonged mechanical ventilation
  Inappropriate antimicrobial therapy
  Transfer to the ICU from another ward

pulmonary superinfection had a 67% mortality rate, whereas patients with primary nosocomial pneumonia had a 38% mortality rate. In earlier studies, Graybill et al[42] observed a 62% mortality rate with superinfection pneumonia, compared with a 40% mortality rate for primary nosocomial lung infection. These data, as well as information from Fagon et al[43] and Trouillet et al,[44] emphasize the important role of prior antibiotics in enhancing mortality, an outcome that is likely the result of secondary infection by more virulent pathogens.

Pathogenesis

General Overview

Pneumonia results when host defenses are overwhelmed by an infectious pathogen. This may occur because the patient has an inadequate immune response, often as the result of underlying comorbid illness, because of anatomic abnormalities (endobronchial obstruction, bronchiectasis), or because of therapy-induced dysfunction of the immune system (corticosteroids, endotracheal intubation).[2,45,46] In addition, there are genetic variations in the immune response, making some patients prone to overwhelming infection because of an inadequate response, and others prone to acute lung injury because of an excessive immune response.[16] In fact, the failure to localize the immune response to the respiratory site of initial infection may explain why develop acute lung injury and sepsis develop in some patients, as the inflammatory response extends to the entire lung and systemic circulation.[47] Pneumonia can even occur in patients who have an adequate immune system if the host defense system is overwhelmed by a large inoculum of bacteria (massive aspiration) or by a particularly virulent organism to which the patient has no preexisting immunity or to which the patient has an inability to form an adequate immune response. With this paradigm in mind, it is easy to understand why infection with virulent pathogens such as viruses (influenza), *Legionella pneumophila*, *Mycoplasma pneumoniae*, *Chlamydophila pneumoniae*, and *Streptococcus pneumoniae* develops in previously healthy individuals. However, it is possible for chronically ill patients to be infected not only by these virulent organisms, but also by organisms that are not highly virulent. Because of host defense impairments, organisms that commonly colonize these patients can cause infection as a result of immune responses that are inadequate. These organisms include enteric Gram-negative bacteria (*Escherichia coli*, *Klebsiella pneumoniae*, *P aeruginosa*, Acinetobacter spp) and fungi (Aspergillus and Candida spp).

Bacteria can enter the lung via several routes, but aspiration from a previously colonized oropharynx is the most common way that pneumonia develops in patients. Patients can also aspirate large volumes of bacteria if they have impaired neurologic protection of the upper airway (stroke, seizure) or if they have GI illnesses that predispose to vomiting. Other routes of entry include inhalation, which applies primarily to viruses *L pneumophila*, and *Mycobacterium tuberculosis*; hematogenous dissemination from extra pulmonary sites of infection (right-sided endocarditis); and direct extension from contiguous sites of infection. In critically ill hospitalized patients, bacteria can also enter the lung from a colonized stomach (spreading retrograde to the oropharynx, followed by aspiration), from a colonized or infected maxillary sinus, from colonization of dental plaque, or they can enter the lung directly via the endotracheal tube (from the hands of staff members). Recent studies[48,49] have shown that the use of nasal tubes (into the stomach or trachea) can predispose to sinusitis and pneumonia, but that a gastric source of pneumonia pathogens in patients receiving ventilation is not common.

The Role of Respiratory Therapy Equipment and Endotracheal Tubes

The endotracheal tube bypasses the filtration and host defense functions of the upper airway and can act as a conduit for direct inoculation of bacteria into the lung. This route may be particularly important if bacteria colonize the inside of the endotracheal tube itself in the form of a biofilm.[50,51] Given the presence of biofilm in endotracheal tubes, it may be tempting to regularly reintubate patients and use a fresh tube, but this approach is not recommended because reintubation is itself a risk factor for VAP.[52] In an effort to minimize the role of the endotracheal tube in pneumonia pathogenesis, efforts are being made to develop new endotracheal tube materials (silver-coated tube) or new tube-cleaning devices (the mucus shaver).

Respiratory therapy equipment and ventilator circuits can play a role in causing VAP.[53,54] One highly contaminated site is the condensate in the tubing; this material can inadvertently be inoculated into patients if the tubing is not handled carefully. Tubing changes every 24 h (rather than every 48 h) served as a risk factor for pneumonia.[55] Although most patients have ventilator tubing changed every 48 h, several studies[56,57] have shown no increased risk of infection if tubing is never changed or changed infrequently. The use of heat moisture exchangers may be one way to avoid this problem, but they have had an inconsistent effect on preventing VAP; however, frequent changes of heat moisture exchangers (ie, every 24 h) have not been shown to have an impact on the incidence of VAP, and heat moisture exchangers should be changed no more frequently than every 48 h.[58]

Clinical Features of Pneumonia

Historical Information

Patients with CAP and an intact immune system generally have classic pneumonia symptoms, but the elderly patient can have a nonrespiratory presentation with symptoms of confusion, falling, failure to thrive, altered functional capacity, or deterioration in a preexisting medical illness, such as congestive heart failure.[59] The absence of clear-cut respiratory symptoms and an afebrile status have themselves been predictors of an increased risk of death. Pleuritic chest pain is also commonly seen in patients with CAP, and in one study,[60] its absence was also identified as a poor prognostic finding.

There are certain clinical conditions associated with specific pathogens in patients with CAP, and these associations should be evaluated when obtaining a history (Table 4).[1] For example, if the presentation is subacute, following contact with birds, rats, or rabbits, then the possibility of psittacosis, leptospirosis, tularemia, or plague should be considered. *Coxiella burnetii* (Q fever) is a concern with exposure to parturient cats, cattle, sheep, or goats; *Francisella tularensis* is a concern with rabbit exposure; hantavirus with exposure to mice droppings in endemic areas;

Chlamydophila psittaci with exposure to turkeys or infected birds; and Legionella with exposure to contaminated water sources (saunas). Following influenza, superinfection with pneumococcus, *S aureus* (including MRSA), and *Haemophilus influenzae* should be considered. With travel to endemic areas in Asia, the onset of respiratory failure after a preceding viral illness should lead to suspicion of a viral pneumonia, which could be severe acute respiratory syndrome (SARS) or avian influenza.[61] Endemic fungi(coccidioidomycosis, histoplasmosis, and blastomycosis) occur in well-defined geographic areas and may present acutely with symptoms that overlap with acute bacterial pneumonia.

Nosocomial pneumonia often presents with less definitive clinical findings, particularly in those who are receiving mechanical ventilation, for whom the clinical diagnosis is made in those with a new or progressive radiographic infiltrate, along with some indication that infection is present (fever, purulent sputum, or leukocytosis). Recently, the Clinical Pulmonary Infection Score

Table 4. *Likely Microbiologic Etiology and Host Epidemiology of CAP and NP/VAP*

Epidemiology	Suspected Pathogen
Community-acquired	
Alcoholism	Pneumococcus (including drug-resistant organisms), anaerobes, H influenzae, K pneumoniae, tuberculosis
Splenic dysfunction (sickle cell disease)	Pneumococcus, H influenzae
COPD	Pneumococcus, H influenzae, M catarrhalis
Recent influenza infection	Pneumococcus, S aureus (including MRSA), H influenzae, enteric Gram-negative organisms
High-risk aspiration	Anaerobes, enteric Gram-negative bacilli
Neutropenia (including chronic corticosteroid therapy)	Gram-negative bacilli (especially P aeruginosa), Aspergillus
HIV infection (risk groups: IV drug abuser, tuberculosis, hemophilia, homosexual)	Pneumococcus, H influenzae, Pneumocystis jirovecii
Rabbit exposure	F tularensis
Exposure to farm animals, parturient cats	C burnetii (Q fever)
Exposure to mouse droppings	Hantavirus
Nursing home-acquired (no prior antibiotics and good functional status)	Pneumococcus (including drug-resistant organisms) and other organisms of CAP
Nursing home-acquired (prior antibiotics or poor functional status)	Gram-negative bacilli (including P aeruginosa, Acinetobacter spp, extended spectrum β-lactam-producing Enterobacteriaceae), S aureus (including MRSA)
Hospital-acquired and VAP	Gram-negative bacilli (including P aeruginosa, Acinetobacter spp, extended spectrum β-lactam-producing Enterobacteriaceae), S aureus (including MRSA)
	Consider local microbiology

(CPIS) has been applied to patients with VAP, and six criteria are scored on a scale from 0 to 2 for each, and pneumonia is diagnosed with a total score of at least 6 (of a maximum of 12).[62] These six criteria are fever, purulence of sputum, WBC count, oxygenation, degree of radiographic abnormality, and the presence of pathogens in the sputum. Many studies have documented that VAP is diagnosed more often clinically than can be confirmed microbiologically, and the diagnosis is further obscured by the fact that most patients receiving mechanical ventilation are colonized by enteric Gram-negative bacteria, and thus the finding of potential pathogens in the sputum has no diagnostic value. In addition, some patients can have purulent sputum and fever without a new infiltrate and have a diagnosis of ventilator-associated tracheobronchitis, an infectious complication of mechanical ventilation that may also require antibiotic therapy, but is not pneumonia.[2]

In taking a history from a patient with nosocomial pneumonia, it is important to identify if there are risk factors present for drug-resistant organisms. For patients receiving ventilation, these include prolonged ICU stay (≥ 5 days), recent antibiotic therapy, and the presence of HCAP.[2,44] In patients with CAP, risk factors for drug-resistant pneumococcus include recent β-lactam therapy, exposure to a child in a day care setting, alcoholism, immune suppression, and multiple medical comorbidities.[1,63]

Physical Examination

One of the most important ways to recognize severe CAP early in the course of illness is to carefully count the respiratory rate.[64,65] In the elderly, an elevation of respiratory rate can be the initial presenting sign of pneumonia, preceding other clinical findings by as much as 1 to 2 days and tachypnea is present in $\geq 60\%$ of all patients, being present more often in the elderly than in younger patients with pneumonia.[65] In addition, the counting of respiratory rate can identify the patient with severe illness, who commonly has a rate > 30 breaths/min. Other vital sign abnormalities are important to document and, as previously discussed, are important in prognostic scoring systems for CAP.

Etiologic Pathogens

CAP

The most common cause of CAP is pneumococcus (S pneumoniae), an organism that is frequently (at least 40% of the time) resistant to penicillin or other antibiotics, leading to the term *drug-resistant S pneumoniae* (DRSP). Fortunately, most penicillin resistance in the United States is still more commonly of the "intermediate" type (penicillin minimum inhibitory concentration [MIC] of 0.1 to 1.0 mg/L) and not of the high-level type (penicillin MIC ≥ 2.0 mg/L).[66] Pneumococcal resistance to other antibiotics is also common, including macrolides and trimethoprim-sulfamethoxazole, but the clinical relevance and impact on outcome of these *in vitro* findings is uncertain, and most experts believe that only organisms with a penicillin MIC of ≥ 4 mg/L lead to an increased risk of death.[67] Recently, the definitions of resistance in the United States have changed for nonmeningeal infection, with sensitive being defined by a penicillin MIC ≤ 2 mg/L, intermediate as MIC of 4 mg/L, and resistant as MIC ≥ 8 mg/L. As mentioned, the clinical impact of resistance on outcomes such as mortality has been difficult to show using older definitions; but with these new definitions of resistance, very few pathogens will be defined as resistant, but those that are may affect outcome.

All patients with severe CAP should be considered to be at risk for DRSP, and, in addition, those admitted to the ICU can have infection with atypical pathogens, which account for up to 20% of infections, either as primary infection or as copathogens. The identity of these organisms varies over time and geography. In some areas, Legionella is a common cause of severe CAP, while in others *C pneumoniae* or *M pneumoniae* predominate.[68] Other important causes of severe CAP include *H influenzae*, *S aureus*, which includes MRSA (especially after influenza), and enteric Gram-negative organisms (including *P aeruginosa*) in patients with appropriate risk factors (particularly bronchiectasis and steroid-treated COPD).

Recently, a toxin-producing strain of MRSA has been described to cause CAP in patients after influenza and other viral infections. This community-acquired MRSA is biologically and genetically distinct from the MRSA that causes nosocomial pneumonia, being more virulent and necrotizing, and associated with the production of the Panton-Valentine leukocidin.[69,70] Viruses can be a cause of severe CAP, including influenza virus, as well as parainfluenza virus and epidemic viruses such as coronavirus (which caused SARS) and avian influenza.[61] Viral pneumonia (SARS and influenza) can lead to respiratory failure, and occasionally tuberculosis or endemic fungi can result in severe pneumonia.

Epidemiologic risk factors for specific pathogens, certain "modifying factors," may be present that increase the likelihood of CAP caused by certain pathogens.[1] Risk factors for DRSP include β-lactam therapy in the past 3 months, alcoholism, age >65 years, immune suppression, multiple medical comorbidities, and contact with a child in a day care setting.[1,63] Risk factors for Gram-negative organisms include residence in a nursing home, underlying cardiopulmonary disease, multiple medical comorbidities, probable aspiration, recent hospitalization, and recent antibiotic therapy. Many of these patients who are at risk for Gram-negative organisms would now be reclassified as having HCAP.[2,13] Some ICU patients are at risk for pseudomonal infection, while others are not. The risk factors for *P aeruginosa* infection are structural lung disease (bronchiectasis), corticosteroid therapy (>10 mg prednisone per day), broad-spectrum antibiotic therapy for >7 days in the past month, previous hospitalization, and malnutrition.[2] Although aspiration has often been considered a risk factor for anaerobic infection, a study[71] of severe CAP in elderly patients with aspiration risk factors found that this population is very likely to have Gram-negative infection, and that, using sensitive microbiologic methods, anaerobes were uncommon. Aspiration is also common in patients with HCAP.

Unusual CAP Pathogens

Several rickettsia can cause CAP, including Q fever (*C burnetii*), which occurs worldwide, Rocky Mountain spotted fever (RMSF), and scrub typhus (*Rickettsia tsutsugamushi*) in Asia and Australia. Transmission typically involves an intermediate vector, often ticks (Q fever and RMSF) or mites (scrub typhus) but also sheep, cows, and contaminated milk (Q fever). These infections have a variable incubation period ranging from days to a few weeks, and are characterized by a febrile syndrome that may have a pneumonic component and a maculopapular rash (Q fever and RMSF).

SARS: In late 2003, a respiratory viral infection caused by a coronavirus emerged in parts of Asia and was termed *SARS*. The illness affected people from a variety of endemic areas in Asia, but was seen in North America when an outbreak occurred in Toronto, Canada. Importantly, as many as 20% of affected patients worldwide were health-care workers, particularly those caring for patients admitted to the ICU. Transmission risk was greatest during emergent intubation, and was also possible during noninvasive ventilation, making this latter modality of therapy contraindicated if SARS is suspected. Infection control may be quite effective in preventing the spread of SARS to health-care workers, and includes the careful handling of respiratory secretions, ventilator circuits, and the use of N-95 respirator masks and careful gowning and gloving. Even more elaborate infection control measures, including personal air exchange units, are needed for health-care workers involved in high-risk procedures such as intubation.

Clinically, patients with SARS present after a 2- to 11-day incubation period with fever, rigors, chills, dry cough, dyspnea, malaise headache, and frequently pneumonia and ARDS. Laboratory data show not only hypoxemia, but also elevated liver function test results In the Toronto experience, about 20% of hospitalized patients were admitted to the ICU, and 15% were received mechanical ventilation. Respiratory involvement typically began on day 3 of the hospital stay, but respiratory failure was not until day 8. The mortality rate for ICU-admitted SARS patients was >30%; and when patients died, it was generally from multiple system organ failure and sepsis. There is no specific therapy, but anecdotal reports have suggested a benefit to the use of pulse doses of steroids, and ribavirin.

Bioterrorism Considerations: Certain airborne pathogens can cause pneumonia as the result of deliberate dissemination by the aerosol route, in the form of a biological weapon, and present a clinical syndrome of CAP. The pathogens that are most likely to be used in this fashion, and that can lead to severe pulmonary infection, are *Bacillus anthracis* (anthrax), *Yersinia pestis* (plague), and *F tularensis* (tularemia).

To date, in the United States, anthrax is the only airborne respiratory agent that was used in a bioterrorism attack. In the fall of 2001, a series of intentional attacks with anthrax led to 11 confirmed cases of inhalational illness. Anthrax is an aerobic Gram-positive, spore-forming bacillus that had rarely led to disease prior to 2001. Particle size is essential in determining the infectiousness of the spores, and a size of 1 to 5 μm is required for inhalation into the alveolar space, but generally infection requires an inoculum size of 8,000 to 40,000 spores. The organisms initially enter alveolar macrophages and are transported to mediastinal lymph nodes, where they can persist and germinate and produce two toxins (lethal toxin and edema toxin); illness follows rapidly after germination. Although respiratory symptoms are often present, anthrax is not a typical pneumonic illness, but rather a disease characterized by hemorrhagic thoracic lymphadenitis, hemorrhagic mediastinitis, and pleural effusion. Although the incubation period of anthrax has varied from 2 to 43 days in prior outbreaks, in the October 2001 series the incubation period was from 4 to 6 days. In the US experience, all patients had chills, fever, and sweats, and most had nonproductive cough, dyspnea, nausea, vomiting, and chest pain. Chest radiographs were abnormal in all of the first 10 patients, and 7 had mediastinal widening, 8 had pleural effusions (generally bloody), and 7 had pulmonary infiltrates. Blood culture findings were positive in all eight patients in whom they were obtained prior to therapy, but sputum culture and Gram stain are unlikely to be positive. In the US attacks, 5 of 11 patients died.

Therapy of anthrax includes supportive management and antibiotics, with possibly some role for corticosteroids if meningeal involvement or mediastinal edema is present. Recommended therapy is ciprofloxacin, 400 mg IV bid or doxycycline, 100 mg IV bid. Until the patient is clinically stable, one to two additional agents should be added, including clindamycin, vancomycin, imipenem, meropenem, chloramphenicol, penicillin, ampicillin, rifampin, and clarithromycin. Therapy should be continued after an initial response with either ciprofloxacin or doxycycline for at least 60 days. Postexposure prophylaxis can be done with ciprofloxacin, or alternatively doxycycline or amoxicillin, for a total of 60 days.

Nosocomial Pneumonia

All patients with nosocomial pneumonia are at risk for infection with a group of bacteria referred to as *core organisms*, which include pneumococcus, *H influenzae*, methicillin-sensitive *S aureus*, and nonresistant Gram-negative organisms (*E coli*, *Klebsiella* spp, Enterobacter spp, Proteus spp, and *Serratia marcescens*). In addition, some patients are also at risk for infection with other organisms, depending on the presence of risk factors such as prolonged hospitalization (≥5 days), prior antibiotic therapy, recent hospitalization (within 90 days), recent antibiotic therapy, residence in a nursing home, or need for long-term care outside the hospital.[2,44] Patients with these risk factors can possibly be infected with MDR Gram-positive and Gram-negative organisms including MRSA, *P aeruginosa*, and Acinetobacter spp. Up to 40% of patients with VAP have polymicrobial infection, involving multiple pathogens.[72]

In patients with VAP, infection with enteric Gram-negative organisms is more common than infection with Gram-positive organisms, although the frequency of MRSA infection is increasing in this population, as is infection with Acinetobacter spp.[73] HCAP patients have been included in the nosocomial pneumonia guidelines as being a group at risk for infection with MDR Gram-positive and Gram-negative organisms; in one study[74] of nursing home patients requiring mechanical ventilation for severe pneumonia, Gram-negative organisms were not present if the patient with severe pneumonia had not received antibiotics in the preceding 6 months and was also of a good functional status (as defined by activities of daily living).

Each hospital, and each ICU within a given hospital, can have its own unique flora and antibiotic susceptibility patterns, and thus therapy needs to be adapted to the organisms in a given institution, which can change over time.[75] In addition, it is especially important to know this information as antibiotic resistance is a common factor contributing to initially inappropriate empiric antibiotic therapy. Choosing the wrong empiric therapy has been a particular problem for organisms such as *P aeruginosa*, Acinetobacter spp, and MRSA.[12] These highly resistant organisms can be present in as many as 60% of patients in whom VAP develops after at least 7 days of ventilation and who have also received prior antibiotic therapy.[2,44]

Diagnostic Issues

Diagnostic testing is performed for two purposes: to define the presence of pneumonia, and to identify the responsible pathogen. In all forms of pneumonia, a chest radiograph is used to identify the presence of a lung infiltrate, but in some clinical settings, especially in suspected VAP, there can be noninfectious causes for the radiographic abnormality. Chest radiographic patterns are generally not useful for identifying the etiology of CAP, although findings such as pleural effusion (pneumococcus, *H influenzae*, *M pneumoniae*, pyogenic streptococci) and cavitation (*P aeruginosa*, *S aureus*, anaerobes, MRSA, tuberculosis) can suggest certain groups of organisms. In those with VAP, bacteria are commonly present in samples of lower respiratory tract secretions, but the presence of a positive culture finding cannot reliably distinguish infection from colonization.

CAP

For patients with CAP, a chest radiograph not only confirms the presence of pneumonia, but can be used to identify complicated and severe illness, if the patient has findings such as multilobar infiltrates, cavitation, or a loculated pleural effusion (suggesting an empyema). CAP patients admitted to the ICU should have a chest radiograph, blood and lower respiratory tract (sputum, endotracheal aspirate, bronchoalveolar lavage, or bronchoscopic specimen) cultures, an arterial blood gas analysis, and routine hematologic and blood chemistry testing. If the patient has a moderate-sized pleural effusion, this should be tapped and the fluid sent for culture and biochemical analysis. Patients with severe CAP should have two sets of blood culture analyses, and these are more likely to be positive if the patient has not received antibiotics at the time of sampling, or if there are signs of systolic hypotension, tachycardia, dehydration, or an elevated WBC count.[76] The presence of

bacteremia may not worsen prognosis, but does allow identification of drug-resistant organisms, and most positive blood culture findings in CAP reveal pneumococcus.

Sputum culture should be accompanied by a Gram stain to guide interpretation of the culture results, but not to focus initial antibiotic therapy. In some situations, Gram stain can be used to broaden initial empiric therapy by enhancing the suspicion for organisms that are not covered in routine empiric therapy (such as *S aureus* being suggested by the presence of clusters of Gram-positive cocci, especially during a time of epidemic influenza). Routine serologic testing is not recommended. However, in patients with severe illness, the diagnosis of Legionella can be made by urinary antigen testing, which is the test that is most likely to be positive at the time of admission, but a test that is specific only for serogroup I infection.[1,77] Examination of concentrated urine for pneumococcal antigen may also be valuable. Bronchoscopy is not indicated as a routine diagnostic test, but may be used to focus the initially broad-spectrum empiric therapy to a simpler regimen, and it is often used if the patient is not responding to initial empiric therapy.[78]

Nosocomial Pneumonia

Nosocomial pneumonia is diagnosed when a patient has been in the hospital for at least 48 to 72 h and then a new or progressive infiltrate develops as shown on chest radiograph, accompanied by at least two of the following three conditions: fever, leukocytosis, and purulent sputum. As mentioned, these clinical findings may be sensitive, but not specific for infection, and efforts to improve the clinical diagnosis of pneumonia have involved the previously mentioned CPIS.[79] Many patients with suspected nosocomial pneumonia can have other diagnoses that can be suggested by the rapidity of the clinical response and by the nature of the clinical findings. These diagnoses include atelectasis and congestive heart failure (very rapid clinical resolution), or in the case of a lack of response to therapy, inflammatory lung diseases, extrapulmonary infection (sinusitis, central line infection, intraabdominal infection), or the presence of an unusual or drug-resistant pathogen. In an effort to make the diagnosis more secure and to avoid the overuse of antibiotics, some investigators have used quantitative sampling of lower respiratory secretions collected either bronchoscopically (BAL, protected specimen brush), or nonbronchoscopically (endotracheal aspirate, nonbronchoscopic catheter lavage), particularly in patients with suspected VAP . When quantitative culture results are collected, some investigators[4,5] have defined the presence of pneumonia by the growth of bacteria at a concentration above a predefined threshold concentration. Although the results can guide therapy decisions, most clinicians use antibiotic therapy, regardless of quantitative culture data, in patients who have clinical signs of sepsis and suspected pneumonia.

All patients with suspected nosocomial pneumonia should have a lower respiratory tract culture collected prior to the start of antibiotic therapy. If this is not a quantitative culture, then a sputum or tracheal aspirate should be obtained and the findings reported "semiquantitatively" as light, moderate, or heavy growth of bacteria.[2,5] A negative culture finding is difficult to interpret if the patient has had initiation or change in antibiotic therapy in the preceding 72 h. However, if either a quantitative or semiquantitative culture finding is negative or does not show a highly resistant pathogen, and antibiotics have not been changed in the past 72 h, then the therapy can often be stopped or focused to a more narrow spectrum.[2,80] One large randomized trial[80] showed no mortality benefit of bronchoscopic quantitative cultures, compared with nonquantitative tracheal aspirate cultures, and no difference in the frequency of de-escalation when comparing the two approaches.

Therapy

Algorithms for initial empiric therapy have been developed for all patients with severe pneumonia, based on the most likely etiologic pathogens in a given patient and clinical setting. If diagnostic testing reveals a specific etiologic pathogen, then therapy can be focused to the results. In addition, as previously mentioned, if an anticipated pathogen is not present in a diagnostic sample, it may be possible to stop empiric coverage of that organism.

General Considerations

Until recently, combination empiric antibiotic therapy for severe pneumonia was universally given by physicians working in ICUs. The rationale for this approach was to provide broad antimicrobial coverage, prevent the emergence of resistance during therapy, and potentially provide synergistic activity if a β-lactam antibiotic was combined with an aminoglycoside (for *P aeruginosa* pneumonia). However, only with bacteremic *P aeruginosa* pneumonia has combination therapy (generally with an aminoglycoside and a β-lactam) been shown to be superior to monotherapy.[80–82] If aminoglycosides are used, it is important to recognize their narrow therapeutic-to-toxic ratio, and their potential for nephrotoxicity, particularly in elderly patients. When peak serum levels have been monitored, levels of >7 μg/mL for gentamicin and tobramycin and >28 μg/mL for amikacin have been associated with more favorable outcomes.[83] Aminoglycosides also penetrate poorly into bronchial secretions, achieving only 40% of the serum concentrations at this site. In addition, antimicrobial activity is reduced at the low pH levels that are common in the bronchial secretions of patients with pneumonia. In one study,[84] the addition of an aminoglycoside to imipenem had no added efficacy for severe nosocomial pneumonia, and only added renal toxicity. In addition, a metaanalysis[82] of the value of adding an aminoglycoside to a β-lactam in critically ill patients, including many with pneumonia, found no therapeutic benefit. It has now become standard to administer aminoglycosides by combining the total 24-h dose into a single dose, rather than in divided doses, but this approach has proved to have little advantage with regard to efficacy or safety.[85] In spite of these findings, if aminoglycosides are used, once-daily dosing is recommended because it is simpler and requires less intensive monitoring (measuring only trough levels).

In the absence of certain high-risk organisms (*P aeruginosa*, Acinetobacter spp, and MRSA), antibiotics that have been effective as monotherapy for severe VAP include imipenem, meropenem, cefepime, ciprofloxacin, high-dose levofloxacin (750 mg/d) and piperacillin/tazobactam.[2,86–90] In the patient with severe pneumonia, it is usually necessary to start therapy with multiple agents; but after tracheal aspirate or other lower respiratory tract culture results become available, it is usually possible to de-escalate to monotherapy, particularly if a highly resistant organism is absent.[80]

Monotherapy should not be used in the following situations: (1) in any patient with severe CAP, for whom the efficacy of this approach has not been demonstrated (which includes no monotherapy with a quinolone); (2) in suspected bacteremic infection with *P aeruginosa*; (3) in the empiric therapy of VAP, if the patient has risk factors for infection with MDR pathogens; (4) if the patient has nosocomial pneumonia and both *S aureus* and *P aeruginosa* are identified in culture as the etiologic pathogens; and (5) possibly not in patients with bacteremic pneumococcal pneumonia and severe illness, in which combination therapy has been associated with a lower mortality than monotherapy. Monotherapy should never be attempted with a third-generation cephalosporin because of the possibility of emergence of resistance during therapy as a result of production of chromosomal β-lactamases by the Enterobacteriaceae group of organisms.[2]

If *P aeruginosa* is a target organism of therapy, then the antipseudomonal β-lactam antibiotics include the penicillins such as piperacillin, azlocillin, mezlocillin, ticarcillin, and carbenicillin; the third-generation cephalosporins such as ceftazidime and cefoperazone; the fourth-generation cephalosporin cefepime; the carbapenems such as doripenem, imipenem, and meropenem; the monobactam aztreonam (which can be used in the penicillin-allergic patient); and the β-lactam/β-lactamase inhibitor combinations ticarcillin/clavulanate and piperacillin/ tazobactam. Other antipseudomonal agents include the quinolone ciprofloxacin, high-dose levofloxacin, and the aminoglycosides (amikacin, gentamicin, tobramycin).

CAP

For patients admitted to the ICU with CAP, initial therapy should be directed at DRSP, Legionella, and other atypical pathogens, enteric Gram-negative organisms, and other selected organisms, based on epidemiologic risk assessment.

Therapy is chosen, depending on whether or not the patient is at risk for *P aeruginosa* infection ("modifying" risk factors previously named). In all the treatment algorithms, no ICU-admitted CAP patient should receive empiric monotherapy, even with one of the new quinolones.[1] In one recent study[91] comparing levofloxacin with a β-lactam/quinolone combination, the single-agent regimen was not shown to be effective for patients in septic shock and for those treated with mechanical ventilation. There are no data showing the efficacy of moxifloxacin as monotherapy for severe CAP.

Recommended therapy for severe CAP in the absence of pseudomonal risk factors should be with a selected IV β-lactam (cefotaxime, ceftriaxone, a β-lactam/β-lactamase inhibitor combination), combined with either an IV macrolide or an IV antipneumococcal quinolone (levofloxacin or moxifloxacin). For patients with pseudomonal risk factors, therapy can be with a two-drug regimen, using an antipseudomonal β-lactam (doripenem, imipenem, meropenem, piperacillin/tazobactam, cefepime) plus ciprofloxacin (the most active antipseudomonal, quinolone) or levofloxacin (750 mg/d); or alternatively with a three-drug regimen using an antipseudomonal β-lactam plus an aminoglycoside plus an IV antipneumococcal quinolone (levofloxacin or moxifloxacin) or a macrolide.[1,92] Penicillin-allergic patients should receive aztreonam with levofloxacin or aztreonam with an aminoglycoside plus an antipneumococcal quinolone or macrolide.

In addition to the antibiotic approach to therapy outlined here, all patients should have coverage for atypical pathogens using either a macrolide or a quinolone in the regimen, based on data that such an approach reduces mortality.[26,27,93] Even in patients with pneumococcal bacteremia, the use of combination therapy (generally with the addition of atypical pathogen coverage to pneumococcal coverage) has been associated with reduced mortality, compared with monotherapy.[93] In addition, certain adjunctive therapies should be considered, including oxygen, chest physiotherapy (if at least 30 mL of sputum daily and a poor cough response), aerosolized bronchodilators, and corticosteroids (if hypotension and possible relative adrenal insufficiency are present). An analysis of the use of activated protein C for patients with septic shock demonstrated that 35% of the patients in the pivotal clinical trial had underlying CAP, and that activated protein C was most effective for those CAP patients with an APACHE II score >25, a PSI class of IV or V, and a CURB-65 score of at least 2. There was also benefit in those with pneumococcal infection and with inadequate therapy, although the benefit was minimal in those treated with adequate therapy.[94] In addition to their value in patients with relative adrenal insufficiency, corticosteroids may be helpful in severe CAP because of their immunomodulating effect. One randomized controlled trial[95] of 48 patients compared hydrocortisone infusion (240 mg/d) with placebo and found that steroid therapy reduced mortality, length of stay, and duration of mechanical ventilation. These findings require other studies to confirm the benefit of this adjunctive therapy. However, if corticosteroids are needed for reasons other than pneumonia, they do not appear to add to mortality risk.

The presence of extrapulmonary infection (such as meningitis), and the identification of certain pathogens (such as bacteremic *S aureus* and *P aeruginosa*) may require longer durations of therapy than the usual 5 to 7 days. Identification of *Legionella pneumophila* pneumonia may require quinolone therapy, and durations as short as 5 days with levofloxacin 750 mg may be effective.[96] Currently there is controversy about the need for empiric therapy directed against community-acquired MRSA. Most experts recommend that this organism should be targeted in patients with severe, necrotizing CAP, but to shut off production of the Panton-Valentine leukocidin toxin that accompanies community-acquired MRSA, it may be necessary to add clindamycin to vancomycin or to use linezolid, as both of these latter agents can inhibit toxin production.[70]

Nosocomial Pneumonia

Antibiotic therapy should be given promptly at the first clinical suspicion of pneumonia, and empiric therapy should be dictated by considering whether the patient is at risk for infection with MDR pathogens, primarily because of the presence of recent antibiotic therapy, a prolonged hospital stay, or the development of infection after residing in a nursing home or other long-term care setting (such as a dialysis center), or if there are other risk factors for HCAP. Patients without risks for MDR pathogens can be treated for the "core pathogens" previously listed, generally with a monotherapy regimen of a second, or non-pseudomonal third-generation cephalosporin, a β-lactam/β-lactamase inhibitor combination, ertapenem, or a quinolone (levofloxacin or moxifloxacin).[2] If the patient is allergic to penicillin, therapy can be with a quinolone or the combination of clindamycin and aztreonam. Probably not all HCAP patients need therapy directed against MDR pathogens, and monotherapy has been successful in patients without MDR risk factors. For HCAP patients, in addition to severe pneumonia, the risk factors for MDR pathogens include recent hospitalization, recent antibiotic therapy, immune suppression, and poor functional status.[71] Patients with severe HCAP and at least one other risk factor should receive empiric therapy directed at MDR pathogens.

In the selection of an empiric therapy regimen, it is necessary to choose an agent that is in a different class of antibiotics than the patient has received in the past 14 days, as repeated use of the same class of antibiotic may drive resistance to that class, especially if the pathogen is *P aeruginosa*.[97] Similar findings have been made for patients with bacteremic pneumococcal pneumonia and CAP, and repeat use of an agent within 3 months may mean that the patient is being treated with an agent to which pneumococcus is more likely to be resistant.[98] In addition, the recent use of quinolones may present a particular problem, because in the ICU recent quinolone therapy may predispose to not only quinolone-resistant organisms, but also to infection with MDR pathogens, extended-spectrum β-lactamase producing Gram-negative organisms, and MRSA.[99]

The concept of "antibiotic rotation" has been studied in patients with VAP and involves using an empiric regimen that is intentionally varied over time to expose bacteria to different antibiotics and thus minimize the selection pressure for resistance. This approach has been effective in reducing the incidence of infection with resistant organisms in some studies.[100] One of the limitations of antibiotic rotation is that it may mean the use of the same regimen repeatedly in the same patient, and this may itself be a risk factor for selecting for resistance. In addition, there are many unanswered questions.[101]

Patients at risk for MDR pathogens generally require combination therapy, rather than monotherapy. The empiric therapy for patients at risk for MDR pathogens should include an aminoglycoside or quinolone (ciprofloxacin or high-dose levofloxacin) plus an antipseudomonal β-lactam (doripenem, imipenem, meropenem, piperacillin/tazobactam, aztreonam, or cefepime). If the patient is at risk for a second ICU-acquired infection (and most are), it may be prudent to use an aminoglycoside for the first episode of infection, reserving the quinolone for any subsequent infection, because of concern about quinolone induction of multidrug resistance, which could limit subsequent therapy options.[102] If the patient is suspected of having MRSA because of a tracheal aspirate Gram stain showing Gram-positive organisms, or because of other risk factors, then a third drug should be added. This could be either linezolid or vancomycin, and recent data[103] have suggested the superiority of linezolid for both survival and clinical cure in patients who have been documented as having MRSA VAP.

If the patient has received a broad-spectrum regimen and the culture findings do not show MDR organisms, then the patient can finish therapy with any of six monotherapy regimens that have been documented to be effective for severe VAP in the absence of MDR organisms: ciprofloxacin, imipenem, meropenem, piperacillin/tazobactam, cefepime, and high-dose levofloxacin. If *P aeruginosa* is present, combination therapy with a β-lactam and aminoglycoside should continue for 5 days, after which the patient can be switched to monotherapy with an agent to which the organism is sensitive.[2] When de-escalation has been used—meaning either the switch to a more narrow spectrum regimen, the use of fewer drugs, or both—mortality in VAP has been reduced, compared to when patients do not have de-escalation.[37,38]

If the lower respiratory tract culture findings are negative, it may be possible to stop therapy (especially if an alternative diagnosis is suspected) or to shorten the duration of therapy. In addition, if culture findings show that the initial empiric regimen was appropriate, and if the patient has a good clinical response (reflected by a drop in the CPIS), then it may be possible to reduce the duration of therapy to as little as 7 to 8 days, although this may not be possible if the etiologic pathogen is *P aeruginosa* or MRSA.[104]

Adjunctive therapeutic measures such as chest physiotherapy, aerosolized bronchodilators, and mucolytic agents are needed in some patients. For select patients who are infected with highly resistant organisms that not responding to systemic antibiotics, it may be valuable to add aerosolized antibiotics (such as gentamicin, tobramycin, colistin, and ceftazidime).[105]

Evaluation of Nonresponding Patients

Nonresponding patients with either CAP or VAP should be evaluated for alternative diagnoses (inflammatory lung disease, atelectasis, heart failure, malignancy, pulmonary hemorrhage, pulmonary embolus, a nonpneumonic infection), a resistant or unusual pathogen (including tuberculosis and fungal infection), a pneumonia complication (empyema, lung abscess, drug fever, antibiotic–induced colitis), or a secondary site of infection (central line infection, intra-abdominal infection). The evaluation of a nonresponding patient should be individualized but may include CT scanning of the chest, pulmonary angiography, bronchoscopy, and occasionally open lung biopsy.

Prevention

Prevention of CAP is important for all groups of patients and includes vaccination with both pneumococcal and influenza vaccines, and cigarette smoking cessation in all at-risk patients. Even for the patient who is recovering from CAP, immunization while in the hospital is appropriate to prevent future episodes of infection. If there is uncertainty about whether the patient has been vaccinated recently, it is probably best to give a pneumococcal vaccination, as repeat administration, even more often than recommended, is not generally associated with an adverse reaction.[106] Hospital-based immunization is recommended. One study[107] found that among 1,633 patients with pneumonia treated in the hospital, 62% had been hospitalized in the preceding 4 years. In addition, 80% of these patients had a high-risk condition that would have qualified them to receive pneumococcal vaccine.

Although no single method is able to reliably prevent nosocomial pneumonia, multiple small interventions may have benefit, especially those focused on modifiable risk factors for infection. Recently, these interventions have been combined into "ventilator bundles," which have been demonstrated to reduce the incidence of VAP if applied carefully.[108,109] Most of these bundles include multiple interventions, so it is difficult to know which individual manipulations are most valuable. Successful bundles have included interventions such as elevation of the head of the bed to 30° (to avoid the risk of aspiration present with the supine position), daily interruption of sedation to attempt weaning, peptic ulcer disease prophylaxis, endotracheal tube suctioning (possibly with a closed-suction system), hand washing, careful oral care, and tight control of blood glucose.[110] In spite of the success of this approach, one recent randomized study[111] has demonstrated a lack of benefit and feasibility of routine elevation of the head of the bed.

Other widely used measures in patients receiving mechanical ventilation are avoidance of large inocula of bacteria into the lung (careful handling of ventilator circuit tubing), mobilization of respiratory secretions (frequent suctioning, use of rotational bed therapy in selected individuals), nutritional support (enteral preferred over parenteral), placing of feeding tubes into the small bowel (to avoid aspiration, which is more likely with stomach tubes), and avoidance of large gastric residuals when giving enteral feeding. In addition, any tube inserted into the stomach or trachea should be inserted through the mouth and not the nose, whenever possible, to avoid obstructing the nasal sinuses, and to prevent nosocomial sinusitis, which can lead to nosocomial pneumonia.[110] A specially adapted endotracheal tube that allows for continuous aspiration of subglottic secretions may interrupt the oropharyngeal-to-tracheal transfer of bacteria and reduce the incidence of pneumonia.[112] Recently, a silver-coated endotracheal tube has been studied and reported to reduce the risk of VAP.[113] Because endotracheal intubation is a risk for pneumonia, noninvasive positive pressure ventilation should be used whenever possible, and this approach is associated with a lower pneumonia risk than traditional mechanical ventilation. There is no specific role for prophylactic systemic or topical antibiotics, but some data suggest that patients with coma due to stroke or head trauma, and those who may have aspirated during an emergent intubation, may benefit from a 24-h course of systemic antibiotics.[114] Selective digestive decontamination has also been studied, but recent data indicate that oral decontamination alone may be effective in preventing VAP, and that the entire regimen is not necessary.[115]

References

1. Mandell LA, Wunderink RG, Anzueto A, et al. Infectious Diseases Society of America/American Thoracic Society consensus guidelines on the management of community-acquired pneumonia in adults. Clin Infect.Dis 2007; 44(suppl 2):S27–S72
2. Niederman MS, Craven DE, Bonten MJ, et al. Guidelines for the management of adults with hospital-acquired, ventilator-associated, and healthcare-associated pneumonia. Am J Respir Crit Care Med 2005; 171:388–416
3. Kaplan V, Clermont G, Griffin MF, et al. Pneumonia: still the old man's friend? Arch Intern Med 2003; 163:317–323
4. Fagon JY, Chastre J, Wolff M, et al. Invasive and noninvasive strategies for management of suspected ventilator-associated pneumonia: a randomized trial. Ann Intern Med 2000; 132:621–630
5. The Canadian Critical Care Trials Group. A randomized trial of diagnostic techniques for ventilator-associated pneumonia. N Engl J Med 2006; 355:2619–2630
6. Torres A, Serra-Batlles J, Ferrer A, et al. Severe community-acquired pneumonia. Epidemiology and prognostic factors. Am Rev Respir Dis 1991; 144:312
7. Pachon J, Prados MD, Capote F, et al. Severe community-acquired pneumonia: Etiology, prognosis, and treatment. Am Rev Respir Dis 1990; 142:369.
8. Ewig S, de Roux A, Bauer T, et al. Validation of predictive rules and indices of severity for community acquired pneumonia. Thorax 2004; 59:421–427
9. Woodhead M, Welch CA, Harrison DA, et al. Community-acquired pneumonia on the intensive care unit: secondary analysis of 17,869 cases in the ICNARC case mix programme database. Crit Care 2006; 10(suppl 2):S1

10. Leroy O, Santre C, Beuscart C. A 5-year study of severe community-acquired pneumonia with emphasis on prognosis in patients admitted to an ICU. Intensive Care Med 1995; 21:24–31

11. Heyland DK, Cook DJ, Griffith L, et al. The attributable morbidity and mortality of ventilator-associated pneumonia in the critically ill patient. The Canadian Critical trials group. Am J Respir Crit Care Med 1999; 159:1249–1256

12. Kollef MH. Inadequate antimicrobial treatment: an important determinant of outcome for hospitalized patients. Clin Infect Dis 2000; 31(suppl 4): S131–S138.

13. Kollef MH, Shorr A, Tabak YP, et al. Epidemiology and outcomes of health-care-associated pneumonia: results from a large US database of culture positive patients. Chest 2005; 128:3854–3862

14. Ruiz M, Ewig S, Torres A, et al. Severe community-acquired pneumonia: risk factors and follow-up epidemiology. Am J Respir Crit Care Med 1999; 160:923–929

15. Nuorti JP, Butler JC, Farley MM, et al. Cigarette smoking and invasive pneumococcal disease. N Engl J Med 2000; 342:681–689

16. Waterer GW, Quasney MW, Cantor RM, et al. Septic shock and respiratory failure in community-acquired pneumonia have different TNF polymorphism associations. Am J Respir Crit Care Med 2001; 163:1599–1604

17. Fine MJ, Smith MA, Carson CA, et al. Prognosis and outcomes of patients with community-acquired pneumonia. A meta-analysis. JAMA 1996; 275:134–141

18. Houck PM, Bratzler DW, Nsa W, et al. Timing of antibiotic administration and outcomes for Medicare patients hospitalized with community-acquired pneumonia. Arch Intern Med 2004; 164:637–644

19. Waterer GW, Kessler LA, Wunderink RG. Delayed administration of antibiotics and atypical presentation in community-acquired pneumonia. Chest 2006; 130:11–15

20. Meteresky ML, Sweeney TA, Getzow MB, et al. Antibiotic timing and diagnostic uncertainty in Medicare patients with pneumonia: is it reasonable to expect all patients to receive antibiotics within 4 hours? Chest 2006; 130:16–21

21. Fine MJ, Auble TE, Yealy DM, et al. A prediction rule to identify low-risk patients with community-acquired pneumonia. N Engl J Med 1997; 336:243–250

22. Lim WS, van der Erden MM, Laing R, et al. Defining community acquired pneumonia severity on presentation to hospital: an international derivation and validation study. Thorax 2003; 58:377–382

23. Aujesky D, Auble TE, Yealy DM, et al. Prospective comparison of three validated prediction rules for prognosis in community-acquired pneumonia. Am J Med 2005; 118:384–392

24. Niederman MS. Making sense of scoring systems in community-acquired pneumonia. Respirology 2009; 14:327–335

25. Ewig S, Ruiz M, Mensa J, et al. Severe community-acquired pneumonia: assessment of severity criteria. Am J Respir Crit Care Med 1998; 158;1102–1108

26. Gleason PP, Meehan TP, Fine JM, et al. Associations between initial antimicrobial therapy and medical outcomes for hospitalized elderly patients with pneumonia. Arch Intern Med 1999; 159:2562–2572

27. Houck PM, MacLehose RF, Niederman MS, et al. Empiric antibiotic therapy and mortality among medicare pneumonia inpatients in 10 Western states: 1993, 1995, and 1997. Chest 2001; 119:1420–1426

28. Marrie TJ, Blanchard W. A comparison of nursing home-acquired pneumonia patients with patients with community-acquired pneumonia and nursing home patients without pneumonia. J Am Geriatr Soc 1997; 45:50

29. Starczewski AR, Allen SC, Vargas E, et al. Clinical prognostic indices of fatality in elderly patients admitted to hospital with acute pneumonia. Age Ageing 1988; 17:181–186

30. Cook DJ, Walter SD, Cook RJ. Incidence of and risk factors for ventilator-associated pneumonia in critically ill patients. Ann Intern Med 1998; 129:433–440

31. Sutherland KR, Steinberg KP, Maunder RJ, et al. Pulmonary infection during the acute respiratory distress syndrome. Am J Respir Crit Care Med 1995; 152:550–556

32. Chastre J, Trouillet JL, Vuagnet A, et al. Nosocomial pneumonia in patients with acute respiratory distress syndrome. Am J Respir Crit Care Med 1998; 157:1165–1172

33. Seidenfeld JJ, Pohl DF, Bell RD, et al. Incidence, site, and outcome of infections in patients with the adult respiratory distress syndrome. Am Rev Respir Dis 1986; 134:12–16

34. Luna CM, Vujacich P, Niederman MS, et al: Impact of BAL data on the therapy and outcome of ventilator associated pneumonia. Chest 1997; 111:676–685

35. Dupont H, Mentec H, Sollet JP, et al. Impact of appropriateness of initial antibiotic therapy on the outcome of ventilator-associated pneumonia. Intensive Care Med 2001; 27:355–362

36. Clec'h C, Timsit JF, De Lassence A, et al. Efficacy of adequate antibiotic therapy in ventilator-associated pneumonia: influence of disease severity. Intensive Care Med 2004; 30:1327–1333

37. Kollef MH, Morrow LE, Niederman MS, et al. Clinical characteristics and treatment patterns among patients with ventilator-associated pneumonia. Chest 2006; 129:1210–1218

38. Soo Hoo GW, Wen E, Nguyen TV, et al. Impact of clinical guidelines in management of severe hospital-acquired pneumonia. Chest 2005; 128:2778–2787

39. Rello J, Sole-Violan J, Sa-borges M, et al. Pneumonia caused by oxacillin-resistant *Staphylococcus aureus* treated with glycopeptides. Crit Care Med 2005; 33:1983–1987

40. Chastre J, Fagon JY. Ventilator-associated pneumonia. Am J Respir Crit Care Med 2002; 165:867–903

41. Rello J, Quintana E, Ausina V, et al. Incidence, etiology, and outcome of nosocomial pneumonia in mechanically ventilated patients, Chest 1991; 100:439–444

42. Graybill JR, Marshall LW, Charache P, et al. Nosocomial pneumonia: a continuing major problem, Am Rev Respir Dis 1973; 108:1130–1140

43. Fagon JY, Chastre J, Hance A, et al. Nosocomial pneumonia in ventilated patients: a cohort study evaluation attributable mortality and hospital stay. Am J Med 1993; 94:281–288

44. Trouillet J-L, Chastre J, Vuagnat A, et al. Ventilator-associated pneumonia caused by potentially drug-resistant bacteria, Am J Respir Crit Care Med 1998; 157:531–539

45. Skerrett SJ, Niederman MS, Fein AM. Respiratory infections and acute lung injury in systemic illness. Clin Chest Med 1989; 10:469–502

46. Campbell GD, Niederman MS, Broughton WA, et al. Hospital-acquired pneumonia in adults: diagnosis, assessment of severity, initial antimicrobial therapy, and preventative strategies: a consensus statement. Am J Respir Crit Care Med 1996; 153:1711–1725

47. Niederman MS, Ahmed QA. Inflammation in severe pneumonia: act locally, not globally. Crit Care Med 1999; 27:2030–2032

48. Niederman MS, Craven DE: Devising strategies for preventing nosocomial pneumonia: should we ignore the stomach? Clin Infect Dis 1997; 24:320–323

49. Holzapfel L, Chastang C, Demingeon G, et al. A randomized study assessing the systematic search for maxillary sinusitis in nasotracheally mechanically ventilated patients: influence of nosocomial maxillary sinusitis on the occurrence of ventilator-associated pneumonia. Am J Respir Crit Care Med 1999; 159: 695–701

50. Sottile FD, Marrie TJ, Prough DS, et al. Nosocomial pulmonary infection: possible etiologic significance of bacterial adhesion to endotracheal tubes, Crit Care Med 1986; 14:265–270

51. Prince AS. Biofilms, antimicrobial resistance, and airway infection. N Engl J Med 2002; 347:1110–1111

52. Torres A, Gatell JM, Aznar E, et al. Re-intubation increases the risk for nosocomial pneumonia in patients needing mechanical ventilation. Am J Respir Crit Care Med 1995; 152:137–141

53. Craven DE, Goularte TA, Make BJ. Contaminated condensate in mechanical ventilator circuits: a risk factor for nosocomial pneumonia. Am Rev Respir Dis 1984; 129:625–628

54. Craven DE, Lichtenberg DA, Goularte TA, et al. Contaminated medication nebulizers in mechanical ventilator circuits. Source of bacterial aerosols. Am J Med 1984; 77:834–838

55. Craven DE, Connolly MG Jr, Lichtenberg DA, et al. Contamination of mechanical ventilators with tubing changes every 24 or 48 hours. N Engl J Med 1982; 306:1505–1509

56. Dreyfuss D, Djedaini K, Weber P, et al. Prospective study of nosocomial pneumonia and of patient and circuit colonization during mechanical ventilation with circuit changes every 48 hours versus no change. Am Rev Respir Dis 1991; 143:738–743

57. Hess D, Burns E, Romagnoli D, et al. Weekly ventilator circuit changes: a strategy to reduce costs without affecting pneumonia rates. Anesthesiology 1995; 82:902–911

58. Djedaini K, Billiard M, Mier L, et al. Changing heat and moisture exchangers every 48 hours rather than 24 hours does not affect their efficacy and the incidence of nosocomial pneumonia. Am J Respir Crit Care Med 1995; 152:1562–1568

59. Metaly JP, Schulz R, Li Y-H, et al. Influence of age on symptoms at presentation in patients with community-acquired pneumonia. Arch Intern Med 1997; 157:1453–1459

60. Fine MJ, Orloff JJ, Arisumi D, et al. Prognosis of patients hospitalized with community-acquired pneumonia. Am J Med 1990; 88:1N–8N

61. Lapinsky SE, Hawryluck L. ICU management of severe acute respiratory syndrome. Intensive Care Med 2003; 29:870–875

62. Luna CM, Blanzaco D, Niederman MS, et al. Resolution of ventilator-associated pneumonia: prospective evaluation of the clinical pulmonary infection score as an early clinical predictor of outcome. Crit Care Med 2003; 31:676–682

63. Clavo-Sánchez AJ, Girón-González JA, López-Prieto D, et al. Multivariate analysis of risk factors for infection due to penicillin-resistant and multidrug-resistant Streptococcus pneumoniae: a multicenter study. Clin Infect Dis 1997; 24:1052–1059

64. Van Eeden SF, Coetzee AR, Joubert JR. Community-acquired pneumonia-factors influencing intensive care admission. S Afr Med J 1988; 73:77–81

65. McFadden JP, Price RC, Eastwood HD, et al. Raised respiratory rate in elderly patients: a valuable physical sign. Br Med J 1982; 284:626–627

66. Doern GV, Richter SS, Miller A, et al. Antimicrobial resistance among Streptococcus pneumoniae in the United States: have we begun to turn the corner on resistance to certain antimicrobial classes? Clin Infect Dis 2005; 41:139–148

67. Feikin DR, Schuchat A, Kolczak M, et al. Mortality from invasive pneumococcal pneumonia in the era of antibiotic resistance, 1995–1997. Am J Public Health 2000; 90:223–229

68. Ruiz M, Ewig S, Torres A, et al. Severe community-acquired pneumonia: risk factors and follow-up epidemiology. Am J Respir Crit Care Med 1999; 160:923–929

69. Francis JS, Doherty MC, Lopatin U, et al. Severe community-onset pneumonia in healthy adults caused by methicillin-resistant Staphylococcus aureus carrying the Panton-Valentine leukocidin genes. Clin Infect Dis 2005 40:100–107

70. Micek ST, Dunne M, Kollef MH. Pleuropulmonary complications of Panton-Valentine leukocidin-positive community-acquired methicillin-resistant Staphylococcus aureus: importance of treatment with antimicrobials inhibiting exotoxin production. Chest 2005; 128:2732–2738

71. El – Solh AA, Pietrantoni C, Bhat A, et al. Microbiology of severe aspiration pneumonia in institutionalized elderly. Am J Respir Crit Care Med 2003; 167:1650–1654

72. Fagon JY, Chastre J, Domart Y, et al. Nosocomial pneumonia in patients receiving continuous mechanical ventilation: prospective analysis of 52 episodes with use of a protected specimen brush and quantitative culture techniques. Am Rev Respir Dis 1989; 139:877–884

73. Gaynes R, Edwards JR, and the National Nosocomial Infections Surveillance System. Overview of infections caused by gram-negative bacilli. Clin Infect Dis 2005; 41:848–854

74. El Solh AA, Pietrantoni C, Bhat A, et al. Indicators of potentially drug-resistant bacteria in severe nursing home-acquired pneumonia. Clin Infect Dis 2004; 39:474–480

75. Rello J, Sa-Borges M, Correa H, et al. Variations in etiology of ventilator-associated pneumonia across four treatment sites. Implications for antimicrobial prescribing practices. Am J Respir Crit Care Med 1999; 160:608–613

76. Metersky ML, Ma A, Bratzler DW, et al. Predicting bacteremia in patients with community-acquired pneumonia. Am J Respir Crit Care Med 2004; 169:342–347

77. Plouffe JF, File TM, Breiman RF, et al. Reevaluation of the definition of Legionnaires' disease: use of the urinary antigen assay. Clin Infect Dis 1995; 20:1286–1291

78. Rello J, Bodi M, Mariscal D, et al. Microbiological testing and outcome of patients with severe community-acquired pneumonia. Chest 2003; 123:174–180

79. Pugin J, Auckenthaler R, Mili N, et al. Diagnosis of ventilator-associated pneumonia by bacteriology analysis of bronchoscopic and nonbronchoscopic "blind" bronchoalveolar lavage fluid, Am Rev Respir Dis 1991; 143:1121–1129

80. The Canadian Critical Care Trials Group. A randomized trial of diagnostic techniques for ventilator-associated pneumonia. N Engl J Med 2006; 355:2619–2630

81. Hilf M, Yu VL, Sharp J, et al. Antibiotic therapy for Pseudomonas aeruginosa bacteremia: outcome correlations in a prospective study of 200 patients, Am J Med 1989; 87:540–546

82. Paul M, Benuri-Silbiger I, Soares-Weiser K, et al. Beta-lactam monotherapy versus beta-lactam-aminoglycoside combination therapy for sepsis in immunocompetent patients: systematic review and meta-analysis of randomised trials. BMJ 2004 2 Mar [Epub ahead of print]

83. Moore RD, Smith CR, Lietman PS. Association of aminoglycoside plasma levels with therapeutic outcome in Gram-negative pneumonia. Am J Med 1984; 77:657–662

84. Cometta A, Baumgartner JD, Lew D, et al. Prospective randomized comparison of imipenem monotherapy with imipenem plus netilmicin for treatment of severe infections in nonneutropenic patients. Antimicrob Agents Chemother 1994; 38:1309–1313

85. Hatala R, Dinh T, Cook DJ. Once-daily aminoglycoside dosing in immunocompetent adults: a meta analysis. Ann Intern Med 1996; 124:717–725

86. Fink MP, Snydman DR, Niederman MS, et al. Treatment of severe pneumonia in hospitalized patients: results of a multicenter, randomized, double-blind trial comparing intravenous ciprofloxacin with imipenem-cilastatin. Antimicrob Agents Chemother 1994; 38:547–557

87. Jaccard C, Troillet N, Harbarth S, et al. Prospective randomized comparison of imipenem–cilastatin and piperacillin–tazobactam in nosocomial pneumonia or peritonitis. Antimicrob Agents Chemother 1998; 42:2966–2972

88. West M, Boulanger BR, Fogarty C, et al. Levofloxacin compared with imipenem/cilastatin followed by ciprofloxacin in adult patients with nosocomial pneumonia: a multicenter, prospective, randomized, open-label study. Clin Ther 2003; 25:485–506

89. Chapman TM, Perry CM. Cefepime: a review of its use in the management of hospitalized patients with pneumonia. Am J Respir Med 2003; 2:75–107

90. Sieger B, Berman SJ, Geckler RW, et al. Meropenem Lower Respiratory Infection Group. Empiric treatment of hospital-acquired lower respiratory tract infections with meropenem or ceftazidime with tobramycin: a randomized study. Crit Care Med 1997; 25:1663–1670

91. Leroy O, Saux P, Bedos JP, et al. Comparison of levofloxacin and cefotaxime combined with ofloxacin for ICU patients with community-acquired pneumonia who do not require vasopressors. Chest 2005; 128:172–183

92. File TM, Niederman MS. Antimicrobial therapy of community-acquired pneumonia. Infect Dis Clin North Am 2004; 18:993–1016

93. Waterer GW, Somes GW, Wunderink RG. Monotherapy may be suboptimal for severe bacteremic pneumococcal pneumonia. Arch Intern Med 2001; 161:1837–1842

94. Laterre PF, Garber G, Levy H, et al. Severe community-acquired pneumonia as a cause of severe sepsis: data from the PROWESS study. Crit Care Med. 2005; 33:952–961

95. Confalonieri M, Urbino R, Potena A, et al. Hydrocortisone infusion for severe community-acquired pneumonia: a preliminary randomized study. Am J Respir Crit Care Med. 2005 ;171:242–248

96. Yu VL, Greenberg RN, Zadeikis N, et al. Levofloxacin efficacy in the treatment of community-acquired legionellosis. Chest 2004; 125:2135–2139

97. Trouillet JL, Vuagnat A, Combes A, et al. *Pseudomonas aeruginosa* ventilator-associated pneumonia: comparison of episodes due to piperacillin-resistant versus piperacillin-susceptible organisms. Clin Infect Dis 2002; 34:1047–1054

98. Vanderkooi OG, Low DE, Green K, Powis et al. Predicting antimicrobial resistance in invasive pneumococcal infections. Clin Infect Dis 2005; 40:1288–1297

99. Nseir S, Di Pompeo C, Soubrier S, et al. First-generation fluoroquinolone use and subsequent emergence of multiple drug-resistant bacteria in the intensive care unit. Crit Care Med 2005; 33:283–289

100. Kollef MH, Vlasnik J, Sharpless L, et al. Scheduled change of antibiotic classes: a strategy to decrease the incidence of ventilator-associated pneumonia. Am J Respir Crit Care Med 1997; 156:1040–1048

101. Niederman MS. Is crop rotation of antibiotics the solution to a resistant problem in the ICU? Am J Respir Crit Care Med 1997; 156:1029–1031

102. Niederman MS. Reexamining quinolone use in the intensive care unit: use them right or lose the fight against resistant bacteria. Crit Care Med 2005; 33:443–444

103. Wunderink RG, Rello J, Cammarata SK, et al. Linezolid vs vancomycin: analysis of two double-blind studies of patients with methicillin-resistant *Staphylococcus aureus* nosocomial pneumonia. Chest 2003; 124:1789–1797.

104. Chastre J, Wolff M, Fagon JY, et al. Comparison of 8 vs 15 days of antibiotic therapy for ventilator-associated pneumonia in adults: a randomized trial. JAMA 2003; 290:2588–2598

105. Michalopoulos A, Kasiakou SK, Mastora Z, et al. Aerosolized colistin for the treatment of nosocomial pneumonia due to multidrug-resistant Gram-negative bacteria in patients without cystic fibrosis. Crit Care 2005; 9:R53–R59

106. Walker FJ, Singleton RJ, Bulkow LR, et al. Reactions after 3 or more doses of pneumococcal polysaccharide vaccine in adults in Alaska. Clin Infect Dis 2005; 40:1730–1735

107. Fedson DS, Harward MP, Reid RA, et al. Hospital-based pneumococcal immunization: epidemiologic rationale from the Shenandoah study. JAMA 1990; 264:1117–1122

108. Zack JE, Garrison T, Trovillion E, et al. Effect of an educational program aimed at reducing the occurrence of ventilator associated pneumonia. Crit Care Med 2002; 30:2407–2412

109. Concanour CS, Peninger M, Domonoske BD, et al. Decreasing ventilator-associated pneumonia in a trauma ICU. J Trauma 2006; 61:122–130

110. Tablan OC, Anderson LJ, Besser R, CDC; Healthcare Infection Control Practices Advisory Committee. Guidelines for preventing health-care-associated pneumonia, 2003. MMWR 2004; 53:1–36

111. Van Nieuwenhoven CA, Vandenbroucke-Grauls C, van Tiel FH, et al. Feasibility and effects of the semirecumbent position to prevent ventilator-associated pneumonia: a randomized study. Crit Care Med 2006; 34:396–402

112. Vallés J, Artigas A, Rello J, et al. Continuous aspiration of subglottic secretions in preventing ventilator-associated pneumonia. Ann Intern Med 1995; 122:179–186

113. Kollef MH, Afessa B, Anzueto A, et al. Silver-coated endotracheal tubes and the incidence of ventilator-associated pneumonia: The NASCENT randomized trial. JAMA 2008; 300:505–513

114. Sirvent JM, Torres A, El-Ebiary M, et al. Protective effect of intravenously administered cefuroxime against nosocomial pneumonia in patients with structural coma. Am J Respir Crit Care Med 1997; 155:1729–1734

115. deSmet AMGA, Kluytmans JAJW, Cooper BS, et al. Decontamination of the digestive tract and oropharynx in ICU patients. N Engl J Med 2009; 360:20–31

Notes

Acute Kidney Injury in the Critically Ill

Richard S. Muther, MD

Objectives:

- Appreciate the impact of acute kidney injury (AKI) not only on acute mortality but also chronic kidney disease
- Develop a systematic diagnostic approach to the various glomerular, interstitial, vascular, and tubular disorders causing AKI
- Learn the preventive, supportive, and renal replacement therapies for critically ill patients with AKI

Key words: acute tubular necrosis; chronic kidney disease; end-stage renal disease; glomerulonephritis; interstitial nephritis; prerenal azotemia; renal replacement therapies

Definition

The incidence and mortality of acute kidney injury (AKI) vary substantially with its definition, which is traditionally based on acute changes in serum creatinine.[1] The RIFLE criteria[2] (Table 1) standardize the definition by identifying the kidney as at risk, injured, or in failure based on either an increase in serum creatinine or a decrease in urine output. Loss of renal function for >30 days may lead to chronic kidney disease (CKD) and either AKI or CKD may result in end-stage renal disease (ESRD).

Three studies validate the classification of AKI defined by the RIFLE criteria in critically ill patients. Hoste et al[3] identified AKI in 67% of 5,383 ICU patients; 12.4% at risk, 26.5% as injured, and 28.1% as renal failure. The mortality progressively increased from 8.8% (hazard ratio [HR], 1.0) with risk, to 11.4% (HR, 1.4) with injury, to 26.7% (HR, 2.7) with failure. Those patients without AKI had an ICU mortality rate of only 5.5%. In another study by Osterman and Chang,[4] risk, injury, and failure were identified in 17.2%, 11%, and 7.6%, respectively, of 41,972 ICU patients. The mortality was 8.4% (HR, 1.0) in those without AKI, 20.9% (HR, 1.4) in those at risk, 45.6% (HR, 1.96) in those with injury, and 56.8% (HR, 1.59) in those with failure. A third study by Bagshaw et al[5] retrospectively found AKI in 36.1% of 120,123 critically ill patients: 16.2% at risk, 13.6% with injury, and 6.3% with failure.

The seemingly minor changes in serum creatinine defining AKI by RIFLE are in fact supported by observational studies. In the largest study, Chertow et al[6] found that even very small changes in serum creatinine (*eg*, 0.3 to 0.4 mg/dL) acutely may significantly increase mortality, length of stay, and the cost of care in 19,982 adult hospitalized patients.

Because the serum creatinine is neither a sensitive nor specific marker of AKI, other biomarkers are generating interest. These include cystatin C, *N*-acetyl-β-D-glucosaminidase, urinary interleukin (IL)-18, kidney injury molecule-1, and neutrophil gelatinase-associated lipocalin (NGAL). For example, in an ICU population, an elevation in serum cystatin C precedes that of serum creatinine by 24 to 48 h and appears to predict not only mortality but also the need for renal replacement therapy (RRT).[7,8] In patients with ARDS, an increase in urinary IL-18 predicts a subsequent (24-h) rise in serum creatinine and is an independent predictor of mortality.[9] In 635 patients presenting to an urban emergency department,

Table 1. *RIFLE Criteria for Diagnosis of Acute Kidney Injury*

Kidney Status	Serum Creatinine Criteria	Urine Output Criteria
Risk	Increase Scr 1.5–2-fold from baseline	<0.5 mL/kg/h for 6 h
Injury	Increase Scr 2–3-fold from baseline	<0.5 mL/kg/h for 12 h
Failure	Increase Scr >3-fold from baseline	<0.3 mL/kg/h for 24 h
	or	or
	Scr >4.0 mg/dL with acute rise ≥0.5 mg/dL	Anuria for 12 h
Loss	Persistent renal failure for >4 wk	
ESRD	Persistent renal failure for >3 mo	

urinary NGAL substantially improved both sensitivity and specificity for detecting AKI and was highly predictive of clinical outcomes.[10] In a trial[11] of pediatric cardiac surgery patients, urinary NGAL increased within 2 h postoperatively (2 to 3 days before an increase in serum creatinine) and correlated with the severity and duration of AKI, length of stay, dialysis requirement, and death. This advancement in diagnostic testing offers the hope of not only early detection of AKI, but also more specific (and successful) treatments.

Epidemiology

The incidence of AKI has increased over the last 25 years both as a percentage of hospitalized patients and of those who are critically ill. Between 1979 and 2002, the National Center for Health Statistics showed an increasing rate of AKI diagnoses among overall hospitalizations and among those "discharged dead" (1.5% in 1979, 15.7% in 2002).[12] Over the same time period, single-center studies found that the incidence of AKI increased in hospitalized patients from 5 to >7% of all hospitalized patients.[13,14]

Two recent multicenter studies focus specifically on critically ill patients. The Program to Improve Care in Acute Renal Disease (PICARD)[15] studied patients admitted to the ICUs of five US academic medical centers. Common etiologies included acute tubular necrosis (ATN) without obvious cause (50%) followed by nephrotoxic ATN (26%), cardiac disease (myocardial infarction, congestive heart failure, cardiogenic shock; 20%), sepsis (19%), unresolved prerenal disease (16%), and liver disease (11%). Mortality ranged from 24 to 62%. In another study,[16] the Beginning and Ending Supportive Therapy for the Kidney (BEST Kidney) group surveyed 54 ICUs in 23 countries. The overall mortality rate was 60.2%. Septic shock was the most common cause (48%), followed by major surgery (34%), cardiogenic shock (27%), hypovolemia (26%), and nephrotoxins (19%). Many patients had multiple causes of AKI.

The PICARD and BEST Kidney studies identified several common predisposing risk factors for AKI, including older age, sepsis, and disease severity (including degree of azotemia and oliguria). Chawla et al[17] also noted hypoalbuminemia, increased A-a gradient, and underlying cancer as risk factors specifically in ICU patients. All studies note a significant incidence of preexisting CKD (approximately 30%) in patients in whom AKI develops.

Despite the high overall mortality rate of AKI, most survivors will recover to dialysis independence, but many are left with significant renal insufficiency (CKD). Up to 30% of these patients will progress to dialysis over the subsequent 3 years (particularly in those with preexisting CKD).[18] Thus, CKD begets AKI, and AKI begets CKD, which may eventually result in ESRD.

Differential Diagnosis

Acute azotemia in the ICUs may result from various artifacts (pseudorenal failure), obstruction to urine flow (postrenal azotemia), decreased renal perfusion (prerenal azotemia), or intrarenal (parenchymal or hemodynamic) disease.

Pseudorenal, Prerenal, and Postrenal Azotemia

Pseudorenal failure occurs when GI bleeding, corticosteroids, tetracyclines, severe catabolic states, or hyperalimentation alter urea metabolism, increasing the BUN without a change in glomerular filtration rate (GFR). Similarly, the serum creatinine level may increase with creatine release from damaged muscles (rhabdomyolysis), blocked renal tubular creatinine secretion (trimethoprim and cimetidine), or interference with the creatinine assay (cefoxitin, acetone, α-methyldopa). Malnutrition and severe muscle wasting may spuriously decrease the plasma urea and creatinine concentrations, respectively. Although the impact of nonrenal factors is relatively small (≤20%), one should always consider these as a potential explanation for acute azotemia (Table 2).

Prerenal azotemia occurs when renal perfusion is compromised by an absolute decrease in extracellular fluid volume ([ECV] eg, hemorrhage, GI fluid losses, burns), a decrease in the "effective" circulating volume (heart failure, ascites), or the accumulation of fluid in a "third space" (eg, pancreatitis, acute abdomen, bowel surgery, muscle trauma). It may occasionally occur with high intraabdominal pressures (>20 mm Hg bladder pressure) after trauma or surgery (abdominal compartment syndrome). Correction of the

Table 2. *Causes of Pseudorenal Failure*

Nonrenal causes of elevated serum urea
  Corticosteroids
  Hyperalimentation
  GI bleeding
Nonrenal causes of elevated serum creatinine
  Increased creatine release from skeletal muscle
    Rhabdomyolysis
  Interference with creatinine assay
    Acetone
    Cefoxitin
    Flucytosine
    Methyldopa
  Blocked tubular creatinine secretion
    Cimetidine
    Trimethoprim

Table 3. *Diagnostic Indices of Prerenal Azotemia and ATN*

Variable	PRA	ATN
BUN/creatinine ratio	20	10
Urine osmolality, mOsm/L	>350	300*
Urine/plasma osmolality ratio	>1.5	1.0
Urine sodium, mEq/L	<20	>30
Fractional excretion of sodium	<1%	>1%
Fractional excretion of urea	<35%	>50%

*PRA = prerenal azotemia.

intravascular volume defect or abdominal pressure should result in improved renal perfusion and resolution of azotemia. In most series, prerenal azotemia has a 90% survival rate. If unrecognized or untreated, ECV depletion can cause ATN and a significantly worse prognosis. In fact, ECV depletion is a very frequent contributor to AKI.

The diagnosis of prerenal azotemia is based on the physical examination demonstrating an alteration of ECV and on several urinary indexes (Table 3). Of these, the fractional excretion of sodium (FENa) is most reliable.[19] The FENa measures the ratio of the sodium excreted (urinary sodium × volume) to the sodium filtered (serum sodium × GFR) by the following formula:

$$FENa = (UNa/SNa) \div (Ucr/Scr) \times 100$$

where U indicates urine; Na, sodium; S, serum; and cr, creatinine. The test can be done on a spot sample of urine and blood. The FENa is <1% when acute azotemia is prerenal but >1% with ATN. A few exceptions must be kept in mind.

Rhabdomyolysis, contrast nephropathy, acute glomerulonephritis, and sepsis are all causes of ATN in which the FENa may be spuriously low, particularly early in the clinical course. In addition, patients with severe heart failure or cirrhosis often have a FENa of <1% despite ATN. Diuretics, glucosuria, or preexisting renal insufficiency will falsely elevate the FENa in a patient with prerenal azotemia. When diuretics elevate the FENa, a fractional excretion of urea of <35% accurately indicates prerenal azotemia.[20] The clinician must be alert to these potential pitfalls of the FENa when approaching the acutely azotemic patient.

In addition to a low FENa and fractional excretion of urea, prerenal azotemia usually causes a low urinary sodium level (<20 mEq/L), high urine osmolality (>350 mOsm/L), and an elevated BUN to creatinine ratio (>20). The urine sediment may show granular casts but is usually devoid of cellular elements. Oliguria is virtually universal unless a diuretic or glucosuria is present. Prerenal azotemia is confirmed if the urinary output improves and the azotemia resolves with the administration of isotonic fluids, improvement in the underlying heart failure, or correction of the third-space defect.

Postrenal azotemia occurs with an obstruction to urine flow. Although anuria is expected, fluctuating or even high urine volumes may result if the blockage is partial. As long as the obstruction is relatively recent (days to weeks) and the serum creatinine level relatively low (<5 mg/dL), correcting the obstruction will usually resolve the azotemia. With urethral or prostatic obstruction, a Foley catheter will suffice. This and a renal ultrasound are required diagnostic steps in any patient with acute azotemia. For patients with one kidney, a CT scan (without contrast) or even a retrograde pyelogram may be necessary to positively exclude obstruction. Upper tract obstruction may require a ureteral stent or percutaneous nephrostomy.

Specific Causes of AKI

After excluding pseudorenal, prerenal, and postrenal azotemia, one must consider the various renal parenchymal or hemodynamic derangements responsible for AKI. These include diseases that primarily affect the glomerulus (glomerulonephritis), interstitium (interstitial nephritis), blood vessels (vascular occlusion or vasculitis), or tubules (ATN; Table 4).

Table 4. *The Common Glomerular, Interstitial, Vascular, and Tubular Causes of AKI**

I. Glomerular
  A. GN
    1. Infectious
      a. Endocarditis
      b. "Shunt" nephritis
      c. Visceral abscess
      d. Hepatitis antigenemia
      e. Poststreptococcal GN
    2. Lupus nephritis
      a. Idiopathic rapidly progressive GN
  B. Glomerular hemodynamics
    1. Hepatorenal syndrome
    2. Angiotensin-converting enzyme inhibitors
    3. NSAIDs
    4. Hypercalcemia
    5. Potent vasodilators (*eg*, nitroprusside)
    6. Abdominal compartment syndrome
II. Interstitial
  A. Allergic interstitial nephritis
  B. Infectious
    1. Pyelonephritis
    2. Viral (cytomegalovirus, measles, mumps)
    3. Rickettsial disease (ehrlichia)
  C. Tumor lysis syndrome
  D. Urate/oxalate deposition nephropathy
  E. Acute phosphate nephropathy
  F. Multiple myeloma
  G. Immune (lupus, Sjögren syndrome)
  H. Infiltrative (sarcoidosis, lymphoma, leukemia)
III. Vascular
  A. Vasculitis
    1. Wegener granulomatosis
    2. Polyarteritis nodosa
    3. Henoch-Schönlein purpura
    4. Hypersensitivity vasculitis
    5. Cryoglobulinemia
  B. Thrombosis/thromboembolism
  C. Cholesterol emboli
  D. Malignant hypertension
  E. Hemolytic uremic syndrome/thrombotic thrombocytopenic purpura
IV. Tubular
  A. Toxins
    1. Aminoglycosides
    2. Platinum
    3. Radiographic contrast
    4. Rhabdomyolysis
    5. Hemolysis
    6. Amphotericin B
  B. Ischemia
    1. Shock
    2. Hemorrhage
    3. Sepsis

*GN = glomerulonephritis.

Glomerular Disease: Fulminant glomerulonephritis due to bacterial endocarditis, lupus erythematosus, staphylococcal septicemia, visceral abscesses, hepatitis B antigenemia, Goodpasture syndrome, or idiopathic rapidly progressive (crescentic) glomerulonephritis is not uncommon in a major ICU. Once considered, these diagnoses are not difficult to make. The urinalysis will show dysmorphic RBCs (those with multiple surface irregularities), RBC casts, pyuria, and moderate-to-heavy proteinuria. Hypertension is variably present. Blood cultures, serologic testing (antinuclear antibody, antineutrophilic cytoplasmic antibodies, hepatitis B surface antigen, and antiglomerular basement membrane antibody), and a search for visceral abscess may be rewarding. An urgent renal biopsy should be strongly considered whenever acute glomerulonephritis is suspected, as aggressive specific therapy (*eg*, plasma exchange, corticosteroids, and/or cyclophosphamide) is often required.

Alterations in glomerular hemodynamics are increasingly recognized as a cause of acute renal failure. These include afferent arteriolar vasoconstriction (hepatorenal syndrome [HRS]) or efferent arteriolar vasodilatation (angiotensin-converting enzyme inhibitors). The latter is usually seen when severe cardiac failure, ECV depletion, or bilateral renal artery stenosis already compromises renal blood flow (RBF). In addition, less well-defined derangements in intrarenal hemodynamics are likely contribute to the AKI of sepsis, potent vasodilators (nitroprusside and nifedipine), and the nonsteroidal antiinflammatory drugs (NSAIDs). In these cases, the urine sediment is usually bland and results of the renal biopsy (if performed) are normal. Recovery of renal function is expected, provided the offending drug is removed or the underlying condition is corrected.

HRS refers to AKI that occurs in the setting of severe liver failure after other obvious causes are excluded. The patient demonstrates avid sodium retention (urinary sodium level, <10 mEq/L; FENa, <1%) and oliguria not responding to ECV expansion. The urine sediment is usually benign. The onset may be insidious or abruptly precipitated by ECV depletion (GI bleeding, diuretics, paracentesis) or sepsis. Because the liver is critical to generation of both urea and creatinine, patients with cirrhosis and ascites are at high risk despite

Acute Kidney Injury in the Critically Ill (Muther

normal serum values. In one study, the incidence of HRS was 18% at 1 year and 39% at 5 years in cirrhotic patients with ascites.[21]

HRS likely results from nitric oxide-induced splanchnic vasodilatation with consequent activation of the renin angiotensin and sympathetic nervous systems. Thus, cardiac output is high and systemic vascular resistance is low ("septic physiology") despite elevated renal vascular resistance. Other theories of pathogenesis include an imbalance of vasoconstrictor/vasodilator prostaglandins (supported by elevated urinary 20-hydroxyeicosatetraenoic acid, a vasoconstrictor prostaglandin), endotoxemia, endothelin-induced renal vasoconstriction, release of false neurotransmitters, or an increase in sympathetic tone pursuant to elevated hepatic sinusoidal pressure.

The preferred treatment of HRS is liver transplantation. As a bridge to transplant, various medical therapies may be tried. Norepinephrine infusion may particularly help patients with a mean arterial pressure of < 60 mm Hg. The sympatholytic agent clonidine may transiently improve GFR. Data on misoprostol and N-acetylcysteine are conflicting. There are promising reports using both terlipressin (an antidiuretic hormone analog) given with albumin infusions[22] and the combination of midodrine and octreotide.[23] Peritoneovenous shunting and the transjugular intrahepatic portosystemic shunt have high complication rates and are generally reserved for refractory patients.

Interstitial Disease: Allergic interstitial nephritis is most commonly due to penicillins, cephalosporins, sulfonamides, diuretics, and NSAIDs, although the list of agents reported to cause the disease is legion. Patients typically have fever, rash, arthralgias, and eosinophilia. Pyuria (sterile) dominates the urinary sediment, although hematuria and proteinuria are also common. Eosinophiluria (best evaluated by Hansel stain) is demonstrated in many cases, often excepting NSAIDs. Other causes of eosinophilia and eosinophiluria associated with AKI (such as atheroemboli or rapidly progressive glomerulonephritis) are usually easily distinguished on clinical grounds. Early steroid therapy improves the recovery of renal function in patients with drug-induced interstitial nephritis.

Tumor lysis syndrome refers to a variety of metabolic complications associated with lymphoreticular or (rarely) solid malignancies. Hyperuricemia (usually >15 mg/dL) and hyperphosphatemia (usually >8 mg/dL) each may cause AKI; the latter usually follows lytic therapy and the former often precedes treatment of the primary malignancy. Hypocalcemia and hyperkalemia often complicate the early clinical course. Patients are usually oligoanuric and the urinary sediment frequently reveals amorphous urates or urate crystals. Urinary alkalinization is not routinely recommended as it may actually enhance renal parenchymal calcium phosphate deposition. ECV expansion with isotonic crystalloid or mannitol has prophylactic benefit. Although allopurinol has not completely eliminated the AKI of tumor lysis, it does help (at high dosages of 600 to 900 mg/d, if possible). Rasburicase, a recombinant urate oxidase, may also be used (unlabeled indication) to prevent hyperuricemia and tumor lysis syndrome.

In addition to the acute precipitation of uric acid in the renal tubules seen with very high (>15 mg/dL) serum levels (uric acid nephropathy), lesser elevations of uric acid may increase the risk for other types of AKI.[24]

Acute phosphate nephropathy is increasingly recognized as a complication of oral sodium phosphate solutions used for bowel preparation prior to colonoscopy.[25] Renal parenchymal deposition of calcium and phosphorus appear responsible not only for AKI but also significant CKD.

Other causes of AKI resulting from interstitial nephritis are less common but include viral or bacterial pyelonephritis, multiple myeloma, uric acid nephropathy, and occasionally infiltrative disorders such as lymphoma, leukemia, and sarcoidosis. Oxalate nephropathy may complicate acute ethylene glycol ingestion (with elevated anion and/or osmolar gaps). The urine sediment in these cases is usually bland, but crystalluria, pyuria, and WBC casts can be seen, even in the absence of infection.

Vascular Disease: Vascular disease is a frequently overlooked cause of AKI. Malignant hypertension causes AKI accompanied by retinopathy, thrombocytopenia, and microangiopathy. Microangiopathy and thrombocytopenia also accompany hemolytic uremic syndrome or thrombotic thrombocytopenic purpura. Renal infarction due to trauma, thrombosis, or thromboembolism causes AKI with fever, hematuria, acute flank pain, ileus, leukocytosis, and an elevated lactate dehydrogenase level, a syndrome that mimics an acute abdomen. Thromboemboli usually arise from the heart in patients with severe left ventricular failure or atrial fibrillation.

Cholesterol emboli syndrome (CES) refers to renal atherosclerotic or cholesterol microemboli that occur following aortic manipulation (surgery or catheterization) or systemic anticoagulation with warfarin. Besides AKI, GI bleeding (due to microinfarcts), livido reticularis of the lower extremities, patchy areas of ischemic necrosis in the toes, hypocomplementemia, and eosinophilia are common. It is important to distinguish CES from a thromboembolic event, as therapeutic anticoagulation is dangerous in patients with the former but necessary for those with the latter.

Renal vasculitis (Wegener granulomatosis, polyarteritis nodosa, hypersensitivity vasculitis, and Henoch-Schönlein purpura) often causes AKI. These disorders are identified by their multisystem manifestations, very active urine sediment (hematuria, pyuria, RBC and WBC casts, and proteinuria), and, in the case of Wegener granulomatosis and polyarteritis nodosa, the presence of antineutrophilic cytoplasmic antibodies in the serum.

Tubular Disease: The most common cause of hospital- and ICU-acquired AKI is ATN,[26] which is broadly divided into toxic and ischemic causes. ATN in the ICU setting is usually attributed to a conspiracy of factors including hypovolemia, poor cardiac output, sepsis, and nephrotoxins.

Among the more common toxins causing ATN are the aminoglycoside antibiotics. Risk factors for aminoglycoside nephrotoxicity include volume contraction, age, hypokalemia, concomitant use of other nephrotoxins, and a short dosing interval. After an initial loading dose (2 to 3 mg/kg), the maintenance dose (1 mg/kg) should be adjusted based on the patient's creatinine clearance ([Ccr] estimated by the formula Ccr = body weight (kg)/serum creatinine) or calculated GFR. Once-daily dosing minimizes nephrotoxicity without compromising therapy. The routine use of peak and trough serum levels does not decrease the likelihood of ATN.

Radiographic contrast agents are more likely to cause AKI in patients who have preexisting renal insufficiency, diabetes mellitus, and poor left ventricular function, or who undergo multiple studies in a 24-h period. The volume of contrast used is directly related to nephrotoxicity. Nonionic and isosmolar contrast appears less nephrotoxic. The best prophylaxis appears to be isotonic sodium chloride or sodium bicarbonate [27] and N-acetylcysteine (1,200 mg po q12h; two doses before and two doses after the procedure).[28] IV mannitol, furosemide (either before or after contrast), dopamine, calcium channel blockers, and fenoldopam do not lessen nephrotoxicity. Theophylline may decrease nephrotoxicity in patients at very high risk, particularly those in whom crystalloid is contraindicated. Prophylactic hemodialysis is ineffective. Hemofiltration does not appear to alter the overall impact of contrast nephrotoxicity. Although most cases are nonoliguric and resolve within a few days, contrast toxicity significantly increases hospital mortality and cost. Patients may require acute dialysis; ESRD is much less likely. CES is potentially a more serious, although less common, renal complication for patients undergoing radiographic contrast studies.

Massive intravascular hemolysis or rhabdomyolysis (Table 5) may produce AKI. Common causes of rhabdomyolysis include drugs (*eg*, heroin, cocaine, statins), major crush injuries, alcohol, seizures, and muscle compression syndromes. All have the potential of producing myoglobinuria and AKI, particularly if ECV depletion or shock exists simultaneously. Hyperkalemia, hyperuricemia, hyperphosphatemia, and hypercreatinemia (low BUN to creatinine ratio) also result. Hypocalcemia often occurs early, but hypercalcemia (as high as 12 to 14 mg/dL) appears during recovery.[29] An elevated creatine phosphokinase level and dark heme-positive urine without RBCs are major diagnostic clues. Prophylaxis against ATN depends on aggressive IV crystalloid. The addition of mannitol and bicarbonate (one-half normal saline solution with 12.5 g of mannitol per liter and 50 mEq of $NaHCO_3$ per liter at 250 to 500 mL/h) may be a useful adjunct.

Renal ischemia may occur after prolonged hypotension, suprarenal aortic or renal artery occlusion (either with clot or clamp), and sepsis. The renal tubular cells are particularly susceptible

Acute Kidney Injury in the Critically Ill (Muther)

Table 5. *Common Causes of Rhabdomyolysis*

I. Trauma
   A. Multiple trauma
   B. Crush injuries
   C. Vascular or orthopaedic injury/surgery
   D. Compression

II. Exertional
   A. Normal muscle
      1. Extreme exertion
      2. Heat exhaustion/heat stroke
      3. Sickle cell/sickle trait
      4. Seizures
      5. Hyperkinetic states
      6. Near drowning
   B. Abnormal muscle
      1. Metabolic myopathies
      2. Mitochondrial myopathies
      3. Malignant hyperthermia
      4. Neuroleptic malignant syndrome

III. Nontraumatic and nonexertional
   A. Alcohol
   B. Drugs and toxins
      1. Colchicine
      2. Statins
      3. Cocaine
      4. Chloroquine
      5. Antiretrovirals (zidovudine and others)
      6. Ipecac
   C. Infections
   D. Electrolyte abnormalities
      1. Hypokalemia
      2. Hypophosphatemia
   E. Endocrinopathies
      1. Diabetic ketoacidosis
      2. Hypothyroidism/hyperthyroidism
      3. Pheochromocytoma
   F. Inflammatory myopathies
   G. Miscellaneous

to ischemic insult because their baseline balance between oxygen supply and demand is tenuous.[30] Thus, whenever systemic or intrarenal blood flow decreases slightly, ischemic insult to the tubular cells may occur. This may help to explain the beneficial effects attributed to loop diuretics shown in some studies. By inhibiting active chloride and sodium transport in the ascending limb of the loop, these agents decrease metabolic work and, therefore, oxygen requirements.

Sepsis is a frequent cause of hospital-acquired AKI, and is particularly common in the critically ill patient. The prognosis appears directly related to the severity of the sepsis. Sepsis causes a simultaneous decrease in systemic vascular resistance and increase in renal vascular resistance, reducing renal plasma flow and GFR.[31] Both circulating and glomerular cells react to endotoxins by producing a variety of cytokines and autacoids, decreasing renal perfusion, and increasing renal tubular cell work. AKI can occur even without systemic hypotension. Fever, leukocytosis, and other overt signs of sepsis may be absent. A mild alteration in mental status or respiratory alkalosis may be the only clinical clue. Oliguria and/or azotemia in this setting should be considered occult septicemia unless disproved.

AKI following cardiac surgery significantly increases ICU and hospital mortality, length of stay, and cost.[32] The risk is increased by age, preexisting CKD, poor left ventricular function, and by the degree of difficulty and pump time.[33] In addition, use of the procoagulant apoprotinin may increase not only the incidence of AKI but also major cardiovascular events and mortality following cardiac surgery.[34] No single prophylactic agent (furosemide, dopamine, *N*-acetylcysteine) has shown benefit. However, a combination cocktail of mannitol, furosemide, and dopamine appeared to abrogate oliguria and the need for dialysis in one small study.[35] Another study[36] suggests a benefit with a combination of atrial natriuretic peptide and furosemide. The best hope for therapeutic advance in this area, however, will likely depend on earlier detection, perhaps by urinary NGAL.[11]

Pathophysiology of AKI

Either a toxic or ischemic insult can initiate an intrarenal cascade that manifests as clinical AKI. The primary renal tubular cellular event appears to be decreased production and increased degradation of adenosine triphosphate, thus increasing local production of phospholipases, hypoxanthine, and adenosine. Phospholipases destabilize tubular cell membranes, causing redistribution of integrin receptors from the basolateral to the luminal surface, decreasing intercellular adhesion. Disruption and shedding of renal tubular cells may then result in intratubular obstruction and back-leak of tubular fluid.

The cells of the thick ascending limb of Henle and the S_3 segment of the proximal tubule appear uniquely susceptible to ischemic injury. Because of marginal medullary blood flow and the unique anatomy of the vasa rectae, these metabolically active cells (responsible for the bulk of sodium transport) normally function in borderline hypoxia[37] such that even minor decrements in perfusion may cause substantial injury. Oxygen free radicals (generated from hypoxanthine and by infiltrating neutrophils) may play a role. Platelet-activating factor released during injury increases vascular permeability and contributes to the infiltration of neutrophils by up-regulating adhesion molecules (intercellular adhesion molecule) on endothelial cells.

Injured renal tubular cells may also release vasoconstrictor prostaglandins, adenosine, endothelin, or other substances that affect intraglomerular hemodynamics (afferent arteriolar vasoconstriction or efferent arteriolar vasodilatation) or glomerular capillary permeability thus decreasing GFR. This phenomenon is known as *tubuloglomerular feedback*. The net result is a prolonged decrement in GFR with varying degrees of urine output. All of these events may occur without an alteration in systemic hemodynamics or even RBF.

Simultaneous with these events causing renal functional decline, other factors appear to mediate a regenerative or repair process.[38] Release of various cytokines from injured cells appears to recruit and activate macrophages, which synthesize growth factors (such as epidermal and transforming growth factors), stimulating renal tubular cell regeneration and recovery. Production of vasodilator prostaglandins and nitric oxide may aid this renal recovery.

Clinically, these pathophysiologic mechanisms produce a brief initial decrease in RBF and GFR, followed by a prolonged (days to weeks) maintenance phase in which GFR remains low but RBF returns to normal. Oliguria may occur during this maintenance period, and dialysis is often necessary. The recovery phase is marked first by increasing urinary volume and finally by return of GFR.

Treatment of AKI

Several therapies for AKI show promise *in vitro* and in animal studies, including diuretics, dopamine, natriuretic peptides, calcium channel blockers, endothelin antagonists, growth factors, and oxygen free radical scavengers. However, application of these therapies in human clinical trials proves disappointing. Therefore, in 2009, the treatment for AKI remains largely preventive and supportive.

Prevention

Because the risk and the mortality of AKI are high in critically ill patients, prevention is the best therapy. Table 6 lists several common risk factors for AKI and suggestions for prophylaxis. Volume expansion can minimize the risk of AKI from radiographic contrast agents, cisplatin, and NSAIDs. *N*-acetylcysteine appears effective in preventing contrast and possibly cisplatin nephrotoxicity. Mannitol may at least partially abrogate the AKI caused by rhabdomyolysis and cisplatin, but not that caused by contrast agents. Limiting the dose and simultaneous exposure appears important in avoiding contrast, aminoglycoside, and cisplatin toxicity. Alkali may limit the nephrotoxicity of contrast, myoglobinuria, and uric acid. Allopurinol or rasburicase should be used before chemotherapy whenever tumor lysis is anticipated. Adjusting the dosing interval for changes in Ccr is important to prevent aminoglycoside toxicity. Polyuria or an increasing creatinine level should prompt additional widening of the dosing interval. Correcting hypokalemia and expanding ECV are also helpful. Although the peak aminoglycoside level correlates with antibacterial effect, there is little evidence that monitoring trough levels minimizes or avoids nephrotoxicity.

Although some data support abdominal decompression with large-volume paracentesis as a means of improving renal perfusion in patients with tense ascites, the clinician should be cautious about paracenteses >1 L, especially without the support of concomitant albumin infusion. Ascitic fluid may rapidly reaccumulate at the expense of intravascular volume, putting the patient at risk because of inadequate preload. Positive end-expiratory pressure (PEEP), as well as high intrathoracic pressure associated with mechanical ventilator support, may compromise cardiac output and renal perfusion. If possible, PEEP should be minimized and ECV expanded in high-risk patients.

Table 6. *Prevention of AKI**

Risk Factor	Strategy for Prevention
Renal hypoperfusion	Avoid nephrotoxins
ECV depletion	Isotonic crystalloids
Hypotension	Replete ECV with crystalloid, colloid; inotropic agents if needed; vasopressors.
Congestive heart failure	Inotropic agents; nesiritide; cautious use of ACEIs
Cirrhosis with ascites	Avoid NSAIDs; colloid if paracenteses; norepinephrine if hypotensive; midodrine and octreotide; peritoneovenous shunt or TIPS?
Third-space ECV	Colloid, isotonic crystalloids
PEEP	Isotonic crystalloids; low tidal volume
Renal artery stenosis	Avoid ACEIs with diuretics
Preexisting azotemia	Avoid ECV depletion; cautious use of nephrotoxins
Sepsis	Avoid ECV depletion; cautious use of nephrotoxins
Nephrotoxins	Avoid ECV depletion and other nephrotoxins
Aminoglycosides	Use alternative agent if possible; lengthen dosing interval; correct hypokalemia
Chemotherapy	Expand ECV; mannitol; *N*-acetylcysteine, possibly theophylline for platinum.
Radiocontrast agents	Limit contrast volume; expand ECV with normal saline or bicarbonate; *N*-acetylcysteine; use nonionic, isoosmolar contrast with preexisting azotemia
Cyclosporine	Calcium channel blockers
NSAIDs	Cautious use in congestive heart failure, cirrhosis, ECV depletion; avoid simultaneous triamterene
Rhabdomyolysis	Expand ECV; mannitol? HCO_3?
Hyperuricemia	Expand ECV; alkalinize urine unless serum phosphorus elevated; allopurinol and/or rasburicase
Electrolyte disorders	
Hypokalemia	Correct
Hypophosphatemia	Correct
Hyperphosphatemia	Avoid calcium therapy; avoid alkalinization; expand ECV; short-term intestinal phosphate binders
Hypercalcemia	Avoid phosphorus therapy; expand ECV; furosemide

*ACEI = angiotensin-converting enzyme inhibitor; TIPS = transjugular intrahepatic portosystemic shunt.

There are animal data to suggest that hyperalimentation may increase the risk of AKI. However, the benefits of nutritional support seem to far outweigh this risk. Minimizing protein intake to between 0.6 and 0.8 g/kg/d during periods of very high risk may be prudent.

Supportive Therapy

Nonoliguric patients presenting with AKI have fewer complications, including a decreased dialysis requirement and improved survival.[39] Although conversion of an oliguric patient to nonoliguric has less certain benefit, it can often be accomplished by repleting volume (if deficient) and using high-dose loop diuretics (*eg*, furosemide, 200 mg IV, or continuous infusions at 10 to 40 mg/h). Loop diuretics may have the theoretical advantage of decreasing tubular cell metabolic activity (thus lessening the oxygen requirement) but do not appear to alter the course of AKI. If used, a loop diuretic should be initiated early and promptly abandoned if an increase in urine volume does not occur within 24 h.

A vasodilator dose of dopamine (1.5 to 2.5 µg/kg/min) may stimulate urine volume, but it does not improve GFR, shorten the duration of AKI, or decrease dialysis requirements.[40] In addition, dopamine may induce significant arrhythmia and possibly intestinal ischemia.

Hyperalimentation preserves lean muscle mass, decreases protein breakdown, improves wound healing, and may improve immune competence. It appears to improve renal tubular cell regeneration in animals with ATN and improve survival in critically ill patients, particularly those with multiple complications.[41] Enteral alimentation is preferred whenever possible. Regardless of the route, the hyperalimentation formula must be individualized and reevaluated daily in patients with AKI. Essential amino acid preparations offer no special advantage.

Potential drug toxicity must be avoided by adjusting antibiotic and other drug dosing in patients with renal failure. This includes potential dietary sources of potassium (salt substitutes, oral tobacco products) and phosphorus (dairy products), as well as the magnesium and aluminum contained in antacids. Decreased renal excretion of normeperidine and N-acetylprocainamide (metabolites) may produce serious toxicity even though their parent drugs (meperidine and procainamide) are metabolized by the liver.[42,43] Finally, decreased protein binding (presumably displaced by uremic toxins) may accentuate the toxicity of morphine and phenytoin in any patient with renal failure.[44,45]

Uremic bleeding is best treated by RBC transfusion, raising the hemoglobin to 10 g/dL. Adjunctive therapies include IV estrogen (0.6 mg/kg/d for 5 days), cryoprecipitate infusion (10 U), and vasopressin (desmopressin acetate, 0.3 µg/kg q12h).[46]

The treatment of hyperkalemia is outlined in Table 7. When the serum potassium is <6 mEq/L, little therapy is required other than discontinuing the occult sources of dietary potassium. As the potassium rises >6 mEq/L and/or peaked T waves appear, volume expansion (as tolerated), loop diuretics, and oral sodium polystyrene sulfonate are appropriate. (Sodium polystyrene sulfonate via rectum is reported to cause colonic necrosis.) Although somewhat slow to act, these treatments actually increase potassium excretion. When more urgent therapy is needed for hyperkalemia (>7 mEq/L), driving potassium intracellularly with glucose and insulin (25 to 50 g of dextrose with 10 to 20 U of regular insulin) and the β-agonist albuterol (5 to 20 mg [1.0 to 4.0 mL] inhaled) is indicated.[47] Albuterol usually works within 30 min, will lower the serum potassium by 0.6 to 1.0 mEq/L, and lasts for ≥2 h. Calcium therapy (10 mEq IV >5 min) is reserved for hyperkalemia-induced heart block, the sine wave, or of course ventricular arrest. Its effect is immediate but short-lived (<30 min). Other maneuvers to remove potassium from the body (such as diuretics or sodium polystyrene sulfonate) must be initiated promptly as well. Dialysis (usually hemodialysis) can also be used to remove potassium.

In addition to the somewhat nephrocentric treatments previously mentioned, one cannot overemphasize the value of general ICU quality care in preventing AKI. In that regard, lower volume ventilation appeared to decrease AKI in the ARDS trial.[48] Intensive insulin therapy also decreases the incidence of AKI in an ICU population.[49] Although renal outcomes were not specifically evaluated in the trial by Rivers et al,[50] early goal-directed therapy for severe sepsis improves many of the most significant risk factors (central venous and mean arterial pressures, central venous oxygen saturation) for the development of AKI.

RRT

Many patients with AKI will recover renal function within days and not require dialysis. However, if the duration of AKI is prolonged, or if hyperkalemia, ECV overload, refractory acidosis, or uremic symptoms (serositis, encephalopathy, bleeding) occur, some form of RRT may be necessary. The major goals of RRT in AKI are to maintain the patient's survival and support

Table 7. *Treatment of Acute Hyperkalemia**

Serum K+	ECG Change	Treatment	Onset	Duration	Mechanism
≥ 6 mEq/L	Peaked T wave	Expand ECV	Hours	Hours	Renal excretion
		Loop diuretic	1–2 h	Hours	Renal excretion
		Sodium polystyrene sulfonate	6–12 h	Hours-days	GI excretion
≥ 7 mEq/L	Prolonged PR and/or widened QRS	Insulin/glucose and inhalation albuterol	15 min 30 min	<5 h	Redistribution
≥ 8 mEq/L	Sine wave	Calcium IV	Minutes	≥1 h	Membrane effect

*The correlation of serum potassium and ECG change is poor.

Table 8. *Available Options for RRT**

Technique	Intermittent	Continuous
PD	Intermittent PD	Continuous cycler PD
HD	Intermittent HD	Continuous HD
		SLED
UF	Intermittent UF	SCUF
HF		CVVH
HDF		CVVHDF

*PD, peritoneal dialysis; HD = hemodialysis; SLED, sustained low-efficiency dialysis; UF, ultrafiltration; SCUF, slow continuous ultrafiltration; HF, hemofiltration; CVVH, continuous venovenous hemofiltration; HDF, hemodiafiltration; CVVHDF, continuous venovenous hemodiafiltration.

nonrenal organ function while awaiting recovery of renal function. Its two main objectives are to control ECV by removing excess fluid (ultrafiltration [UF]), and to control azotemia by removing excess solute. Depending on a patient's needs, these two objectives can be accomplished separately or simultaneously, intermittently or continuously, by peritoneal or hematogenous access. The available options for RRT are outlined in Table 8.

Peritoneal dialysis (PD) plays a relatively minor role as a RRT in the ICU. Nevertheless, it offers several advantages including simplicity, hemodynamic stability, and freedom from anticoagulation. Peritoneal access is achieved through a surgically or percutaneously placed catheter. Automated cyclers easily accomplish the exchange of dialysate. Even with frequent dialysate exchanges and very hypertonic dialysate (4.25 g/dL of dextrose), PD clearance of solute (Curea approximately 18 mL/min) and UF rates (6 to 8 L/d) are limited. The intraperitoneal volume of dialysate can compromise respiration, and glucose loads and protein losses can be excessive. Therefore, PD appears better suited for the less catabolic, less uremic, and relatively normovolemic patient. I use it almost exclusively in patients previously on PD with a superimposed illness requiring ICU admission.

Intermittent hemodialysis (IHD) remains the most frequently used RRT in the United States. Patient blood and dialysate, separated by a semipermeable membrane, run countercurrently through an artificial dialyzer in an extracorporeal circuit. A percutaneously placed, dual-lumen central venous catheter allows blood flows (Qb) of 300 to 400 mL/min. Solute removal is accomplished by diffusion down an electrochemical gradient maintained by continuous dialysate flow (Qd) of 500 to 800 mL/min. UF is driven by the transmembrane pressure. The membrane permeability (a product of pore size and surface area) limits the molecular size of solute clearance and the rate of UF at any given transmembrane pressure. Typical membranes used for IHD restrict clearance to relatively small solutes (molecular weight <5,000 d) manifested by urea clearances of 200 to 250 mL/min. Volume removal is limited only by signs or symptoms of acute volume depletion as UF rates begin to exceed 1.0 L/h. The major clinical benefit of IHD is rapid solute clearance.

The hemodialysis membrane is not simply a passive structure but, depending on its composition, may induce significant biochemical effects. For example, cellulose-based dialysis membranes (cellulose acetate, cuprophane) can activate complement, induce coagulation factor XII, and induce functional defects in neutrophils.[51] This may increase susceptibility to infection, cause leukoagglutination, exacerbate renal injury, and delay recovery from AKI. Excellent clinical studies[52] demonstrate not only a lower rate of recovery from AKI but also a higher patient mortality when these so-called bioincompatible membranes are compared with "synthetic" membranes (eg, polysulfone, polyamide, polyacrylonitrile, polymethyl methacrylate) in the treatment of AKI. This mandates the use of synthetic, biocompatible membranes for all extracorporeal RRT in the ICU.

Although the issues of bioincompatibility relate to all forms of extracorporeal RRT, other problems are unique to IHD. Rapid solute removal can cause confusion, disorientation, and other mental status changes termed *disequilibrium syndrome*. Hypoxemia (a decrease as much as a 10-mm Hg decrease in Pao_2) is expected. Air embolism and bleeding can occur with any central venous access catheter. The most frequent complication of IHD is hypotension. In a patient with AKI, in whom the kidney has lost the ability to autoregulate blood flow, even mild hypotension can induce oliguria, produce significant renal ischemia, and delay functional recovery. Other serious difficulties may arise if cerebral, myocardial, splanchnic, and peripheral perfusion are compromised.

Several factors contribute to hemodialysis-induced hypotension, including rapid UF, rapid solute loss (decreasing intravascular osmolality, resulting in extracellular-to-intracellular fluid shift), changes in cardiac output and systemic vascular resistance, and the use of acetate as a dialysate buffer. These effects can be minimized by slowing Qb, lengthening dialysis times, using intradialytic hypertonic crystalloids or colloids IV, temporarily suspending dialysate flow ("bypass"), lowering the dialysate temperature to 35°C, and buffering with HCO_3-based dialysate. Nevertheless, hypotension remains the major potential complication of IHD and is the major incentive for use of continuous renal replacement therapies.

Isolated UF (ie, without simultaneous dialysis [diffusion]) can provide substantial fluid losses without hypotension. The absence of dialysate flow limits solute removal to the minimum generated by convection alone. This protects intravascular volume while producing several liters of net UF daily. This technique can be used emergently to treat acute pulmonary edema or as an adjunct to IHD, enhancing fluid removal either immediately adjacent to or isolated from a dialysis treatment. Slow continuous ultrafiltration (SCUF) is particularly suited to a patient who has excessive IV fluid requirements with marginal urinary output, eg, a patient with severe cardiac or hepatic disease who needs parenteral nutrition. However, because of its inability to simultaneously control azotemia, SCUF has largely been replaced by continuous hemofiltration techniques.

Hemofiltration (HF) overcomes the inability of SCUF to effectively remove solute. The permeability of the membrane filter is increased to the point where sieving coefficients approach 1 for most molecules up to a molecular weight of 25,000 d. Therefore, 1 L of ultrafiltrate equals 1 L of clearance for those molecules (ie, clearance rate equals UF rate). Because the therapy is continuous, the quantity of UF enables solute clearance to approach and even surpass that of IHD on a daily (> 40L) or weekly basis. Of course, this massive rate of UF threatens hemodynamic stability. Therefore, replacement fluid is necessary as a substitute for ultrafiltrate. These two changes—increased membrane permeability and the need for replacement fluid—distinguish HF from SCUF.

Replacement fluid is a simple crystalloid solution adjusted for the patient's individual needs.

Generally, calcium, magnesium, and bicarbonate are added to 0.45 to 0.9% saline solution based on frequent laboratory evaluation (every 6 to 12 h). Potassium and phosphorus also require replacement. The rate of administration depends on the patient's ECV and is adjusted to achieve the desired net hourly UF (net UF = actual UF − replacement volume). Replacement fluid can be administered either before or after filter. Predilution improves UF rates and thus solute clearance, and lessens the need for anticoagulation. On the other hand, as UF volumes increase, logistics usually necessitate both pre- and postfilter infusion of replacement fluid. High volumes of room-temperature replacement fluid may induce hypothermia.

As solute clearance is equal to the UF rate, the efficacy of HF as a treatment is directly dependent on the daily UF volume. Increasing UF volume to 35 mL/kg/h will control azotemia in all but the most severely catabolic patients. If necessary, this convective clearance can be supplemented with a diffusive component by simply adding dialysate flow through. The dialysate used is either a lactate-based PD solution or a basic crystalloid solution with bicarbonate added. Dialysate flow rates (usually 1 to 2 L/h) are much lower than with IHD. Adding this diffusion component transforms HF to hemodiafiltration (HDF). However, at UF rates demonstrated to favorably influence survival (35 mL/kg/h), HDF is rarely, if ever, required. No trials are available to judge the value of this diffusive component added to hemofiltration.

Continuous arteriovenous HF or HDF using the patient's own arteriovenous pressure gradient has largely been replaced by continuous venovenous hemofiltration (CVVH) or continuous venovenous hemodiafiltration (CVVHDF) requiring a blood pump. CVVH/CVVHDF avoids an arterial puncture and because it is pump driven, Qb is usually higher and more constant. This improves UF rates (and therefore clearance rates) and may modify the need for anticoagulation, although anticoagulation is required for these and all extracorporeal RRTs. Continuous heparin (infused prefilter) or regional citrate anticoagulation are both acceptable.

The very porous membrane used for HF allows convective transport not only of small molecules such as urea, but also of larger molecules (so-called *middle molecules*) thought to contribute to the chronic uremic syndrome. Whether this has any impact on acute renal failure or its survival is unknown. Perhaps the most intriguing feature of HF is its ability to remove even larger molecules (by filtration or adsorption), such as the proinflammatory cytokines tumor necrosis factor, IL-1, and IL-6. As mentioned, this offers the hope that HF may abrogate the systemic inflammatory response so often a feature of multiorgan failure and be useful as a primary therapy of sepsis, independently of its ability to treat renal failure. However, despite the removal of anti-inflammatory mediators, plasma levels of these cytokines usually remain constant, likely because of increased synthesis.[53] This might be overcome when short-term ultra-high-volume HF (35 L/4 h) is used as a "salvage" therapy for patients with refractory septic shock.[54] Nevertheless, to date there is no convincing evidence to support the use of HF as a treatment of sepsis alone.

Slow Low-Efficiency Dialysis: Several adjustments to IHD can improve its inherent hemodynamic instability. These include slowing blood and dialysate flow rates to 200 mL/min. Longer treatment times avoid the decrease in of solute clearance. Nocturnal hemodialysis employs these principles in patients with ESRD who, by dialyzing for 8 h per night, 6 to 7 nights per week, significantly improve not only solute clearance but also ECV control, mineral balance, and nutritional parameters while avoiding hypotensive episodes. This technique is gaining wider acceptance as a treatment for AKI as well.[55] Termed *sustained low-efficiency dialysis* (SLED) or *extended daily dialysis*, it is usually applied for 8 to 12 h/d, thus avoiding immobilization and the inevitable interruptions to continuous RRT (*eg*, surgery, procedures, radiology). SLED easily achieves significant solute clearance and control of hypervolemia with hemodynamic stability.

Recent attention has focused of the question of dialysis dose or intensity. Schiffl et al[56] demonstrated improved survival with IHD daily vs every other day. Ronco et al[57] showed a survival benefit with CVVH UF rates at 35 or 45 mL/kg/h vs 20 mL/kg/h. Paganini et al[58] directly correlated survival with the dose of RRT regardless of which RRT treatment was used. This study was particularly enlightening as it evaluated the influence of severity of illness on AKI requiring dialysis.

At the extremes of illness (where patients either universally recovered or universally died despite therapy), dialysis dose appeared to have no effect. In the middle ranges of severity of illness, however, the dose of dialysis had a significant impact on survival.

A study by Palevsky et al[59] clarifies that this dosing effect on survival has limits. Critically ill patients randomized to more intensive IHD, SLED, or CVVHDF had no survival (60 day) or renal recovery (28 day) advantage over those less intensively treated, as long as a weekly Kt/V urea of ≥ 4.0 (IHD or SLED) or filtrate volume of 30 mL/Kg/h (CVVHDF) is achieved. (Kt/V urea is an index of dialysis adequacy directly related to blood flow rate, the size of the artificial dialyzer and the time on dialysis, and inversely related to patient size.)

To date, no study clearly demonstrates an advantage of any particular RRT over another.[60–62] With no clear survival advantage established, the clinician is free to target a particular RRT to any given patient. When rapid solute control is necessary (*eg*, in a patient with severe hyperkalemia [rhabdomyolysis] or hyperuricemia [tumor lysis]), IHD is most suitable. UF without dialysis (intermittently or SCUF) is best if volume overload without azotemia is the primary clinical problem. For hypotensive patients, we prefer either CVVH (particularly with sepsis and multisystem organ failure) or SLED. CVVH is also indicated when hepatic failure or head trauma complicate AKI. We primarily apply PD in the ICU only to those patients previously using PD who are not compromised by abdominal or respiratory problems. With extracorporeal techniques, filters with biocompatible or synthetic membranes should always be used. Regardless of the particular RRT selected, the clinician must ensure an adequate dose of dialysis.

Prognosis and Recovery

In most clinical series, mortality from AKI continues to average 50%. Mortality rate in nonoliguric patients may be as low as 25%; with oliguric AKI requiring RRT, it approaches 70%. The major determinants of outcome include preexisting renal function, precipitating event, the severity of comorbid conditions, and the number of complications. AKI associated with ventilatory failure, sepsis, trauma, abdominal catastrophe, and burns carries a mortality rate of 70 to 90%, but the mortality rate is 25 to 30% for patients with AKI caused by aminoglycosides, radiographic contrast, or other drug reactions.[63,64] Mortality approaches 100% if three or more major organ systems have failed simultaneously. Mortality is highest in the very young and very old. The dose of dialysis (solute removal) appears to directly improve survival, while the severity of azotemia and the choice of dialysis modality do not. Again, the use of biocompatible dialysis membranes improves survival in those patients requiring dialysis.

Infection is the most common cause of death and is usually due to overwhelming sepsis from resistant Gram-negative bacteria or yeast. Other common causes of death are cardiovascular compromise (*eg*, strokes and myocardial infarction), respiratory failure (often with nosocomial pneumonia), and GI bleeding.

If the patient with AKI survives, recovery is usually prompt and sufficient to achieve dialysis independence (although as many as 50% of patients are left with some degree of CKD). Oliguria (if present) averages 10 to 14 days. Urinary volume recovers gradually during the next 3 to 7 days. Fluid therapy is needed to support this obligatory diuretic phase. Although the BUN and creatinine levels continue to rise during this phase, dialysis can usually be discontinued. Renal recovery usually occurs within 30 days; rarely, a patient requires 60 to 90 days to recover. In one large series,[65] 95% of survivors regained renal function, almost all within 30 days. Those patients who have delayed or no recovery are usually older, have preexisting renal insufficiency, or suffer severe ischemic insults to the kidney.

References

1. Hoste EA, Schurgers M. Epidemiology of acute kidney injury: how big is the problem? Crit Care Med 2008; 36:S146–S151

2. Bellomo R, Ronco C, Kellum JA, et al. Acute renal failure: definitions, outcome measures, animal models, fluid therapy and information technology needs. The Second International Consensus Conference of the Acute Dialysis Quality Initiative (ADQI) Group. Crit Care 2004; 8:R204–R212

3. Hoste EA, Clermont G, Kersten A, et al. RIFLE criteria for acute kidney injury are associated with hospital mortality in critically ill patients: a cohort analysis. Crit Care 2006 May 12 [Epub ahead of print]

4. Osterman M, Chang RW. Acute kidney injury in the intensive care unit according to RIFLE. Crit Care Med 2007; 35:1837–1843

5. Bagshaw SM, George C, Bellomo R, et al. A comparison of the RIFLE and AKIN criteria for acute kidney injury in critically ill patients. Nephrol Dial Transplant 2008; 23:1569–1574

6. Chertow GM, Burdick E, Honour M, et al. Acute kidney injury, mortality, length of stay, and costs in hospitalized patients. J Am Soc Nephrol 2005; 16:3365–3370

7. Herget-Rosenthal S, Marggraf G, Husing J, et al. Early detection of acute renal failure by serum cystatin C. Kidney Int 2004; 66:1115–1122

8. Dharnidharka VR, Kwon C, Stevens G. Serum cystatin C is superior to serum creatinine as a marker of kidney function: a meta-analysis. Am J Kidney Dis 2002; 40:221–226

9. Parikh CR, Abraham E, Ancukiewicz M, et al. Urine IL-18 is an early diagnostic marker for acute kidney injury and predicts mortality in the intensive care unit. J Am Soc Nephrol 2005; 16:3046–3052

10. Nickolas TL, O'Rourke MJ, Yang J, et al. Sensitivity and specificity of a single emergency department measurement of urinary neutrophil gelatinase-associated lipocalin for diagnosing acute kidney injury. Ann Intern Med 2998; 148:810–819

11. Bennett M, Dent CL, Ma Q, et al. Urine NGAL predicts severity of acute kidney injury after cardiac surgery. Clin J Am Soc Nephrol 2008; 3:665–673

12. Xue JL, Daniels F, Star RA, et al. Incidence and mortality of acute renal failure in medicare beneficiaries. J Am Soc Nephrol 2006; 17:1135–1142

13. Hou SH, Bushinsky DA, Wish JB, et al. Hospital acquired renal insufficiency; a prospective study. Am J Med 1983; 74:243–248

14. Nash K, Hafeez A, Hou SH. Hospital acquired renal insufficiency. Am J Kidney Dis 2002; 39:930–936

15. Mehta RL, Pascual MT, Soroko S, et al. Spectrum of acute renal failure in the intensive care unit: the PICARD experience. Kidney Int 2004; 66:1613–1621

16. Uchino S, Kellum JA, Bellomo R, et al. Acute renal failure in critically ill patients: a multinational, multicenter study. JAMA 2005; 294:813–818

17. Chawla LS, Abell L, Mazhari R, et al. Identifying critically ill patients at high risk for developing acute renal failure: a pilot study. Kidney Int 2005; 68:2274–2280

18. Ishani A, Xue JL, Himmelfarb J, et al. Acute kidney injury increases risk of ESRD among eldery. J Am Soc Nephrol 2009; 20:223–228

19. Diamond JR, Yoburn DC. Nonoliguric acute renal failure associated with a low fractional excretion of sodium. Ann Intern Med 1982; 96:597–600

20. Diskin CJ, Stokes TJ, Dansby LM, et al. The evolution of the fractional excretion of urea as a diagnostic tool in oliguric states. Am J Kidney Dis 2008; 51:869–970

21. Gines A, Escorsell A, Gines P, et al. Incidence, predictive factors, and treatment of the hepatorenal syndrome with ascites. Gastroenterology 1993; 105:229–236

22. Uriz J, Gines P, Cardenas A, et al. Terlipressin plus albumin infusion: an effective and safe therapy of hepatorenal syndrome. J Hepatol 2000; 33:43–48

23. Wong F, Pantea L, Sniderman K. Mdodrine, octreoride, albumin, and TIPS in selected patients with cirrhosis and type 1 hepatorenal syndrome. Hepatology 2004; 40:55–64

24. Ejaz AA, Mu W, Kang D-H, et al. Could uric acid have a role in acute renal failure? Clin J Am Soc Nephrol 2007; 2:16–21

25. Markowitz GS, Stokes MB, Radhakrishnan J, et al. Acute phosphate nephropathy following oral sodium phosphate bowel purgative: an underrecognized cause of chronic renal failure. J Am Soc Nephrol 2005; 16:3389–3396

26. Liano F, Pascual J. Epidemiology of acute renal failure: a prospective, multicenter, community-based study. Kidney Int 1996; 50:811–818

27. Merten GJ, Burgess WP, Gray LV, et al. Prevention of contrast-induced nephropathy with sodium bicarbonate: a randomized controlled trial. JAMA 2004; 291:2328–2334

28. Marenzi G, Assanelli E, Marana I, et al. N-acetylcysteine and contrast induced nephropathy in primary angioplasty. N Engl J Med 2006; 354:2773–2782

29. Hadjis T, Grieff M, Locknat D, et al. Calcium metabolism in acute renal failure due to rhabdomyolysis. Clin Nephrol 1993; 39:22–27

30. Brezis M, Rosen SN. Hypoxemia of the renal medulla: its implications for disease. N Engl J Med 1995; 332:647–655

31. Schrier RW, Wang W. Acute renal failure and sepsis. N Engl J Med 2004; 351:159–169

32. Lassnigg A, Schmidlin D, Mouhieddine M et al. Minimal changes of serum creatinine predict prognosis in patients after cardiothoracic surgery: a prospective cohort study. J Am Soc Nephrol 2004; 15:1597–1605

33. Thakar CV, Arrigain S, Worley S, et al. A clinical score to predict acute renal failure after cardiac surgery. J Am Soc Nephrol 2005; 16:163–169

34. Mangano DT, Tudor IC, Dietzel C. The risk associated with aprotinin in cardiac surgery. N Engl J Med 2006; 354:353–365

35. Sirivella S, Gielchinsky I, Parsonnet V. Mannitol, furosemide and dopamine infusion in postoperative renal failure complicating cardiac surgery. Ann Thorac Surg 2000; 69:501–506

36. Sward K, Valsson F, Odencrants P, et al. Recombinant human atrial natriuretic peptide in ischemic acute renal failure: a randomized placebo controlled trial. Crit Care Med 2004; 32:1310–1315

37. Bonventre JV. Mechanisms of ischemic acute renal failure. Kidney Int 1993; 43:1160–1178

38. Toback FG. Regeneration after acute tubular necrosis. Kidney Int 1992; 41:226–246

39. Anderson RJ, Linas SL, Berns AS, et al. Nonoliguric acute renal failure. N Engl J Med 1977; 296:1134–1138

40. Friedrich JO, Adhikari N, Herridge MS, et al. Meta-analysis: low-dose dopamine increases urine output and does not prevent renal dysfunction or death. Ann Intern Med 2005; 142:510–524

41. Fiaccadori E, Lombrdi M, Leonardi S, et al. Prevalence and clinical outcome associated with preexisting malnutrition in acute renal failure: a prospective cohort study. J Am Soc Nephrol 1999; 10:581–593

42. Szeto HH, Inturrisi CE, Saal S, et al. Accumulation of normeperidine, an active metabolite of meperidine, in patients with renal failure or cancer. Ann Intern Med 1977; 86:738–741

43. Bauer LA, Black D, Gensler A, et al. Influence of age, renal function and heart failure on procainamide clearance and N-acetylprocainamide serum concentrations. Int J Clin Pharmacol Ther Toxicol 1989; 27:213–216

44. Aronoff GR, Berns JS, Brier ME, et al. Drug prescribing in renal failure: dosing guidelines for adults. 4th ed. Philadelphia, PA: American College of Physicians, 1999

45. Borga O, Hoppel C, Odar-Cederlof I, et al. Plasma levels and renal excretion of phenytoin and its metabolites in patients with renal failure. Clin Pharmacol Ther 1979; 26:306–314

46. Soundararajan R, Golper TA. Medical management of the dialysis patient undergoing surgery [CD-ROM]. Wellesley, MA: UpToDate, 2009

47. Montoliu J, Lens XM, Revert L. Potassium-lowering effect of albuterol for hyperkalemia in renal failure. Arch Intern Med 1987; 147:713–717

48. ARDSNet: Ventilation with lower tidal volumes as compared with traditional tidal volumes for acute lung injury and the acute respiratory distress syndrome. N Engl J Med 2000; 342:1301–1308

49. Schetz M, Vanhorebeek I, Wouters PJ, et al. Tight blood glucose control is renoprotective in critically ill patients. J Am Soc Nephrol 2008; 19:571–578

50. Rivers E, Nguyen B, Havstad S, et al. Early goal-directed therapy for the treatment of severe sepsis and septic shock. N Engl J Med 2001; 345:1368–1377

51. Cheung AK. Biocompatibility of hemodialysis membranes. J Am Soc Nephrol 1990; 1:150–161

52. Himmelfarb J, Tolkoff Rubin N, Chandran P, et al. A multicenter comparison of dialysis membranes in the treatment of acute renal failure requiring dialysis. J Am Soc Nephrol 1998; 9:257–266

53. De Vriese AS, Colardyn FA, Philippe JJ, et al. Cytokine removal during continuous hemofiltration in septic patients. J Am Soc Nephrol 1999; 10:846–853

54. Honore PM, Jamez J, Wauthier M, et al. Prospective evaluation of short term, high volume isovolemic hemofiltration on the hemodynamic course and outcome in patients with intractable circulatory failure resulting from septic shock. Crit Care Med 2000; 28:3581–3587

55. Marshall MR, Golper TA, Shaver MJ, et al. Sustained low-efficiency dialysis for critically ill patients requiring renal replacement therapy. Kidney Int 2001; 60:777–785

56. Schiffl H, Lang SM, Fischer R. Daily hemodialysis and the outcome of acute renal failure. N Engl J Med 2002; 346:305–310

57. Ronco R, Bellomo R, Homel P, et al. Effects of different doses in continuous veno-venous haemofiltration on outcomes of acute renal failure: a prospective randomized trial. Lancet 2000; 355:26–30

58. Paganini EP, Tapolyai M, Goormastic M, et al. Establishing a dialysis therapy patient outcome link in intensive care unit acute dialysis for patients with acute renal failure. Am J Kidney Dis 1996; 28(suppl 3):S81–S96

59. Pavelsky PM, Zhang JH, O'Connor TZ, et al. Intensity of renal support in critically ill patients with acute kidney injury. N Engl J Med 2008; 359:7–20

60. Swartz RD, Messana JM, Orzol S, et al. Comparing continuous hemofiltration with hemodialysis in patients with severe acute renal failure. Am J Kidney Dis 1999; 34:424–432

61. Mehta RL, McDonald B, Gabbai FB, et al. A randomized clinical trial of continuous versus intermittent dialysis for acute renal failure. Kidney Int 2001; 60:1154–1163

62. Cho KC, Himmelfarb J, Paganini E, et al. Survival by dialysis modality in critically ill patients with acute kidney injury. J Am Soc Nephrol 2006; 17:3132–3138

63. Spurney RF, Fulkerson WJ, Schwab SJ. Acute renal failure in critically ill patients: prognosis for recovery of kidney function after prolonged dialysis support. Crit Care Med 1991; 19:8–11

64. McCarthy JT. Prognosis of patients with acute renal failure in the intensive care unit: a tale of two eras. Mayo Clin Proc 1996; 71:117–126

65. Morgera S, Kraft AK, Siebert G, et al. Longterm outcomes in acute renal failure patients treated with continuous renal replacement therapies. Am J Kidney Dis 2002; 40:275–279

Antibiotic Therapy in Critical Illness

Michael S. Niederman, MD, FCCP

Objectives:

- Define the mechanism of action of common antibiotics
- Review principles of pharmacokinetics and pharmacodynamics of antibiotic use
- Define strategies of antibiotic use in the critically ill to minimize antibiotic resistance
- Use pneumonia to illustrate principles of antibiotic use
- Discuss antibiotic resistance and the role of antibiotic therapy in pathogenesis and management

Key words: antibiotic resistance; bactericidal; drug penetration; minimum inhibitory concentration; pharmacokinetics; pneumonia

---

Antibiotics are the foundation of therapy for infections in the critically ill, but the approach to their use varies with the type of infection present (community-acquired pneumonia [CAP], systemic sepsis, health-care-related or nosocomial pneumonia), as well as with the age of the affected patient, the presence of various comorbid illnesses, and risk factors for infection by specific pathogens. For most patients, initial therapy is aimed at a broad spectrum of potential pathogens and is empiric because the infecting pathogen is often not known. Therapy can be more specifically focused on the basis of results of diagnostic tests. In some cases, initial empiric therapy must be continued because no etiologic pathogen is identified. When a pathogen is defined, the term *appropriate* refers to the use of at least one antimicrobial agent that is active *in vitro* against the etiologic pathogen.[1] The term *adequate* includes not only appropriate therapy, but also the use of that agent in the correct dose, via the right route, given in a timely fashion, and with penetration to the site of infection.

Timely and appropriate antibiotic therapy can improve survival in patients with CAP and nosocomial pneumonia (hospital-acquired pneumonia [HAP]), as well as with sepsis, and the benefits are most evident in patients who are not otherwise terminally ill.[1–4] In the setting of CAP, effective initial antibiotic therapy is associated with a marked improvement in survival, compared with ineffective initial therapy, particularly in patients with severe illness.[2,5] Data on patients with severe CAP provide the most convincing argument for the use of empiric therapy. In several studies,[1–3] identification of the pathogens causing severe CAP did not lead to an improved survival rate, while the use of a broad-spectrum, empiric regimen directed at likely pathogens reduced mortality. In patients with HAP and ventilator-associated pneumonia (VAP), survival is improved with the use of antibiotics to which isolated pathogens are susceptible, compared with empiric, nonspecific therapy.[1,2] In both forms of respiratory infection, the timing of appropriate therapy has also been identified as a determinant of outcome. Delays of at least 24 h in starting therapy are an important mortality risk factor in VAP.[1,4] In the therapy for treatment of sepsis, each hour of delay in starting antibiotic therapy raises mortality by as much as 7 to 8%.

Even with the use of the correct agents, not all patients recover. The fact that some HAP patients die in spite of microbiologically appropriate therapy is a reflection of the degree of antibiotic efficacy, as well as a reflection of host response capability (which may, in part, have a genetic determination), and the fact that not all deaths are the direct result of infection.[6]

In this discussion, the principles underlying antibiotic use are examined, followed by a discussion of the commonly used antibiotics for critically ill patients, with a focus on respiratory tract infections. The therapy for treatment of severe pneumonia can be used as a paradigm to demonstrate the principles of antibiotic therapy for treatment of critically ill patients. Although the focus of this discussion will be on empiric antibiotic therapy, the principles of antibiotic penetration and concentration in the lung are summarized in Table 1.

Table 1. *Principles of Antibiotic Therapy for HAP*

Prompt empiric therapy, especially in the setting of septic shock: initiate when there is clinical suspicion of infection
  Obtain a lower respiratory tract culture (sputum, tracheal aspirate, protected brush, BAL) prior to initiation of antibiotic therapy; samples can be obtained bronchoscopically or nonbronchoscopically, cultured quantitatively or semiquantitatively.

Use a narrow-spectrum agent for patients only at risk for infection with core pathogens and with no risk factors for multidrug-resistant pathogens
  Options include ceftriaxone, ampicillin/sulbactam, ertapenem, levofloxacin, or moxifloxacin; for penicillin allergy, use a quinolone or the combination of clindamycin and aztreonam.

Use combination therapy with a broad-spectrum regimen, containing at least two antimicrobials in patients with risk factors for multidrug-resistant pathogens; specific choices should be guided by a knowledge of local microbiology patterns
  Use an aminoglycoside or an antipneumococcal quinolone (ciprofloxacin or high-dose levofloxacin) plus an antipseudomonal β-lactam such as cefepime, ceftazidime, doripenem, imipenem, meropenem, or piperacillin-tazobactam; if there is concern about MRSA, add either linezolid or vancomycin

Use the correct therapy in recommended doses (see text and Table 3)

Choose an empiric therapy that uses agents from a different class of antibiotics than the patient has received in the past 2 weeks

Try to de-escalate to monotherapy after initial combination therapy, after reviewing culture data and clinical response
  If *P aeruginosa*, consider stopping the aminoglycoside after 5 days and finish with a single agent to which the organism is sensitive
  If a nonpseudomonal infection, switch to a single agent that the organism is sensitive to, using either imipenem, meropenem, cefepime, piperacillin/tazobactam, ciprofloxacin, or high-dose levofloxacin

The drug of choice for Acinetobacter is a carbapenem, but colistin should be considered if there is carbapenem resistance; tigecycline monotherapy in this setting is not recommended.

Consider linezolid as an alternative to vancomycin in patients with proven MRSA VAP, and in those with renal insufficiency, and in those receiving other nephrotoxic medications (such as an aminoglycoside)
  Consider adjunctive aerosolized aminoglycosides in patients with highly resistant Gram-negative pathogens

---

Principles of Antibiotic Use

Mechanisms of Action

Antibiotics interfere with the growth of bacteria by undermining the integrity of their cell wall or by interfering with bacterial protein synthesis or common metabolic pathways. The terms *bactericidal* and *bacteriostatic* are broad categorizations, and may not apply for a given agent against all organisms, with certain antimicrobials being bactericidal for one bacterial pathogen but bacteriostatic for another.[7] Bactericidal antibiotics kill bacteria, generally by inhibiting cell wall synthesis or by interrupting a key metabolic function of the organism. Agents of this type include the penicillins, cephalosporins, aminoglycosides, fluoroquinolones, vancomycin, daptomycin, rifampin, and metronidazole. Bacteriostatic agents inhibit bacterial growth, do not interfere with cell wall synthesis, and rely on host defenses to eliminate bacteria. Agents of this type include the macrolides, tetracyclines, sulfa drugs, chloramphenicol, linezolid, and clindamycin. The use of specific agents is dictated by the susceptibility of the causative organism(s) in a given location to individual antibiotics. However, when neutropenia is present, or if there is accompanying endocarditis or meningitis, the use of a bactericidal agent is preferred.

Antimicrobial activity is often described by the terms *minimum inhibitory concentration* (MIC) and *minimum concentration needed to cause a 3-logarithmic decrease (99.9% killing) in the size of the standard inoculum* (generally all pathogenic bacteria are killed at this concentration). MIC defines the minimum concentration of an antibiotic that inhibits the growth of 90% of a standard-sized inoculum, leading to no visible growth in a broth culture. At this concentration, not all the bacteria have necessarily been killed. MIC is used to define the sensitivity of a pathogen to a specific antibiotic, under the assumption that the concentration required for killing (the MIC) can be reached in the serum *in vivo*. However, these terms must be interpreted cautiously in the treatment of specific infections, because the clinician must consider the MIC data in light of the penetration of an agent into the site of infection, with some agents achieving serum levels that are higher at certain sites of infection and lower at other sites.

In recent years, most respiratory infections have been dominated by concerns of antimicrobial resistance, and a new term has emerged, the *mutant prevention concentration* (MPC).[8] MPC is defined as the lowest concentration of an antimicrobial that prevents bacterial colony formation from a culture containing $> 10^{10}$ bacteria. At concentrations lower than MPC, spontaneous mutants can persist and be enriched among the organisms that remain during therapy. The concept has been most carefully studied with pneumococcus and the fluoroquinolones. In general, the MPC is higher than the MIC, implying that it is possible to use an antimicrobial to successfully treat an infection but not to prevent the remaining organisms (which are not causing illness) from emerging as resistant, and persisting and spreading to other patients.

Penetration Into the Lung (Considerations in Treating Pneumonia)

The concentration of an antibiotic in the lung depends on the permeability of the capillary bed at the site of infection (the bronchial circulation), the degree of protein binding of the drug, and the presence or absence of an active transport site for the antibiotic in the lung.[8,9] In the lung, the relevant site to consider for antibiotic penetration is controversial and not clearly defined. Sputum and bronchial concentrations may be most relevant for bronchial infections, while concentrations in lung parenchyma, epithelial lining fluid, and cells such as macrophages and neutrophils are probably more important for parenchymal infections. The localization of the pathogen may also be important, and intracellular organisms such as *Legionella pneumophila* and *Chlamydophila pneumoniae* may be best eradicated by agents that achieve high concentrations in macrophages. Local concentrations of an antibiotic must be considered in light of the activity of the agent at the site of infection. For example, antibiotics can be inactivated by certain local conditions. Aminoglycosides have reduced activity at acidic pH levels, which may be present in infected lung tissues. In addition, high local concentrations of antibiotic can mitigate against certain bacterial resistance mechanisms such as production of destructive bacterial enzymes (such as β-lactamases), altered permeability of the outer bacterial cell wall, and pumping (efflux) of the antimicrobial from the interior of the bacterial cell.

The concentration of an antibiotic in lung parenchyma depends on its penetration through the bronchial circulation capillaries. The bronchial circulation has a fenestrated endothelium, so antibiotics penetrate in proportion to their molecular size and protein binding, with small molecules that are not highly protein-bound passing readily into the lung parenchyma. When inflammation is present, penetration is further improved. For an antibiotic to reach the epithelial lining fluid, it must pass through the pulmonary vascular bed, which has a nonfenestrated endothelium. This presents an advantage for lipophilic agents, which are generally not inflammation dependent, and include chloramphenicol, the macrolides (including the azalides and ketolides), linezolid, clindamycin, the tetracyclines, the quinolones, and trimethoprim (TMP)-sulfamethoxazole (SMX). Agents that are poorly lipid soluble are inflammation dependent and include the penicillins, cephalosporins, aminoglycosides, vancomycin, carbapenems, and monobactams.

Some general categories of antibiotic penetration have been established (Table 2). Drugs that penetrate well into the sputum or bronchial tissue include the quinolones, the newer macrolides and azalides (azithromycin and clarithromycin), the ketolides, the tetracyclines, clindamycin, and TMP-SMX. On the other hand, the aminoglycosides, vancomycin, and to some extent the β-lactams, penetrate less well into these sites. With

Table 2. *Penetration of Antibiotics into Respiratory Secretions*

Good penetration: lipid soluble, concentration not inflammation dependent

Quinolones
New macrolides: azithromycin, clarithromycin
Ketolides
Tetracyclines
Clindamycin
TMP-SMX

Poor penetration: relatively lipid insoluble, inflammation dependent for concentration in the lung

Aminoglycosides
β-Lactams
Penicillins
Cephalosporins
Monobactams
Carbapenems

the use of once-daily aminoglycoside dosing, high peak serum concentrations can be achieved, but the alveolar lining fluid concentration in patients with pneumonia is only 32% of the serum level over the first 2 h; however, the two sites have more similar concentrations later in the dosing interval.[10] Because aminoglycosides require high peak concentrations for optimal killing, their poor penetration with systemic administration often makes this impossible, suggesting a potential role for delivery by the aerosol route (discussed later).

Antibiotic Pharmacokinetics and Pharmacodynamics

Pharmacokinetics refers to the absorption, distribution, and elimination of a drug in the body, and the information can be used to describe the concentration in serum. Pharmacokinetics also includes the study of the concentration at other sites of the body, including the site of infection and the relationship between drug concentrations and their pharmacologic or toxic effect.[8] For antibiotics, this means the relationship of antibiotic concentrations at the site of infection, compared with the MIC of the target organism.

The way in which an antibiotic reaches the site of infection, considering the frequency of administration and dose administered, can affect its ability to kill bacteria, thus defining a close relationship between pharmacokinetics and pharmacodynamics. Some agents are bactericidal in relation to how long they stay above the MIC of the target organism (time-dependent killing), while others are effective in relation to the peak concentration achieved (concentration-dependent killing).[8] If antibiotic killing is time dependent, dosing schedules should be chosen to achieve the maximal time above the MIC of the target organism, such as continuous infusion or prolonged release. Antibiotics of this type include the β-lactams (penicillins and cephalosporins), carbapenems, aztreonam, macrolides, and clindamycin. The rate of killing is saturated once the antibiotic concentration exceeds four times the MIC of the target organism. In spite of these considerations, for many organisms, the concentration of the antibiotic only needs to be above the MIC for 40 to 50% of the dosing interval, and possibly for as

little as 20 to 30% of the interval in the case of carbapenems. For the time-dependent killing drugs listed previously, the pharmacodynamic parameter that best predicts clinical efficacy is the time above the MIC.

When killing is concentration dependent, activity is related to how high a concentration is achieved at the site of infection and how great is the area under the curve (AUC)—the drug concentration plotted vs time—in relation to the MIC of the target organism. Alternatively, the action of these agents can be described by how high the peak serum concentration (Cmax) is in relation to the organism MIC. Classic agents of this type include the aminoglycosides and the fluoroquinolones, but the ketolides are also concentration-dependent antibiotics.[8] For these types of agents, the optimal killing of bacteria is defined by the ratio of AUC to MIC, often referred to as the *area under the inhibition curve*, or the AUIC. The target AUIC for Gram-negative bacteria is ≥ 125, whereas for most antibiotics that treat pneumococcus, the AUIC is at least 30. For both the aminoglycosides and quinolones, some studies[8a] have shown that efficacy can also be defined by the ratio of peak serum concentrations to MIC (Cmax/MIC), aiming for a target of 12 for quinolones against pneumococcus. Optimal use of these agents would entail infrequent administration but with high doses, which is the underlying principle behind the once-daily administration of aminoglycosides. With once-daily aminoglycoside dosing regimens, the patient achieves a high peak concentration (maximal killing) and a low trough concentration (minimal nephrotoxicity), relying on the "postantibiotic effect" (PAE) to maintain the efficacy of the antibiotic after the serum (or lung) concentrations fall below the MIC of the target organism. If an antibiotic has a PAE, it is capable of suppressing bacterial growth even after its concentration falls below the MIC of the target organism. Even though most agents exhibit a PAE against Gram-positive organisms, a prolonged PAE against Gram-negative bacilli is achieved by the aminoglycosides and fluoroquinolones.[8]

Some investigators[7] have suggested that antibiotic therapy be chosen on the basis of another property of certain agents: their ability to stimulate inflammation and cytokine production in

Antibiotic Therapy in Critical Illness (Niederman)

response to the presence of the bacterial cell wall lysis products that they generate. It has been known for many years that certain antibiotics liberate bacterial cell wall products that can interact with cytokine-producing cells, stimulating the production of high levels of cytokines such as tumor necrosis factor. In theory, this could lead to the development, or worsening, of the sepsis syndrome in patients immediately after therapy for pneumonia is started, a phenomenon seen in the therapy for treatment of *Pneumocystis jiroveci* pneumonia and pneumococcal meningitis, leading to recommendations to use corticosteroids with antibiotics when treating these infections. Other than in these situations, it is unclear if cytokine release is clinically relevant: if an antibiotic has a high affinity for bacterial penicillin-binding protein 3, it may kill slowly and lead to filamentous cell wall products that are potent stimuli for cytokine release. On the other hand, agents that kill rapidly and do not interact with penicillin-binding protein 3 are associated with lower levels of *in vitro* stimulation of cytokine production by host inflammatory cells. In addition to these considerations, the use of antibiotics that inhibit protein synthesis (linezolid, clindamycin) may have an advantage in toxin-mediated illnesses, such as those caused by certain strains of *Staphylococcus aureus*, when compared with cell-wall active bactericidal antibiotics.[11]

Features of Specific Antimicrobials

Macrolides (Including Azalides)/Tetracyclines

Macrolides are bacteriostatic agents that bind to the 50S ribosomal subunit of the target bacteria and inhibit RNA-dependent protein synthesis. The macrolides have traditionally had good activity against pneumococci, as well as atypical pathogens (C *pneumoniae*, *Mycoplasma pneumoniae*, Legionella), but the older erythromycinlike agents are not active against *Haemophilus influenzae*, and have poor intestinal tolerance, so that prolonged therapy is difficult. The new agents in this class include azithromycin (also referred to as an *azalide*) and clarithromycin, and have better intestinal tolerance than erythromycin. These agents have enhanced activity against *H influenzae*

(including β-lactamase–producing strains), although on an MIC basis azithromycin is more active. Erythromycin is active against *Moraxella catarrhalis*, although the new agents have enhanced activity against this pathogen.

Azithromycin can be used in its IV form for patients with severe pneumonia but should be administered at 500 mg/d, with the duration defined by the clinical course of the patient, but usually for 7 to 10 days.[2] Because of its IV administration, the serum levels achieved have been adequate for therapy for treatment of bacteremic pneumococcal pneumonia.[12] Clinical studies[13,14] of CAP have consistently shown a mortality benefit of using macrolide therapy, usually in conjunction with a β-lactam, but the mechanism for this favorable effect is not known. Speculation has included the possibility of atypical pathogen coinfection, a possibility supported by studies[2,3] that have found the benefit of the addition of a macrolides to vary over the course of time. Another explanation has been that macrolides have anti-inflammatory effects, which may explain their benefit in improving quality of life in patients with cystic fibrosis. Macrolides have a myriad of other effects, including the interference with "quorum sensing" between bacteria, which could inhibit the *in vivo* proliferation of *Pseudomonas aeruginosa* after colonization has occurred.

Although macrolides remain an important therapeutic option for community respiratory tract infections, pneumococcal resistance is becoming increasingly common, being present in as many as 35 to 40% of all pneumococci, especially in patients who have received an agent of this class in the past 3 months.[15] In addition, macrolide resistance can also coexist with penicillin resistance, and as many as 30 to 40% of penicillin-resistant pneumococci are also erythromycin-resistant. The clinical relevance of these *in vitro* findings remains to be defined. However, there are two forms of pneumococcal macrolide resistance, one involving efflux of the antibiotic from the bacterial cell, and the other involving altered ribosomal binding of the antibiotic. The former mechanism is associated with much lower levels of resistance than the latter, and is present in two-thirds of the macrolide-resistant pneumococci in the United States. Fortunately, the latter form of resistance is less common because, if present, it is unlikely that macrolide therapy for pneumococcal infection would be effective.[16]

The tetracyclines are also bacteriostatic agents that act by binding the 30S ribosomal subunit and interfering with protein synthesis. These agents can be used in CAP as an alternative to macrolides because they are active against *H influenzae* and atypical pathogens. In the United States, however, pneumococcal resistance to tetracyclines may be approaching 20%, and may exceed 50% among organisms with high-level penicillin resistance.

Ketolides

This new class of antimicrobials is a semi-synthetic derivative of the macrolides, with a 14-member ring structure and the substitution of a keto group at the C3 site. These agents act to inhibit ribosomal protein synthesis in bacteria by binding to two different sites on the 50S ribosomal subunit, and because of enhanced binding affinity and the binding to multiples sites, may be able to avoid some of the resistance problems associated with the macrolides.[17] In addition, this class of antibiotics has a poor affinity for the pneumococcal efflux pump. Because of these characteristics, ketolides are active against pneumococci that are macrolide-resistant by either the efflux or ribosomal mechanism. Ketolides are also active against *H influenzae*, but *in vitro* activity is not quite as high as with azithromycin. No agents in this class are currently available.

TMP-SMX

This combination antibiotic has been used as a mainstay for therapy for treatment of *P jiroveci* pneumonia, but has limited value in other severe infections. It has bactericidal activity against pneumococcus, *H influenzae*, and *M catarrhalis*, but not against atypical pathogens. It has become less popular because of the emergence of pneumococcal resistance at rates of at least 30%, because 80 to 90% of organisms that are penicillin resistant are also resistant to TMP-SMX. The sulfa component of the drug inhibits the bacterial enzyme responsible for forming the immediate precursor of folic acid, dihydropteroic acid. TMP is synergistic with the sulfa component because it inhibits the activity of bacterial dihydrofolate reductase.

TMP-SMX is available in a fixed combination of 1:5 (TMP:SMX), and is dosed as either 80/400 mg or 160/800 mg orally bid for 10 days, but the dosage should be adjusted in renal failure. An IV preparation is also available. Side effects generally result from the sulfa component and include rash, GI upset, and occasional renal failure (especially in elderly patients).

β-Lactam Antibiotics

These bactericidal antibiotics have in common the presence of a β-lactam ring, which is bound to a five-membered thiazolidine ring in the case of the penicillins and to a six-membered dihydrothiazine ring in the case of the cephalosporins. Modifications in the thiazolidine ring can lead to agents such as the penems (doripenem, imipenem, ertapenem, and meropenem), while absence of the second ring structure characterizes the monobactams (aztreonam). These agents can also be combined with β-lactamase inhibitors such as sulbactam, tazobactam, or clavulanic acid to create the β-lactam/β-lactamase inhibitor drugs. These agents extend the antimicrobial spectrum of the β-lactams by providing a substrate (sulbactam, clavulanic acid, tazobactam) for the bacterial β-lactamases, thereby preserving the antibacterial activity of the parent compound. β-Lactam antibiotics work by interfering with the synthesis of bacterial cell wall peptidoglycans by binding to bacterial penicillin-binding proteins.

The penicillins include the natural penicillins (penicillin G and V), the aminopenicillins (ampicillin, amoxicillin), the antistaphylococcal agents (nafcillin, oxacillin), the antipseudomonal agents (piperacillin, azlocillin, mezlocillin, ticarcillin), and the β-lactam/β-lactamase inhibitor combinations (ampicillin/sulbactam, amoxicillin/clavulanate, piperacillin/tazobactam, and ticarcillin/clavulanate). Among the antipseudomonal penicillins, piperacillin is the most active agent.

The cephalosporins span from first to fourth generation. The earlier agents were generally active against Gram-positive organisms but did not extend activity to the more complex Gram-negative organisms, or anaerobes, and were susceptible to destruction by bacterial β-lactamases. The newer-generation agents are generally more specialized, with broad-spectrum activity, and with more mechanisms to resist breakdown by bacterial enzymes. The second-generation and newer agents are resistant to bacterial β-lactamases, but recent data suggest that cefuroxime may not be an optimal pneumococcal agent if resistance is present in a patient with bacteremic CAP.[18] On the other hand, the third-generation agents such as ceftriaxone and cefotaxime are reliable and active against penicillin-resistant pneumococci, while ceftazidime is not reliable against pneumococcus but is active against *P aeruginosa*. The third-generation agents may induce β-lactamases among certain Gram-negative organisms (especially the Enterobacteriaceae spp), and thus promote the emergence of resistance during monotherapy. The fourth-generation agent cefepime is active against pneumococci and *P aeruginosa*, but is also less likely to induce resistance among the Enterobacteriaceae than the third-generation agents. Ceftobiprole is a new agent in development that appears to be active against both *P aeruginosa* and methicillin-resistant *S aureus* (MRSA), but was not effective in the therapy for treatment of ventilator-associated pneumonia in one clinical trial.

Imipenem, doripenem, and meropenem are the broadest spectrum agents in this class, being active against Gram-positive organisms, anaerobes, and Gram-negative organisms including *P aeruginosa*. They have shown efficacy for patients with severe pneumonia, both CAP and HAP, as well as a variety of nonpulmonary (intraabdominal) infections. On an MIC basis, doripenem is the most active agent in this class against *P aeruginosa*. A nonpseudomonal carbapenem, ertapenem, is also available and has been used effectively in the therapy for treatment of CAP. Aztreonam is a monobactam that is so antigenically different from the rest of the β-lactams that it can be used in penicillin-allergic patients. It is only active against Gram-negative organisms, having a spectrum very similar to the aminoglycosides.

Because β-lactams kill bacteria in a time-dependent fashion, clinical trials[8] have been conducted using either continuous or prolonged (>3 to 4 h) infusions of these agents. To date, these trials have not shown superiority, but they have shown safety and efficacy, using continuous infusions of penicillins, cefepime, and piperacillin/tazobactam and prolonged infusions of doripenem and meropenem.

Fluoroquinolones

These bactericidal agents act by interfering with bacterial DNA gyrase and/or topoisomerase IV, leading to impaired DNA synthesis repair, transcription, and other cellular processes, resulting in bacterial cell lysis. DNA gyrase is only one form of a bacterial topoisomerase enzyme that is inhibited by quinolones, and activity against other such enzymes is part of the effect of a variety of quinolones. The earlier quinolones (such as ciprofloxacin and ofloxacin) are active primarily against DNA gyrase, which accounts for their good activity against Gram-negative organisms. The newer agents (gemifloxacin, levofloxacin, and moxifloxacin) bind both DNA gyrase and topoisomerase IV, and have extended their activity to Gram-positive organisms, including drug-resistant *Streptococcus pneumoniae* (DRSP). Resistance to quinolones can occur through mutations in the topoisomerase enzymes, by altered permeability of the bacterial cell wall, or by efflux of the antibiotic from the inside of the bacteria.[19] The quinolones kill in a concentration-dependent fashion, and thus optimal antibacterial activity can be achieved with infrequent dosing and with high peak concentrations and high ratios of either AUC/MIC or Cmax/MIC. In addition, because quinolones have a PAE against both Gram-positive and Gram-negative organisms, they can continue to kill even after local concentrations fall below the MIC of the target organism. These properties make the quinolones well suited to infrequent dosing, with the ideal being once-daily dosing, particularly given the relatively long half-life of the newer compounds. On the basis of the AUC/MIC ratio for pneumococcus, the most active agents are gemifloxacin and moxifloxacin, which are up to four times more active than levofloxacin. The only factor limiting a switch to once-daily dosing for all quinolones is the toxicity associated with high doses of some agents (such as ciprofloxacin), particularly concerns related to neurotoxicity and possible seizures.

In the therapy for treatment of respiratory infections, quinolones have the advantage of excellent penetration into respiratory secretions and inflammatory cells within the lung, achieving local concentrations that often exceed serum levels. In addition, these agents are highly bioavailable with oral administration, and thus similar serum and tissue levels can be reached if administered orally or IV, promoting early transition from IV to oral therapy in responding patients.

The fluoroquinolones have excellent antimicrobial activity against β-lactamase producing *H influenzae* and *M catarrhalis*, but the newer agents (gemifloxacin, levofloxacin, and moxifloxacin) extend the activity of the quinolones by having enhanced Gram-positive activity, as well as by being more active against *C pneumoniae* and *M pneumoniae*, compared with older agents. The new agents are also highly effective against *L pneumophila*, and may be the drug of choice for this organism, with cure rates of >90% even in patients with severe CAP.[20] However, if *P aeruginosa* is the target organism (as it is in certain patients with CAP and HAP), then only ciprofloxacin (750 mg bid po or 400 mg q8h IV) or levofloxacin (750 mg/d po or IV) are active enough for clinical use.[1] When levofloxacin is used for patients with severe CAP, the recommended dose to assure pneumococcal efficacy is also 750 mg/d.

Pneumococcal resistance to quinolones is uncommon, but many organisms contain mutations that may lead to future resistance emergence, and the use of the most active agents (defined *in vitro*) may have an advantage to avoid future resistance. One potent risk factor for pneumococcal resistance and failure of therapy is repeated therapy with a quinolone in a 3-month period. Other risk factors for quinolone resistance among pneumococci are recent hospitalization and residence in a nursing home.

One major distinction among these new quinolones is their profile of toxic side effects. A number of agents have been removed from clinical use (temafloxacin) because of toxicities such as QT prolongation (grepafloxacin), phototoxicity (sparfloxacin), hypoglycemia (gatifloxacin), and liver necrosis (trovafloxacin). The side effects of the other new agents have generally been acceptable, but as with any therapy, the risks of use should be weighed against the benefits. A study[21] comparing moxifloxacin with levofloxacin in elderly hospitalized patients with CAP, with a high frequency of heart disease, showed comparable safety, including a low frequency for both drugs of cardiac arrhythmias and *Clostridium difficile*-related diarrhea. Currently there are no well-performed studies of severe CAP showing efficacy of any of the quinolones as monotherapy, although in nosocomial pneumonia, monotherapy has been tested and shown to be effective, provided that the patient does not have *P aeruginosa* infection.

Aminoglycosides

These bactericidal agents act by binding to the 30S ribosomal subunit of bacteria, thus interfering with protein synthesis. Aminoglycosides have primarily a Gram-negative spectrum of activity and are usually used in combination with other agents targeting difficult organisms such as *P aeruginosa* or other resistant Gram-negative organisms. When combined with certain β-lactam agents, they can achieve antibacterial synergy against *P aeruginosa*. Amikacin is the least susceptible to enzymatic inactivation by bacteria, while tobramycin is more active than gentamicin against *P aeruginosa*. Aminoglycosides penetrate poorly into lung tissue, and can be inactivated by acid pH, which is common in pneumonic lung tissue. Thus, in clinical trials[1,22] of nosocomial pneumonia therapy, the use of an aminoglycoside with a β-lactam was no more effective than a β-lactam alone, and the combination regimen was not more effective in preventing the emergence of pseudomonal resistance during therapy than was the monotherapy regimen with a β-lactam. In the treatment of bacteremic pseudomonal pneumonia, aminoglycoside combination therapy may be more effective than monotherapy. A meta-analysis[22] has suggested that the use of combination therapy with an aminoglycoside is of limited value; it may simply add to the risk of nephrotoxicity, and may not prevent the emergence of resistance during therapy.

As previously discussed, aminoglycosides kill in a concentration-dependent fashion, and can be dosed once daily to optimize killing while minimizing toxicity (primarily renal insufficiency). In clinical practice, this has not been proven to occur, and once-daily dosing is comparable in efficacy and nephrotoxicity to multiple-dose regimens.[23] When aminoglycosides are used, it is necessary to monitor serum levels to minimize the occurrence of acute renal failure. Peak concentrations correlate with efficacy, but the utility of monitoring levels in patients treated with once-daily regimens has not been established. Trough concentrations are monitored to minimize toxicity and probably should be followed regardless of dosing regimen. Because of poor penetration into tissues, some investigators have used nebulized aminoglycosides for the therapy for treatment of Gram-negative pneumonia, as will be discussed.

New Agents Active Against MRSA

In the past several years, MRSA has emerged as an important pathogen in patients with a variety of severe infections, particularly VAP and skin and soft-tissue infections, and recently has been described as a potential pathogen in patients with necrotizing postinfluenza CAP. In the past, vancomycin was the agent used most commonly for this pathogen. However, there have been concerns about limited efficacy of vancomycin, primarily because of its poor penetration into respiratory secretions, its potential synergistic nephrotoxicity with aminoglycosides, and its inability to inhibit toxin production by organisms such as community-acquired MRSA. Because of this latter concern, some have suggested that clindamycin should be added to vancomycin if a patient with toxin-producing MRSA infection is being treated. Linezolid is the first agent in a new antibiotic class, the oxazolidinones, and is active against MRSA; it may also block the production of antibacterial toxins, such as the Panton-Valentine leukocidin, which can be produced by community-acquired MRSA strains. The oxazolidinones act to inhibit bacterial protein synthesis by binding to the 50S ribosomal subunit and preventing the binding of transfer RNA and the formation of the 70S initiation complex.

Linezolid is not only active against MRSA, but also against DRSP and vancomycin-resistant enterococci (both *Enterococcus faecium* and *Enterococcus faecalis*). The agent has high bioavailability, and thus serum levels are the same with oral or IV therapy. Renal and nonrenal clearance occurs, and dosing adjustment is not needed for patients with renal failure. Efficacy has been shown for HAP and CAP, but one recent analysis[24] suggested that linezolid may be superior to vancomycin for the therapy for treatment of VAP that is proven to be caused by MRSA. Side effects are not common and include nausea, diarrhea, anemia, and thrombocytopenia and neuropathy

(especially with prolonged use). It is also a weak monoamine oxidase inhibitor.

Quinupristin/dalfopristin has been tested in patients with VAP and was not as effective against MRSA as vancomycin, in spite of good *in vitro* activity. There are several other agents in various stages of development that have activity against MRSA, but they are not yet proven to be useful for the therapy for respiratory tract infections. Among these new agents is daptomycin, which has been shown to be inactivated by pulmonary surfactant, thus explaining its lack of efficacy in pneumonia therapy trials. Daptomycin is an effective therapy for MRSA bacteremia, including endocarditis, possibly because of its bactericidal action. Tigecycline is available for nonrespiratory tract infections, and its efficacy in the therapy for treatment of pneumonia is not yet known, although it does have *in vitro* activity against MRSA and many Gram-negative organisms, including Acinetobacter spp, but not *P aeruginosa*. Other agents currently in development are dalbavancin and telavancin. Available trial data with telavancin have shown efficacy in the therapy for treatment of MRSA and methicillin-susceptible *S aureus* nosocomial pneumonia.

Aerosolized Antibiotics for Respiratory Tract Infections

Local administration of antimicrobials has been used in the therapy for treatment of bronchiectasis, especially in the setting of cystic fibrosis, and in the therapy for treatment of VAP.[25] This approach is used to enhance the delivery of agents to the site of respiratory infection, especially for antibiotics that penetrate poorly into the lung. Direct delivery of antibiotics is usually achieved by nebulization, and this approach not only achieves high intrapulmonary concentrations, but may do so with low systemic absorption, and thus a reduced risk of systemic toxicity. The use of this approach in mechanically ventilated patients has been proposed for patients with either infectious tracheobronchitis or VAP, as both infections can involve highly resistant Gram-negative bacteria, and the local delivery of antibiotics may effectively treat some pathogens that cannot be eradicated by systemic therapy.

In patients receiving mechanical ventilation, local antibiotic administration, by instillation or nebulization, has been used to prevent pneumonia, but this is not a recommended approach because even when it has been successful, there has been concern about the emergence of multidrug-resistant (MDR) Gram-negative organisms in those in whom infection subsequently develops, and these organisms may be difficult to treat. Most studies[25-27] in this population have involved either the aminoglycosides or polymyxin B. Only one prospective randomized trial[26] has examined the impact of the adjunctive use of locally instilled tobramycin with IV agents in the management of VAP. Although the addition of endotracheal tobramycin did not improve clinical outcome compared with placebo, microbiologic eradication was significantly greater in the patients receiving aerosolized antibiotics.

In spite of these data, sporadic small and uncontrolled series[27,28] have shown that when patients have VAP due to MDR *P aeruginosa* or Acinetobacter spp, aerosolized aminoglycosides, polymyxin, or colistin may be helpful as adjunctive therapy to systemic antibiotics. One side effect of aerosolized antibiotics has been bronchospasm, which can be induced by the antibiotic or the associated diluents present in certain preparations. A specially formulated preparation of tobramycin for aerosol administration was designed to avoid this complication.

Although the optimal method of administration of aerosol therapy is unknown, most studies[25,28,29] have shown that nebulization can be effective and achieve more uniform distribution than direct instillation. When aerosol therapy is used in patients receiving mechanical ventilation, it must be carefully synchronized with the ventilator cycle, and the optimal delivery device is not yet defined. In an animal model, investigators[29] found that using an ultrasonic nebulizer placed in the inspiratory limb of the ventilator circuit, proximal to the "Y-connector," up to 40% of the administered dose can be retained in the lung, achieving tissue concentrations 10 times higher than can be achieved with comparable doses given systemically, and with minimal systemic absorption. To optimize delivery, inspiratory time may need to be as high as 50% of the ventilatory cycle, and routine humidification should be stopped during antibiotic administration. In patients receiving ventilation, the ventilator may need to be set with a tidal volume of 8 to 10 mL/kg, with no humidification system in use during the application of the ultrasonic nebulizer, which should be set to deliver 8 L/min.

Principles of Antibiotic Use

CAP

Selection of Initial Therapy for Severe CAP: In the ICU population, all individuals should be treated for DRSP and atypical pathogens, but only those with appropriate risk factors (such as bronchiectasis, prolonged corticosteroid therapy for COPD, malnutrition, recent hospital stay, or prolonged antibiotics) should have coverage for *P aeruginosa*. As mentioned, quinolone monotherapy has not been established as safe or effective for these patients, and monotherapy should not be used in any ICU-admitted CAP patient. Those without pseudomonal risk factors should be treated with a selected IV β-lactam (cefotaxime, ceftriaxone, or ampicillin/sulbactam), combined with either an IV macrolide or an IV quinolone. For patients with pseudomonal risk factors, therapy can be with a two-drug regimen, using an antipseudomonal β-lactam (cefepime, doripenem, imipenem, meropenem, piperacillin/tazobactam) plus ciprofloxacin or high-dose levofloxacin, or alternatively, with a three-drug regimen, using an antipseudomonal β-lactam plus an aminoglycoside plus either an IV nonpseudomonal quinolone or macrolide. If the patient is penicillin allergic, aztreonam can be used with an aminoglycoside and a quinolone or macrolide.

In addition to the general approach to therapy outlined here, patients with CAP need timely administration of initial antibiotic therapy. Retrospective data have shown a reduced mortality for admitted patients with CAP who are treated within 4 to 6 h of arrival to the hospital, compared with those who are treated later.[3] However, it is uncertain if these outcomes are related to the timing of therapy or whether the timeliness of antimicrobial administration is a surrogate marker of other relevant factors. In patients with septic shock, each hour of delay in initiating therapy is associated with a 7 to 8% increase in mortality. In the empiric therapy for treatment of CAP, there is a limited need for routine therapy against MRSA;

however, a new strain of this organism has been described to cause a severe, necrotizing form of CAP after influenza.[11] Although the frequency of this organism is still low, vigilance is needed to see how common it becomes in the future. The algorithms presented here suggest that all patients should receive empiric therapy that provides coverage for atypical pathogens. As mentioned, this recommendation is based on outcome studies,[13,14,30] and may be explained by a high frequency of atypical pathogen coinfection. In fact, even with bacteremic pneumococcal pneumonia, mortality is reduced when a β-lactam is used with a macrolide, compared to when it is used as monotherapy.

HAP

How To Initiate Responsible Empiric Therapy: Many studies[1,4,31] have documented that mortality in HAP is increased if initial empiric therapy is incorrect, or if there is a delay in the initiation of therapy (Table 2). In the American Thoracic Society/Infectious Diseases Society guideline for HAP, the terms *appropriate* and *adequate* therapy were defined. Appropriate refers to the use of an antibiotic that is active *in vitro* against the identified pathogen; the adequate refers to not only using an antibiotic to which the organism is sensitive, but also using that therapy without delay, in the right doses, having it penetrate to the site of infection, and using combination therapy if needed. For example, for critically ill patients with normal renal function who were effectively treated for nosocomial pneumonia in clinical trials, the correct doses of common antibiotics include the following: cefepime, 1 to 2 g every 8 to 12 h; imipenem, 500 mg q6h or 1 g q8h; doripenem, 500 mg q8h (as a 1- or 4-h infusion); meropenem, 1 g q8h; piperacillin-tazobactam, 4.5 g q6h; levofloxacin, 750 mg/d, or ciprofloxacin, 400 mg q8h; vancomycin, 15 mg/kg q12h, leading to a trough level of 15 to 20 mg/L; linezolid, 600 mg q12h; and aminoglycosides of 7 mg/kg/d of gentamicin or tobramycin, and 20 mg/kg of amikacin (Table 3).[1] However, it is still a challenge to use antibiotics adequately, without using them too widely, and thus promoting antibiotic resistance, which is often driven by antibiotic use. Thus, the guideline emphasizes the need for a "de-escalation" strategy of usage, which generally

Table 3. *Proper Doses of Common Antibiotics in the Critically Ill With Normal Renal Function*

Drug	Dosage
β-Lactams	
Cefepime	1–2 g q8–12h
Ceftazidime	2 g q8h
Ceftriaxone	2 g/d
Imipenem	1 g q8h or 500 mg q6h
Meropenem	1 g q6–8h
Doripenem	500 mg q8h (1 h- or 4-h infusion)
Piperacillin/tazobactam	4.5 g q 6h
Aminoglycosides	
Gentamicin or tobramycin	7 mg/kg/d or amikacin 20 mg/kg/d
Antistaphylococcal agents (MRSA)	
Vancomycin	15 mg/kg q12h
Linezolid	600 mg q12h
Quinolones	
Ciprofloxacin	400 mg q8h
Levofloxacin	750 mg/d

urges prompt broad-spectrum empiric therapy whenever there is a clinical suspicion of infection in order to avoid a delay of therapy, combined with a commitment to focus, narrow the spectrum, reduce the duration of therapy, or stop therapy once culture and clinical response information become available. Several studies[1] have shown that it is possible to effectively treat VAP with 6 to 8 days of therapy, provided that the initial therapy is appropriate. The optimal duration of therapy for infections caused by *P aeruginosa* and MRSA is still uncertain, but prolonged therapy may be no better than short-duration therapy in the absence of bacteremia.

Algorithms for Initial Empiric Therapy: Once there is a clinical suspicion of HAP, the antibiotic choice falls into either a narrow spectrum of therapy or a broad-spectrum regimen, directed at MDR pathogens. The narrow-spectrum approach is used if the patient has a pneumonia that started in the first 4 days of hospitalization and there are no other risk factors for MDR pathogens. These risk factors include recent antibiotic therapy within the past 90 days, immunosuppressive illness or therapy (corticosteroids or chemotherapy), admission to a unit with a high rate of MDR organisms, recent hospitalization for ≥2 days within the past 90 days, residence in a nursing home or long-term care facility (*ie*, the presence of health-care–associated pneumonia), or regular visits to a hospital clinic or hemodialysis center. All others receive a broad-spectrum therapy approach.[1]

The narrow-spectrum therapy is usually a monotherapy with ceftriaxone, ampicillin/sulbactam, ertapenem, levofloxacin, or moxifloxacin. If the patient is penicillin allergic, a quinolone can be used, or the patient can be given the combination of clindamycin and aztreonam. When the patient has risk factors for MDR pathogens, the recommended therapy is to use either an aminoglycoside or an antipseudomonal quinolone (ciprofloxacin or levofloxacin) in combination with an antipseudomonal β-lactam (cefepime, ceftazidime, imipenem, meropenem, or piperacillin-tazobactam). If there are concerns about MRSA because of risk factors, a high local prevalence, or the presence of Gram-positive organisms on a Gram stain of lower respiratory tract secretions, then a third agent, either linezolid or vancomycin, should be added. Current data suggest that an aminoglycoside may be the preferred initial agent over a quinolone because quinolones can induce cross resistance to multiple antibiotics, thus limiting the ability to treat subsequent ICU infections. If quinolones are not used for a first episode of infection, there may be more options available if the patient develops a second infection while in the hospital.

The use of combination therapy is controversial, and as previously mentioned, there are limited data to show that the use of an aminoglycoside with a β-lactam is more effective than β-lactam monotherapy. Dual therapy may have value if the patient is neutropenic or if pseudomonal bacteremia is present, but both situations are uncommon. Thus, the most compelling reason for using empiric combination therapy in patients with suspected MDR pathogens is to provide a broad enough spectrum of agents to increase the likelihood that the initial therapy was appropriate. Once the organism is identified, it is possible to de-escalate, and if an aminoglycoside was used with a β-lactam, the maximal benefit may have been achieved after 5 days of dual therapy, and thus the aminoglycoside can usually be stopped at that point.[32] Similarly, if a nonresistant Gram-negative organism is identified, therapy can be with a single agent; those that have been shown to be effective for critically ill patients receiving mechanical ventilation are ciprofloxacin, levofloxacin, imipenem, meropenem, piperacillin/tazobactam, and cefepime.[1] Thus, it is usually possible to de-escalate to monotherapy with one of these agents as soon as culture data become available, or after 5 days of dual therapy with an aminoglycoside if *P aeruginosa* has been identified.

Other Principles of Antibiotic Usage for HAP: In general, it is necessary to use an agent as empiric therapy that is in a different class of antimicrobials than the patient has received recently. A number of studies[1,33] of HAP have demonstrated that recent therapy with an antibiotic (within the past 2 weeks) predicts a greater frequency that pathogens such as *P aeruginosa* will be resistant to the agents recently used. This applies to β-lactams as well as to quinolones.[33] In addition, as previously mentioned, some studies[33,34] have shown that quinolones promote not only Gram-negative resistance to quinolones but also to β-lactams, and that their use can cause resistance to many types of β-lactam antimicrobials. In the management of HAP, as clinical and microbiologic data become available, it is often possible to de-escalate therapy in the form of using less drugs, using agents of narrower spectrum, stopping therapy, or reducing the duration of therapy. The key decision point for manipulating therapy is on days 2 to 3, when a decision can be made about whether or not the patient is improving. This decision is made by assessing clinical features such as fever, leukocytosis, purulence of secretions, radiographic patterns, and oxygenation. In general, the best clinical predictor of response is improvement in oxygenation, which usually occurs by day 3 in survivors of VAP, but not in nonsurvivors.[35] If the patient is improving, then cultures should be checked, and efforts made to de-escalate and shorten duration of therapy. In some instances, all signs of pneumonia are gone by days 2 to 3, respiratory culture findings are negative, and, in retrospect, the diagnosis was heart failure or atelectasis, and antibiotics can be completely stopped.[36]

Therapy for Other Infections: Empiric therapy for treatment of other common nonrespiratory infections is summarized in Table 4.

Table 4. *Empiric Therapy for Common Nonrespiratory Sepsis*

Source unknown

    Organisms: *S aureus* (especially if IV line), Gram-negative organisms, fungi (steroids, prior antibiotics)

    Therapy: dual pseudomonal ± oxacillin, vancomycin, or alternatives (linezolid, daptomycin)

Intraabdominal source: secondary peritonitis

    Organisms: Gram-negative organisms, anaerobes, enterococci (latter two more with secondary vs primary infection)

    Therapy: piperacillin/tazobactam, ertapenem, ampicillin/sulbactam, moxifloxacin or ciprofloxacin, levofloxacin, or cefepime plus metronidazole

Life-threatening

Imipenem or meropenem or

Ampicillin plus metronidazole plus ciprofloxacin or levofloxacin or antipseudomonal aminoglycoside

Antibiotic Resistance

There are four basic mechanisms of resistance:

1. Decreased permeability of microbial cell wall. This is an important mechanism for Gram-negative resistance and is caused by alteration of porin channels.

2. Production of destructive enzymes, such as β-lactamases. This is the major mechanism for Gram-negative resistance and can combine with altered permeability in specific organisms. β-Lactamases can be type I or extended spectrum, and are commonly produced by organisms like *P aeruginosa* and the Enterobacteriaceae. Resistance to third-generation cephalosporins is often mediated by this mechanism.

3. Alteration of the target site of action, such as the penicillin-binding proteins, the DNA gyrase (quinolones), and RNA polymerase. This is an important mechanism for Gram-positive resistance. For pneumococcus, resistance can occur to β-lactams by alteration of the penicillin-binding proteins, and to macrolides by alteration of the ribosomal target of action. This type of macrolide resistance is coded by the *erm* gene, and confers a high level of resistance, much higher than if resistance is caused by an efflux mechanism (see following discussion).

4. Active efflux of the antibiotic, which can occur in Gram-positive and Gram-negative organisms, but is an important mechanism of macrolide resistance in pneumococci., encoded for by the *mef* gene.

Antimicrobial Control Programs

Antimicrobial control programs—such as guidelines, standards, prior authorization policies, and performance measures—primarily focus on limiting antibiotic use.[37] Several studies evaluating antibiotic control programs have not demonstrated reduced resistance rates. This may relate to the fact that other variables besides antibiotic use in ICUs determine the presence of resistance in the hospital. The type of antimicrobial control program that is used in a given hospital may be best dictated by knowledge of local antibiotic usage and resistance patterns. For example, if antibiotic usage is controlled and appropriate, and a single strain of a highly resistant pathogen is present, then there may be a need for more intensive infection-control efforts. On the other hand, if usage is high and inappropriate, and many strains of resistant pathogens are prevalent, control of antibiotic usage may be the most pressing need. Antibiotic rotation is another form of antibiotic control, but its benefit is uncertain. The principles for antimicrobial stewardship have been compiled into a guideline, with the focus on prospective audit and feedback of antibiotic use, de-escalation of broad-spectrum therapy, proper dosing, and the development of local guidelines for antibiotic use, based on a knowledge of local microbiology.[37] Restriction of antibiotics was not a highly recommended strategy.

However, as previously mentioned, as the importance of using broad-spectrum regimens when initiating empiric therapy has been stressed, it is equally important for clinicians to narrow or discontinue therapy when more data on the patient's clinical progress and the microbiologic data become available. This practice has been termed *de-escalation* and can involve focusing from broad-spectrum to narrow therapy, from multiple to single agents, and even discontinuing antibiotics if patients do not have proven infection. In the ICU, combination therapy may be needed for certain resistant pathogens such as *P aeruginosa*, or mixed infections involving resistant Gram-positive and Gram-negative organisms. Once the clinical response has been observed and culture data are available, the patient's therapy can often be switched to fewer antibiotics that are targeted to the cultures. The ability to shorten duration of therapy for nonfermenting Gram-negative bacteria, such as *P aeruginosa*, is uncertain. Some preliminary data suggest that de-escalation is not associated with increased mortality and that it may actually reduce mortality in patients with VAP.

References

1. Niederman MS, Craven DE, Bonten MJ, et al. Guidelines for the management of adults with hospital-acquired, ventilator-associated, and health-care-associated pneumonia. Am J Respir Crit Care Med 2005; 171:388–416

2. Niederman MS, Mandell LA, Anzueto A, et al. Guidelines for the management of adults with community-acquired lower respiratory tract infections: diagnosis, assessment of severity, antimicrobial therapy and prevention. Am J Respir Crit Care Med 2001; 163:1730–1754

3. Houck PM, Bratzler DW, Nsa W, et al. Timing of antibiotic administration and outcomes for Medicare patients hospitalized with community-acquired pneumonia. Arch Intern Med 2004; 164:637–644

4. Luna CM, Vujacich P, Niederman MS, et al. Impact of BAL data on the therapy and outcome of ventilator-associated pneumonia. Chest 1997; 111:676–685

5. Leroy O, Santré C, Beuscart C, et al. A five-year study of severe community-acquired pneumonia with emphasis on prognosis in patients admitted to an intensive care unit. Intensive Care Med 1995; 21:24–31

6. Heyland DK, Cook DJ, Griffith L, et al. The attributable morbidity and mortality of ventilator-associated pneumonia in the critically ill patient: the Canadian Critical Trials Group. Am J Respir Crit Care Med 1999; 159:1249–1256

7. Finberg RW, Moellering RC, Tally FP, et al. The importance of bactericidal drugs: future directions in infectious disease. Clin Infect Dis 2004; 39:1314–1320

8. Andes D, Anon J, Jacobs MR, et al. Application of pharmacokinetics and pharmacodynamics to antimicrobial therapy of respiratory tract infections. Clin Lab Med 2004; 24:477–502

8a. Preston SL, Drusano FL, Berman AL. Pharmacodynamics of levofloxacin: a new paradigm for early clinical trails. JAMA 1998; 279:125–129

9. Honeybourne D. Antibiotic penetration into lung tissues. Thorax 1994; 49:104–106

10. Panidis D, Markantonis SL, Boutzouka E, et al. Penetration of gentamicin into alveolar lining fluid of critically ill patients with ventilator-associated pneumonia. Chest 2005; 128:545–552

11. Micek ST, Dunne M, Kollef MH. Pleuropulmonary complications of Panton-Valentine leukocidin-positive community-acquired methicillin-resistant *Staphylococcus aureus*: importance of treatment with antimicrobials inhibiting exotoxin production. Chest 2005; 128:2732–2738

12. File TM, Niederman MS. Antimicrobial therapy of community-acquired pneumonia. Infect Dis Clin North Am 2004; 18:993–1016

13. Gleason PP, Meehan TP, Fine JM, et al. Associations between initial antimicrobial therapy and medical outcomes for hospitalized elderly patients with pneumonia. Arch Intern Med 1999; 159:2562–2572

14. Houck PM, MacLehose RF, Niederman MS, et al. Empiric antibiotic therapy and mortality among Medicare pneumonia inpatients in 10 Western states: 1993,1995,1997. Chest 2001; 119:1420–1426

15. Vanderkooi OG, Low DE, Green K, et al. Predicting antimicrobial resistance in invasive pneumococcal infections. Clin Infect Dis 2005; 40:1288–1297

16. Rothermel CD. Penicillin and macrolide resistance in pneumococcal pneumonia: does *in vitro* resistance affect clinical outcome? Clin Infect Dis 2004; 38(suppl 4):S346–S349

17. Lonks JR, Goldmann DA. Telithromycin: a ketolide antibiotic for treatment of respiratory tract infections. Clin Infect Dis 2005; 40:1657–1664

18. Yu VL, Chiou CC, Feldman C, et al. An international prospective study of pneumococcal bacteremia: correlation with *in vitro* resistance, antibiotics administered, and clinical outcome. Clin Infect Dis 2003; 37:230–237

19. Richter SS, Heilmann KP, Beekman SE, et al. The molecular epidemiology of *Streptococcus pneumoniae* with quinolone resistance mutations. Clin Infect Dis 2005; 40:225–235

20. Yu VL, Greenberg RN, Zadelkis N, et al. Levofloxacin efficacy in the treatment of community-acquired legionellosis. Chest 2004; 125:2135–2139

21. Anzueto A, Niederman MS, Pearle J, et al. Community-acquired pneumonia recovery in the elderly (CAPRIE): efficacy and safety of moxifloxacin therapy versus that of levofloxacin therapy. Clin Infect Dis 2006; 42:73–81

22. Paul M, Benuri-Silbiger I, Soares-Weiser K, et al. Beta-lactam monotherapy versus beta-lactam-aminoglycoside combination therapy for sepsis in immunocompetent patients: systematic review and metaanalysis of randomised trials. BMJ 2004, March [Epub ahead of print]; doi:10.1136/bmj.520995.63

23. Hatala R, Dinh T, Cook DJ. Once-daily aminoglycoside dosing in immunocompetent adults: a metaanalysis. Ann Intern Med 1996; 124:717–725

24. Wunderink RG, Rello J, Cammarata SK, et al: Linezolid vs vancomycin: analysis of two double-blind studies of patients with methicillin-resistant *Staphylococcus aureus* nosocomial pneumonia. Chest 2003; 124:1789–1797

25. Badia JR, Soy D, Adrover M, et al. Deposition of instilled versus nebulized tobramycin and imipenem in ventilated intensive care unit patients. J Antimicrob Chemother 2004; 54:508–514

26. Brown RB, Kruse JA, Counts GW, et al. Double-blind study of endotracheal tobramycin in the treatment of Gram-negative bacterial pneumonia: the Endotracheal Tobramycin Study Group. Antimicrob Agents Chemother 1990; 34:269–272

27. Michalopoulos A, Kasiakou SK, Mastora Z, et al. Aerosolized colistin for the treatment of nosocomial pneumonia due to multidrug-resistant Gram-negative bacteria in patients without cystic fibrosis. Crit Care 2005; 9:R53–R59

28. Palmer LB, Smaldone GC, Chen JJ, et al. Aerosolized antibiotics and ventilator-associated tracheobronchitis in the intensive care unit. Crit Care Med 2008; 36:2008–2013

29. Goldstein I, Wallet F, Robert J, et al. Lung tissue concentrations of nebulized amikacin during mechanical ventilation in piglets with healthy lungs. Am J Respir Crit Care Med 2002; 165:171–175

30. Martinez JA, Horcajada JP, Almela M, et al. Addition of a macrolide to a B-lactam–based empirical antibiotic regimen is associated with lower inpatient mortality for patients with bacteremic pneumococcal pneumonia. Clin Infect Dis 2003; 36:389–395

31. Iregui M, Ward S, Sherman G, et al. Clinical importance of delays in the initiation of appropriate antibiotic treatment for ventilator-associated pneumonia. Chest 2002; 122:262–268

32. Gruson D, Hilbert G, Vargas F, et al. Strategy of antibiotic rotation: long-term effect on incidence and susceptibilities of Gram-negative bacilli responsible for ventilator-associated pneumonia. Crit Care Med 2003; 31:1908–1914

33. Trouillet JL, Vuagnat A, Combes A, et al. *Pseudomonas aeruginosa* ventilator-associated pneumonia: comparison of episodes due to piperacillin-resistant versus piperacillin-susceptible organisms. Clin Infect Dis 2002; 34:1047–1054

34. Nseir S, Di Pompeo C, Soubrier S, et al. First-generation fluoroquinolone use and subsequent emergence of multiple drug-resistant bacteria in the intensive care unit. Crit Care Med 2005; 33:283–289

35. Luna CM, Blanzaco D, Niederman MS, et al. Resolution of ventilator-associated pneumonia: prospective evaluation of the clinical pulmonary infection score as an early clinical predictor of outcome. Crit Care Med 2003; 31:676–682

36. Hoffken G, Niederman MS. Nosocomial pneumonia: the importance of a de-escalating strategy for antibiotic treatment of pneumonia in the ICU. Chest 2002; 122:2183–2196

37. Dellit TH, Owens RC, McGowan JE, et al. Infectious Diseases Society of America and the Society for Healthcare Epidemiology of America guidelines for developing an institutional program to enhance antimicrobial stewardship. Clin Infect Dis 2007; 44:159–177

Notes

Electrolyte Disorders: Derangements of Serum Sodium, Calcium, Magnesium, and Potassium

Richard S. Muther, MD

Objectives:

- Review the basic physiology affecting sodium, water, calcium, magnesium, and potassium balance
- Recognize the common critical care syndromes and causes of deranged serum cation levels
- Become facile with the short-term treatment of disordered cation balance

Key words: hypercalcemia; hyperkalemia; hypermagnesemia; hypernatremia; hyperosmolality; hypocalcemia; hypokalemia; hypomagnesemia; hyponatremia; hypoosmolality

Sodium

Water balance is measured by changes in osmolality. The term *osmolality* refers to the number of osmotically active particles (osmoles) per liter of solution. (Osmolarity is expressed per kilogram). *Hypoosmolality* indicates an excess of water relative to osmoles; *hyperosmolality* indicates water deficiency. The serum osmolality (in milliosmols per liter) can be calculated by the following formula:

$$\text{Serum osmolality} = 2\,(Na^+ + K^+) + (glucose/18) + (urea/2.8)$$

where Na is sodium and K is potassium; glucose and urea are given in milligrams per deciliter. The molecular weight of glucose is 180; of urea, 28. Conversion from milligrams per deciliter to milliosmols per liter yields 18 and 2.8.

One can see that serum osmolality is primarily due to the serum concentrations of sodium and potassium (and their accompanying anions), glucose, and urea. Of these, the serum sodium concentration is the most powerful, accounting for nearly 95% of serum osmolality. Therefore, in most clinical circumstances, the serum sodium can be used as a surrogate for osmolality. The serum sodium concentration has no direct relationship to the total body sodium concentration but, rather, is an indicator of water balance relative to total body sodium concentration.

The term *tonicity* refers to the osmotic force (ie, the ability to move water across a semipermeable membrane) exerted by osmotically active particles. Hypotonic solutions will lose water to an isotonic solution, and hypertonic solutions will gain water from an isotonic solution. Not all osmoles are equivalent in tonicity. For example, urea, because of its low molecular weight, readily crosses cell membranes and exerts no tonic force. Glucose will induce water movement from most cells (although not from the brain). The major extracellular osmole, sodium, is responsible for the variation in serum tonicity in most cases and, as such, is largely responsible for the extracellular fluid volume (ECV). Therefore, an excess of body sodium causes water movement from the intracellular space into the extracellular space and obligates an increase in ECV, though not an increase in sodium concentration.

Hyponatremia is not always equivalent to hypoosmolality (Fig 1). By stimulating water movement into the ECV, hyperglycemia physiologically lowers the serum sodium concentration by 1.6 mEq per 100 mg/dL glucose, causing hyponatremia with hyperosmolality. The same is true for hypertonic mannitol. Other molecules increasing serum osmolality, such as ethanol, isopropyl alcohol, ethylene glycol, and methanol, do not cause hyponatremia because of their small size and high membrane permeability (ie, they do not create an osmotic force [or tonicity]). They will, however, cause an osmolar gap defined as a difference of >20 mOsm/L between the calculated and measured serum osmolality (Table 1). Hyperproteinemia (usually >10 g/dL) and hyperlipidemia cause an increase in the solid phase of the blood volume, causing "hyponatremia" as the sodium present is indexed to an artificially increased volume. The serum osmolality does not change. This pseudohyponatremia usually accounts for

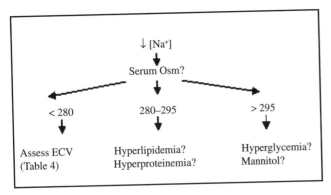

Figure 1. The term *pseudohyponatremia* applies when hyponatremia does not reflect hypoosmolality.

Table 1. *Differential Diagnosis of an Elevated Osmolar Gap**

With Anion-Gap Acidosis	Without Acidosis
Ethylene glycol	Isopropyl alcohol
Methanol	Diethyl ether
Formaldehyde	Mannitol
GFR <10 mL/min	Severe hyperproteinemia
Paraldehyde	Severe hyperlipidemia

*Osmolar gap = measured − calculated osmolality. Calculated serum osmolality = 2(Na$^+$ + K$^+$) + glucose (in milligrams per deciliter)/18 + BUN (in milligrams per deciliter)/2.8.

Table 2. *Characteristics of Sodium and Water Balance**

Characteristics	Sodium	Water
Distribution	Extracellular volume	TBW
Assessment	Physical examination	Serum osmolality
	Urinary Na, FENa	Serum sodium
		UOsm and COsm
Regulation	GFR	Thirst
	Aldosterone	ADH
	Third factors	Renal handling of water

*UOsm = urinary osmolality; COsm = osmolar clearance.

relatively small changes in serum sodium concentration (*eg*, 1 mEq sodium per 460 mg/dL lipid).

In most clinical situations (pseudohyponatremia excepted), the serum sodium concentration is directly related to the serum osmolality such that hyponatremia indicates an excess and hypernatremia indicates a deficiency of water relative to total body sodium concentration. The characteristics of body sodium and water balance are outlined in Table 2.

Regulation of Sodium Balance

As the major extracellular cation and osmole, sodium largely determines ECV. Changes in total body sodium concentration are reflected as changes in the ECV and are best assessed clinically by physical findings. Therefore, rales, jugular venous distention, edema, and an S3 gallop indicate excess ECV and body sodium. Tachycardia, hypotension, flat neck veins in the supine position, dry mucous membranes, and skin tenting indicate ECV and body sodium depletion. In neither case will the serum sodium concentration

necessarily change. Thus, neither the total body sodium concentration nor the ECV is directly related to the serum sodium concentration.

Ordinarily, renal sodium loss balances dietary sodium intake. The renal excretion of sodium is dependent on the glomerular filtration rate (GFR), aldosterone, and a variety of "third factors" that affect the renal tubular reabsorption of filtered sodium. These include natriuretic peptides (atrial natriuretic peptide and brain natriuretic peptide), the renin angiotensin system, norepinephrine, prostaglandins, and intraglomerular and peritubular Starling forces. The GFR in turn is dependent on renal blood flow, the transglomerular capillary hydrostatic and oncotic pressures, and the permeability of the glomerular capillary wall. The afferent and efferent glomerular arteriolar sphincters largely determine intraglomerular Starling forces (transglomerular capillary hydrostatic pressure and transglomerular capillary oncotic pressure). Aldosterone enhances distal tubular sodium reabsorption coupled to a hydrogen ion (H$^+$) and potassium secretion. Normally, approximately 99% of filtered sodium is reabsorbed. The 1% of excreted sodium is best measured by the fractional excretion of sodium (FENa).

Regulation of Water Balance

Thirst, antidiuretic hormone (ADH), and the kidneys control water balance. Hypothalamic receptors for hyperosmolality and hypovolemia stimulate thirst and ADH secretion. While hyperosmolality is the more common stimulus, hypovolemia is a more potent stimulus for ADH release. Therefore, a hypovolemic patient will continue to secrete ADH despite hypoosmolality and

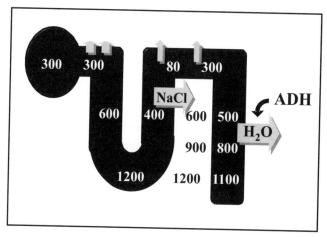

Figure 2. The renal handling of water. Water reabsorption (urinary concentration) requires the presence of ADH and a concentrated medullary interstitium provided by active Na^+ and Cl^- reabsorption in the ascending limb of Henle. Water excretion (urinary dilution) occurs in the absence of ADH. GFR and proximal tubular reabsorption affect urinary concentration and dilution by controlling the delivery of glomerular filtrate to the loop and distal nephron. (Numbers reflect osmolality.)

hyponatremia. ADH exerts its primary effect by activating vasopressin V_2 receptors, which allow water reabsorption across the collecting tubule, thus concentrating the urine (Fig 2). This passive reabsorption of water is dependent on the presence of a more highly concentrated renal medullary interstitium caused by active sodium and chloride reabsorption from the ascending limb of Henle. Sodium (but not water) reabsorption from the late ascending limb and early distal tubule dilutes the filtrate and generates free water. Free water excretion occurs in the absence of ADH. Both the GFR and proximal tubular reabsorption rate affect free water excretion (urine dilution) and reabsorption (urine concentration) as these factors control the quantity of glomerular filtrate delivered to the downstream nephron segments.

Clinical Disorders of Sodium Balance (Disorders of the ECV)

ECV Depletion: Hemorrhage, GI sodium loss, or renal sodium loss can deplete the ECV. Usually, the sodium loss is isotonic. For example, the sodium concentration in diarrhea is approximately 120 mEq/L. In emesis, depending on the pH, it varies from 60 to 120 mEq/L. Coupled with insensible losses, therefore, the serum sodium changes little in most cases where GI sodium loss

depletes the ECV. In fact, the predominant electrolyte disturbance is hypokalemia, which is associated with metabolic acidosis in cases of diarrhea, metabolic alkalosis with vomiting, or a balanced acid-base status in which diarrhea and vomiting coexist.

Diuretics are the most common cause of renal salt wasting. Again, these are isotonic losses, which are usually not associated with changes in the serum sodium concentration. Certainly, severe hyponatremias are reported with the use of diuretics, but these are idiosyncratic (in the case of thiazide diuretics) or are associated with an underlying disorder of sodium retention such as heart failure. Hypoaldosteronism will cause renal sodium loss and isotonic ECV depletion. If coupled to glucocorticoid deficiency, mild hyponatremia can occur. Various renal tubular defects can also cause "salt-losing" nephropathy. This is not uncommon, but it is usually relatively mild with several types of chronic interstitial nephritis. Very rare causes of renal sodium loss include Bartter syndrome and renal tubular acidosis (RTA). Again, the volume lost in these cases is approximately isosmolar, so that serum sodium concentration is either unchanged or mildly decreased. The major clinical feature is ECV depletion, which is determined by physical examination. The urinary sodium concentration (or FENa) is the best way to distinguish GI from renal sodium loss.

Basic fluid therapy for ECV depletion is isotonic crystalloid or colloid. The Saline versus Albumin Fluid Evaluation (or SAFE) study found no difference in organ dysfunction, ICU or hospital days, and ventilator or dialysis days when comparing the use of crystalloid and colloid for fluid resuscitation. The volume of replacement can be estimated by a percentage of total body water (TBW). Mild, moderate, or severe volume losses approximate 5%, 10%, or 15% of TBW, depending on the rapidity with which they occurred. (The effect of sodium is on TBW, although its distribution is extracellular.) [Table 3]. When blood and/or colloid are needed, they are converted to "crystalloid equivalents" at a ratio of 3:1. The rate of replacement depends on the degree of hemodynamic instability.

ECV Expansion: The classic causes of ECV excess are the following "edematous disorders": congestive heart failure (CHF); cirrhosis (with ascites); and nephrosis (nephrotic syndrome). Renal failure (decreased GFR) and hyperaldosteronism are other causes of sodium retention. Physical findings of ECV excess such as rales, jugular venous distension, ascites, and edema are usually present. When mild, the serum sodium concentration is usually normal in these syndromes. When hyponatremia occurs, it is a marker of disease severity and an independent predictor of mortality.

Several mechanisms are responsible for the renal sodium retention seen in patients with these edematous disorders. The GFR is often low as a result of poor cardiac output or decreased oncotic pressure. Aldosterone excess, and its effect on increases in distal tubular sodium reabsorption, is a secondary result. Increased levels of circulating or regionally generated angiotensin II cause preferential constriction of the efferent glomerular sphincter, lowering the hydrostatic pressure while raising the oncotic pressure in the peritubular capillary, thus enhancing proximal renal tubular sodium retention. These factors override the increased production and effects of natriuretic peptides such that the urinary sodium concentration and FENa are extremely and inappropriately low. The basic fluid therapy for patients with ECV excess is salt and water restriction.

Clinical Disorders of Water Balance

Hyponatremia: Hyponatremia is present in 6 to 22% of general hospitalized patients, but in as many as 30% of ICU patients, and is a significant predictor of mortality. The degree of hyponatremia directly correlates with the severity of both CHF and parenchymal liver disease. As a surrogate for serum osmolality, the serum sodium concentration reflects changes in water balance relative to total body sodium concentration. Therefore, after excluding pseudohyponatremia, one can best approach hyponatremia based on the patient's ECV (Table 4).

Hyponatremia occurs with ECV depletion whenever free water intake accompanies GI or renal sodium loss. The most common example is a GI illness with continued oral or IV water (without salt) replacement. Another example is

Table 3. *Signs and Symptoms of ECV Depletion Roughly Correlate to a Percentage of TBW**

Variables	ECV Depletion		
	Mild	Moderate	Severe
TBW depletion	5%	10%	15%
Symptoms	"Dry"	Lethargy	Stupor
Heart rate, beats/min	80	100	120
BP	Normal	Orthostatic	Shock
Jugular vein	Normal	<5 cm H_2O	Flat
Skin	Normal		Tenting

*The severity of symptoms and the urgency of replacement are affected by the acuity of the underlying disease.

Table 4. *Differential Diagnosis of Hyponatremia and Hypoosmolality**

Variables	Hypovolemia (↓ ECV)	Euvolemia (Normal ECV)	Hypervolemia (↑ ECV)
Diagnoses	Vomiting, diarrhea, and fistula (UOsm, >300 mOsm/L; UNa, <20mEq/L)/ diuretics, hypoaldosteronism, RTA, "salt losing," and CSW (UOsm, 300 mOsm/L; UNa, >20 mEq/L)	Polydipsia and malnutrition (UOsm, <100 mOsm/L; UNa, >30 mEq/L)/ SIADH, hypothyroid, and hypocortisol (UOsm, >100 mOsm/L; UNa, >30 mEq/L)	CHF, cirrhosis/ascites, nephrotic syndrome, renal failure (UOsm, >300 mOsm/L†; UNa, <10 mEq/L†)
Other findings	Hypokalemia: vomiting, diarrhea, diuretics, and RTA Hyperkalemia: hypoaldosteronism Metabolic alkalosis: vomiting and diuretics Metabolic acidosis: diarrhea and hypoaldosteronism	Hypokalemia: SIADH and polydipsia Hyperkalemia: hypocortisol Hypouricemia	
Fluid therapy	Isotonic saline	Restrict H_2O	Restrict H_2O and saline

*CSW = cerebral salt wasting; ↓ = decrease; ↑ = increase. See Table 2 for other abbreviations not used in the text.
† Excludes renal failure.

diuretic-associated hyponatremia. Although it is usually mild, severe hyponatremia can occur, particularly with thiazide-type diuretics. Thiazides limit free water excretion by inhibiting distal tubular sodium reabsorption. ECV depletion appropriately stimulates ADH secretion and water reabsorption, contributing to the hyponatremia. Loop diuretics, on the other hand, gradually diminish the medullary interstitial solute and osmolarity, thereby limiting the osmolar gradient for water reabsorption so that hyponatremia is less commonly a side effect of these agents. Elderly women and patients taking nonsteroidal antiinflammatory drugs (NSAIDs) are particularly prone to thiazide-induced hyponatremia. Polydipsia and hypokalemia contribute to the pathogenesis. Treatment is to discontinue therapy with thiazides, restrict water, and replace potassium.

Cerebral salt wasting may cause ECV depletion and hyponatremia. This syndrome usually follows an acute CNS catastrophe or surgery, and is likely due to the release of natriuretic peptides and secondary ADH secretion.

Isotonic saline solution is indicated for those patients with moderate-to-severe volume depletion. Care must be taken to avoid too rapid a correction of hyponatremia. Because ADH secretion is abrogated as saline solution is replaced, a physiologic water diuresis will correct the hyponatremia promptly. Administration of hypertonic saline solution is rarely necessary.

Exercise-induced hyponatremia occurs in as many as 15% of participants in high-endurance activities such as marathons and triathlons. It is likely related to a conspiracy of factors including sodium losses in the sweat, excess free water intake (related to a racing time of >4 h) and the nonosmotic stimulation of ADH. It is more frequent in woman and users of nonsteroidals antiinflammatory drugs. Treatment is reserved for symptomatic patients and may require therapy with isotonic or hypertonic saline solution, depending on the patient's ECV status.

Hyponatremia with a normal ECV occurs whenever the addition of free water to the ECV exceeds the renal capacity to excrete water. In healthy patients, 10 to 15 L of water intake is required to cause significant hyponatremia. Extreme polydipsia (called *psychogenic polydipsia*)

is rare, but hyponatremia can occur with significantly less water intake if ADH secretion is stimulated or its renal tubular effect is enhanced by certain drugs (Table 5). Chronic malnutrition or "low osmolar syndrome" is a much less dramatic cause of hyponatremia. These disorders will have appropriately dilute urine (specific gravity, <1.010; urinary osmolality, <200). The drug "Ecstasy" (3,4 methyldioxymethamphetamine) can cause acute hyponatremia by simultaneously stimulating both thirst and ADH secretion.

The syndrome of inappropriate ADH (SIADH) also causes hyponatremia in euvolemic patients. In fact, edema is an exclusion criterion for SIADH, as are hypothyroidism and glucocorticoid deficiency. Features include hypoosmolality with relatively high urinary osmolality (less than maximally dilute urine or >100 mOsm/L) and hyponatremia with relatively high urinary sodium (>30 mEq/L). Excluding the edematous disorders (ie, heart, liver, and kidney disease) is also a prerequisite for the diagnosis of SIADH.

Table 5. *Differential Diagnosis of SIADH*

Diagnosis	Description
Drugs	Amitriptyline
	Bromocriptine
	Carbamazepine
	Chlorpropamide
	Cisplatin
	Cyclophosphamide
	3,4 methyldioxymethamphetamine (Ecstasy)
	Haloperidol
	Monoamine oxidase activity inhibitors
	Methylenedioxymethamphetamine
	NSAIDs
	Serotonin reuptake inhibitors (eg, fluoxetine)
	Thioridazine
	Thiothixene
	Vincristine/vinblastine
Malignancy	Small cell lung
	Other lung
	Pancreas
	Several others
CNS diseases	Cerebrovascular accident
	Infection
	Trauma
Pulmonary	Pneumonia
	Atelectasis
	Asthma
	Pneumothorax
Major surgery	Transphenoidal

Although malignancy (particularly in the lung) is a common and important cause of SIADH, nearly one third of patients with lung cancer and hyponatremia have no evidence of ectopic ADH production. The ectopic production of atrial natriuretic peptide may be responsible in some of these patients. Fluid restriction will worsen the hyponatremia, and, unlike patients with SIADH, these patients will improve with the IV administration of saline solution.

The basic fluid therapy for polydipsia or SIADH is sodium and water restriction. Drugs that inhibit the ADH effect are useful therapeutic adjuncts. These include demeclocycline, phenytoin, lithium, and loop diuretics (by limiting medullary interstitial osmoles).

Vasopressin receptor antagonists, which are now available for the treatment of euvolemic hyponatremia (eg, SIADH), may also have application in patients with refractory hyponatremia of CHF and cirrhosis. The inhibition of the V_2 (renal collecting tubule) receptor induces an aquaresis without significant sodium or potassium loss and without neurohumoral activation. However, a negative feedback increase in vasopressin levels may lead to unopposed stimulation of V_1 receptors (ie, vascular smooth muscle, myocardium, and liver) with negative effects (ie, ventricular remodeling, and coronary or intestinal vasospasm in patients with CHF) or positive effects (ie, decreased portal pressure and variceal bleeding in patients with cirrhosis). Conivaptan, an IV V_1/V_2 receptor antagonist and the only approved agent in this class, may abrogate these negative cardiac and hemodynamic effects. It increases free water clearance and serum sodium concentration in patients with SIADH and CHF. Tolvaptan and savavaptan (not yet available) are oral selective V_2 receptor antagonists, which increase serum sodium levels and improve mental function in patients with CHF. Neither agent has had an effect on mortality.

Hyponatremia commonly accompanies and is a marker of severity of CHF. The decrease in "effective" intravascular volume stimulates thirst, increases ADH secretion, limits GFR, and enhances proximal renal tubular reabsorption of sodium and water, thus limiting the delivery of glomerular filtrate to the diluting ascending limb. The result is increased intake and limited excretion of free water. Hyponatremia is also commonly seen in patients with cirrhosis (particularly those with ascites) and nephrotic syndrome. The urinary sodium concentration is low (<20 mEq/L), and the urinary osmolarity is high (>300 mOsm/L), mimicking ECV depletion, although with very different physical findings. Basic fluid therapy for these disorders is salt and water restriction with diuretics.

Hypernatremia: Because thirst provides excellent protection against hyperosmolality, hypernatremia is unusual unless access to water is impaired. Therefore, hypernatremic patients are usually elderly, have a decreased mental status, or are in some way incapacitated. The fact that hypernatremia mandates hypertonicity ensures cellular dehydration, particularly of the brain. Therefore, hypernatremic patients are usually quite ill. Because hypernatremia is synonymous with hyperosmolality, a water deficit relative to sodium is always present. Therefore, an approach to the hypernatremic patient based on his or her salt balance (ECV) is appropriate (Table 6, Fig 3).

Hypernatremia in patients with decreased ECV occurs with the administration of osmotic cathartic and diuretic agents. The osmotic effect ensures that water will be lost without an excess of sodium (because of the presence of a nonsodium osmole). This occurs with the presence of lactulose or sorbitol in the intestinal tract, or in the urine in patients with hyperglycemia; mannitol; low-molecular-weight proteins (from hyperalimentation); and urea (postobstructive diuresis). The osmotic effect also causes variable salt depletion. Fluid therapy for these patients, therefore, requires water (to correct the free water deficit) and isotonic saline solution (to correct the decreased ECV).

Euvolemia with hypernatremia indicates the isolated loss of free water. This can occur with massive insensible losses such as severe sweating or hyperventilation, or, rarely, with primary hypodipsia. The most common cause of euvolemic hypernatremia, however, is diabetes insipidus (DI). These patients have an inappropriately low ADH level (central DI) or a blunted ADH effect (nephrogenic DI). The urinary osmolality is inappropriately low (<300 mOsm/L) despite hypernatremia. Patients with central DI will respond to the parenteral administration of ADH by increasing urinary osmolality and decreasing urinary volume. Both central

Electrolyte Disorders: Derangements of Serum Sodium, Calcium, Magnesium, and Potassium (Muther,

Table 6. *Differential Diagnosis of Hypernatremia**

Variables	Hypovolemia (↓ ECV)	Euvolemia (Normal ECV)	Hypervolemia (↑ ECV)
Diagnoses	GI loss: vomiting, diarrhea, and fistula (UOsm, >800 mOsm/L; UNa, <20 mEq/L)/renal loss: hyperglycemia, mannitol, high-protein feedings, and postobstructive diuresis (UOsm, 300–800 mOsm/L; UNa, >30 mEq/L)	Sweating and hypodipsia (UOsm, >800 mOsm/L; UNa, <20 ≥/L)/central DI and nephrogenic DI (UOsm, <300 mOsm/L†; UNa, <20 mEq/L)	Hypertonic NaHCO₃, hypertonic saline solution, sea water ingestion (UOsm, >800 mOsm/L; UNa, >30 mEq/L)
Other findings	Hypokalemia: vomiting, diarrhea, diuresis; metabolic alkalosis: vomiting	UOsm after AVP: central DI, 400–800 mOsm/L†; nephrogenic DI, no change	
Fluid therapy	Combined water and saline solution	Water	Water

*AVP = aqueous vasopressin, 5 U subcutaneously. See Tables 2 and 4 for other abbreviations not used in the text.
†Urine osmolality varies with partial vs complete DI.

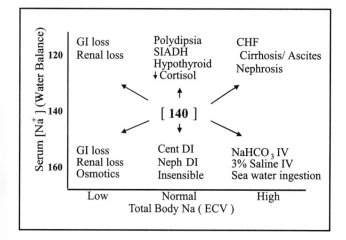

Figure 3. Differential diagnosis of hyponatremia and hyponatremia based on water balance relative to total body sodium (ECV). Cent = central; Neph = nephrogenic.

Table 7. *Differential Diagnosis of Central and Nephrogenic DI*

Central DI	Nephrogenic DI
Trauma	Drugs
Neurosurgery	Lithium
Transphenoidal	Demeclocycline
Pituitary infarction	Amphotericin
Sheehan	Cisplatin
Cerebrovascular accident	Glyburide
Shock	Hypercalcemia
Neoplasm	Hypokalemia
Meningitis/encephalitis	Tubulointerstitial nephritis
Drugs	Obstructive uropathy
Phenytoin	Diuretic-phase acute tubular
Ethanol	necrosis
Familial	

and nephrogenic DI can occur in either partial or complete forms and, therefore, with a broad range of urinary osmolalities following water deprivation or ADH. The differential diagnosis of both central and nephrogenic DI is listed in Table 7.

The rarest clinical salt and water problem is hypernatremia with increased ECV. This occurs with the massive administration of hypertonic bicarbonate or hypertonic saline solution, or rarely in those persons who have experienced salt or salt-water ingestion. The urinary osmolality is high, and the patients are appropriately excreting increased amounts of urinary sodium. Treatment is obviously to restrict the salt and administer free water and diuretics as needed.

Figure 3 plots the common derangements of body salt (disorders of the ECV) and water

(disorders of serum osmolality). Most of the clinical syndromes seen in critically ill patients are actually combinations of separate salt (ECV) and water problems. When this occurs, it is helpful to approach each patient as if there are two separate problems. First, define the nature and treatment of the ECV problem. Next, identify the water (osmolality) problem and its treatment. Finally, sum up and administer the therapies. This approach will simplify even the most severe derangement of fluid and electrolytes.

Treatment Issues

Serum osmolality is the major determinant of brain water and therefore of brain volume (Fig 4). Abrupt hypoosmolality causes brain

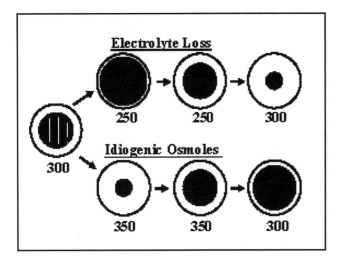

Figure 4. Acute change in serum osmolality effects intracerebral swelling or shrinkage. Within days, a new steady state is reached by brain electrolyte loss (in response to hypoosmolality) or the generation of osmoles (in response to hyperosmolality). A too rapid correction of serum osmolality will similarly effect a change in cerebral volume.

edema; abrupt hyperosmolality causes brain shrinkage. The more rapidly this occurs, the more likely it is that symptoms will occur and the more urgent is the need for therapy. Over time, adaptation to changes in osmolality occurs. With chronic hypoosmolality, the brain loses electrolytes (osmolytes), thus lowering intracellular osmolality to that of plasma. With hyperosmolality, the brain will generate osmoles (idiogenic osmoles), thus raising intracerebral osmolality. Both adaptations tend to return brain osmolality toward plasma osmolality and brain volume toward normal as a new steady state is reached. Any subsequent change in plasma osmolality (*ie*, those induced by therapy) will cause brain swelling or shrinkage once again. Potential complications of this include altered mental status, seizures, coma, or the most serious complication, central pontine myelinolysis. Therefore, slow correction is the rule for severe degrees of either hyponatremia or hypernatremia.

For asymptomatic patients with hyponatremia, simple water restriction and observation are adequate. If the patient is hyponatremic and ECV depleted, isotonic saline solution can be administered. Again, because ADH secretion is volume sensitive, a too rapid correction can occur as the saline solution is administered; thus, frequent monitoring of serum Na levels is required.

For patients who are severely symptomatic with hyponatremia, the administration of hypertonic (3%) saline solution is indicated to increase the serum Na by not >0.5 to 1 mEq/L/h and not >8 mEq/L in a 24-h period. One can calculate the sodium deficit in these patients as follows:

$$\text{Na deficit} = (\text{desired Na} - \text{current Na}) \times \text{TBW}$$

TBW is approximately 60% of body weight in men, and 50% of body weight in women and in the elderly. Using this formula, a 70-kg man with a serum Na concentration of 103 mEq/L would need 504 mEq of Na to raise his serum Na concentration to 115 mEq/L (12 mEq/L $\times$ 42 L). This is approximately 3.3 L of isotonic saline solution (154 mEq/L). To avoid central pontine myelinolysis, correction should not exceed 8 mEq/L/d. Again, close observation for the occurrence of a too rapid correction or signs of fluid overload is mandatory in these patients.

For hypernatremia, the water deficit can be calculated as follows:

$$\text{Water deficit} = ([\text{current Na} + \text{target Na}] - 1) \times (0.6 \times \text{body weight [in kilograms]})$$

For example, a 60-kg man with a serum Na concentration of 175 mEq/L needs 9 L of free water to correct his serum Na concentration to 140 mEq/L (*ie*, $[175 + 140] - 1 \times 36$ L = 9 L). As with hyponatremia, correction should not exceed 0.5 to 1 mEq/L/h and not >12 mEq/L in a 24-h period in severely hypernatremic patients.

An excellent approach to fluid therapy for either hyponatremia or hypernatremia is to determine the effect of 1 L of a given fluid on the serum [Na$^+$] concentration as outlined by the following formula:

$$\text{Change [Na}^+\text{]} = ([\text{infusate Na}^+ + \text{K}^+] - \text{serum [Na}^+\text{]})/(\text{TBW} + 1)$$

In our above example, 1 L of a 5% dextrose solution in water would decrease the patient's serum [Na$^+$] concentration by 4.7 mEq/L ($[0 - 175] + 37 = 4.7$). By this formula, it would require 7.5 L to decrease his serum Na$^+$ concentration from 175 to 140 mEq/L. This formula easily adjusts for any potassium administered. Use of this formula requires knowledge of the Na$^+$ content of commonly prescribed IV fluids. These are

Table 8. *Sodium Content and Percentage Distribution Into the ECV of 1 L of Crystalloid Solutions*

Infusate	Na+, mEq	% in ECV
Dextrose 5% in water	0	40
0.2% normal saline solution	34	55
0.45% normal saline solution	77	73
Lactated Ringer solution	130	97
0.9% normal saline solution	154	100

outlined in Table 8, along with their percentage distribution into the ECV.

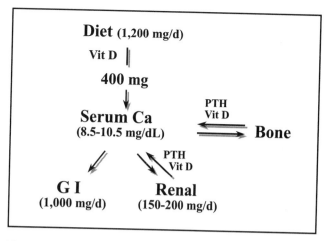

Figure 5. Calcium balance.

Calcium

Calcium balance is depicted in Figure 5. Approximately 400 mg (30 to 35% of an average daily intake of 1,200 mg) is absorbed from the intestinal tract. The daily excretion of this amount occurs in the urine and stool (150 to 200 mg/d in each). Vitamin D is the major factor controlling absorption. The fat-soluble vitamin D3 is absorbed from the diet, 25-hydroxylated in the liver (to calcifediol), and 1-hydroxylated by the kidney to 1,25 dihydroxy vitamin D (calcitriol), which is the active form of the vitamin. Parathyroid hormone (PTH) and hypophosphatemia primarily stimulate the formation of calcitriol. Malabsorption, liver disease, and renal disease may cause vitamin D deficiency.

PTH preserves serum calcium by stimulating osteoclast resorption of bone, increasing renal tubular reabsorption of filtered calcium, and stimulating the production of calcitriol, which enhances the intestinal absorption of calcium. PTH secretion is stimulated by ionized hypocalcemia, and is suppressed by hypercalcemia and hypomagnesemia. It is primarily the combined action of PTH and vitamin D on bone that controls the serum calcium concentration.

In the blood, approximately 40 to 50% of calcium is in the ionized or physiologically active form. In critically ill patients, total serum calcium concentration is a poor predictor of ionized calcium. Albumin binding, alkalosis, and the presence of chelators, such as citrate, phosphate, or lactate, can significantly influence the ionized fraction with relatively little alteration of the total calcium level (Table 9). In fact, the term *pseudohypercalcemia* refers to the elevation of serum total calcium levels due to hyperalbuminemia. Similarly, low levels of serum albumin will lower serum total calcium levels. In neither case will the active or ionized calcium level change. This direct relationship of total calcium to albumin can be quantitated as follows: Δalbumin of 1 g/dL = Δtotal calcium of 0.8 g/dL. The direct measurement of ionized calcium by an ion-specific electrode is now widely available and offers a much more accurate assessment of serum calcium levels in critically ill patients.

Table 9. *Common Clinical Conditions That Dissociate Total (TCa) and Ionized (ICa) Calcium**

Condition	TCa	ICa	Explanation	Degree
Hypoalbuminemia	↓	N	Decreased protein binding	ΔAlb 1.0 mg/dL = ΔTCa 0.8 mg/dL
Hyperalbuminemia	↑	N	Increased protein binding	ΔAlb 1.0 mg/dL = ΔTCa 0.8 mg/dL
Multiple myeloma	↑	N	Ca binding to globulin	
Respiratory alkalosis	N	↓	Increased albumin binding	ΔpH 0.1 = ΔICa 0.16 mg/dL
Hyperparathyroidism	N	↑	Decreased albumin binding	
Hyperphosphatemia	N	↓	Chelation	
Hypercitratemia	N	↓	Chelation	

*TCa = total calcium; ICa = ionized calcium; N = normal; Alb = albumin. See Table 4 for other abbreviations not used in the text.

Table 10. *Common Causes of Hypercalcemia*

Cause	Description
Increased GI absorption	Vitamin D intoxication
	Ectopic vitamin D
	Lymphoma
	Sarcoidosis
	Histoplasmosis
	Tuberculosis
Increased bone resorption	Primary
	hyperparathyroidism
	Ectopic PTH and PTHrP
	Osteolytic metastases
	Multiple myeloma
	(osteoclast-activating
	factor)
	Immobilization
	Posthypocalcemic
	(*eg,* rhabdomyolysis)
Increased renal reabsorption	Hyperparathyroidism
	Thiazide diuretics

Hypercalcemia

Hypercalcemia (Table 10) can occur with excessive GI absorption (*eg,* milk alkali syndrome and excess vitamin D) or with increased renal reabsorption of filtered calcium (*eg,* hyperparathyroidism and thiazides). However, clinically significant hypercalcemia most often occurs with accelerated bone resorption. In hyperparathyroidism, direct osteoclast activation by PTH causes hypercalcemia. PTH or PTH-related peptides (PTHrPs) can also be produced by several malignancies (*eg,* in the lung, ovary, kidney, or bladder). Osteoclast-activating factor, which is produced by myeloma cells, also causes hypercalcemia. Hypercalcemia caused by the direct lytic involvement of bone is seen with several cancers (*ie,* breast and prostate). Immobilization can cause hypercalcemia by increasing bone resorption, particularly in young patients or those with Paget disease. Hypercalcemia is common in the recovery phase of rhabdomyolysis-induced acute renal failure. Severe hypercalcemia (>14 mg/dL [3.5 mmol/L]) usually requires a combination of factors, including excessive osteoclast-stimulated bone resorption, increased renal tubular calcium reabsorption (due to PTH, PTHrP, or volume depletion), and immobilization. This combination is most often seen in patients with malignancy in the ICU setting.

The clinical manifestations of hypercalcemia include anorexia, constipation, and abdominal pain progressing to weakness, lethargy, obtundation, and even coma as the serum calcium concentration increases to 16 mg/dL. Polyuria due to nephrogenic DI may produce volume depletion, which in turn stimulates renal tubular calcium reabsorption and aggravates hypercalcemia. Renal insufficiency is common with acute and/or severe hypercalcemia. A shortened QT interval, bradycardia, and heart block may occur, particularly in patients receiving therapy with digitalis.

The treatment of mild hypercalcemia (<12 mg/dL) may require only simple hydration, restriction of dietary calcium, and treatment of the underlying disease. As the serum calcium concentration increases to >12 mg/dL or the patient becomes symptomatic, specific anticalcemic therapy may be required (Table 11). IV saline solution (3 to 4 L/d) and furosemide (80 to 160 mg/d) can produce a modest decrement in serum calcium levels

Table 11. *Treatment of Hypercalcemia**

Therapy	Dose	Onset	Duration	Efficacy, mg/dL	Toxicity
NS	3–6 L/d	Hours	Hours	1–2	Excess ECV
Furosemide	80–160 mg/d	Hours	Hours	1–2	ECV depletion
Hydrocortisone	200 mg/d	Hours	Days	Mild†	↑BP, ↓K, ↑glucose
Calcitonin	4–8 U/kg	Hours	Hours	1–2	Nausea, thrombopenia
Mithramycin	25 µg/kg	12 h	Days	1–5	Marrow, liver, kidney
Pamidronate	30–90 mg/wk	Days	1–4 wk	1–5	Fever
Zolendrate‡	4–8 mg	Days	Weeks	1–5	
Gallium	200 mg/m²	Days	Days to weeks	1–5	Fever

*NS = normal saline solution. See Table 4 for other abbreviations not used in the text.
†Effective for hypercalcemia of vitamin D excess or ectopic vitamin D syndromes.
‡Preferred bisphosphonate.

Electrolyte Disorders: Derangements of Serum Sodium, Calcium, Magnesium, and Potassium (Muther)

by enhancing renal calcium excretion. When using saline solution and furosemide, one should achieve a minimum urinary output of 100 mL/h. Corticosteroids (hydrocortisone, 200 to 300 mg/d IV, or prednisone, 40 to 80 mg/d po) are effective when hypercalcemia is caused by excess vitamin D (*eg*, vitamin D intoxication, sarcoidosis, or lymphoma) or multiple myeloma.

More aggressive treatment is required for serum calcium concentrations of >14 mg/dL. Although relatively weak, calcitonin (4 to 8 U/kg q6 to 12h) can work within hours to lower the serum calcium concentration. Calcitonin is also a potent analgesic and therefore particularly suited for patients with bone pain. Usually, treatment with mithramycin (25 µg/kg IV) or the bisphosphonates (etidronate, 7.5 mg/kg IV; pamidronate, 30 to 90 mg IV; or zoledronic acid, 4 to 8 mg IV) will also be necessary. Mithramycin will begin to lower serum calcium concentration within hours, with its nadir effect at 48 to 72 h. The effect typically persists for several days, but repeat dosing is often necessary. The effect of bisphosphonate therapy is usually slower but more prolonged, with a nadir in serum calcium level at 7 days and a duration of several weeks. Zolendronic acid (4 to 8 mg IV) is likely superior to pamidronate and is now the preferred therapy for most cases of moderate-to-severe hypercalcemia. A constant infusion of gallium nitrate (200 mg/m^2/d for 5 days) will normalize serum calcium concentrations in 70 to 80% of hypercalcemic patients. The onset, however, is relatively slow, and the nadir is usually at 8 to 10 days. The use of gallium is limited by its nephrotoxicity. The use of oral phosphate (too weak) and IV phosphate (too dangerous) is no longer recommended for the treatment of hypercalcemia. Hemodialysis or peritoneal dialysis with a zero-calcium dialysate is rarely necessary but can be used to treat severe hypercalcemia.

Hypocalcemia

Hypocalcemia (Table 12) can be seen with vitamin D deficiency, PTH deficiency or resistance, or binding by various intravascular or tissue chelators. The malabsorption of calcium and vitamin D most commonly occurs as a result of small-bowel resection or inflammation (*eg*, Crohn disease). Liver disease (decreased synthesis of calcifediol) or renal

Table 12. *Common Causes of Hypocalcemia*

Causes	Description
Decreased GI absorption	Vitamin D deficiency
	Malabsorption
	Hepatic failure
	Renal failure
	Malabsorption syndromes
Decreased bone resorption	Hypoparathyroidism
	Postthyroidectomy
	Familial hypomagnesemia
	Sepsis
	Burns
	Pancreatitis
	Rhabdomyolysis
	PTH resistance
	Hypomagnesemia
	Pseudohypoparathyroidism
	Osteoblastic metastases
Intravascular or tissue chelation	Citrate
	Transfusion
	Anticoagulation
	Albumin
	Fat embolus
	Hyperphosphatemia
	Burns
	Rhabdomyolysis
	Tumor lysis
	Renal failure

disease (decreased synthesis of calcitriol) may also cause vitamin D deficiency. Hypoparathyroidism most often occurs postthyroidectomy but rarely is due to a familial multiglandular condition. Suppression of PTH release is usually due to hypomagnesemia but may accompany severe hypermagnesemia, sepsis, burns, pancreatitis, or rhabdomyolysis. Hypomagnesemia also causes PTH resistance. Rapid or massive blood or plasma transfusion may cause calcium chelation by citrate, an effect that is also seen when citrate is used as an alternative anticoagulant for hemodialysis. The most common calcium chelator, however, is phosphorus, and this hypocalcemic syndrome may occur in patients with major tissue damage (*eg*, burns or rhabdomyolysis), tumor lysis syndrome, or acute and chronic renal failure.

The clinical signs of hypocalcemia include perioral paresthesia, muscular spasms, tetany, and even seizures. Chvostek and Trousseau signs do not usually develop unless the serum calcium concentration falls below 6 mg/dL. Several studies have suggested that ionized hypocalcemia and elevated PTH levels are associated with an increased mortality. Prolongation of the QT interval is common. Bradycardia and hypotension are indications for emergent therapy.

Because the treatment of hypocalcemia with calcium alone is only transiently effective, one must identify and correct the underlying cause. Mild or asymptomatic hypocalcemia requires only an increase in dietary calcium. The administration of calcium (100 to 200 mg IV over 10 min followed by constant infusion at a rate of 100 mg/h) should be reserved for symptomatic patients or those with serum calcium concentrations of <6 mg/dL. Therapy with calcium gluconate (90 mg elemental calcium per 10 mL ampoule) is preferred to limit vein irritation and extravasation. Calcium infusion should be avoided in patients with severe hyperphosphatemia. The serum calcium level should initially be monitored every 4 h. Once the serum calcium concentration is >7 mg/dL, it usually can be maintained with oral calcium supplements (0.5 to 1.0 g tid). The addition of vitamin D3 (25,000 to 50,000 U three times weekly), calcifediol (25-[OH]D3; 50 to 300 μg/d), or calcitriol (1,25 (OH)2 D3; 0.25 to 1 μg/d) will be necessary in those patients with vitamin D deficiency. Thiazide diuretics increase proximal tubular calcium reabsorption by inducing intravascular volume contraction and can serve as a therapeutic adjunct. Finally, the hypocalcemia of magnesium depletion cannot be corrected until magnesium losses are replaced.

Magnesium

One third of the daily dietary magnesium requirement of approximately 360 mg (30 mEq) is absorbed (Fig 6). Renal excretion accounts for most of the daily magnesium loss, but some GI secretion occurs as well. Like calcium, magnesium is primarily an intracellular cation that is stored in bone (55%) and skeletal muscle (30%). Less than 1% of total body magnesium is in the extracellular fluid (ECF). Unlike calcium, however, no hormones control the magnesium balance, and serum magnesium is not readily exchangeable with tissue stores. Therefore, the loss of magnesium can lead rather quickly to hypomagnesemia, and there is little protection against hypermagnesemia when renal excretion is impaired.

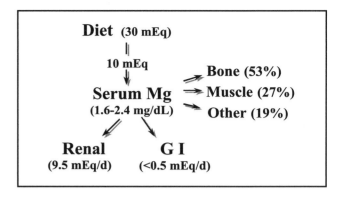

Figure 6. Magnesium balance.

Table 13. *Clinical Manifestations of Hypomagnesemia/Hypermagnesemia Related to the Serum Level*

Serum Level, mg/dL	Manifestations
>12	Muscle paralysis, complete heart block, cardiac arrest
>7	Somnolence, respiratory depression, hypocalcemia, bradycardia, and hypotension
>4	Lethargy and hyporeflexia
1.6–4	Usually asymptomatic
<2	Normomagnesemic magnesium depletion
<1.6	Weakness, anorexia, hypokalemia, and hypocalcemia
<1.2	Tetany, positive Chvostek and Trousseau signs, wide QRS, and peaked T
<0.8	Convulsions, prolonged PR, and ventricular arrhythmia

Hypermagnesemia

Hypermagnesemia occurs primarily in patients with renal insufficiency or in those receiving excess magnesium by IV route (treatment of pre-eclampsia), rectal route (magnesium-containing enemas), or oral route (antacids and laxatives). The latter occurs more commonly when absorption is enhanced by GI inflammation (*eg*, ulcer, gastritis, or colitis). Excess dietary magnesium will not cause hypermagnesemia unless renal function is impaired.

The signs and symptoms of hypermagnesemia are related to the plasma level (Table 13). Lethargy and hyporeflexia can occur at levels >4 mg/dL. Respiratory depression, bradycardia, and hypotension are usually seen at levels >7 mg/dL. A serum magnesium level of >12 mg/dL can cause muscle paralysis, complete heart block, and cardiac arrest. In these cases, IV calcium (100 to 200 mg of elemental calcium over 5 to 10 min) can be life saving. Dialysis can also be used when renal function is impaired. Milder symptoms and magnesium levels of <8 mg/dL require only volume expansion and the discontinuing of exogenous magnesium.

Hypomagnesemia

Hypomagnesemia occurs in 12% of hospitalized patients, but in 40 to 60% of ICU patients. It predicts excess mortality in acutely ill and postoperative adult patients, and in neonates with ventilatory failure. The treatment of hypomagnesemia improves survival in some studies of endotoxic shock (rats), patients with acute myocardial infarction (MI), and postoperative patients with left ventricular dysfunction.

GI and renal losses account for most cases of magnesium depletion (Table 14). Extreme diarrhea or malabsorption can readily deplete serum magnesium; prolonged vomiting or gastric secretion induces hypomagnesemia more gradually. Because of obligate daily losses of magnesium in the stool and urine, a 1- to 2-week period of not eating or not receiving magnesium in IV fluids will cause hypomagnesemia in most patients.

Renal magnesium wasting occurs with excessive diuresis (IV fluids, postobstructive, and diuretic phase of acute renal failure), with the use of diuretic drugs (loop and thiazide diuretics), and with the use of several other drugs (Table 14). Renal magnesium loss can easily be distinguished from GI losses by demonstrating an elevated fractional excretion of magnesium (>1.5%) in a hypomagnesemic patient. The calculation must account for the plasma (P) protein binding of magnesium as follows:

$$FeMg = (UMg \times Pcr \times 100)/[(0.7 \times PMg) \times Ucr]$$

where UMg is urinary magnesium, Pcr is plasma creatinine, PMg is plasma magnesium, Ucr is urinary creatinine, and FeMg is the fractional excretion of magnesium.

Hypomagnesemia can result with increased cellular uptake from several causes, including refeeding, insulin therapy, or tissue injury (rhabdomyolysis). Acute pancreatitis can cause hypomagnesemia by saponification.

Table 14. *Common Causes of Hypomagnesemia*

Causes	Description
GI losses	Malabsorption
	Diarrhea
	Gastric suction
	Prolonged dietary restriction
Renal losses	Excessive IV fluids
	Postobstructive diuresis
	Recovery-phase acute tubular necrosis
	Drugs
	Diuretics
	Aminoglycosides
	Alcohol
	Amphotericin
	Cyclosporine
	Platinum
	Ketoacidosis
	Bartter syndrome
	Renal tubular acidosis
Increased cellular uptake	Refeeding
	Recovery from hypothermia
	Insulin
	Rapid tumor growth
	Rhabdomyolysis
	Pancreatitis

The clinical manifestations of magnesium depletion are roughly correlated with the plasma level of magnesium (Table 13). Weakness, anorexia, and neuromuscular irritability can progress to respiratory depression and convulsions in severe cases. The cardiac toxicity is highly dependent on concurrent myocardial perfusion such that severe arrhythmias may occur with seemingly mild hypomagnesemia in the setting of acute MI. Hypokalemia (due to renal potassium wasting) and hypocalcemia (due to altered PTH resistance and release) occurs in as many as 40% of magnesium-deficient patients (trication deficiency). Neither the hypokalemia nor hypocalcemia of magnesium deficiency can be corrected without magnesium repletion. In fact, hypokalemia and hypocalcemia in the ICU patient often can be corrected with magnesium administration, even in normomagnesemic patients (*ie*, normomagnesemic magnesium depletion).

The treatment of hypomagnesemia includes correcting the underlying GI or renal cause. Serious complications such as ventricular ectopy, hypokalemia, or hypocalcemic tetany require IV magnesium sulfate (1 g [8 mEq] IV immediately

Table 15. *Treatment of Hypomagnesemia*

Serum Mg, mg/dL	Clinical Situation	Treatment	Elemental Mg		
			mg	mmol/L	mEq
≥1.6	Chronic depletion	Magnesium oxide, 400 mg bid	241	10	20
≥1.6	Prolonged IV fluids	MgSO₄, 4 g/d IV	400	16	32
1.2–1.6	Minimal signs/symptoms	MgSO₄, 8 g/d IV	800	32	64
<1.2	Hyperreflexia, myoclonus	MgSO₄, 6 g IV q6–8h	600	25	50
<1.2	Ventricular arrhythmias	MgSO₄, 2 g IV over 15 min	200	8	16

followed by 6 g over 24 h). Because serum levels normalize before tissue stores are replenished, renal losses of magnesium usually continue, necessitating daily magnesium replacement (6 to 8 g of magnesium sulfate) for 3 to 5 days. Milder cases of hypomagnesemia can be treated by slow-release tablets (Table 15). Amiloride will increase magnesium absorption in the cortical collecting tubule and is an excellent adjunct to magnesium therapy.

The use of magnesium to prevent arrhythmias and improve survival in patients with acute MI remains controversial and is not routinely recommended. However, in high-risk patients, 16 mEq (8 mmol/L or 192 mg) of magnesium IV infused over 5 to 15 min prior to reperfusion (thrombolysis or angioplasty) with 128 mEq (64 mmol/L or 1,536 mg) infused over the ensuing 24 h appears to decrease the incidence of arrhythmia and left ventricular dysfunction, and to improve mortality. It is contraindicated in patients with a greater than first-degree heart block or bradycardia, as magnesium can delay atrioventricular conduction.

Potassium

Although only 2% of total body potassium is in the ECF, serum potassium is in dynamic equilibrium with intracellular stores. Movement into and out of cells is controlled by the adrenergic nervous system, insulin, and alterations in pH. Daily dietary intake (100 mEq) is matched by daily renal excretion (90 mEq) and GI excretion (10 mEq). Like calcium and magnesium, alterations in serum potassium levels are best explained by changes in intake, cellular shift, and renal excretion (Fig 7).

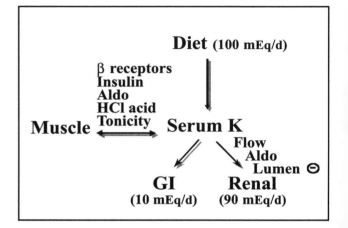

Figure 7. Potassium balance. Aldo = aldosterone.

Hyperkalemia

The causes of hyperkalemia are outlined in Table 16. The release of potassium when blood clots *in vitro* is termed *pseudohyperkalemia*. Patients with severe leukocytosis (>100,000) or thrombocytosis (>400,000) are particularly prone to this phenomenon. This diagnosis is confirmed by a simultaneously drawn serum potassium level (red-top) and plasma potassium level (green-top). Pseudohyperkalemia can also result from variations in the phlebotomy technique used.

Because the kidney is able to substantially increase potassium excretion (up to 300 mEq daily), excess dietary potassium rarely causes hyperkalemia. However, in patients with even mild renal impairment, excessive potassium intake may be an important cause of hyperkalemia. Besides oral potassium supplements, occult sources of potassium include potassium penicillin, salt substitutes, stored blood, and oral (chewed) tobacco products.

Hyperkalemia is often due to the release of cellular potassium. Nonselective β-blockers

Table 16. *Common Causes of Hyperkalemia*

Causes	Description
Pseudohyperkalemia	Thrombocytosis
	Leukocytosis
	Phlebotomy
	Prolonged tourniquet
	Fist clenching
Excess intake (usually only with renal insufficiency)	Potassium supplements
	Salt substitutes
	Potassium penicillin
	Stored blood
	Oral tobacco products
Intracellular-to-extracellular shift	β_2-Blockers
	Aldosterone deficiency
	Insulin deficiency
	Hypertonicity
	Succinylcholine
	Hyperchloremic acidosis
	Cell lysis
	Tumor lysis syndrome
	Hemolysis
	Rhabdomyolysis
Decreased renal excretion	Decreased GFR (<5 mL/min)
	Decreased tubular secretion
	Hypoaldosteronism
	Primary
	Hyporeninemic
	Heparin
	ACEIs/ARBs
	Tubulointerstitial nephritis
	Analgesic nephropathy
	Pyelonephritis
	Sickle-cell nephropathy
	Renal transplant nephropathy
	Obstructive nephropathy
Drugs	Amiloride
	Spironolactone
	Triamterene
	Cyclosporine
	Tacrolimus
	Trimethoprim
	Pentamidine
	NSAIDs
	Digitalis toxicity

(*eg*, propranolol) may elevate serum potassium levels by this mechanism. Aldosterone deficiency increases serum potassium levels by causing an intracellular-to-extracellular potassium shift and by decreasing renal excretion. Insulin deficiency and hypertonicity (*eg*, hyperglycemia) independently cause a cellular-to-serum shift of potassium, which explains the hyperkalemia (and the prompt resolution with therapy) that is so often seen in patients with diabetic ketoacidosis. Hyperchloremic acidosis (but not organic acidoses

[*eg*, ketoacidosis or lactic acidosis]) is also associated with hyperkalemia due to cellular shifts. In these cases, the serum potassium level increases by an average of 0.5 mEq/L for each 0.1 decrement in pH. Finally, cell lysis can present a potentially huge potassium burden to the ECF. Thus, life-threatening hyperkalemia can be seen with rhabdomyolysis, tumor lysis syndrome, massive hemolysis, and occasionally with succinylcholine administration, particularly with simultaneous renal insufficiency.

The most common causes of true hyperkalemia are related to decreased renal excretion. Because the renal tubules not only reabsorb nearly all potassium filtered at the glomerulus, but also secrete most of the 90 mEq of potassium that is excreted daily, hyperkalemia rarely develops from renal failure (*ie*, low GFR) *per se*. Rather, "renal hyperkalemia" is usually due to some defect in tubular potassium secretion. The tubular secretion of potassium requires aldosterone, good-functioning distal and collecting tubular cells, and an adequate delivery of filtered sodium and water to these nephron segments. Thus, any cause of hypoaldosteronism (*eg*, hyporeninemia, isolated aldosterone deficiency, angiotensin-converting enzyme inhibitors [ACEIs] or angiotensin-receptor blockers [ARBs], and heparin therapy) predisposes the patient to hyperkalemia. Hyperkalemia frequently accompanies tubulointerstitial renal diseases (particularly chronic pyelonephritis, analgesic nephropathy, sickle-cell disease, transplant rejection, and obstructive uropathy) despite the relative preservation of renal function (GFR, >20 mL/min). The failure to simultaneously secrete hydrogen ion allows hyperchloremic (non-anion-gap) acidosis frequently to accompany hyperkalemia (type IV RTA). Finally, several drugs cause hyperkalemia by inhibiting tubular potassium secretion. In addition to potassium-sparing diuretics (*ie*, spironolactone, triamterene, and amiloride), cyclosporine, tacrolimus, high-dose trimethoprim, pentamidine, NSAIDs, and ACEIs all share this potential complication.

The acceptance of ACEI/ARBs, spironolactone, and eplerenone as standard therapies for CHF has increased the incidence of severe hyperkalemia in this group of patients. Although the incidence of hyperkalemia (>6 mEq/L) in the Randomized Aldactone Evaluation Study (or RALES)

Table 17. *Treatment of Hyperkalemia*

Serum K, mEq/L	ECG Δ	Treatment	Onset	Duration	Mechanism
<6	None	Avoid NSAIDs			
		Restrict dietary K			
<6	Peaked T	ECV expansion	Hours		
	Prolonged PR	Loop diuretic IV	1–2 h	Hours	Renal excretion
		Kayexalate po	2–4 h	Hours	GI excretion
<7	Widened QRS	Glucose/insulin IV	Minutes	Hours	Redistribution
		Albuterol (inhaled)	Minutes	Hours	Redistribution
		NaHCO₃ IV*	Minutes	Hours	Redistribution
<8	Sine wave	Calcium	1–3 min	<1 h	Cardiac

*Most useful with simultaneous hyperchloremic acidosis.

was only 5%, patients with renal insufficiency (creatinine level, >2 mg/dL) were excluded. An incidence of hyperkalemia of 15 to 20% is more likely when heart failure is complicated by diabetes and renal insufficiency, and is treated with ACEI/ARBs and spironolactone.

The toxicity of hyperkalemia is neuromuscular and cardiac. Paresthesias and weakness may progress to flaccid paralysis. ECG changes include peaked T waves in the precordial leads followed by decreased R-wave amplitude, widened PR interval, and widened QRS complex, and finally loss of the P wave and the development of the sine wave. Heart block or ventricular standstill may occur at any point. The correlation between the serum potassium level and the ECG findings is quite variable.

The treatment of hyperkalemia is outlined in Table 17. When the serum potassium concentration is <6 mEq/L, little therapy is required other than discontinuing the occult sources of dietary potassium that are listed in Table 16. As the potassium concentration rises to >6 mEq/L and/or peaked T waves appear, volume expansion (as tolerated), and therapy with loop diuretics and oral sodium polystyrene sulfonate powder (Kayexalate; sanofi-aventis; Bridgewater, NJ) are appropriate. (Oral sodium polystyrene sulfonate powder administered via the rectum is reported to cause colonic necrosis.) Although somewhat slow to act, these treatments actually increase potassium excretion. When more urgent therapy is needed for hyperkalemia (potassium level, >7 mEq/L), driving potassium intracellularly with glucose and insulin (25 to 50 g of dextrose

with 10 to 20 U of regular insulin) or the β-agonist albuterol (5 to 20 mg [1.0 to 4.0 mL] inhaled) is indicated. Albuterol usually works within 30 min, will lower the serum potassium level by 0.6 to 1.0 mEq/L, and lasts for ≥2 h. Calcium therapy (10 mEq IV infused over 5 min) is reserved for hyperkalemia-induced heart block, widened QRS complex, a sine wave, or, of course, ventricular arrest. Its effect is immediate but short-lived (<60 min). Other maneuvers to remove potassium from the body (eg, diuretics or oral sodium polystyrene sulfonate powder) must be promptly initiated as well. Dialysis (usually hemodialysis) can also be employed to remove potassium.

Hypokalemia

The causes of hypokalemia are listed in Table 18. Significant GI loss of potassium is usually colonic (eg, diarrhea or cathartic abuse) and is accompanied by a hyperchloremic acidosis. Although gastric juice contains very little potassium (10 mEq/L), vomiting or gastric suction often causes hypokalemia due to concurrent volume contraction, secondary hyperaldosteronism, and renal potassium wasting. (This also explains the renal hydrogen ion secretion and the seemingly "paradoxical aciduria" of contraction alkalosis.) GI binding of potassium by long-term clay ingestion (geophagia) can also cause hypokalemia.

Hypokalemia caused by an extracellular-to-intracellular shift usually accompanies the refeeding of severely malnourished patients or the correction of vitamin B12 deficiency. Hypokalemia may also complicate therapy with

Table 18. *Common Causes of Hypokalemia*

Causes	Description
GI losses	Diarrhea
	Cathartics
	Enteric fistula
	Villous adenoma
	Oral sodium polystyrene sulfonate powder (Kayexalate; Sanofi)
	Clay ingestion (geophagia)
Extracellular-to-intracellular shift	Insulin therapy
	Refeeding
	β-Agonists
	Cesium chloride
	Periodic paralysis
Renal losses	Primary hyperaldosteronism
	Adrenal adenoma
	Cushing syndrome
	Renin secreting tumors
	Glucocorticoid-remediable hyperaldosteronism
	Secondary hyperaldosteronism
	Vomiting/gastric suction
	Renal artery stenosis
	Exogenous steroids
	Licorice
	Nonabsorbable anions
	Carbenicillin
	Ticarcillin
	Piperacillin
	Ketones
	Increased urine flow/sodium delivery
	Diuretics
	Renal tubular acidosis
	Ibuprofen overdose
	Bartter syndrome
	Gittleman syndrome
	Magnesium depletion

β-agonists or insulin. Cesium chloride, which is sold as an alternative cancer therapy, can cause severe hypokalemia and ventricular arrhythmias.

Renal artery stenosis (secondary hyperaldosteronism) causes hypokalemia due to urinary potassium loss. Renal wastage is also seen when non-reabsorbable anions (*eg*, carbenicillin) are filtered into the urine, increasing distal potassium secretion. Any process increasing tubular flow (*eg*, diuretics, diuretic phase of acute renal failure, or postobstructive diuresis) will enhance tubular potassium secretion. RTA (type I and II) and Bartter syndrome are rare causes of renal hypokalemia. Hypomagnesemia is a more common cause of hypokalemia due to renal potassium loss (exact mechanism unknown).

Hypokalemia may cause a wide range of clinical manifestations. Muscle weakness (including respiratory muscles), myalgias, cramps, and even rhabdomyolysis can occur. Gastroparesis, ileus, and constipation are common features. Hypokalemia may also cause nephrogenic DI, renal phosphate wasting, and acidification defects due to decreased ammonia production. The most serious hypokalemia toxicity, however, is cardiac. Isolated premature ventricular contractions, ventricular tachycardia, delayed conduction, enhancement of digitalis toxicity, and various ECG changes (*ie*, U waves, flat T waves, ST-segment depression, and atrioventricular block) may all occur.

Potassium replacement can be accomplished via the enteral or IV route. Potassium with chloride or other anions (citrate, bicarbonate, or phosphate) is effective orally or via a gastric tube and can be administered with impunity as long as renal function is normal. With more severe degrees of hypokalemia or in patients who are symptomatic from hypokalemia, rapid correction may be accomplished IV. When the potassium level is >2 mEq/L and there are no ECG changes, infusion of 10 mEq/h is sufficient; an infusion of 40 mEq/h can be given with cardiac monitoring if the serum potassium level is <2 mEq/L. Peripheral infusions should be concentrated to ≤60 mEq/L and administered through as large a vein as possible. Central infusions are best administered into the superior vena cava. One must remember the necessity of treating coexistent magnesium depletion in hypokalemic patients.

Bibliography

Sodium

Adrogue HJ, Madias NE. Hyponatremia. N Engl J Med 2000; 342:1581–1589

Adrogue HJ, Madias NE. Hypernatremia. N Engl J Med 2000; 342:1493–1499

Chute JP, Taylor E, Williams J, et al. A metabolic study of patients with lung cancer and hyponatremia of malignancy. Clin Cancer Res 2006; 12:888–896

Faber MD, Kupin WL, Heilig CW, et al. Common fluid electrolyte and acid-base problems in the intensive care unit: selected issues. Semin Nephrol 1994; 14:8–22

Rai A, Whaley-Connel A, McFarlane S, et al. Hyponatremia, arginine vasopressin receptor dysregulation, and vasopressin receptor antagonism. Am J Nephrol 2006; 26:579–589

Rose BD. Hypoosmolal states. In: Clinical physiology of acid-base and electrolyte disorders. 4th ed. New York, NY: McGraw-Hill, 1994; 651–694

SAFE Study Investigators. A comparison of albumin and saline for fluid rescussitation in the intensive care unit. N Engl J Med 2004; 350:2247–2256

Schrier RW, Gross P, Gheorghiade M, et al. Tolvaptan, a selective oral vasopressin V_2-receptor antagonist, for hyponatremia. N Engl J Med 2006; 355:2099–2112

Zaloga GP, Kirby RR, Bernards WC, et al. Fluids and electrolytes. In: Civetta JM, Taylor RW, Kirby RR, eds. Critical care. 3rd ed. Philadelphia, PA: JB Lippincott, 1997; 413–441

Calcium

Akmal M, Bishop JE, Telfer N, et al. Hypocalcemia and hypercalcemia in patients with rhabdomyolysis with and without acute renal failure. J Clin Endocrinol Metab 1986; 63:137–142

Belezikian JP. Management of acute hypercalcemia. J Clin Endocrinol Metab 1993; 77:1445–1449

Binstock ML, Mundy GR. Effect of calcitonin and glucocorticoids in combination on the hypercalcemia of malignancy. Ann Intern Med 1980; 93:269–272

Major P, Lortholary A, Hon J, et al. Zolendronic acid is superior to pamidronate in the treatment of the hypercalcemia of malignancy: a pooled analysis of two randomized controlled clinical trials. J Clin Oncol 2001; 19:558–567

Stewart AF. Clinical practice: hypercalcemia associated with cancer. N Engl J Med 2005; 352:373–379

Suki WN, Yium JJ, Von Minden M, et al. Acute treatment of hypercalcemia with furosemide. N Engl J Med 1970; 283:836–840

Magnesium

Alfrey AC. Normal and abnormal magnesium metabolism. In: Schrier RW, ed. Renal and electrolyte disorders. 4th ed. Boston, MA: Little Brown, 1992; 371–404

Broner CW, Stidham GL, Westenkirchner DF, et al. Hypermagnesemia and hypocalcemia as predictors of high mortality in critically ill pediatric patients. Crit Care Med 1990; 18:921–928

Rubeiz GJ, Thill-Baharozian M, Hardie D, et al. Association of hypomagnesemia and mortality in acutely ill medical patients. Crit Care Med 1983; 21:203–209

Salem M, Munoz R, Chernow B. Hypomagnesemia in critical illness: a common and clinically important problem. Crit Care Clin 1991; 7:225–252

Woods KL, Fletcher S. Long-term outcome after intravenous magnesium sulfate in inspected acute myocardial infarction: the second Leister intravenous magnesium intervention trial (LIMIT-2). Lancet 1994; 343:816–819

Potassium

Allon M, Copkney C. Albuterol and insulin for treatment of hyperkalemia in hemodialysis patients. Kidney Int 1990; 38:869–872

DeFronzo RA. Hyperkalemia and hyporeninemic hypoaldosteronism. Kidney Int 1980; 17:118–134

Fulop M. Serum potassium in lactic acidosis and ketoacidosis. N Engl J Med 1979; 300:1087–1089

Gabow PA, Peterson LN. Disorders of potassium metabolism. In: Schrier RW, ed. Renal and electrolyte disorders. 4th ed. Boston, MA: Little Brown, 1992; 231–285

Hamill RJ, Robinson LM, Wexler HR, et al. Efficacy and safety of potassium infusion therapy in hypokalemic critically ill patients. Crit Care Med 1991; 19: 694–699

Kruse JA, Carlson RW. Rapid correction of hypokalemia using concentrated intravenous potassium chloride infusions. Arch Intern Med 1990; 150:613–617

Palmer BF. Managing hyperkalemia caused by inhibitors of the rennin-angiotensin-aldosterone system. N Engl J Med 2004; 351:585–592

Schepkens H, Vanholder R, Billiouw JM, et al. Life-threatening hyperkalemia during combined therapy with angiotensin converting enzyme inhibitors and spironolactone: an analysis of 25 cases. Am J Med 2001; 110:438–441

Notes

Notes

Notes

Notes

Notes

Notes

Notes

Notes